You're Wrong, I'm Right

Corey S. Scher · Anna Clebone
Sanford M. Miller · J. David Roccaforte
Levon M. Capan
Editors

You're Wrong, I'm Right

Dueling Authors Reexamine Classic Teachings in Anesthesia

Springer

Editors
Corey S. Scher, MD
Clinical Professor of Anesthesiology, Department of Anesthesiology
Perioperative Care and Pain Medicine, New York University School of Medicine
New York, NY
USA

Anna Clebone, MD
Assistant Professor, Department of Anesthesia and Critical Care
The University of Chicago
Chicago, IL
USA

Sanford M. Miller, MD
Clinical Professor of Anesthesiology (Emeritus), Former Assistant Director of Anesthesiology, Bellevue Hospital Center
Retired from Department of Anesthesiology, Bellevue Hospital Center
New York University School of Medicine
New York, NY
USA

J. David Roccaforte, MD
Clinical Associate Professor of Anesthesiology and Surgery, Department of Anesthesiology
Bellevue Hospital Center, Perioperative Care and Pain Medicine, New York University School of Medicine, Surgical Intensive Care Unit
New York, NY
USA

Levon M. Capan, MD
Department of Anesthesiology
Perioperative Care and Pain Medicine, Vice Chair Faculty Promotion Associate Director Anesthesia Service Bellevue Hospital Center
New York, NY
USA

ISBN 978-3-319-43167-3 ISBN 978-3-319-43169-7 (eBook)
DOI 10.1007/978-3-319-43169-7

Library of Congress Control Number: 2016947744

Printed on acid-free paper

This Springer imprint is published by Springer Nature
The registered company is Springer International Publishing AG Switzerland

To all of my hearts, Lisa, Ryan, Danielle, Oliver, and Dakota

—Corey S. Scher

To my wonderful husband, Keith Ruskin

—Anna Clebone

To my wife, Marcia, who has stood with me for 61 years

—Sanford M. Miller

Preface

Our journals are designed for critical readers to determine whether the best freshly published papers will become essential for practice or not. As anesthesiologists work more hours, with fewer resources and sicker patients than ever before, it is truly a challenge to maintain currency. For many, reading on the subject of anesthesia does not take priority while juggling a personal and professional life. Investing in print copies or gaining Internet access to journals in our field is low on the to-do list.

Anesthesiologists love to talk to fellow anesthesiologists about cases. Even the most dour clinicians will come to life when another anesthesiologist says, "You will never believe what happened to me in the operating room last week." It is readily transparent than many clinicians are holding onto clinical paradigms that were learned in residency that are, at a minimum, now controversial and sometimes no longer true.

There has been a veritable explosion over the last 20 years of high-quality research in anesthesiology, pain medicine, and critical care. The merit of each journal is quantitatively determined by its "Impact Factor"—the frequency that its articles are cited in other papers or reports. The impact of anesthesiology and its related fields has soared by over 65 % in the past 5 years. Fully overwhelming evidence now influences the clinical care of patients in our field and is the reason for this gain. Despite new statistical measures, project design, and editorial approval, many clinicians are holding onto practice parameters that are outdated or irrelevant. The process of practice change involves 3 steps. With the introduction of a new practice parameter, the provider goes through: (1) denial, (2) understanding that there is controversy, and (3) after more time than should be needed, acceptance.

The editors of this book made a bold attempt at creating a book that is targeted at every clinician in the field, whether they stay current or not. We present 126 cases, broken down by subspecialty, where the author has a "split personality." After a case is presented, the author forcefully represents 2 adversarial positions: a pro stance and a con stance. In each case, the authors speak freely, having checked their academic title at the door. During a freewheeling discussion, the case authors alternate between talking off the cuff and presenting current evidence. The book is meant as an easy read that can be opened up at any page. Each case is only a few pages long and can capture the attention of the reader for as long as needed. This is not meant to be a reference book. Simply stated, the cases are meant to be entertaining and a "fun read."

In almost every clinical arena, concepts that we thought were written in stone are on the road to becoming myths. Examples include the utility of cricoid pressure, the use of normal saline, left uterine displacement, and the neurotoxicity of inhaled anesthetics in young children. These are just the tip of the iceberg of controversial topics recently debated in our high-impact journals. Large database analyses on an increasingly large number of topics demand a change in practice.

Another objective of this book is to help the reader take a small step toward currency. The informal presentation of topics is what we believe is the most accessible way to convey new information to a large number of readers. This is how information is most frequently shared in the "real world" both inside and outside of medicine. We believe that this book accomplishes this goal of information sharing, and that most of the cases in the book address the most relevant controversies in anesthesiology today.

The pro–con approach offers advantages over other methods of teaching. These cases can be presented to residents in a manner similar to the Socratic method. In our experience, residents do prefer to be taught using a case-based method. Long intervals exist in the operating room during which minimal activity occurs, although vigilance must still be maintained. Case-based discussions are a perfect way to spend this time. This book is essentially a library for a teacher who is looking for high-quality case-based topics.

The enthusiasm of the authors of each case was the most satisfying aspect of this book. The quality of each case demonstrates that sentiment. Each case author is to be commended for the wisdom and skillful writing contributed to these cases. While we are grateful for everyone involved in getting this work to print, we will be most grateful if the readers simply enjoy this book and use it as a road to currency and an important mode of teaching anesthesia.

New York, USA Corey S. Scher
Chicago, USA Anna Clebone

Contents

Contributors

Elina Abramchayeva, DO Department of Anesthesiology, Mount Sinai West St. Luke's Hospital, New York, NY, USA

Sharon E. Abramovitz, MD Department of Anesthesiology, New York Presbyterian Hospital—Weill Cornell Medicine, New York, NY, USA

A. Elisabeth Abramowicz, MD Department of Anesthesiology, New York Medical College, Westchester Medical Center, Valhalla, NY, USA

Sherryl Adamic, BA, MSA Department of Anesthesiology, University Hospitals of Cleveland, Cleveland, OH, USA; Mentor, OH, USA

Olga N. Albert, MD Department of Anesthesiology, Perioperative and Pain Medicine, Stanford University Medical Center, Stanford, CA, USA

Brooke Albright-Trainer, MD Department of Anesthesiology, Hunter Holmes McGuire VA Medical Center, Richmond, VA, USA

David Amar, MD Department of Anesthesiology and Critical Care Medicine, Memorial Sloan Kettering Cancer Center, New York, NY, USA

Melissa M. Anastacio, MD Department of Surgery, Medstar Washington Hospital Center, Washington, DC, USA

Magdalena Anitescu, MD, Ph.D Department of Anesthesia and Critical Care, University of Chicago Medicine, Chicago, IL, USA

John L. Ard, Jr MD Department of Anesthesiology, New York University Langone Medical Center, New York, NY, USA

Arthur Atchabahian, MD Department of Anesthesiology, New York University School of Medicine, New York, NY, USA

Jeffrey Bernstein, MD Department of Anesthesiology, Montefiore Medical Center—Weiler Division, Bronx, NY, USA

Himani V. Bhatt, DO, MPA Cardiothoracic Division, Department of Anesthesiology, Mount Sinai Medical Center, New York, NY, USA

Matt Bilbily, MD Department of Anesthesiology, Kingston General Hospital, Kingston, ON, Canada

Ian H. Black, MD Department of Surgery, Cheyenne VA Medical Center, Cheyenne, WY, USA

Brian Blasiole, MD, Ph.D Department of Anesthesiology, Children's Hospital of Pittsburgh of UPMC, Pittsburgh, PA, USA

Steven D. Boggs, MD, MBA Department of Anesthesiology, James J. Peters VA Medical Center and the Mount Sinai Hospital, Bronx, NY, USA; Department of Anesthesiology, Icahn School of Medicine at Mount Sinai, Manhattan, NY, USA

Jan Boublik, MD, Ph.D Department of Anesthesiology, Perioperative and Pain Medicine, Stanford School of Medicine, Stanford University, Stanford, CA, USA; Somers, NY, USA

Nicholas J. Bremer, MD Division of Pain Medicine, Department of Anesthesiology, Columbia University Medical Center, New York, NY, USA

Ethan O. Bryson, MD Departments of Anesthesiology and Psychiatry, Icahn School of Medicine at Mount Sinai, New York, NY, USA

Mark Burbridge, MD Department of Anesthesia, Stanford University Medical Center, Stanford, CA, USA

Francisco Calixto, MD Department of Anesthesiology, Tulane Medical Center, New Orleans, LA, USA

Levon M. Capan, MD Department of Anesthesiology, Perioperative Care and Pain Medicine, New York University School of Medicine, New York, NY, USA

M. Megan Chacon, MD Department of Anesthesiology, University of Nebraska Medical Center, Omaha, NE, USA

Floria Chae, MD Department of Anesthesiology, Perioperative Care and Pain Medicine, New York University Langone Medical Center, New York, NY, USA

Judy Chang, MD Department of Anesthesiology, Perioperative Care and Pain Medicine, New York University Langone Medical Center, New York, NY, USA

Jerry Y. Chao, MD Department of Anesthesiology, Montefiore Medical Center, The University Hospital for Albert Einstein College of Medicine, Bronx, NY, USA

Junping Chen, MD, Ph.D Department of Anesthesiology, Mount Sinai St. Luke's and Mount Sinai West Hospital, New York, NY, USA

David S. Cheng, MD Department of Orthopedic Surgery/Physical Medicine and Rehabilitation, Rush University, Chicago, IL, USA

Howard Ching, MD Department of Anesthesiology, NYU Langone Medical Center, New York, NY, USA

Katherine Chuy, MD Department of Anesthesiology, Perioperative Care and Pain Medicine, New York University Langone Medical Center, New York, NY, USA; Englewood Cliffs, NJ, USA

Anna Clebone, MD Department of Anesthesia and Critical Care, The University of Chicago, Chicago, IL, USA

Christopher J. Curatolo, MD, MEM Department of Anesthesiology, Icahn School of Medicine at Mount Sinai, New York, NY, USA

Manoj Dalmia, MD Department of Anesthesiology, Perioperative Care and Pain Management, New York Langone Medical Center, New York, NY, USA

Alaeldin A. Darwich, MD Department of Anesthesiology, New York Presbyterian Hospital —Weill Cornell Medicine, New York, NY, USA

Juan Davila-Velazquez, MD Department of Anesthesiology, Montefiore Medical Center—Weiler Division, Bronx, NY, USA

Paul Delahoussaye, MD Department of Anesthesiology, Louisiana State University Health Sciences Center, New Orleans, LA, USA

Christopher DeNatale, MD Department of Anesthesiology, Perioperative Care and Pain Medicine, New York University Langone Medical Center, New York, NY, USA

Shawna Dorman, MD Department of Anesthesia, New York University Langone Medical Center- Hospital for Joint Diseases, New York, NY, USA

Dalia H. Elmofty, MD Department of Anesthesia and Critical Care, University of Chicago, Chicago, IL, USA

Olga Eydlin, MD Department of Anesthesiology, Perioperative Care and Pain Medicine, New York University School of Medicine, New York, NY, USA

Scott A. Falk, MD Department of Anesthesiology and Critical Care, Hospital of the University of Pennsylvania, Philadelphia, PA, USA; Voorhees, NJ, USA

Jonathan V. Feldstein, MD Department of Anesthesiology, New York University Langone Medical Center, New York, NY, USA

Antonio Gonzalez Fiol, MD Department of Anesthesiology, Rutgers, New Jersey Medical School, Newark, NJ, USA; Secaucus, NJ, USA

Cedar J. Fowler, MD, Ph.D, MPH Department of Anesthesiology, Perioperative and Pain Medicine, Stanford University, Stanford, CA, USA

Elizabeth A.M. Frost, MBChB, DRCOG Icahn Medical Center at Mount Sinai, New York, NY, USA; Purchase, NY, USA

Andrew Goldberg, MD Department of Anesthesiology, Icahn School of Medicine at Mount Sinai, New York, NY, USA

Mark M. Goldfinger, MD, FAAP Department of Anesthesiology and Perioperative Medicine, University Hospitals Case Medical Center, Rainbow Babies and Children's Hospital, Cleveland, OH, USA

Michelle N. Gonta, MD Department of Anesthesiology, Perioperative Care and Pain Medicine, New York University Langone Medical Center, New York, NY, USA

Stephanie R. Goodman, MD Department of Anesthesiology, Columbia University Medical Center, New York Presbyterian – Columbia, New York, NY, USA

Dennis Grech, MD Department of Anasthesiology, Rutgers New Jersey Medical School, Newark, NJ, USA

Ryan T. Gualtier, MD Department of Anesthesiology, New York University Langone Medical Center, New York, NY, USA

Nicole R. Guinn, MD Department of Anesthesiology, Duke University Medical Center, DUMC, Durham, NC, USA

Caitlin J. Guo, MD, MBA Department of Anesthesiology, Perioperative Care and Pain Medicine, New York University Langone Medical Center, New York, NY, USA

Benjamin Heller, MD Department of Anesthesiology, Icahn School of Medicine at Mount Sinai, New York, NY, USA

John Hui, MD Department of Anesthesiology, Montefiore Medical Center, Albert Einstein College of Medicine, Bronx, NY, USA; Department of Anesthesiology, Mayo Clinic, Rochester, MN, USA

Angela Renee Ingram, MD Department of Anesthesiology, Children's Hospital of Pittsburgh of UPMC, Pittsburgh, PA, USA

Mark R. Jones, BA Department of Surgery, Harvard Medical School, Brigham and Women's Hospital, Boston, MA, USA

Madelyn Kahana, MD Department of Anesthesiology, Montefiore Medical Center, Bronx, NY, USA

David Kam, MD Department of Anasthesiology, Perioperative Medicine, and Pain Management, University of Miami, Miami, Fl, USA

Misuzu Kameyama, DO Department of Anesthesiology, Perioperative Care and Pain Medicine, New York University Langone Medical Center, New York, NY, USA

Alan David Kaye, MD, Ph.D Department of Anesthesiology, Louisiana State University Health Sciences Center, University Medical Center, New Orleans, LA, USA

Samir Kendale, MD Department of Anesthesiology, Perioperative Care and Pain Medicine, New York University Langone Medical Center, New York, NY, USA

M. Fahad Khan, MD, MSc, MSPH Department of Anesthesiology, Perioperative Care and Pain Medicine, New York University School of Medicine, New York, NY, USA

Irene Kim, MD Department of Neurosurgery, New York University Langone Medical Center, New York, NY, USA

Jinu Kim, MD Department of Anesthesiology, Mount Sinai West St. Luke's Hospital, New York, NY, USA

Simon Kim, BA, MD Department of Anesthesiology, Bellevue Hospital, New York, NY, USA; Department of Anesthesiology and Perioperative Care, University of California Irvine, Orange, CA, USA

Joseph Kimmel, BSE, MD Department of Anesthesiology, Perioperative Care and Pain Medicine, New York University Langone Medical Center, New York, NY, USA

Daniel Kohut, MD Department of Anesthesiology, New York University Langone Medical Center, New York, NY, USA

Anna Korban, MD Department of Anesthesiology, Rutgers, New Jersey Medical School, South River, NJ, USA

Tomas J. Kucera, MD, MS Attending Physician, Advanced Pain Management, Madison, WI, USA

Agnes McNamara Lamon, MD Department of Anesthesiology, Mt. Sinai Roosevelt Hospital, New York, NY, USA; Durham, NC, USA

Joseph Thomas Largi, MD Department of Anesthesiology, Perioperative Care and Pain Medicine, New York University School of Medicine, New York, NY, USA

James Leonard, MD Department of Anesthesiology, Perioperative Care and Pain Medicine, New York University Langone Medical Center, New York, NY, USA

Alexandra Lewis, MD Department of Anesthesiology and Critical Care Medicine, Memorial Sloan Kettering Cancer Center, New York, NY, USA

Thor Lidasan, MD Department of Anesthesiology, Perioperative Care and Pain Medicine, Bellevue Hospital Center, New York, NY, USA

Jennifer L. Liedel, MD Division of Pediatric Critical Care, Department of Pediatrics, Albert Einstein College of Medicine, Children's Hospital at Montefiore, Bronx, NY, USA

Elana B. Lubit, Ph.D, MD Department of Anesthesiology, New York University School of Medicine/Bellevue Hospital Center, New York, NY, USA

Brent J. Luria, MD Department of Anesthesiology, Perioperative Care and Pain Medicine, New York University Langone Medical Center, New York, NY, USA

Anuj Malhotra, MD Department of Anesthesiology, Pain Management, Icahn School of Medicine at Mount Sinai, New York, NY, USA

Suzanne K.W. Mankowitz, MD Department of Anesthesiology, Columbia University Medical Center, New York, NY, USA; Teaneck, NJ, USA

Glenn E. Mann, MD Department of Anesthesiology, Montefiore Medical Center, The University Hospital for Albert Einstein College of Medicine, Bronx, NY, USA

Olga Ferreira Martins, MD Department of Anesthesiology, Perioperative Care and Pain Medicine, New York University Langone Medical Center, New York, NY, USA

Sanford M. Miller, MD New York University School of Medicine, New York, NY, USA; Department of Anesthesiology, Bellevue Hospital Center, New York, NY, USA

Rebekah Nam Department of Anesthesiology, New York University Langone Medical Center, New York, NY, USA

Michael J. Naso, MD Philadelphia, PA, USA

Kristina Natan, MD Northern Valley Anesthesiology, Shirley, NY, USA

Howard Nearman, MD, MBA Department of Anesthesiology and Critical Care, Hospital of the University of Pennsylvania, Philadelphia, PA, USA; Department of Anesthesiology and Perioperative Medicine, University Hospitals Case Medical Center, Cleveland, OH, USA

Peter J. Neuburger, MD Department of Anesthesiology, Perioperative Care and Pain Medicine, New York University School of Medicine, New York University Langone Medical Center, New York, NY, USA

Jennie Y. Ngai, MD Department of Anesthesiology, Perioperative Care and Pain Medicine, New York University School of Medicine, NYU Anesthesia Associates, New York, NY, USA

Barbara Orlando, MD Department of Anesthesiology, Mount-Sinai West Hospital, New York, NY, USA; Scarsdale, NY, USA

Hersh Patel, MD, MBA Department of Anesthesiology, New York University Langone Medical Center, New York, NY, USA; Monmouth Junction, NJ, USA

Preet Patel, MD Department of Anesthesiology and Pain Management, Rutgers Robert Wood Johnson Medical School, New Brunswick, NJ, USA

Rahul Pathak, MD Department of Anesthesiology, Perioperative Care and Pain Medicine, New York University School of Medicine, New York, NY, USA

Arati Patil, MD Department of Anesthesiology, Perioperative Care and Pain Medicine, New York University Langone Medical Center, New York, NY, USA

Sheetal Patil, MD Department of Anesthesia and Pain Management, University of Chicago, Chicago, IL, USA

Minda L. Patt, MD Department of Anesthesiology, New York Presbyterian Hospital, Weill Cornell Medicine, New York, NY, USA

Sergey Pisklakov, MD Department of Anesthesiology, Montefiore Medical Center, Albert Einstein College of Medicine, Bronx, NY, USA

David Porbunderwala, MD Department of Anesthesiology, New York University Langone Medical Center, New York, NY, USA

Amit Prabhakar, MD, MS Department of Anesthesiology, Louisiana State University Health Sciences Center, New Orleans, LA, USA

Glen D. Quigley, MD, MBA Department of Anesthesiology, Lankenau Medical Center, Wynnewood, PA, USA

Omar Rashid Qureshi, DO Department of Anesthesia and Critical Care, University of Chicago Medical Center, Chicago, IL, USA

Saad Rasheed, MD Department of Anesthesiology, New York University, New York, NY, USA

James Riopelle, MD Department of Clinical Anesthesiology, Louisiana State University Health Sciences Center, New Orleans, LA, USA

Lisa Q. Rong, MD Department of Anesthesiology, Weill Cornell Medical Center, NYP, New York, NY, USA

Dmitry Rozin, MD Department of Anesthesiology, Montefiore Medical Center, Bronx, NY, USA

Lori Russo, MD Department of Anesthesiology, NYU Langone Medical Center, New York, NY, USA

Migdalia Saloum, MD Department of Anesthesiology, Mt. Sinai West/Mt. Sinai St. Luke's, New York, NY, USA; Brooklyn, NY, USA

Corey S. Scher, MD Department of Anesthesiology, Perioperative Care and Pain Medicine, New York University School of Medicine/Langone Medical Center, New York, NY, USA

Elliot S. Schwartz, BA, MD Department of Anesthesiology and Perioperative Medicine, University Hospital, Case Western Reserve University, Cleveland, OH, USA

Samion Shabashev, MD Department of Anesthesia, New York University Langone Medical Center, New York, NY, USA

Nirali Shah-Doshi, MD Department of Anesthesia and Critical Care, The University of Chicago Medical Center, Chicago, IL, USA

Chirag D. Shah, MD, JD Department of Physical Medicine and Rehabilitation, Rush University Medical Center, Chicago, IL, USA

David Shapiro, MD Department of Anesthesiology, Icahn School of Medicine at Mount Sinai, New York, NY, USA

Beamy Sharma, MBA, MD Department of Anesthesiology, Perioperative Care and Pain Medicine, New York University Langone Medical Center, New York, NY, USA

Paul Shekane, MD Department of Anesthesiology, New York University Langone Medical Center, New York, NY, USA

Alexander Sinofsky, MD Department of Anesthesiology, New York University Langone Medical Center, New York, NY, USA; Louisville, KY, United States

Patrick B. Smollen, MD Department of Anesthesiology, Perioperative Care, and Pain Medicine, New York University Langone Medical Center, New York, NY, USA

Jamey Jermaine Snell, MD Department of Anesthesiology, Perioperative and Pain Medicine, Boston Children's Hospital/Harvard Medical School, Boston, MA, USA

Michale Sofer, MD Department of Anesthesiology, Perioperative Care and Pain Medicine, New York University Langone Medical Center, New York, NY, USA

Nader Soliman, MD Department of Anesthesiology, New York University, New York, NY, USA; Los Angeles, CA, USA

Kiwon Song, MD Department of Anesthesiology, Perioperative Care and Pain Medicine, New York University Langone Medical Center, New York, NY, USA

Tiffany Sou, MD Department of Anesthesiology, New York University Langone Medical Center, New York, NY, USA

Lee Stein, MD Department of Anesthesiology, New York University/Bellevue, New York, NY, USA

Agathe Streiff, MD Department of Anesthesiology, Mount Sinai St. Luke's and Mount Sinai West Hospital, New York, NY, USA

Kenneth M. Sutin, MD Department of Anesthesiology, Perioperative Care and Pain Medicine, NYU School of Medicine, New York, NY, USA

Suzuko Suzuki, MD Department of Anesthesiology, New York University Langone Medical Center/Hospital for Joint Diseases, New York, NY, USA

Christopher Y. Tanaka, MD Department of Anesthesiology, Montefiore Medical Center, Albert Einstein College of Medicine, Bronx, NY, USA

Mohan Tanniru, MD MIS, School of Business Administration Oakland University, Rochester, MI, USA

Jonathan Teets Department of Anesthesiology, Perioperative Care and Pain Medicine, NYU School of Medicine, New York, NY, USA

Shruthima Thangada, MD Department of Anesthesiology, New York University Langone Medical Center, New York, NY, USA

Jacob Tiegs, MD Department of Anesthesiology, Perioperative Care & Pain Medicine, New York University School of Medicine, New York, NY, USA

Robert Trainer, DO, MBA Department of Anesthesiology, Hunter Holmes McGuire VA Medical Center, Richmond, VA, USA

Paul A. Tripi, MD, FAAP Department of Anesthesiology and Perioperative Medicine, University Hospitals Case Medical Center, Rainbow Babies and Children's Hospital, Cleveland, OH, USA

Mitchell H. Tsai, MD, MMM Department of Anesthesiology, University of Vermont Medical Center, Burlington, VT, USA

Kevin Turezyn, BA, MD Department of Anesthesiology, New York University Langone Medical Center, New York, NY, USA; Long Island City, NY, USA

Uchenna O. Umeh, MD Department of Anesthesiology, Perioperative Care and Pain Medicine, New York University Langone Medical Center/Hospital for Joint Disease, New York, NY, USA; Queens Village, NY, USA

Lucia Daiana Voiculescu, MD Department of Anesthesiology, Perioperative Care and Pain Medicine, New York University School of Medicine, New York, NY, USA

Cindy J. Wang, MD Department of Anesthesiology, New York-Presbyterian Hospital/Weill Cornell Medicine, New York, NY, USA

Cynthia Wang, MD Department of Anesthesiology and Pain Management, University of Texas Southwestern Medical Center, Dallas, TX, USA

Melville Q. Wyche III, MD Department of Anesthesiology, Louisiana State University Health Sciences Center School of Medicine, New Orleans, LA, USA

Angela Zangara, BSN RN, MSN FNP Department of Anesthesia, New York University School of Medicine, New York, NY, USA; Brooklyn, NY, USA

Jeron Zerillo, MD Department of Anesthesiology, Division of Liver Transplantation, Icahn School of Medicine at Mount Sinai, New York, NY, USA

Part I
General

1 Should Recent Clinical Trials Change Perioperative Management in Patients with Cardiac Risk Factors?

Corey S. Scher

Case

A 75-year-old man with a known history of an ischemic cardiomyopathy presents for resection of a presumed malignant liver tumor. He had 2 cardiac stents placed in the last year and a half. His medications include spironolactone, lisinopril, pioglitazone, and atorvastatin. He also takes 81 mg aspirin per day. A recent cardiac catheterization showed that his stents were wide open and there was evidence of diffuse, cardiac arterial disease not amenable to stenting or surgery. His ejection fraction is 32 %, and there is diastolic dysfunction on his echocardiogram.

Question

What is the best plan for anesthetic management in a patient with multiple cardiac risk factors?

CON: I think I have all of the information I need to go ahead with a general anesthetic, a preoperative thoracic epidural and an awake arterial line before induction. I will use pulse pressure variation (PPV) to determine fluid status and use either hetastarch or albumin if he ends up on the steep portion of the Starling curve where it is essential to give fluids. A PPV >13 % means that stroke volume is changing with inspiration and expiration; these oscillations imply a decrease in preload. It follows that a patient with PPV of >13 % will be fluid responsive [1]. I would not hydrate to a PPV less than 13 % as there is a risk of fluid overload and congestive heart failure. I would go lightly on the crystalloids and be a bit heavy-handed on blood products or colloid to improve stroke volume. In addition, I will get a colleague to help me out with a trans-esophageal echocardiogram (TEE).

C.S. Scher (✉)
Department of Anesthesiology, Perioperative Care and Pain Medicine, New York University School of Medicine, New York, NY 10016, USA
e-mail: coreyscher@gmail.com

PRO: I think that your plan is more than reasonable; I am curious how this plan evolved. I think there is more that you can offer the patient to improve his care based on essential clinical trials. To begin with, I think the patient would have benefited if he had been on a statin. The CARE trial (Cholesterol And Recurrent Events) clearly showed that lowering low-density lipoproteins (LDL) with a statin lowered the risk of a cardiac event in patients with documented cardiac disease [2]. It is essential to note that this was not an anesthesia study but simply a study on the value of statins on both lipids and heart disease. There were fewer myocardial infarctions in the statin group compared to placebo. Statin use led to a lower incidence of infarction and stroke when interventions such as stents or surgery were chosen. More and more proof exists over time that taking perioperative statins is protective against complications [2]. While the relative success of the CARE trial was attributed to lowering LDL and its associated plaque formation, it is possible that the statin might have impacted the amount of inflammation in the coronary arteries.

CON: Every patient should be managed on a case-by-case approach. Although the CARE trial is interesting, I would not delay the case for preoperative management of his lipoproteins. If he reported good exercise tolerance and general function, I would go ahead today. The cancer surgery will certainly be more beneficial to this patient's survival. The evidence for giving statins at the time of surgery is muddled, as the study is old and cardiac stents are a clearer prophylactic paradigm than statins.

PRO: I think you should also add a beta-blocker to your patient's regimen. The POISE trial (Perioperative Ischemic Evaluation) [3] was a randomized controlled trial exploring the impact of perioperative beta-blockers on cardiac death, non-fatal myocardial infarctions, and non-fatal cardiac arrest. In the trial, metoprolol was found to decrease the risk of non-fatal myocardial infarction, while making the risk of stroke and mortality higher [3]. I have been using

C.S. Scher et al. (eds.), *You're Wrong, I'm Right*, DOI 10.1007/978-3-319-43169-7_1

beta-blockers for years and have never seen a case of stroke due to hypoperfusion, but I only use beta-blockers in patients with persistent hypertension and not in cases of hypovolemia. I titrate my dose carefully. An individual evaluation should be performed for each patient to determine the risk–benefit ratio of using beta-blockade. I would clearly use it in this case.

PRO: I do like that the patient is on spironolactone.

CON: Why is that a factor? You would have to make up a reason to convince me.

PRO: There is good evidence for aldosterone inhibitors in patients with systolic heart failure [4].

CON: However, the evidence from patients with *heart failure and a preserved ejection* fraction (HFpEF), such as yours, is limited. In patients with HFpEF, the function of spironolactone was considered [5]. The outcomes of patients hospitalized for HFpEF who received spironolactone were compared to those who did not. The post-hospital mortality rate and readmissions at 1 year were analyzed. With a multivariate survival analysis, 1212 patients with HFpEF with a mean age of 79 years were studied. The majority had hypertensive heart disease (50.7 %). For patients with HFpEF, the administration of spironolactone was associated with an increase in all-cause readmission, perhaps due to the higher rate of hyperkalemia.

PRO: The Aldo-DHF randomized controlled trial, the Treatment of Preserved Cardiac Function Heart Failure with an Aldosterone Antagonist trial [4] and its echocardiography sub-study showed improvements in echocardiographic measures of diastolic function in patients on spironolactone. In the first of these trials, hospitalization for heart failure was significantly reduced with spironolactone therapy; there was no difference in the primary outcome of cardiovascular death. In patients who are at high risk, there may be a reduction in cardiovascular mortality. The final word is not yet in, but the evidence is increasing in favor of using spironolactone for stable heart failure patients.

CON: Sounds like the cost–benefit is evolving in favor of blocking aldosterone, even with the risk of hyperkalemia.

How do I avoid fluid overload, though? I do not want to overload this patient. I will titrate normal saline boluses based on pulse pressure variation.

PRO: Fluid administration is a loaded topic. It makes no sense to give normal saline (NS) because these patients invariably end up with a hyperchloremic metabolic acidosis, which is associated with increased morbidity and mortality [6].

I will also say, from all that I have read in the last 2 years, colloids aren't great either.

CON: So what have you been reading that made you come to that conclusion? In my mind, it is clear that less volume is needed and the patients look better after colloid resuscitation.

PRO: Let us not confuse opinions with facts. Finally there are some strong data that there is very little place for colloid resuscitation. In a fairly recent meta-analysis by Perel et al. [7], the author states, "There is no evidence from randomized controlled trials that resuscitation with colloids reduces the risk of death, compared to resuscitation with crystalloids, in patients with trauma, burns or following surgery. Furthermore, the use of hydroxyethyl starch might increase mortality. As colloids are not associated with an improvement in survival and are considerably more expensive than crystalloids, it is hard to see how their continued use in clinical practice can be justified" [7]. Enough said on this issue, as thousands of patients were included in the 78 trials analyzed.

CON: I am starting to agree, as I have not seen any randomized controlled trials with strong data for colloids. I am now second-guessing my clinical practice.

There is something else that is bugging me. While colloids appear to not be useful, is there a difference between crystalloids?

PRO: Actually that is an essential question. Balanced salt solutions such as plasmalyte, lactated Ringers, and Normosol-R are superior to normal saline for resuscitation. I am going to go on record declaring that normal saline no longer has a place in modern medicine. Simply stated, the title of a paper in Anesthesia and Analgesia in 2013 by McCluskey et al. [6] says it all, "Hyperchloremia after noncardiac surgery is independently associated with increased morbidity and mortality: a propensity-matched cohort study." The stuff is outright toxic. After a liter, you start to go down the wrong path. I cannot think of a case where it would be advantageous. Some are scared to give balanced salt solutions, with their small amounts of potassium, to renal failure patients; I have found that in clinical practice this is a nonissue. For resuscitation, hypertonic saline, 5–7 %, is increasingly used, because it is hyperoncotic and can be used as a volume expander. Hypertonic saline draws fluid into the intravascular space, and very little is needed to get the job done. Although a concern, hypernatremia is only rarely seen after a 100 cc infusion. A single 100 cc bag of 5 % saline can bridge a patient to transfusion when blood is not available or is not ready. Still, caution must be exercised, as hypernatremia can be associated with significant morbidity or even mortality.

CON: I have resuscitated hundreds of patients over 30 years with normal saline and have never had a problem.

PRO: Maybe you just don't follow up well with how your patients do postoperatively.

CON: I'll meet you in the alley after I finish this liver segment resection. Do you have any more pearls of wisdom for that case, Sir Professor?

PRO: In liver lobe resections, with the excellent surgical team that we have, we place 1 large-bore IV and a blood pressure cuff. A thoracic epidural is placed under fluoroscopic guidance.

CON: No arterial line?! And with no central line, how do you measure central venous pressure (CVP)? The surgeons always want the CVP on the low side to prevent engorgement of the liver while they are cutting it. The arterial line is also essential in a potential hemorrhage.

PRO: Simply stated, the CVP does not correlate with filling of the heart as determined by TEE. If you give a small dose of phenylephrine to any patient, the CVP will increase with no change in filling pressures [8].

Massicotte et al. published a paper that is conclusive for my practice [8]. In it, they ask, "do right ventricular end-diastolic volume (RVEDV) and intrathoracic blood volume (ITBV) by TEE represent cardiac preload better than central venous pressure (CVP) and pulmonary capillary wedge pressure (PCWP)?" Left ventricular end-diastolic volume (LVEDV) is the real measure of cardiac preload, and LVEDV was compared to these other measures.

It was demonstrated that a variety of factors, like the use of positive end-expiratory pressure (PEEP) and vasopressors, had a significant impact on CVP but a small effect on LVEDV (true cardiac preload). When the CVP is high, it is inconceivable that you could lower it with any technique other than phlebotomy—which you would never want to do in a liver resection [8]. Simply stated, maybe, and I emphasize maybe, CVP could be valuable in trending. If a central vein is very distensible, adding volume may not increase CVP and if the vein used, by nature, is not distensible, small changes in volume may increase the CVP significantly without any impact on preload.

And how would you manage this patient's diabetes?

PRO: There are many of us who practice anesthesia and do not know what to look for in postoperative visits. If it is not in our anesthesiology journals, it does not mean it does not exist.

The patient is on pioglitazone, an oral agent for diabetes. "Optimal Glucose Management in the Perioperative Period" is an excellent paper [9] from the surgical literature on a topic that I was "soft" on. In the past I would not cancel a case for a blood sugar of 200. In fact, these borderline glucose levels only climb as the case proceeds. Hyperglycemia is defined as glucose greater than 189 mg/dl. Factors contributing to poor control include "counterregulatory hormones, hepatic insulin resistance, decreased insulin-stimulated glucose uptake, use of dextrose-containing intravenous fluids, and enteral and parenteral nutrition" [9]. Hyperglycemia in the perioperative period is associated with increased morbidity and decreased survival. Both morbidity and mortality around the time of surgery are decreased by ideal glucose management. I now measure glucose with a venous sample and send it off to the laboratory with a request for immediate results or obtain an arterial or venous blood gas, which gives you a response within minutes. I would now characterize my behavior surrounding hyperglycemia as "intense."

CON: Would you go through this "intense" therapy for a glucose of 200?

PRO: With surgical stimulation and the accompanying cortisol release, the glucose only goes up, and yes, anything above 180 receives intense insulin therapy. There has to be a line somewhere, that is the trigger point. There are so many pros and cons in what appears to be a routine case. Let us look at some of them after consulting our colleagues in our department.

CON: We need to chat more. I am ready to go into the operating room. Despite the impressive database you have in your mind, I will do this case just like I always have.

Summary

These papers might change the way you practice. Staying current is essential as so much of the literature from the time that I was a resident is simply not true anymore. Although not every study will stand the test of time, it is worth examining and discussing the latest literature with your colleagues, for the ultimate benefit of the patients you care for every day.

References

1. Luecke T, Roth H, Herrmann P, Joachim A, Weisser G, Pelosi P, Quintel M. Assessment of cardiac preload and left ventricular function under increasing levels of positive end-expiratory pressure. Intensive Care Med. 2004;30(1):119–26.
2. Sacks FM, Pfeffer MA, Moye LA, Rouleau JL, Rutherford JD, Cole TG, et al. The effect of pravastatin on coronary events after myocardial infarction in patients with average cholesterol levels. Cholesterol and Recurrent Events Trial investigators. N Engl J Med. 1996;335(14):1001–9.
3. POISE Study Group, Devereaux PJ, Yang H, Yusuf S, Guyatt G, Leslie K, Villar JC, et al. Effects of extended-release metoprolol succinate in patients undergoing non-cardiac surgery (POISE trial): a randomized controlled trial. Lancet. 2008;371(9627):1839–47.
4. Edelmann F, Gelbrich G, Duvinage A, Stahrenberg R, Behrens A, Prettin C, et al. Differential interaction of clinical characteristics with key functional parameters in heart failure with preserved ejection fraction—results of the Aldo-DHF trial. Int J Cardiol. 2013;169 (6):408–17.
5. Bulluck H, Fröhlich GM, Mohdnazri S, Gamma RA, Davies JR, Clesham GJ, et al. Mineralocorticoid receptor antagonist pretreatment to MINIMISE reperfusion injury after ST-elevation myocardial infarction (the MINIMISE STEMI Trial): rationale and study design. Clin Cardiol. 2015;38(5):259–66.
6. McCluskey SA, Karkouti K, Wijeysundera D, Minkovich L, Tait G, Beattie WS. Hyperchloremia after noncardiac surgery is independently associated with increased morbidity and mortality: a propensity-matched cohort study. Anesth Analg. 2013;117(2):412–21.
7. Perel P, Roberts I, Ker K. Colloids versus crystalloids for fluid resuscitation in critically ill patients. Cochrane Database Syst Rev 2013; 2:CD000567.
8. Massicotte L, Perrault MA, Denault AY, Klinck JR, Beaulieu D, Roy JD, et al. Effects of phlebotomy and phenylephrine infusion on portal venous pressure and systemic hemodynamics during liver transplantation. Transplantation. 2010;89(8):920–7.
9. Evans CH, Lee J, Ruhlman MK. Optimal glucose management in the perioperative period. Surg Clin North Am. 2015;95(2):337–54.

Should Real-Time Ultrasound Guidance Be Routinely Used for Central Venous Catheter Placement?

2

James Leonard

Case

A cardiac anesthesia fellow on his first day had just intubated a 67-year-old male undergoing an on-pump 2-vessel coronary artery bypass grafting. The patient had a history of peripheral vascular disease, type 2 diabetes, hypertension, and recent non–ST-segment elevation myocardial infarction (NSTEMI). The fellow had just finished positioning and prepping the patient for a right internal jugular central venous catheter (CVC) placement when his attending walked back into the room and noticed the ultrasound equipment next to the patient's head.

"Wait a second, why do you have this in the room?" the attending asked.

"Ultrasound-guided central line placement was done by everyone at the residency program I was trained at," the fellow replied.

"I've been placing central lines for 30 years, have never used ultrasound, and have never had a complication. If you know your landmarks, you should be able to insert the catheter successfully every time without the use of ultrasound."

Question

Should real-time ultrasound guidance be routinely used for central venous catheter placement?

PRO: The overwhelming majority of central venous catheters (CVCs) are placed in 1 of 3 locations: the internal jugular (IJ), subclavian, or femoral veins using either the landmark technique or the real-time ultrasound-guided technique.

J. Leonard (✉)
Department of Anesthesiology, Perioperative Care and Pain Medicine, New York University Langone Medical Center, 550 First Avenue, New York, NY 10016, USA
e-mail: james.leonard@nyumc.org

While there are many techniques utilizing landmarks for IJ cannulation, the most commonly described method relies on directing the needle between the medial and lateral heads of the sternocleidomastoid muscle, lateral to the carotid artery, and advancing the needle toward the ipsilateral nipple in order to cannulate the vein. For subclavian vein cannulation, the patient is positioned in Trendelenburg, the shoulders are extended, and the needle is inserted 1 cm lateral to the middle third of the clavicle. The needle is walked under the clavicle, directed toward the sternal notch, and slowly advanced until cannulation occurs. For femoral vein cannulation, the femoral artery is palpated and the needle is directed medially to the arterial pulsation 1–2 cm below the inguinal ligament until cannulation occurs.

Ultrasound-guided techniques have been described for IJ, subclavian, and femoral vein CVC placement. Based upon available evidence, ultrasound guidance for IJ CVC placement is the most strongly supported of the 3 sites. Meta-analyses of randomized trials including both adults and infants demonstrated the following benefits of ultrasound guidance versus the landmark technique: a significantly higher rate of successful placement in both adults and infants (99 versus 78 %), a reduction in failed IJ cannulation on the first attempt (33 versus 57 %), fewer total numbers of attempts in adults and infants (1.5–2 fewer mean needle passes), and a reduction in complications, including arterial puncture, in both adults and infants (from 16 to 5 % and from 30 to 6 %, respectively) [1, 2].

CON: The cardiac anesthesia attending allowed the fellow to proceed with ultrasound-guided right IJ CVC placement. Upon ultrasound examination of the right IJ vein, significant intravascular clot was found. Examination of the left IJ revealed a similar level of clot.

"We should attempt a right subclavian line placement," the attending remarked to the fellow. "Should we use ultrasound for that as well?".

Evidence in support of ultrasound guidance is decidedly less robust for femoral and subclavian CVC placement

C.S. Scher et al. (eds.), *You're Wrong, I'm Right*, DOI 10.1007/978-3-319-43169-7_2

compared to IJ placement. With regard to femoral vein cannulation, 1 randomized controlled trial found a higher first-attempt success rate and fewer required needle passes with ultrasound guidance compared to the landmark technique in pediatric patients [3]. For subclavian vein cannulation, a randomized controlled trial of more than 400 mechanically ventilated patients in medical intensive care units reported fewer insertion attempts, higher success rates, reduced access time, and fewer arterial punctures and hematomas when using ultrasound guidance compared with the anatomic landmark approach [4].

PRO: The fellow was familiar with the available evidence regarding ultrasound use in subclavian vein cannulation and knew that his attending was testing his depth of knowledge.

"While I have less experience with ultrasound for subclavian vein CVC placement, I don't think you could be faulted for utilizing it. Overall, ultrasound is a safe technique, and there aren't any complications unique to ultrasound-guided vascular access compared to landmark-guided access that I'm aware of. If you feel comfortable with the technique, why wouldn't you use it?" the fellow replied.

CON: "You bring up something very important there," the attending noted. "The level of benefit of these ultrasound-guided techniques is probably highly operator-dependent."

Indeed, the attending may have a point. When discussing the relative strengths and weaknesses of their study on ultrasound-guided subclavian vein cannulation, Fragou and colleagues conceded that "the benefits of the ultrasound method may not accrue until after a significant learning period and its learning curve may be highly operator-dependent" [4]. This operator-dependent learning curve should therefore be taken into account when ultrasound-guided techniques are utilized.

The fellow and attending proceeded with successful landmark-guided right subclavian central line placement and noted an excellent venous waveform upon connecting the CVC to the transducer.

"Should we get a chest X-ray in the recovery room to confirm the position of the catheter?" the attending asked.

While radiographic confirmation of femoral vein CVC placement is not routinely performed, a variety of modalities have been described to confirm IJ or subclavian catheter placement. Manometry was found in a retrospective analysis to detect arterial punctures not identified by blood flow and color [5]. A randomized controlled trial showed that continuous electrocardiography is efficacious in identifying correct catheter tip placement compared with not using the technique [6]. Observational studies have noted that both fluoroscopy and chest radiography are beneficial in identifying the catheter tip's position after CVC placement. However, in cases where fluoroscopy has been used for catheter placement (such as in the IR suite), a post-procedure chest X-ray is unnecessary unless the suspicion for complications such as pneumothorax is high. More recently, investigators have questioned the need for routine post-procedure chest X-rays for uncomplicated right IJ catheters placed on the first attempt, as the incidence of complications and catheter malposition in this situation is very low [7].

Summary

The available evidence strongly supports the use of ultrasound guidance in IJ CVC placement. This recommendation is reinforced in the 2012 American Society of Anesthesiologists (ASA) Practice Guidelines on Central Venous Access [8], which also states that ultrasound guidance may be used when the subclavian or femoral vein is selected for cannulation. Furthermore, these guidelines recommend the use of waveform manometry or pressure measurement to confirm venous placement of the catheter prior to use. Methods for confirming proper catheter tip position include fluoroscopy, chest radiography, or continuous electrocardiography. While unnecessary when the catheter is placed under fluoroscopy, a post-procedure chest X-ray is still recommended to confirm correct intraoperative placement of IJ and subclavian CVCs, although recent studies have questioned the utility of routine postoperative chest X-rays for uncomplicated right IJ CVC insertions.

References

1. Hind D, Calvert N, McWilliams R, Davidson A, Paisley S, Beverley C, et al. Ultrasonic locating devices for central venous cannulation: meta-analysis. BMJ. 2003;327(7411):361.
2. Calvert N, Hind D, McWilliams RG, Thomas SM, Beverley C, Davidson A. The effectiveness and cost-effectiveness of ultrasound locating devices for central venous access: a systematic review and economic evaluation. Health Technol Assess. 2003;7(120):1–84.
3. Aouad MT, Kanazi GE, Abdallah FW, Moukaddem FH, Turbay MJ, Obeid MY, Siddik-Sayyid SM. Femoral vein cannulation performed by residents: a comparison between ultrasound-guided and landmark technique in infants and children undergoing cardiac surgery. Anesth Analg. 2010;111:724–8.
4. Fragou M, Gravvanis A, Dimitriou V, Papalois A, Kouraklis G, Karabinis A, Saranteas T, Poularas J, Papanikolaou J, Davlouros P, Labropoulos N, Karakitsos D. Real-time ultrasound-guided subclavian vein cannulation versus the landmark method in critical care patients: a prospective randomized study. Crit Care Med. 2011;39:1607–12.
5. Ezaru CS, Mangione MP, Oravitz TM, Ibinson JW, Bjerke RJ. Eliminating arterial injury during central venous catheterization using manometry. Anesth Analg. 2009;109:130–4.

6. Gebhard RE, Szmuk P, Pivalizza EG, Melnikov V, Vogt C, Warters RD. The accuracy of electrocardiogram-controlled central line placement. Anesth Analg. 2007;104:65–70.
7. Lessnau KD. Is chest radiography necessary after uncomplicated insertion of a triple-lumen catheter in the right internal jugular vein, using the anterior approach? Chest. 2005;127:220.
8. American Society of Anesthesiologists Task Force on Central Venous Access, Rupp SM, Apfelbaum JL, Blitt C, Caplan RA, Connis RT, Domino KB, et al. Practice guidelines for central venous access: a report by the American Society of Anesthesiologists Task Force on Central Venous Access. Anesthesiology. 2012;116(3): 539–73.

A Patient with Chronic Kidney Disease Is Coming to the Operating Room for an Emergent Procedure, Which Intravenous Fluid Do You Plan to Give Her?

3

Jacob Tiegs and Arthur Atchabahian

Case

A 56-year-old female with stage 3 chronic kidney disease (CKD) has been diagnosed with acute appendicitis. She has mild hypertension that went undiagnosed for a few years but is now controlled on medication, the name of which she cannot remember. She denies any other medical problems and has no allergies. She states she still makes urine and that she is followed by her nephrologist closely, but unfortunately her renal function has slowly been worsening over the last year. She appears euvolemic and normotensive. You are the anesthesiologist on call and are preparing the operating room for the case, but which IV fluid do you plan to give her?

Question

Which intravenous (IV) fluid choice is best for patients with chronic kidney disease? Does it make a difference if they still produce urine or are anuric?

PRO: You notice, as the patient is being transported to the holding area, that an IV is in place and she has been receiving 0.9 % saline (normal saline). The anesthesia technician says he needs to run to central supply to get more normal saline bags because you are out of them in the operating room (OR). You plan on switching her IV fluid to Plasma-Lyte 148 in the meantime.

J. Tiegs (✉)
Department of Anesthesiology, Perioperative Care & Pain Medicine, New York University School of Medicine, 550 First Avenue, New York, NY 10016, USA
e-mail: jacobtiegs@gmail.com

A. Atchabahian
Department of Anesthesiology, New York University School of Medicine, 301 East 17th St. Room C2-222, New York, NY 10003, USA
e-mail: arthur.atchabahian@gmail.com; Arthur.Atchabahian@nyumc.org

CON: As you are obtaining consent from the patient, a colleague of yours who is taking OB call comes by the OR to see if anything is going on. He says the only patient on L&D just delivered and he wanted to come by to see if you needed help. You tell him briefly about the case and mention you are a little worried about her kidney disease. He reminds you it is stage 3 chronic kidney disease (CKD) and that her glomerular filtration rate (GFR) is still 30–59, and that she makes urine. He says he would not worry too much about it and that he would continue the normal saline she is currently receiving. When you ask why he would choose normal saline, he says "because she is already on it!"

PRO: You reply, "But aren't you worried about the supra-physiologic concentration of chloride in normal saline? It can lead to hyperchloremia and metabolic acidosis, which can potentially cause renal vasoconstriction and worsening GFR."

Your colleague doesn't know that you had just been cleaning out your office and found your stack of 2012 JAMAs. In the journal, Yunos et al. found that the use of a chloride liberal fluid (such as 0.9 % saline) was associated with an increased risk of acute kidney injury and need for renal replacement therapy when compared with a chloride restrictive fluid (such as Hartmann's solution or Plasma-Lyte 148) [1].

You tell your colleague, "I am leaning towards using Plasma-Lyte for this case because of the JAMA article."

CON: You colleague is impressed with your scholarly knowledge; however, he remarks "I too read that article and I believe they studied patients in the ICU, not in the OR. A patient is usually in the OR for a much shorter time than one who is in the ICU."

You note that this is a valid point but feel Yunos' findings cannot be ignored [1].

Your colleague breaks your train of thought with a question, "Wouldn't you be worried using Plasma-Lyte and causing hyperkalemia? It has potassium in it."

PRO: With any patient at risk for renal disease or with existing chronic renal failure, it is important to avoid hyperkalemia.

C.S. Scher et al. (eds.), *You're Wrong, I'm Right*, DOI 10.1007/978-3-319-43169-7_3

However, you remind you colleague that Plasma-Lyte only contains 5 mmol/L of potassium. You state you would have to give a very large volume to increase someone's potassium purely with Plasma-Lyte. Also, most of the potassium in the body is intracellular, and hyperkalemia is more likely to be caused by shifts across cell membranes than by the exogenous administration of small amounts of potassium. In addition, a Cochrane review by Burdett et al. [2] found no difference in postoperative potassium levels between patients receiving buffered (4.02 mmol/L) versus non-buffered (4.03 mmol/L) solutions in their review, and another clinical study by Khajavi et al. [3] found that serum potassium was significantly lower in renal transplant patients given lactated Ringer's versus normal saline. Because of this you feel hyperkalemia is not a particularly strong concern.

However, you are still very much worried about the hyperchloremic metabolic acidosis that can occur with the administration of normal saline. You review the chloride composition of both normal saline, 0.9 %, and Plasma-Lyte 148. Normal saline contains 154 mmol/L of chloride, while Plasma-Lyte 148 contains 100 mmol/L. A normal chloride value on a basic metabolic panel (BMP) is around 96–106 meq/L. It has been well described that hyperchloremic acidosis may cause renal artery vasoconstriction and decrease GFR. But you explain to your colleague "that not only does this acidosis affect kidney function, it also causes an extracellular shift of potassium which would increase overall potassium levels." For these reasons, you really want to avoid normal saline infusion, especially in this patient with impaired renal function who is already at risk.

You decide to bring the patient to the OR and start the case. You have also decided to use Plasma-Lyte as your IV fluid choice. The case is underway and you are given a morning break, during which time you quickly look up the topic on PubMed. You find another article by Shaw et al. that states the use of normal saline in patients after open abdominal surgery was associated with a higher incidence of renal failure requiring dialysis and increased electrolyte abnormalities compared with patients receiving calcium-free balanced crystalloids (Plasma-Lyte), further supporting your decision to not continue the normal saline the patient was receiving on arrival to the OR [4]. You call the anesthesia tech and tell him not to worry about restocking the bags of normal saline.

CON: As the case continues, everything is going along well except her blood pressure begins to drift. You have augmented her BP with small amounts of vasopressors, but believe what she really needs is intravascular volume expansion. At this time, your colleague comes into the room to see how the case is going and to see if you need a lunch break. He notices the downward blood pressure trend and says why not give a colloid such as hydroxyethyl starch (HES) solution. He states it would help expand her intravascular volume while also minimizing the amount of fluid you give to this renally impaired patient.

PRO: Although you appreciate your colleague's advice, you feel that it would not be the best care for the patient.

You tell him, "There have been numerous studies, most notably the SAFE and CRISTAL trials, that have found no difference in morbidity and mortality using colloids versus crystalloids [5, 6]."

In fact, you feel that HES would be a particularly bad choice for your patient. You tell him in addition, a recent study by Kashy et al. found that the use of HES in non-cardiac surgery resulted in a 21 % increased risk of acute kidney injury (AKI) compared with only crystalloids [7]. This effect was dose-dependent, meaning that the more HES a patient received, the greater his chance of developing AKI. Not only that, but patients who received HES also had a higher likelihood of needing renal replacement therapy. You tell your colleague you want to give Plasma-Lyte for volume replacement in this patient and that you only need a quick break. You do not want to be gone too long because you are beginning not to trust your co-worker's clinical judgment.

You come back from your break and are relieved to see your colleague has given the patient a 500 cc bolus of Plasma-Lyte and the blood pressure has responded. As the case is finishing, you begin to wonder if your decisions about intravenous fluid and volume replacement would have been different if your patient had acute kidney injury or was anuric. But you do not believe you would have changed anything. That same Cochrane review you looked at earlier also found no statistical difference between the two groups (patients who received buffered versus non-buffered IV solutions) with regard to urine output or changes in post-operative creatinine levels or creatinine clearance [2]. But in light of the other facts presented here, you feel confident a low chloride crystalloid solution would still be optimal.

As in any clinical situation, each decision you make needs to be patient dependent. Each patient is different, and there is no cookie-cutter approach to any situation. The patient's vital signs and the scenario should guide your decision-making process. But you realize the principles from this case also apply to most patients with impaired renal function. If you believe a patient's hypotension is due to decreased intravascular volume, you should give volume. And as we have discussed, that volume should likely be a low chloride crystalloid such as Plasma-Lyte or lactated Ringer's. In most cases, you should not give fluid just for the purpose of increasing urine output. This holds true for patients with acute kidney injury or chronic kidney disease, whether they make urine or are anuric. The goal is to keep your patient euvolemic and of course not to fluid overload them, but you do not want them hypovolemic either.

Summary

The next day you do a postoperative check on your patient and note she is doing quite well. Her abdominal pain is gone, and she feels much better. Importantly, her renal function remains at baseline. From now on, you will be using a low chloride crystalloid solution for your IV fluid choice in all of your patients with kidney disease. However, more investigation is warranted into which crystalloid (Plasma-Lyte versus Lactated Ringer's) is best for renally impaired patients. Also, there is not currently much research about intravenous fluid choice in patients with existing chronic renal insufficiency or chronic kidney disease. Most of the studies investigate the development of acute kidney injury in the presence of different IV fluids. Studies looking at fluid choice in patients with chronic renal insufficiency would help guide clinicians with these patients whom we often see in the operating room.

References

1. Yunos NM, Bellomo R, Hegarty C, Story D, Ho L, Bailey M. Association between a chloride-liberal vs chloride-restrictive intravenous fluid administration strategy and kidney injury in critically ill adults. JAMA. 2012;308:1566–72.
2. Burdett E, Dushianthan A, Bennett-Guerrero E, Cro S, Gan TJ, Grocott MP, James MF, Mythen MG, O'Malley CM, Roche AM, Rowan K. Perioperative buffered versus non-buffered fluid administration for surgery in adults (Review). Cochrane Database Syst Rev. 2012;12:CD004089.
3. Khajavi MR, Etezadi F, Moharari RS, Imani F, Meysamie AP, Khashayar P, Najafi A. Effects of normal saline vs. Lactated Ringer's during renal transplantation. Ren Fail. 2008;30:535–9.
4. Shaw AD, Bagshaw SM, Goldstein SL, Scherer LA, Duan M, Schermer CR, Kellum JA. Major complications, mortality, and resource utilization after open abdominal surgery: 0.9 % saline compared to Plasma-Lyte. Ann Surg. 2012;255:821–9.
5. Finfer S, Bellomo R, Boyce N, French J, Myburgh J, Norton R, SAFE Study Investigators. A comparison of albumin and saline for fluid resuscitation in the intensive care unit. N Engl J Med. 2004;350:22.
6. Annane D, Siami S, Jaber S, Martin C, Elatrous S, Declère AD, Preiser JC, Outin H, Troché G, Charpentier C, Trouillet JL, Kimmoun A, Forceville X, Darmon M, Lesur O, Reignier J, Abroug F, Berger P, Clec'h C, Cousson J, Thibault L, Chevret S, CRISTAL Investigators. Effects of fluid resuscitation with colloids vs crystalloids on mortality in critically ill patients presenting with hypovolemic shock. The CRISTAL randomized trial. JAMA. 2013;310:1809–17.
7. Kashy BK, Podolyak A, Makarova N, Dalton JE, Sessler DI, Kurz A. Effect of hydroxyethyl starch on postoperative kidney function in patients having noncardiac surgery. Anesthesiology. 2014;121:730–9.

Just Say NO to Nitrous!

4

Corey S. Scher

Case

A 65-year-old man is having an open prostatectomy. His ejection fraction is 30 % due to previous myocardial infarctions. He has multiple coronary artery stents for his extensive coronary artery disease. In addition he is in rate-controlled atrial fibrillation treated with metoprolol and flecainamide. The patient is advised to have a neuraxial anesthetic but he declines. The risks and benefits of a general anesthetic are explained to the patient, and it is decided to give a small dose of sevoflurane with the addition of nitrous oxide and fentanyl to pick up the "slack." The case is discussed in morning conference, and the majority of providers do not agree with the use of nitrous oxide.

Question

Has the evidence finally arrived that it no longer helps the patient to use nitrous oxide?

PRO: In your mind, is the nausea and vomiting associated with nitrous oxide the reason that you prefer not to use it?

CON: After doing anesthesia for 30 years, I am convinced that it could be an issue, especially in ambulatory anesthesia where the last patient to go home is the patient who had nitrous oxide. I do agree that the results of most studies are somewhat non-committal on the postoperative nausea and vomiting (PONV) issue.

PRO: When talking about nausea and vomiting, the term "emetogenic" must be applied. Without a doubt, the chemotherapeutic agent cis-platinum is highly emetogenic, because in normal clinical doses, most patients get sick. Nitrous oxide is always bundled in with inhaled anesthetics and narcotics, and it is clinically hard to sort out. The majority of patients that do receive this daily generic anesthetic do not get sick. Simply stated, nitrous is not strongly emetogenic. I am sure I read a paper a few months ago that concluded that if you were on nitrous for less than an hour, then nitrous would not be a factor in PONV [1]. I know what you are going to say next. By the time the patient is prepped and draped, at least an hour goes by so what is the point?

CON: I do think that you are understating the role of nitrous oxide in PONV. In addition, there is a culture among the surgeons who believe that nitrous oxide distends bowel. Whether it is a fact or not, I do not use it in closed-space cases such as obstructed bowel, ear cases, and eye cases as it always generates an argument that I can avoid by simply not using it. The surgeons do not want to listen to my arguments that in ear cases, nitrous oxide is only a problem if the Eustachian tube is blocked. In eye cases, unless air becomes trapped intraocularly, creating a bubble that could expand, nitrous oxide will not cause a problem.

PRO: There are big-ticket items more important than PONV that we have to settle between us. In a multivariate analysis, the risk of chronic postsurgical pain was decreased in patients who received nitrous oxide [2]. This is a game changer for me. It is common knowledge that chronic pain after surgery is not uncommon and everything that can be done should be done to prevent starting up this malicious cycle. In addition, severe pain in the first postoperative week, wound complications, and abdominal incisions increase the risk of chronic pain.

In the ENIGMA trial, "chronic postsurgical pain was common after major surgery…intraoperative nitrous oxide administration was associated with a reduced risk of chronic postsurgical pain" [3].

Of equal if not more importance is that in many patients, such as those with sleep apnea, higher doses of narcotics are not ideal. Nitrous will lower the intraoperative narcotic

C.S. Scher (✉)
Department of Anesthesiology, Perioperative Care and Pain Medicine, New York University School of Medicine, New York, NY 10016, USA
e-mail: coreyscher@gmail.com

C.S. Scher et al. (eds.), *You're Wrong, I'm Right*, DOI 10.1007/978-3-319-43169-7_4

requirement, increasing safety and potentially decreasing the risk of hypopnea in the postoperative period.

CON: Does the literature make that recommendation or is that just "your common sense"?

PRO: My common sense tells me until we have reason not to; nitrous allows you to give a full anesthetic with a major upside that cannot be ignored. You are one of the many in our field who stopped reading after residency.

CON: I do read. To the best of my knowledge, the ENIGMA trial strongly suggested that nitrous oxide oxidizes the cobalt ion on vitamin B12, inactivating methionine synthase causing a dose-dependent increase in plasma homocysteine concentrations for days after surgery. So you think I do not read! Acutely increased homocysteine concentrations impair endothelial function, induce oxidative stress, and potentially destabilize coronary artery plaques [3]. The use of nitrous is associated with an increased long-term risk of myocardial infarction. If this does not make you stop using nitrous, nothing will [3].

PRO: You do read! You read only the abstract. This was the ENIGMA 1 trial, a flawed retrospective study that was replaced by the ENIGMA 2 trial. The newer trial was done by the same authors but prospectively with a different design targeted at the weaknesses of the ENIGMA 1 trial. Are you familiar with that trial or even better, the differences in the 2 project designs?

CON: When someone mentions the word retrospective, it is assumed that it is flawed. I have seen many prospective studies that have perfect stats and yet are still not believable. A meta-analysis is better because it should take into account the diversity of variables in many populations. Analyzing patient-by-patient rather than study-by-study when the meta-analysis is performed is even better.

PRO: Let me show you the differences in the two designs. In the ENIGMA 1 trial, 2050 surgical patients aged 18 and older and were retrospectively randomized to either 70 % nitrous oxide in 30 % oxygen or oxygen and air. Case reports and records were reviewed. Perioperative care was the decision of each anesthesiologist. The primary end point was duration of stay in the hospital. Slightly more than 50 % of patients were lost to lack of follow-up. Simply stated, the study was very much out of control and underpowered. The patients were analyzed, and the postoperative myocardial infarction rate was only slightly increased in patients given nitrous oxide. In the small number of patients who had homocysteine levels drawn, there was little difference between the two groups. Surveillance for myocardial infarction and stroke were inconsistent by the patient's doctors. I think this paper was published as an introduction to the ENIGMA 2 trial, which was much less flawed. If you do not read the paper and only focus on the abstract, your opinions on nitrous would be ill based and the nitrous dial would be turned off for good.

CON: I am not a very good critical reader. What specific design enhancers were in trial 2 that were not in trial 1?

PRO: ENIGMA 2 was an international randomized, assessor-blinded trial in patients at least 45 years old (better than 18) with known or suspected coronary artery disease having major non-cardiac surgery. The investigators are mostly the same as in the first trial. An automated telephone service randomly assigned patients, stratified by site, to receive general anesthesia with or without nitrous oxide. While providers were not blinded, the patients and assessors were. Of the 7112 patients enrolled, 3543 patients received nitrous and 3509 did not. The primary outcomes assessed were a composite of death and cardiovascular events (non-fatal myocardial infarction, cardiac arrest, pulmonary embolism, and stroke). Postoperative myocardial infarction was defined as a raised biomarker, plus at least 1 of the following: symptomatic ischemia, pathologic EKG waves, EKG findings of ischemia, a coronary artery intervention, a new regional wall motion abnormality on ECHO, and autopsy findings of infarction [4]. There were no differences in any item looked at with all cardiovascular primary outcomes equal at 8 %. No difference was found in wound infection and PONV. The sample size is huge, parameters to be measured were well defined and follow-up is well defined. I feel relieved that the use of nitrous oxide has little if any relationship to postoperative cardiovascular events.

CON: There are still unresolved issues. I have always been taught that nitrous is detrimental to the myelin sheath in nerves. We have all been taught this in medical school, yet we totally ignore this issue, which may or may not be significant. What is your take on this?

PRO: Vitamin B12 (cyanocobalamin) is a component of 2 biochemical reactions: succinyl coenzyme A's transformation into L-methylmalonyl coenzyme A and the methylation of homocysteine creating methionine. It is the transmethylation reaction that is required for DNA synthesis and for the upkeep of the myelin sheath via methylation of myelin basic protein. In order for vitamin B12 to be active, the cobalt within it must stay in its reduced form (Co+). Irreversible oxidation of cobalt occurs with exposure to nitrous oxide, making vitamin B12 useless.

If your patient has severe vitamin B12 deficiency to start with, it follows that nitrous oxide exposure could cause further, even permanent decreases in neurologic function, or even death [5]. There are several case reports of sub-acute degeneration of the spinal cord related to this issue. The frequency is unknown but I would not use nitrous oxide in those with a diagnosis of pernicious anemia where B12 is not absorbed or in patients who are anorexic with concomitant cachexia.

CON: After listening to your 3 teaching points, I have not changed my thoughts on nitrous. I have vomited in the dentist chair from nitrous. I am concerned that on any given day someone could be getting nitrous with a low B12 level. Additionally, the randomized single blind study is just that, a single study.

Summary

Clinicians choose to believe what they want to with regard to the literature in our journals. By no means are these 3 teaching points the end of the controversy. At the end of the day, if you do not use nitrous oxide, then you do not have to worry about these concerns. Some may choose to keep in mind that nitrous oxide has a long history as an anesthetic, starting in December 1844, when Horace Wells performed the first dental operations with the gas in Hartford, Connecticut. Additionally, nitrous oxide may assist with narcotic sparing and therefore decrease the risk of postoperative apnea, especially in the elderly, young pediatric, and fragile patients. The potential role of nitrous oxide in preventing postoperative pain is yet another area well worth additional research.

References

1. Peyton PJ, Wu CY. Nitrous oxide-related postoperative nausea and vomiting depends on duration of exposure. Anesthesiology. 2014;120(5):1137–45.
2. Chan MT, Wan AC, Gin T, Leslie K, Myles PS. Chronic postsurgical pain after nitrous oxide anesthesia. Pain. 2011;152 (11):2514–20.
3. Leslie K, Myles PS, Chan MT, Forbes A, Paech MJ, Peyton P, et al. Nitrous oxide and long-term morbidity and mortality in the ENIGMA trial. Anesth Analg. 2011;112(2):387–93.
4. Myles PS, Leslie K, Chan MT, Forbes A, Peyton PJ, Paech MJ, et al. ANZCA Trials Group for the ENIGMA-II investigators. The safety of addition of nitrous oxide to general anesthesia in at-risk patients having non-cardiac surgery (ENIGMA-II): a randomised, single-blind trial. Lancet. 2014;384(9952):1446–54.
5. Flippo TS, Holder WD Jr. Neurologic degeneration associated with nitrous oxide anesthesia in patients with vitamin B12 deficiency. Arch Surg. 1993;128(12):1391–5.

Closed-Loop Anesthesia: Wave of the Future or No Future?

5

Cedar J. Fowler and Howard Ching

Case

A healthy 30-year-old male presents for a laparoscopic appendectomy. He undergoes induction uneventfully, and the case is underway when you feel the sudden urge to go to the bathroom. You contact your colleague who grudgingly arrives to give you a break. She says to you, "I wish we had an automatic system to manage the anesthetic for these healthy patients so we could take breaks whenever we wanted." You respond by saying, "Even if we did have a closed-loop anesthesia system, we would still need to be here to manage and monitor our anesthetic."

Questions

What is closed-loop anesthesia and is it a good idea to consider? Is it feasible in today's clinical practice?

What Is Closed-Loop Anesthesia?

Before describing closed-loop anesthesia, we should talk about closed-loop systems. An example of a closed-loop system is a thermostat. A user can set the desired room temperature, and the thermostat will control the heating and cooling systems to achieve the set temperature. A closed-loop system has a variable the user would like to control (room temperature) and a target value for the variable (thermostat temperature). The crucial piece is the feedback control system that tells the system how to achieve the target value based on the control value. In the case of the thermostat, should it turn on the heater or air conditioner? A closed-loop anesthesia system is more complex and would allow for the administration of anesthesia to different individuals. The target variables in closed-loop anesthesia can be any of the monitors we use on a daily basis, such as heart rate and blood pressure. The bispectral index (BIS) monitor also gives us a possible surrogate for the level of hypnosis in a patient. The variables that the system would control can be anything from IV fluids to IV medications.

C.J. Fowler
Department of Anesthesiology, Perioperative and Pain Medicine, Stanford University, 300 Pasteur Drive, Department of Anesthesia, H3580, Stanford, CA 94305-5640, USA
e-mail: cedar@stanford.edu

H. Ching (✉)
Department of Anesthesiology, NYU Langone Medical Center, New York, NY 10016, USA
e-mail: howard.ching@nyumc.org

PRO: Automation has become increasingly prevalent in our lives, playing a greater role with each passing year. We have become comfortable with automation controlling the temperature in our homes and ensuring our safety in air travel. We are also likely to see even more automation in our automobiles as the major car companies are reported to be planning self-driving cars by 2020. Thus, public comfort and acceptance of automation is likely to increase in the near future.

CON: Automation can take away my independence and potentially my job. If I use an approved system and a patient has a bad outcome, who is ultimately responsible? I'm not sure if I feel comfortable putting my medical license on the line by using a machine.

PRO: Currently, there are no commercially available closed-loop anesthesia systems and definitely not one that could control every aspect of anesthesia care for a patient. So you are not at risk of losing your job. A few systems are in the research phase, and most studies are still trying to tease out the risks versus benefits of using a closed-loop system. The focus in the literature appears to be on closed-loop fluid resuscitation and systems capable of monitoring and controlling hypnosis and analgesia. If the technology is able to prove itself, then it is possible that using closed-loop anesthesia may be necessary in order to keep your job and to comply with hospital outcome measures and reimbursement, as OR events become increasingly integrated into the EMR system and easier to benchmark. Data supporting this are

C.S. Scher et al. (eds.), *You're Wrong, I'm Right*, DOI 10.1007/978-3-319-43169-7_5

already being reported in the literature. A decision support system to identify critical events in patients under spinal anesthesia found that it resulted in significantly fewer episodes of hypoxemia as well as a decrease in the time to detect and treat critical events compared to manual control [1]. This randomized controlled trial also noted that the manual control group was 25 % less likely to identify a critical event than the decision support system.

A multicenter Indian trial found that closed loop was better able to maintain BIS and heart rate than manual control. They used a closed-loop anesthesia delivery system that used BIS as the control variable and propofol infusion as its feedback control. Here too, they noted greater variability among the different study sites in the manual control group than under the closed-loop system [2]. With regard to closed-loop fluid resuscitation, a recent clinical trial found better compliance with closed-loop goal-directed fluid therapy (GDFT) than with manual control. They also found that the automated system did not significantly change the workload of the anesthesiologist when compared to non-GDFT practice [3].

The good news is that pharmacology and physiology are not going to change, and closed-loop systems should be easily integrated into our practice when the time comes. These systems still require a skilled anesthetist to operate them, while allowing us more freedom to perform higher-level clinical tasks.

CON: I will forever be able to make better clinical decisions than a program because I bring years of clinical experience and medical knowledge whenever I administer an anesthetic. Those systems you just mentioned only monitor and control 1 aspect of anesthesia care. If I am already responsible for total anesthesia and patient care how does this help me? Can't I just setup my own propofol infusion that requires minimal intervention? Why would I need this system?

PRO: That's true, you do have much more knowledge and skill than a closed-loop system, but I think you should be applying your experience to higher-level tasks, especially with more complicated and sick patients. As a more practical example, McGill University is working on a closed-loop system they call McSleepy that monitors hypnosis via BIS and analgesia with Analgoscore, a previously proven home-grown surrogate marker for antinociception. Their system monitors 3 aspects of anesthesia care. McSleepy provides hypnosis with propofol, analgesia with remifentanil, and muscle relaxation with rocuronium. They found that McSleepy maintained hypnosis and antinociception closer to the desired goals significantly more often than manual administration of total intravenous anesthesia [4].

The studies we previously mentioned demonstrate that computer systems excel at repetitive, "attention-based" tasks, do not suffer from decreased vigilance, and also allow standardization from OR to OR.

CON: Great, so a computer can keep a target variable within a specific range better than I can, so what? Anesthesia isn't just a numbers game.

PRO: You're absolutely right, so you would still need to be present to monitor the patient and perform higher-level functions, leaving the more repetitive tasks to the closed-loop system.

CON: So you're saying that these systems would be more like copilots rather than autopilots?

PRO: Yes.

CON: I think I can live with that; ultimately I'll still be able to monitor my own patients and provide medical care. I guess I won't have to worry too much about it until they develop a robot that can also intubate and put in IVs…

PRO: Interestingly, that too may not be too far off [5] … until then, I'll see you when I get back from the bathroom.

References

1. Zaouter C, Wehbe M, Cyr S, Morse J, Taddei R, Mathieu P, Hemmerling TM. Use of a decision support system improves the management of hemodynamic and respiratory events in orthopedic patients under propofol sedation and spinal analgesia: a randomized trial. J Clin Monit Comput. 2013;28:41–7.
2. Puri G, Mathew P, Biswas I, Dutta A, Sood J, Gombar S, et al. A multicenter evaluation of a closed-loop anesthesia delivery system. Anesth Analg. 2016;122(1):106–14.
3. Rinehart J, Lilot M, Lee C, Joosten A, Huynh T, Canales C, Imagawa D, Demirjian A, Cannesson M. Closed-loop assisted versus manual goal-directed fluid therapy during high-risk abdominal surgery: a case–control study with propensity matching. Crit Care. 2015;19(19):94.
4. Hemmerling T, Arbeid E, Wehbe M, Cyr S, Taddei R, Zaouter C. Evaluation of a novel closed-loop total intravenous anaesthesia drug delivery system: a randomized controlled trial. Br J Anaesth. 2013;110:1031–9.
5. Tighe P, Badiyan S, Luria I, Lampotang S, Parekattil S. Robot-assisted airway support. Anesth Analg. 2010;111:929–31.

6 Should Acute Respiratory Distress Syndrome (ARDS) Preventative Ventilation Be Standard in the Adult Operating Room?

Samir Kendale

Case

Dr. X is leaving for the night after starting anesthesia for a laparoscopic cholecystectomy. Dr. Y comes into the operating room (OR) to take over the case. The patient is a 70 kg, 5′3″, 45-year-old female with a history of hypertension. The surgery is being performed under general endotracheal anesthesia. Dr. X has set the ventilator to volume control, at a tidal volume of 700 mL, respiratory rate of 12, fraction of inspired oxygen (FiO2) of 50 %, and positive end-expiratory pressure (PEEP) of 0. After Dr. X has completed his turnover of the case, Dr. Y reaches over to the ventilator and reduces the tidal volume to 400 mL. Dr. X asks Dr. Y why he has changed the ventilator settings.

Question

Should acute respiratory distress syndrome (ARDS) preventative ventilation be standard in the adult operating room?

PRO: Don't you read journals? Intensive care unit (ICU) physicians have been using low tidal volumes to reduce the mortality of their ARDS patients for years now. We should be doing the same for our patients in the OR. High tidal volumes can induce lung injury, including volutrauma and barotrauma.

CON: But how do we know if the same reduced tidal volume strategy is going to have any effect on surgical patients?

PRO: Because the mechanisms of injury to the lung are the same, we can assume that the excessive stretch on the lungs is going to cause ventilator-induced damage. The ventilator should be set to 6–8 mL/kg of ideal body weight. There was a prospective trial that confirmed this, and patients on smaller tidal volumes had a reduced occurrence of acute respiratory failure and a reduced hospital length of stay [1]. At the very least, even if you aren't using a lung-protective strategy, you should have used ideal body weight to determine this patient's ventilator settings.

CON: I'll give you that one. This patient's ideal body weight is closer to 50 kg, so my ventilator settings should have been set based on that. You haven't answered my question though; that study was in patients with an intermediate to high risk of postoperative pulmonary complications [1]. How does that translate to our general anesthesia population, in which most patients do not have injured lungs and are not at high risk of pulmonary complications? See, I do read journals.

PRO: Well, even with open abdominal surgery, in patients that did not have an increased risk of postoperative pulmonary complications a protective ventilation strategy results in improved pulmonary function tests and higher oxygen saturation [2].

CON: So it may be beneficial in abdominal surgery, but we don't know about other surgical procedures. We have traditionally used higher tidal volumes to prevent hypoxia and atelectasis, especially in laparoscopic cases where the pneumoperitoneum may worsen atelectasis. There was that one prospective study that showed no benefit to low tidal volumes in upper abdominal surgery [3].

PRO: That study was not clear about the use of PEEP. We should be using PEEP in combination with low tidal volumes to prevent hypoxia and atelectasis. This may aid in avoidance of inflammation in the lungs from the repetitive opening and closing of alveoli. Not using PEEP in a lung-protective strategy, actually, may result in increased mortality [4].

S. Kendale (✉)
Department of Anesthesiology, Perioperative Care and Pain Medicine, New York University Langone Medical Center, 550 First Avenue, New York, NY 10016, USA
e-mail: samir.kendale@nyumc.org

C.S. Scher et al. (eds.), *You're Wrong, I'm Right*, DOI 10.1007/978-3-319-43169-7_6

CON: OK. How much PEEP do we need to use?

PRO: Um…I don't know exactly.

CON: Right. Because the Protective Ventilation Using High Versus Low PEEP (PROVHILO) trial demonstrated that there was an increase in hemodynamic instability and hypotension with the institution of high levels of PEEP [5].

PRO: That trial compared a PEEP of 12 cmH_2O with a PEEP of ≤ 2 cmH_2O. Those may not be the appropriate values to explore because they are so disparate. And the Intraoperative Protective Ventilation (IMPROVE) trial showed benefit from the use of 6–8 cmH_2O PEEP [6].

CON: Just PEEP and low tidal volume? There will still be areas of the lung that will not be distended and consequently poorly aerated.

PRO: Obviously, we will use recruitment maneuvers as well, as that will allow the PEEP to maintain the lung volume once it has been expanded.

CON: Recruitment maneuvers may not be enough to improve postoperative lung function in morbidly obese patients who undergo laparoscopic gastric bypass surgery [7]. If recruitment maneuvers are not useful in that population that is highly susceptible to postoperative atelectasis, then what's the point?

PRO: It depends on what parameters we want to look at. Perhaps if alternate outcomes are assessed, we may find what the exact benefit is. We also may need to find the exact group of patients and the right components and combinations of lung-protective strategies.

CON: So you're saying we should probably use a lung-protective strategy with PEEP and recruitment maneuvers in a certain subset of patients. That subset may be patients with a high likelihood of postoperative pulmonary complications. It may be patients having open abdominal surgery. It may be patients having only major surgery. It may be some specific combination of these factors, but it also may harm patients if used in the wrong population.

PRO: Yes, that is correct.

CON: We also don't know how much PEEP to use or whether or not to use recruitment maneuvers, and in what population these will be most effective.

PRO: Well, yes, that's also true, but we do know it definitely has a significant impact in a specific subset of patients.

CON: We should just use our clinical judgment then?

PRO: Most likely, at this point, yes. We should consider whether a patient is at risk of pulmonary complications and whether any intraoperative events are going to increase this risk, and then decide what our ventilation strategy will be. I think that, though, most likely a comprehensive approach involving low tidal volume, PEEP, and recruitment maneuvers will prove to be beneficial to a large number of patients.

References

1. The Acute Respiratory Distress Syndrome Network Ventilation with lower tidal volumes as compared with traditional tidal volumes for acute lung injury and the acute respiratory distress syndrome. N Engl J Med. 2000;342(18):1301–8.
2. Severgnini P, Selmo G, Lanza C, Chiesa A, Frigerio A, Bacuzzi A, et al. Protective mechanical ventilation during general anesthesia for open abdominal surgery improves postoperative pulmonary function. Anesthesiology. 2013;118:1307–21.
3. Treschan TA, Kaisers W, Schaefer MS, Bastin B, Schmalz U, Wania V, et al. Ventilation with low tidal volumes during upper abdominal surgery does not improve postoperative lung function. Br J Anaesth. 2012;109:263–71.
4. Levin MA, McCormick PJ, Lin HM, Hosseinian L, Fischer GW. Low intraoperative tidal volume ventilation with minimal PEEP is associated with increased mortality. Br J Anaesth. 2014;113: 97–108.
5. Hemmes SN, Gama de Abreu M, Pelosi P, Schultz MJ, PROVE Network Investigators for the Clinical Trial Network of the European Society of Anaesthesiology. High versus low positive end-expiratory pressure during general anaesthesia for open abdominal surgery (PROVHILO trial): a multicentre randomised controlled trial. Lancet. 2014;384(9942):495–503.
6. Futier E, Constantin JM, Paugam-Burtz C, Pascal J, Eurin M, Neuschwander A, et al. A trial of intraoperative low-tidal-volume ventilation in abdominal surgery. N Engl J Med. 2013;369(5): 428–37.
7. Defresne AA, Hans GA, Goffin PJ, Bindelle SP, Amabili PJ, DeRoover AM, et al. Recruitment of lung volume during surgery neither affects the postoperative spirometry nor the risk of hypoxaemia after laparoscopic gastric bypass in morbidly obese patients: a randomized controlled study. Br J Anaesth. 2014;113 (3):501–7.

I Gave Rocuronium 3 Hours Ago, Do I Need to Reverse?

7

Daniel Kohut and Kevin Turezyn

Case

A 58-year-old woman with chronic low back pain secondary to nerve impingement presents for lumbar laminectomy and fusion. The patient has a history of coronary disease treated with a stent 3 years ago, as well as obesity and moderate chronic obstructive pulmonary disease (COPD) from smoking. Transcranial motor evoked potential monitoring will be performed during the procedure to assess motor function, so neuromuscular blocking drugs cannot be given during the case. One dose of rocuronium, 30 mg, is given at the surgeon's request to aid the initial dissection, and no further muscle relaxation is administered for the rest of the operation. Three hours later, the patient is breathing spontaneously with good tidal volumes, seemingly ready for extubation. Your attending walks in and asks if the patient has been reversed.

Question

Should a dose of neuromuscular blockade reversal be given?

CON Doc, rocuronium is an intermediate acting non-depolarizing agent. It reaches peak effect within several minutes and lasts for approximately 45–90 min. The patient is able to produce adequate tidal volumes on her own with the endotracheal tube in place. She is also able to sustain a head lift of >5 s. These parameters are generally accepted as indications that a patient is strong enough to maintain adequate ventilation. Therefore, I don't think she needs any reversal.

PRO Your facts are correct, but how do you really know that the patient's muscle strength is truly back to her baseline, or at least close to it? Being able to take "normal" tidal volumes doesn't give us much information, as up to 80 % of her receptors may still be occupied! Even if she is able to sustain a 5-s head lift, up to 50 % of her receptors may still be occupied. Are you still comfortable extubating without any reversal?

CON I see what you're saying, which is why I also used a twitch monitor. I placed the leads on the patient's lateral forehead over her facial nerve and found that she has a train-of-four (TOF) ratio >0.9. In addition to this, she has no evidence of fade on sustained tetanus. Together, these 2 signs indicate that the patient has no residual paralysis and that the endotracheal tube can be removed without providing medication for reversal.

PRO OK, but you are aware of how bad we as clinicians are at accurately assessing TOF ratios quantitatively, right? I'd be slightly more comfortable if you used double-burst suppression, which consists of 2 short 50 Hz stimuli separated by 750 ms. The strength of the first twitch is comparable to the strength of the first TOF twitch, and the strength of the second is comparable to the fourth twitch in TOF. It's much easier to assess the difference in strength between 2 rather than the first and last of 4 twitches.

In addition, the fact that you are using facial muscles to assess muscle strength is also concerning. The orbicularis oculi and the corrugator supercilii are both fairly resistant to neuromuscular blockade; therefore, when you observe 4 twitches there, the patient may only have 2 or 3 at the

D. Kohut (✉) · K. Turezyn
Department of Anesthesiology, New York University Langone Medical Center, 550 First Avenue, New York, NY 10016, USA
e-mail: Daniel.Kohut@nyumc.org

K. Turezyn
e-mail: kevin.Turezyn@nyumc.org

D. Kohut
480 2nd Avenue, Apt. 9C, New York, NY 10016, USA

K. Turezyn
43-10 Crescent Street, Apt. 2507, Long Island City, NY 11101, USA

C.S. Scher et al. (eds.), *You're Wrong, I'm Right*, DOI 10.1007/978-3-319-43169-7_7

adductor pollicis, for example. It has been shown recently that using a twitch monitor on facial muscles is associated with an increased incidence of postoperative residual neuromuscular block in the PACU [1].

Ideally, we should use a more quantitative metric to assess neuromuscular blockade, such as acceleromyography. With this technique, a piezoelectric myograph is attached to the stimulated muscle and is used to measure the force produced by the electrical stimulus. The acceleromyography then calculates the TOF ratio, providing the clinician with an objective value. Murphy et al. showed that acceleromyography was superior to the subjective TOF technique in preventing PACU complications such as the need for further airway interventions and the incidence of oxygen desaturation [2]. The problem with such devices, though, is that most clinicians aren't aware of how to use them. Every patient's response must be calibrated and normalized prior to administering any neuromuscular blocker, as assessing the quantitative TOF with a non-calibrated device is essentially useless.

CON Wow, Doc, you're like a walking journal! OK, so you're not satisfied with my assessment of this patient's muscle strength, but I'd like to mention a few things about the reversal you seem to be pushing for. Neuromuscular reversal drugs are not benign. Even when a patient is given an appropriate weight-based dose, it has variable physiologic effects. The increased parasympathetic output that results from acetylcholinesterase inhibition by neostigmine can lead to bradycardia, causing hypotension. Worse, it can occasionally lead to unstable junctional or ventricular rhythms. In order to prevent this, neostigmine is usually given with a dose of an anticholinergic agent. This often causes patients to become tachycardic. While this is usually benign, it can produce hemodynamic instability in patients with aortic stenosis. It can also affect the ratio of myocardial oxygen demand to perfusion in patients like ours who have a history of coronary disease, leading to myocardial ischemia.

PRO You are indeed correct! But tachycardia and bradycardia are both treatable, and it is also important in patients with severe cardiac disease to prevent post-op respiratory complications.

CON Well, Doc…that's where it gets really tricky! Not only can neostigmine have adverse hemodynamic affects, but recent studies have also shown that it can have adverse respiratory effects! One moderate-sized prospective study showed an increase in post-op atelectasis in patients given neostigmine. This same study showed even larger effects, including an increased incidence of pulmonary edema as well as longer hospital and PACU stays when patients were given high-dose neostigmine [3]. While the exact reasons for this are unclear, it is hypothesized that neostigmine may actually have a paradoxical affect on respiration when given to patients who have spontaneously achieved full recovery. It is believed that it may decrease respiratory muscle strength and increase upper airway collapse, leaving patients more prone to respiratory complications.

PRO Well, it seems we're at an impasse. On the one hand we can extubate the patient without any reversal and risk having postoperative weakness and all its associated complications, while on the other hand we risk untoward hemodynamic effects of neostigmine, and even increased muscle weakness. Ah, what the hell, let's just pull the tube and just keep a close eye on her in PACU.

References

1. Thilen SR, Hansen BE, Ramaiah R, Kent CD, Treggiari MM, Bhananker SM. Intraoperative neuromuscular monitoring site and residual paralysis. Anesthesiology. 2012;117:964–72.
2. Murphy GS, Szokol JW, Marymont JH, Greenberg SB, Avram MJ, Vender JS, Nisman M. Intraoperative acceleromyographic monitoring reduces the risk of residual neuromuscular blockade and adverse respiratory events in the postanesthesia care unit. Anesthesiology. 2008;109:389–98.
3. Sasaki N, Meyer MJ, Malviya SA, Stanislaus AB, MacDonald T, Doran ME, Igumenshcheva A, Hoang AH, Eikermann M. Effects of neostigmine reversal of nondepolarizing neuromuscular blocking agents on postoperative respiratory outcomes. Anesthesiology. 2014;121:959–68.

How Do You Recognize and Treat Perioperative Anaphylaxis?

8

Amit Prabhakar, Melville Q. Wyche III, Paul Delahoussaye, and Alan David Kaye

Case

A 60-year-old female is scheduled to have an elective umbilical hernia repair. Preoperative evaluation revealed a past medical history of hypertension, obesity, and well-controlled type II diabetes mellitus. Her home medications include lisinopril, 10 mg, once a day, and metformin, 1000 mg, twice a day. The surgical history includes 2 previous cesarean sections and an elective abdominoplasty done at an outside facility. The patient reported no history of complications associated with her prior anesthetic exposure and no history of allergies. Physical examination was relevant for a moderately obese female with good dentition and a Mallampati 2 airway. The patient was given an ASA classification of 2.

On the day of surgery, the patient's vital signs were stable and NPO status was confirmed. She was given midazolam, 2 mg, prior to being moved to the operating room. Once in the operating room, the patient was attached to standard ASA monitors and had several minutes of preoxygenation prior to induction. She was induced with 2 % lidocaine, 100 mg; propofol, 150 mg; and succinylcholine, 120 mg, for a rapid sequence intubation. Direct laryngoscopy was attempted twice; however, the vocal cords were not visualized because of an anterior larynx. An Eschmann catheter was then used to assist in securing the airway. The patient was then put on 2 % sevoflurane, and given vecuronium, 4 mg, and cefazolin, 2 g, at the surgeon's request.

During the perioperative period, the patient was noted to have labile blood pressure, ranging from 75–110/40–80. In an attempt to maintain a mean arterial pressure (MAP) of 70, 100 µg boluses of phenylephrine were given intermittently. Despite the blood pressure fluctuations, all other vital signs remained stable throughout the procedure.

Upon completion of the surgery, the patient was given glycopyrrolate, 0.8 mg, and neostigmine, 4 mg, for reversal of neuromuscular blockade. The patient met the recommended criteria for extubation. She was following commands, breathing spontaneously with a tidal volume of approximately 500 mL, and was able to maintain a head lift for 5 s.

Immediately after extubation, the patient's blood pressure increased to 220/115 and epistaxis was seen. Simultaneously she began to have difficulty breathing independently and her tongue was noted to be enlarged. The decision was made to re-intubate the patient because of impending obstructive respiratory failure. Direct laryngoscopy with the Eschmann stylet was attempted, but was unsuccessful due to extremely edematous upper airway tissue. Video laryngoscopy with an Eschmann was then attempted twice and was also unsuccessful because of edema and swelling. The patient's oxygen saturation dropped to 80 %. After communicating with the surgeons, the decision was made to prevent further harm and perform an emergency tracheostomy.

Emergency tracheostomy was performed, and the patient's oxygen saturation increased to 99 %. However, the blood pressure remained labile during the tracheostomy and multiple 10 µg doses of epinephrine were required to maintain a MAP of 50–60. After the definitive airway was established, a transthoracic echocardiogram was done to rule

A. Prabhakar
Department of Anesthesiology, Louisiana State University Health Sciences Center, 1542 Tulane Ave., Suite 653, New Orleans, LA 70112, USA
e-mail: Amitprabhakar7@gmail.com; aprab1@lsuhsc.edu

M.Q. Wyche III
Department of Anesthesiology, Louisiana State University Health Sciences Center School of Medicine, 1542 Tulane Avenue, Suite 659, New Orleans, LA 70112, USA
e-mail: mwych1@lsuhsc.edu

P. Delahoussaye
Department of Anesthesiology, Louisiana State University Health Sciences Center, 1542 Tulane Ave., New Orleans, LA 70112, USA
e-mail: pdelah@lsuhsc.edu

A.D. Kaye (✉)
Department of Anesthesiology, Louisiana State University Health Sciences Center, Room 656, 1542 Tulane Ave., New Orleans, LA 70112, USA
e-mail: alankaye44@hotmail.com

C.S. Scher et al. (eds.), *You're Wrong, I'm Right*, DOI 10.1007/978-3-319-43169-7_8

out a cardiovascular etiology. The echocardiogram showed an ejection fraction >55 %, no wall motion abnormalities, and volume depletion. Intraoperative bronchoscopy was also performed and showed edema of the trachea and mainstem bronchi. The patient was stabilized and transferred to the ICU for further resuscitation.

Question

How do you recognize and treat perioperative anaphylaxis?

PRO: Perioperative anaphylaxis is a rare and potentially lethal event that requires quick recognition by the clinician. The incidence of perioperative anaphylaxis is estimated to be 1 in 10,000–20,000 anesthetic procedures [1, 2]. According to the National Institute of Allergy and Anaphylaxis Network symposium, anaphylaxis is defined as "a serious allergic reaction that is rapid in onset and may cause death" [3]. This is a difficult case because she had a negative surgical history, so you really wouldn't expect anything as bad as full blown anaphylaxis.

CON: While statistically rare, the true incidence of anaphylaxis is likely underreported because the majority of reactions go unrecognized because they are mild and transient. As an anesthesiologist, you can never assume anything. You are expected to be the person in the room who can quickly identify and solve the problem when others can't.

PRO: Well, if you do suspect anaphylaxis you should be aware of the typical signs of a severe allergic reaction. Those include erythema, edema, pruritus, hypotension, tachycardia, and bronchial and gastrointestinal smooth muscle constriction [1].

CON: Yes, but everything is much trickier for a patient under general anesthesia. The majority of these signs and symptoms are masked by anesthesia. The patient is often fully covered with a sterile drape, so cutaneous signs may not be seen initially [1]. Blood pressure is often lower than normal during anesthesia due to various anesthetic agents. Thus, the anesthesia provider may just treat it as decreased vascular tone and give a small dose of a vasopressor. Also, fluctuations in blood pressure are expected in patients with hypertension because of an altered autoregulatory curve. And obviously an intubated patient won't be able to tell you that they are itching. Clinicians should be wary of refractory hypotension with minimal response to vasopressors and increasing peak inspiratory pressures.

PRO: So then the initial diagnosis has to be presumptive and based upon astute clinical judgment. This is important because life-threatening anaphylaxis can progress within minutes of initial presentation. To review, there are 4 different types of hypersensitivity reactions and they present differently. Type I is an IgE-mediated response that leads to histamine release from mast cells causing vasodilation, bronchospasm, and cardiovascular collapse in severe cases. This type of reaction is common with drugs and is the most likely one to be encountered in the operating room. Type II is an IgG-mediated reaction that occurs when preformed antibodies bind to an antigen and activate the complement cascade. A type III hypersensitivity reaction is when an antibody–antigen complex forms and causes an immune response. Type IV hypersensitivity reactions involve T cell-mediated cytokine release in response to a previously encountered antigen.

CON: The initial diagnosis can be presumptive, but it is imperative to establish a definitive diagnosis once the patient is stabilized. This is crucial because there are no preemptive therapeutic strategies to prevent anaphylaxis in the future. The patient should undergo extensive allergy testing to help identify the triggering agent [1]. While a definitive diagnosis is dependent on testing, there are several markers you can look for that support a diagnosis of anaphylaxis. Preformed histamine is released by both basophils and mast cells in response to activation and cell degranulation. Histamine usually has a half-life of 15–20 min [4]. However, in severe anaphylactic reactions histamine levels can remain elevated for up to 2 h, likely because of saturation of enzymatic metabolism [4]. Serum tryptase levels can also be measured within 2 h of a suspected reaction with elevated levels supporting mast cell activation and anaphylaxis [4].

PRO: The anesthesiologist must also be aware of the potential triggers of anaphylaxis. The most of common causes of hypersensitivity reactions and anaphylaxis in the perioperative period include drugs, latex products, and intravenous fluids. The most common drugs associated with anaphylaxis are antibiotics, neuromuscular blockers, hypnotic agents, and rarely, opiates.

CON: Studies have shown that neuromuscular blocking agents are the most common offending drugs, with an incidence of 50–70 % [5, 6]. The second most common trigger is latex, which has been reported to account for 16.9 % of perioperative anaphylactic reactions [5, 7]. The third most common cause of anaphylaxis in the operating room includes antibiotics such as β-lactams and vancomycin [5]. The patient in our case received preoperative cefazolin and midazolam, and vecuronium on induction. The surgery team also used latex gloves. As you can see there is a myriad of possible triggers and allergy testing for this patient is still ongoing.

Summary

Anaphylaxis is a severe allergic reaction that can progress to a life-threatening condition within minutes of initial presentation. Acute management of the patient includes conventional emergency supportive measures. These include boluses of intravenous fluid and epinephrine to counteract refractory hypotension, β-2 agonists to reverse bronchospasm, and corticosteroids with or without histamine-1 receptor antagonists to mitigate cytokine release. While an immediate definitive diagnosis is not possible, the clinician must be cognizant of the acute presentation and treatment of anaphylaxis in the perioperative setting. Once the patient is stabilized, definitive diagnosis and management require a coordinated effort by anesthesiologists, allergists, and the surgery team.

References

1. Riou B. Anaphylaxis and anesthesia. Anesthesiology. 2009;111:1141–50.
2. Dewachter P, Mouton-Faivre C. What investigation after an anaphylactic reaction during anesthesia? Curr Opin Anaesthesiol. 2008;21:363–8.
3. Sampson HA, Muñoz-Furlong A, Campbell RL, Adkinson NF Jr, Bock SA, Branum A, et al. Second symposium on the definition and management of anaphylaxis: summary report—Second National Institute of Allergy and Infectious Disease/Food Allergy and Anaphylaxis Network symposium. J Allergy Clin Immunol. 2006;117:391–7.
4. French Society of Anesthesiology and Intensive Care Medicine. Reducing the risk of anaphylaxis during anesthesia. Ann Fr Anesth Reanim. 2002;21(suppl 1):7–23.
5. Reisacher WR. Anaphylaxis in the operating room. Curr Opin Otolaryngol Head Neck Surg. 2008;16:280–4.
6. Mertes PM, Laxenaire MC. Allergy and anaphylaxis in anaesthesia. Minerva Anestesiol. 2004;70:285–91.
7. Mertes PM, Alla F, Laxenaire MC. Anaphylactic and anaphylactoid reactions occurring during anesthesia in France in 1999–2000. Anesthesiology. 2003;99:536–45.

9 Is Monitored Anesthesia Care (MAC) Safe for All Cases?

Kenneth M. Sutin and Jonathan Teets

Case

Before surgery, the surgeon comforts his anxious patient, "I can do this (choose one: biopsy, face lift, endoscopy, hand procedure) with local anesthesia and a little sedation." The surgeon reassures the patient, "No, I never use general anesthesia, that would be far too risky for such a simple procedure. You'll be in and out before you know it."

The Problem

Boxed into a small corner with no egress, you are the anesthesia provider du jour assigned for this "simple procedure" with sedation and monitored anesthesia care (MAC). You review the patient's record; his internist's preoperative consult indicates that during anesthesia you should avoid hypoxemia and hypotension. Since his Lap-Band surgery, the patient is now only mildly overweight and his sleep apnea has improved. His well-groomed full beard nicely conceals his retrognathia.

Time for Surgery

In the operating room (OR), you commence sedation with a mildly intoxicating cocktail of fentanyl, midazolam, and propofol at 50 mcg/kg/min. Also, you monitor nasal exhaled CO_2 and administer 2 L/min O_2 by nasal cannula to maintain a satisfactory saturation on the pulse oximeter (SpO_2).

All is well until the surgeon indicates, "The patient is still moving, can't you give more propofol?"

You respond, "Yes, I can, but if I do, the patient might stop breathing!"

The surgeon quips, "You're not going to last long around here. If you can't do this, get me someone who can."

Reluctantly, you give more sedation, a little more fentanyl, and then raise the propofol infusion to 100 mcg/kg/min. A few minutes pass and the patient is calm. Soon, the SpO_2 dips to 88 %, you dial up O_2 flow rate; the saturation improves until it falls again, abruptly! You raise the drapes, attempt mask ventilation, but hear only squeaks of air leaking around the patient's face. You fail to insert an LMA, and since the patient is no longer moving, you attempt tracheal intubation as the patient vomits, the pulse oximeter utters a few more deep bass notes, the heart rate slows, then there's a PEA arrest, and you call a code in OR #13.

The surgeon grouses, "My patient better be OK or this is the last day you will ever practice anesthesia!"

Fortunately, this story deserves a happy ending: You successfully intubate the trachea and the patient winds up doing fine. The surgeon cancels the case. Clearly, this could never happen in real life? Does this scenario sound remotely familiar?

Question

Should we make the surgeon happy "at all costs" by following the anesthetic plan he has already promised to the patient?

PRO: MAC with sedation is common and used for millions of procedures every year in the USA. The surgeon is the one who brings in the business, they are HIS patients. At least with an anesthesiologist present, the patient is continually monitored by an individual who is only performing the anesthetic. More and more commonly, surgeons, proceduralists, and dentists are administering "sedation" by themselves at the same time they are performing the procedure. By the careful proceduralists, this amount of sedation is carefully titrated and limited—but not every surgeon is careful!

K.M. Sutin (✉) · J. Teets
Department of Anesthesiology, Perioperative Care and Pain Medicine, NYU School of Medicine, 550 First Avenue, New York, NY 10016, USA
e-mail: kenneth.sutin@nyumc.org; kensutin@yahoo.com

C.S. Scher et al. (eds.), *You're Wrong, I'm Right*, DOI 10.1007/978-3-319-43169-7_9

CON: That's a terrible scenario too, but it doesn't mean that the surgeon should be able to push the anesthesiologist into doing something that is bad for the patient.

MAC is simply dangerous in some cases. When the level of sedation transitions from moderate to deep (defined below), and when supplemented with oxygen, anesthesiologists (rather their patients) may be treading on thin ice. Sure, whether by virtue of skill or good fortune, almost all patients do fine; except, that is, for those who do not. And when they don't, their stories are memorialized in the pages of New York's most prominent medical journal: the *New York Times*. This is MAC's pachyderm in the pantry. When things go wrong, patients transition from hypoventilation to respiratory arrest not with an explosion, but in silence; thus, the signs of apnea can easily be missed if vigilance wavers even for a minute. Never forgotten, however, are the disastrous consequences of delayed or ineffective airway intervention—cardiac arrest, brain damage, and death. Since most patients tolerate deep levels of "conscious" sedation, surgeons and anesthesia providers are readily lulled into a false sense of security that conscious sedation is safe and therefore appropriate in all cases.

Impact of Sedative Agents

Medications commonly used to achieve sedation produce dose-related hypoventilation. They decrease both respiratory rate and tidal volume by a right shift (opioids) or a decrease in slope (benzodiazepines, propofol) of the ventilatory response to $PaCO_2$. When sedative agents are combined, they act synergistically to accelerate oxygen desaturation, hypopnea, and/or apnea [1]. Furthermore, especially when sedation is prolonged, there is progressive atelectasis and a decreased functional residual capacity (FRC). Finally, the individual response to sedation is not always predictable; we have cared for some patients in whom, despite our best intention to achieve moderate sedation, the response is unpredictable and bimodal, vacillating between the extremes of agitation and apnea.

Level of Sedation

The American Society of Anesthesiologists has formally defined increasing levels of sedation as: minimal, moderate, deep, and general anesthesia [2]. The key distinctions for our purpose are that at moderate levels of sedation, patients remain responsive to mild stimulation, airway intervention is not required, and spontaneous ventilation is adequate, while at a deep level of sedation, patients are less responsive to stimulation, they may require airway intervention, and spontaneous ventilation may be insufficient. To limit the consequences of hypoventilation, it is reasonable to avoid prolonged deep sedation unless the airway is controlled.

SpO_2 Monitoring

Anesthesia providers employ a reliable noninvasive tool to measure arterial oxygen saturation (SaO_2)—the pulse oximeter (SpO_2). Unfortunately, we do not often employ noninvasive devices to assess arterial CO_2 ($PaCO_2$), although such devices are commercially available. It is fortuitous that SaO_2 will decrease when the patient is hypoventilating, and in this way, we can take advantage of the pulse oximeter to indirectly assess respiratory depression, but only when the patient is breathing room air!

Capnography

During sedation, anesthesiologists frequently monitor oral or nasal end-tidal CO_2 (or the capnography waveform) to measure respiratory rate, to assess for airway obstruction, and to exclude apnea; for these purposes capnography is effective. However, the absolute value of $EtCO_2$ always underestimates $PaCO_2$, and the gap between the 2 widens with progressive hypoventilation. During conscious sedation, where the tidal volume is not easily measured or predictable, the absolute value of the $EtCO_2$ is prone to misinterpretation. Thus, capnography is useful only to confirm the presence of ventilation and circulation, but not whether either is sufficient.

Room Air Oxygen and the Pulse Oximeter

Since noninvasive $PaCO_2$ measures are not commonly employed, let's examine instead how the arterial saturation measured by a pulse oximeter might be of assistance. Although a detailed analysis is beyond our scope, a few calculations will suffice. One can estimate the consequence of increasing $PaCO_2$ on SpO_2 from the following equations.

Assume:

$$PaO_2 = FiO_2 * (P_{atm} - P_{H2O}) - PaCO_2/RQ - Ps$$

where P_{atm} = 760 mm Hg, P_{H2O} = 47 mm Hg, RQ = 0.8, Ps = shunt.

The Hill equation estimates SaO_2 from PaO_2, (at pH = 7.4, T = 37 °C) [3]:

$$SaO_2 = (23,400 * (PaO_2^3 + 150 * PaO_2)^{-1} + 1)^{-1}$$

Finally, assuming negligible levels of carboxy- and methemoglobin:

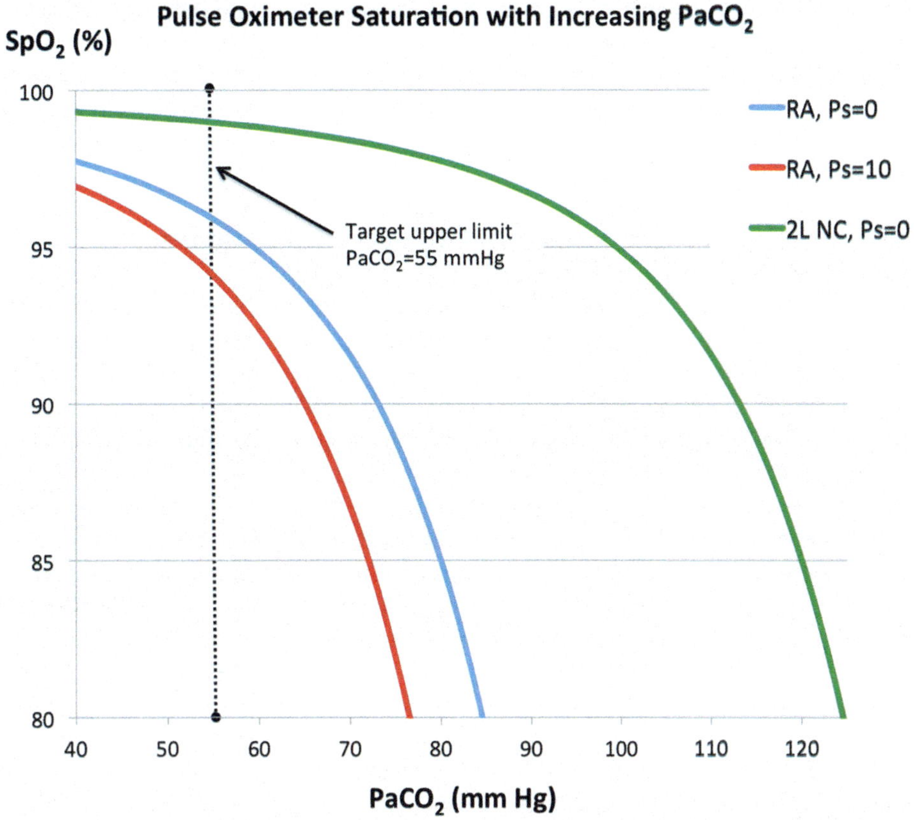

Fig. 9.1 Pulse oximeter saturation with increasing $PaCO_2$

$$SpO_2 = SaO_2$$

For the purposes of our discussion, let's consider that a reasonable decrease in ventilation is achieved when the $PaCO_2$ climbs to 55 mm Hg, and exceeding that number might encroach on potentially dangerous levels of respiratory depression. Further, we will limit this discussion to relatively healthy adult patients and specifically exclude those with respiratory insufficiency, sleep apnea, or oxygen dependency. Applying these formulas, we will estimate the impact of increasing $PaCO_2$ on SpO_2, at specific values of FiO_2 and shunt (Ps). See Fig. 9.1.

For a healthy adult, let's assume there is no shunt; thus, Ps = 0. On room air (RA, FiO_2 = 21 %), the SaO_2 will be $\geq$96 % until the $PaCO_2$ rises above 54 mm Hg. This becomes our safe target: to maintain the saturation at $\geq$96 %. At a $PaCO_2$ of 55 mm Hg, the PaO_2 is still a comfortable 81 mm Hg.

If our patient has some atelectasis, how will that impact these calculations? Let's assume atelectasis introduces a small shunt, Ps = 10 mm Hg. Again, breathing room air, when the $PaCO_2$ reaches our target 55 mm Hg, the saturation will be 94 % and the PaO_2 will be a bit more concerning 71 mm Hg. Thus, compared to a patient with no shunt, the presence of a shunt causes the SpO_2 to read a lower saturation for any given increment in $PaCO_2$, and, provided that we carefully monitor SpO_2, this affords an enhanced margin of safety.

Next, we will estimate the impact of oxygen delivered at 2 L/min by nasal cannula and assume this generates a PiO_2 of 200 mm Hg. Intuitively, we might expect such a small amount of enriched oxygen to have only a minor impact, but that is not the case. Again, we will assume Ps = 0. With enriched O_2, the SpO_2 will remain $\geq$97 % until the $PaCO_2$ rises to 88 mm Hg! At our target for tolerable $PaCO_2$ of 55 mm Hg: (1) SpO_2 will be 98.9 % and will not properly signal when we have achieved our endpoint for moderate hypoventilation, while (2) the PaO_2 is a luxurious 131 mm Hg! This observation that supplemental oxygen can abolish the utility of the pulse oximeter to detect hypoventilation is not a new finding [4]. One final example, assuming a large shunt, Ps = 50 mm Hg, while breathing 2L O_2 NC the SPO_2 drops below 96 % only after the $PaCO_2$ climbs to 55 mm Hg (not shown in graph). Next, we will look at the impact of atelectasis and decreased FRC to see how this fits with our model.

Atelectasis

Small tidal volumes predispose to atelectasis and thus increase shunt. Although a 10 mm Hg shunt is quite small, only on RA is its impact readily detectable by a decrease in SpO_2, and this can be promptly remedied by asking the patient to perform a recruitment maneuver (take a deep breath or cough). In contrast, with enriched inspired O_2, even very significant atelectasis (shunt) may persist undetected by the SpO_2.

FRC

Although decreases in FRC are generally invisible to SpO_2 monitoring, FRC becomes critical during periods of apnea or hypopnea (AH), and these events are common [5]. The reasoning is simple; for a given volume of FRC, the greater the FiO_2, the more residual O_2 is available within the FRC, and the longer the duration of AH until SpO_2 desaturation occurs. In fact, some argue this is advantageous and sedated patients should breathe 100 % O_2 to better tolerate longer periods of AH without SpO_2 desaturation. However, rather than blindly tolerate AH, we suggest it is safest to avoid AH altogether and, if it occurs, to detect it at its earliest onset to expedite proper interventions. As shown earlier, when supplemental O_2 is used, the SpO_2 may still read a high value while $PaCO_2$ climbs dangerously high, so that if or when AH occurs, it does so in the presence of a preexisting respiratory acidosis.

The implication is clear, to help prevent oversedation, one can provide room air O_2 and titrate sedation to a mild decrease in SpO_2. If sedation is still inadequate, rather than giving supplemental O_2, which masks hypoventilation resulting from moderate or deep sedation, first consider obtaining a controlled airway (face mask, LMA, or endotracheal tube) and provide positive pressure ventilation and enriched oxygen as appropriate.

It was well said by Dr. Carl Hug almost a decade ago, "MAC should stand for maximum anesthesia caution, not minimal anesthesia care!" [6].

Many if not most of the severe complications associated with conscious sedation are due to respiratory depression, and for the most part, these are preventable [7].

We propose that employing only RA may provide an extra margin of safety and help to prevent oversedation and potential adverse consequences. If you have previously used enriched oxygen for conscious sedation, when you first employ RA, you will likely be surprised by just how frequently SpO_2 desaturations occur with customary sedative doses (that you likely thought were safe). Employing RA and carefully following every beat and tone of the pulse oximeter enables medications to be titrated to an acceptable (mild) decrease in SPO_2; this can help maintain an adequate respiratory drive and prevent excessive respiratory depression. There is another benefit of room air; because enriched oxygen is the most important factor contributing to OR fires, the risk of fire is decreased.

Summary

Perhaps Joseph Priestley (credited with the discovery of oxygen) said it best in 1776, "…the air which nature has provided for us is as good as we deserve!" When the necessary sedation produces excess depression (e.g., SpO_2 desaturation, loss of airway reflexes, unarousability, airway obstruction, or apnea), consider early intervention to control the airway and ventilation. Finally, our role as consultant anesthesiologists requires us to educate our colleagues about the potential risks associated with moderate or deep sedation, especially when the patient presents with risk factors such as sleep apnea, difficult airway, or a full stomach, or when a patient's individual response to sedation is unpredictable or unacceptable.

References

1. Bailey PL, Pace NL, Ashburn MA, Moll JW, East KA, Stanley TH. Frequent hypoxemia and apnea after sedation with midazolam and fentanyl. Anesthesiology. 1990;73(5):826–30.
2. American Society of Anesthesiologists Task Force on S, Analgesia by N-A. Practice guidelines for sedation and analgesia by non-anesthesiologists. Anesthesiology. 2002;96(4):1004–17.
3. Severinghaus J. Simple, accurate equations for human blood O2 dissociation computations. J Appl Physiol Respir Environ Exerc Physiol. 1979;46(3):599–602.
4. Fu ES, Downs JB, Schweiger JW, Miguel RV, Smith RA. Supplemental oxygen impairs detection of hypoventilation by pulse oximetry. Chest. 2004;126(5):1552–8.
5. Anand GW, Heuss LT. Feasibility of breath monitoring in patients undergoing elective colonoscopy under propofol sedation: a single-center pilot study. World J Gastrointest Endosc. 2014;6 (3):82–7.
6. Hug CC Jr. MAC should stand for Maximum Anesthesia Caution, not Minimal Anesthesiology Care. Anesthesiology. 2006;104 (2):221–3.
7. Bhananker SM, Posner KL, Cheney FW, Caplan RA, Lee LA, Domino KB. Injury and liability associated with monitored anesthesia care: a closed claims analysis. Anesthesiology. 2006;104(2):228–34.

Does Electrophysiology Really Have to Reprogram My Patient's Pacemaker Prior to Electroconvulsive Therapy?

10

Ethan O. Bryson

Case

A new hire fresh out of residency, Dr. Jacobs was assigned to cover the electroconvulsive therapy (ECT) service for the morning. Despite never having done this during her training, she was confident in her ability to manage the brief period of general anesthesia required for each case. "Really," she thought, "How complicated could it be?"

The first case on the schedule was an 86-year-old man with a long history of major depressive disorder (MDD) who was presenting for ECT, having failed several medication trials over the previous 2 years. His prominent symptoms included emotional numbing, lack of motivation, lassitude, and passive suicidal ideation. His medical history was significant for long-standing hypertension (HTN), coronary artery disease (CAD), and chronic obstructive pulmonary disease (COPD). An echocardiogram and stress test had been performed 2 years prior and, according to a note from the patient's cardiologist, this man had diffuse coronary artery disease with an ejection fraction of 20 % for which an implantable cardioverter-defibrillator (ICD) had been placed.

Nothing in the chart indicated the type of implanted device, and the patient did not have his device identification card. Dr. Jacob interviewed the patient, conducted an airway examination, reviewed the available information in the chart, and wondered:

Question

Does electrophysiology (EP) really have to reprogram my patient's pacemaker prior to electroconvulsive therapy?

Realizing she did not know the answer, Dr. Jacobs consulted 2 of her senior colleagues: Dr. Perez, who had completed a fellowship in cardiothoracic anesthesia and currently served as the chief of the cardiothoracic (CT) anesthesia service, and Dr. Singh, the chief of service and coordinator responsible for anesthesia services. The 3 physicians reviewed the available information together and discussed their options.

PRO: Dr. Perez commented first. "Since it is unclear what type of device this patient has, the prudent thing to do is to have the electrophysiology service interrogate it and, if necessary, reprogram it."

CON: After thoughtfully considering Dr. Perez's comments, Dr. Singh replied, "Maybe in a perfect world, but you know as well as I do that our EP service is not going to come to the ECT suite any time soon and this is the first of 20 patients on the day's schedule. Besides, we already know from the chart that this patient has an ICD. Why not just put a magnet over the pulse generator and be done with it?"

PRO (Dr. Perez): "If this device is a simple ICD then I might agree with you, because it is safe to assume that a magnet will deactivate an ICD's ability to detect and treat a malignant arrhythmia. But what if it is a pacemaker? Then we have no idea how the pacemaker will respond to a magnet" [1].

CON (Dr. Singh): "Wait a minute, Dr. Perez, how do we know that this patient has a pacemaker? I was under the impression that this was an ICD placed for a low ejection fraction."

PRO (Dr. Perez): "All ICD devices are also potentially pacemakers, in that they all retain the ability to overdrive pace tachyarrhythmias or pace asystole if needed after a defibrillatory shock" [2].

CON (Dr. Singh): "Granted, but if this patient is not pacemaker-dependent, does it matter?"

E.O. Bryson (✉)
Departments of Anesthesiology and Psychiatry, The Icahn School of Medicine at Mount Sinai, 1 Gustave L. Levy Place, Box 1010, New York, NY 10029, USA
e-mail: ethan.bryson@mountsinai.org

C.S. Scher et al. (eds.), *You're Wrong, I'm Right*, DOI 10.1007/978-3-319-43169-7_10

Having reached a point where it was obvious that more information was needed to safely manage this patient's anesthetic care, the 3 brought the patient into the treatment area where he could be attached to the electrocardiogram (ECG) and other monitors. A 5-lead setup was used, and on the monitor pacing spikes were clearly visible in both lead II and precordial lead 5.

PRO (Dr. Perez): "Well now, it seems that our patient is, in fact, pacemaker dependent, and this makes things a bit more complicated. Dr. Jacob it's a good thing you called us."

CON (Dr. Singh): "Dr. Perez, I'm still not convinced that all of this is necessary. What exactly are we trying to do here? The anesthesia required for ECT is only a brief period of general anesthesia, what could possibly go wrong?"

PRO (Dr. Perez): "The potential adverse outcomes we are trying to avoid include physical damage to the device, including lead fracture or repositioning resulting in device failure, changes in device function such as inadvertent reprograming, inappropriate defibrillator activation, and inadvertent reset to backup mode. Any one of these changes could be catastrophic for this patient as he clearly retains insufficient intrinsic cardiac pacing" [1].

CON (Dr. Singh): "I understand that these are clearly adverse events we should try to avoid, but really, how likely are any of these things to happen? Doesn't placing a magnet over the device present a greater risk than the procedure itself?"

PRO (Dr. Perez): "This patient will receive a significant electrical stimulus as part of the treatment, strong enough to induce a therapeutic seizure. The stimulus itself has the potential to generate electromagnetic interference (EMI) strong enough to interfere with the proper functioning of the device" [2].

CON (Dr. Singh): "Yes, but any electromagnetic interference that is greater than 15 cm from the device has a minimal chance of interfering with device function. This includes interference from the ECT stimulus, or even interference from the use of a peripheral nerve monitor" [2].

PRO (Dr. Perez): "True. However, we still have to recognize that simply placing a magnet over the device when the patient is pacemaker dependent will not reliably protect the device from reprograming."

CON (Dr. Singh): "All right then, contact the EPS service and have this patient's device interrogated, and Dr. Jacobs, please have the next patient brought into the treatment area so we can move things along while we sort this issue out."

Summary

When a patient with a cardiac implanted electrical device presents for ECT, the next question should always be: "What type of device is it?" For patients with a simple pacemaker who are not pacemaker dependent, simply having a magnet available in case of device failure is sufficient. If the patient is pacemaker dependent, consider reprograming to asynchronous mode with either a programmer or a magnet. If the patient has an ICD, it should be deactivated with either a programmer or a magnet. Remember, however, that if the device is deactivated it is essential to have backup external defibrillation available. If the patient is pacemaker dependent, a magnet will not put the pacemaker into asynchronous mode and consultation with EPS for reprograming is indicated. In any case, always have backup external pacing available in case of device failure.

References

1. Bryson EO, Kellner CK, Popeo D, Briggs M, Pasculli R. AICD in electroconvulsive therapy (ECT). J Electroconvuls Ther. 2015;31(1): e22.
2. Stone ME, Salter B, Fischer A. Perioperative management of patients with cardiac implantable electronic devices. Br J Anaesth. 2011;107(S1):i16–i126.

When Can Transesophageal and Trans-Thoracic Echocardiography Be Useful in a Non-Cardiac Case?

11

Lisa Q. Rong

Case

An 83-year-old man with a history of hypertension, hyperlipidemia, and previous transient ischemia attack without any residual neurological deficits is brought to the operating room for urgent hip arthroplasty to repair a traumatic femoral neck fracture. He has an exercise tolerance of 2–3 blocks that is limited by knee and back pain. His EKG demonstrates sinus tachycardia at 105 beats per minute, left axis deviation, and left ventricular hypertrophy. His chest X-ray demonstrates mild pulmonary congestion, and lab values reveal a hemoglobin concentration of 8.5 g/dl, normal electrolytes with elevated creatinine of 1.4 mg/dl. His vital signs in the operating room are HR 105, BP 179/80, RR 18, Sp02 of 96 % on 2 L of nasal cannula. After routine induction of anesthesia, the patient remains hypotensive despite 2 liters of fluid resuscitation and frequent boluses of phenylephrine. An arterial line, another large bore IV, and a phenylephrine drip is started with marginally improved blood pressure. An arterial blood gas demonstrates a stable hemoglobin of 8.0 g/dl. The anesthesiologist, who is basic transesophageal echocardiography (TEE) certified, places a TEE probe to evaluate the cause of the persistent hypotension. The TEE examination demonstrates a dilated left atrium and global systolic hypokinesis of the left ventricle with estimated ejection fraction of 30–35 %. Inotropic support is initiated, patient is taken to the catheterization laboratory for coronary angiogram, and the surgery is postponed to after the optimization of his cardiac status.

Questions

Was this an appropriate use of intraoperative TEE? Was the non-cardiac anesthesiologist capable of making the correct diagnosis? Could a pulmonary artery (PA) catheter be equally or more appropriate in this setting? Would a trans-thoracic echo prior to induction have led to postponement of the case and avoided altogether the postinduction hemodynamic instability?

PRO: This was definitely an appropriate use of intraoperative echocardiography. Many studies have shown the utility of "rescue" intraoperative TEE for both the diagnosis and appropriate intervention that was potentially life saving. Recent guidelines in 2010 by the American Society of Anesthesiologists (ASA) and the Society of Cardiovascular Anesthesiologists (SCA) recommend the use of TEE in patients who are undergoing non-cardiac surgery and exhibit persistent hypotension or hypoxia despite intervention [1]. Schillcutt et al. looked at patients with similar characteristics and situations as our patient in a case study and found that "all patients had an explainable diagnosis for hemodynamic instability on echocardiographic examination" with the most common diagnosis consisting of left heart dysfunction, right heart dysfunction, hypovolemia, and myocardial ischemia [2].

CON: The recommendations by the ASA and SCA are category 2B and 3B evidence, meaning that there are no randomly controlled trials, or a significant body of evidence pointing to both the utility and cost-effectiveness of TEE intraoperatively. Most of the trials that demonstrate benefit of TEE are present in emergency medicine and critical care literature [3–6], and the guidelines are heavily based on expert opinion [7]. The article mentioned by Shillcutt et al is a retrospective study that includes TEE and transthoracic echocardiography (TTE) in a small number of patients ($N = 31$) [2]. Moreover, there were no standardized guidelines as to when, or how echocardiography could be used. The study did not require standardized imaging planes or qualifications of the echocardiographer—they included anesthesiologists, cardiac anesthesiologists, and cardiologists. It is unclear even whether or not it was in the scope of

L.Q. Rong (✉)
Department of Anesthesiology, Weill Cornell Medical Center, NYP, 525 East 68 th Street, New York, NY 10065, USA
e-mail: lisarong@gmail.com

C.S. Scher et al. (eds.), *You're Wrong, I'm Right*, DOI 10.1007/978-3-319-43169-7_11

practice of a basic TEE trained anesthesiogist to diagnose left ventricular dysfunction.

PRO: The study quoted by Schillcutt was done in 2012, and is one of the newer studies in the anesthesia literature demonstrating the usefulness in diagnosis and early intervention based on TEE [2]. Guidelines delineating standard views and the scope of practice for the non-cardiac trained anesthesiologist on basic intraoperative TEE were published in 2013 [8]. The guidelines state that the goals are "intraoperative monitoring rather than specific diagnosis, except in emergent situations, diagnoses requiring intraoperative cardiac surgical intervention or postoperative medical/surgical management must be confirmed by an individual with advanced skills in TEE or by an independent diagnostic technique" [8]. Given that the case above was an urgent situation, the basic echocardiography is within his/her scope of practice to recognize "specific diagnoses that may require advanced imaging skills and competence." Furthermore, basic echocardiographers are able to diagnosis cardiac dysfunction qualitatively with a visual estimation of systolic function. Though imprecise, visual estimation allows a basic echocardiographer to identify those patients who might benefit from inotropic treatments. Multiple publications support the use of TEE in patients with severe hemodynamic disturbances and unknown ventricular function [2–5]. Even simple imaging of the 6 midpapillary segments from the TG midpapillary SAX view may be enough for an important, intervenable diagnosis [8].

CON: Though it may be necessary in emergent situations for a basic echocardiographer to place a TEE probe, the main purpose of his or her skill set is for non-diagnostic intraoperative monitoring. As stated earlier, in an ideal controlled situation, it is prudent to call someone with advanced echocardiographic skills to confirm the diagnosis. In the same vein, the recent American Society of Echocardiography (ASE) guidelines for the Use of Echocardiography as a Monitor for Therapeutic Intervention in Adults in 2015 emphasize the need for an advanced level 2 or above training experience to use TEE as a quantitative monitoring tool, regardless of the clinical scenario for which it is being applied [7]. It also states that "basic clinical trials are lacking on the use of echocardiography in guiding trauma management or other critical care and surgical applications" and the authors recommend "additional clinical trials be performed that document the utility of both TTE and TEE as dynamic monitoring modalities to aid in the treatment of several acute medical and surgical conditions" [7]. This brings back the earlier point that there is no proven utility of echocardiography versus another diagnostic tool such as a PA catheter in emergent situations.

PRO: To address more of the PA catheter versus TEE echo debate: There is a reason why PA catheters have fallen out of favor. They have not been found to improve survival or decrease length of stay in hospitalized patients in large randomized controlled trials in critically ill populations such as chronic heart failure and sepsis [9]. PA catheters are invasive and associated with multiple potential complications such as bleeding, infection, pneumothorax, arrhythmia, and pulmonary artery rupture. They can also be inaccurate due to waveform artifacts, damping, tricuspid regurgitation, and calculated thermodilution cardiac output may vary with respiration and volume status [9]. Furthermore, transesophageal echocardiography is faster and less invasive method that can provide more information on valvular function and diastolic dysfunction compared to other hemodynamic measurement tools such as the pulmonary artery catheter.

CON: Though TEE is relatively safe, it remains associated with complications such as severe odynophagia, dental injury, upper gastrointestinal hemorrhage, and esophageal perforation. There are contraindications to TEE, including signs of GI disease (severe dysphagia, odynophagia, reflux, hematemesis) or history of pathology, recent surgery [3]. TEE also requires more highly trained personnel; whereas a PA catheter can be placed by a general anesthesiologist, a TEE probe requires at least a level one TEE performer to place and interpret the TEE findings. A PA catheter might be more practical than a TEE in the postoperative, intensive care unit monitoring of the patient because it provides instantaneous, continuous monitoring that does not require additional highly trained personnel to perform and interpret the results of the TEE. Therefore, the PA catheter remains a good alternative to TEE to evaluate acute hemodynamic especially in cases where advanced echocardiographers are not present, there are contraindications to TEE, or there is a need for postoperative continuous monitoring.

Pro and Con Concessions

Most diagnoses are made from history and physical examination. This patient had a starting saturation of 96 % on supplemental oxygen. A room air saturation was never obtained. Everything else in the case scenario was suggestive of acute worsening of heart failure, and an oxygen saturation significantly lower than 96 % on room air may have prompted a preoperative trans-thoracic echo (TTE), which is much less invasive than either a TEE or a PA catheter. The patient could then have been optimized prior to induction of anesthesia. Sometimes the best use of a life preserver is to avoid falling overboard in the first place.

Due to the ease and cost-effectiveness of focused TTE, there has been significant interest evaluating high-risk patients for possible undiagnosed cardiopulmonary disease that might alter intraoperative anesthetic management. There is literature suggesting users can be proficient in focused TTE, including the evaluation of left ventricular function and valvular function, and basic use of color Doppler, relatively quickly. A recent observational study by Canty et al. [3] found that a focused preoperative TTE changed the management in patients older than 65 or patients with suspected cardiac disease over 50 % of the time (either escalation or de-escalation of care). It mentions the limitations and scope of the focused TTE; it does not replace the complete TTE, but can give more clinical information than physical exam, a so-called "ultrasound-assisted examination."

The concept of focused TTE can be applied to our patient to determine whether or not the examination would have escalated anesthetic care (arterial line placement or vasopressor support) or led to the postponement of the case. In the study, significant findings that lead to surgical delay existed in 2 out of the 100 patients, they were severe mitral regurgitation with pulmonary hypertension and aortic stenosis with an empty left ventricle [3]. These findings would likely have not been present in someone with diastolic dysfunction, and the case would likely not have been delayed. Diastolic dysfunction alone might not prompted additional monitoring, but the presence of an arterial line could have minimized or prevented hemodynamic collapse.

The patient's hypoxia could have been multifactorial due to atelectasis, intrinsic lung disease, pulmonary embolism, etc., and not completely secondary to heart failure, but a focused TTE is reasonable in a high-risk patient to assess for cardiac causes of hypoxia. The major point of the case is that echo is dynamic and preoperative echo could have been helpful but also could have been relatively normal, and rescue TEE still might have been necessary to diagnose acute changes in cardiac function intraoperatively.

References

1. Thys DM, Abel MD, Brooker RF, Cahalan MK, Connis RT, Duke PG, et al. Practice guidelines for perioperative transesophageal echocardiography: an updated report by the American Society of Anesthesiologists and the Society of Cardiovascular Anesthesiologists task force on transesophageal echocardiography. Anesthesiology. 2010;112:1084–96.
2. Shillcutt SK, Markin NW, Montzingo CR, Brakke TR. Use of rapid "rescue" perioperative echocardiography to improve outcomes after hemodynamic instability in noncardiac surgical patients. J Cardiothoracic Vasc Anesthesia. 2012;26:362–70.
3. Canty DJ, Royse CF, Kilpatrick D, Bowman L, Royse AG. The impact of focused transthoracic echocardiography in the pre-operative clinic. Anesthesia. 2012;67(6):618–25.
4. Kallmeyer IJ, Collard CD, Fox JA, Body SC, Shernan SK. The safety of intraoperative transesophageal echocardiography: a case series of 7200 cardiac surgical patients. Anesth Analg. 2001;92 (5):1126–30.
5. Memtsoudis SG, Rosenberger P, Loffler M, Eltzschig HK, Mizuguchi A, Shernan SK, Fox JA. The usefulness of transesophageal echocardiography during intraoperative cardiac arrest in non-cardiac surgery. Anesth Analg. 2006;102:1653–7.
6. Rebel A, Klimkina O, Hassan ZU. Transesophageal echocardiography for the noncardiac surgical patient. Int Surg. 2012;97:43–55.
7. Porter TR, Shillcutt SK, Adams MS, Desjardins G, Glas KE, Olson JJ, et al. Guidelines for the use of echocardiography as a monitor for therapeutic intervention in adults: a report from the American Society of Echocardiography. JASE. 2015;28:40–56.
8. Reeves ST, Finley AC, Skubas NJ, Swaminathan M, Whitley WS, Glas KE, Council on Perioperative Echocardiography of the American Society of Echocardiography, Society of Cardiovascular Anesthesiologists, et al. Basic perioperative transesophageal echocardiography examination: a consensus statement of the American Society of Echocardiography and the Society of Cardiovascular Anesthesiologists. J Am Soc Echocardiogr. 2013;26(5):443–56.
9. Sandham JD, Hull RD, Brant RF, Knox L, Pineo GF, Doig CJ, et al. A randomized, controlled trial of the use of pulmonary artery catheters in high-risk surgical patients. N Engl J Med. 2003;348:5–14.

Should Antifibrinolytics Be Used in Patients Undergoing Total Joint Replacements?

12

Suzuko Suzuki

Case

In the preoperative testing clinic, I meet a thin elderly woman who is scheduled to have a revision of her left total hip replacement. I call her into my office and she walks slowly with a cane. A quiet "unh" punctuates each step she takes. The 3-m distance never seemed so far. She had a history of breast cancer in remission after a mastectomy and chemotherapy 5 years ago. She also has thalassemia trait. In her previous surgeries, she required blood transfusions. I look over the blood test results and note that her hemoglobin is 11 gm/dl and hematocrit 34 %. Her blood type and screen shows the presence of antibodies to the surface antigens to her red blood cells.

She sits across from me with hopeful eyes and says, "My surgeon said there is this miracle drug that minimizes bleeding and I can have my hip replaced again, this time without needing blood transfusions."

Question

Should antifibrinolytics be used in patients undergoing total joint replacements?

Tranexamic acid (TXA) is used in cardiac surgeries and some orthopedic surgeries. A quick PubMed search for "tranexamic acid AND total hip replacement" produces a long but manageable list of literature. Skimming a few meta-analyses, there appears an almost unanimous favorable conclusion on the use of TXA for blood conservation [1, 2]. A Cochrane Review from 2011 concluded that antifibrinolytics reduced the rate of blood transfusions [3]. It also warned about the increased rate of myocardial infarction (MI) with aprotinin, while it did not contain a similar warning against TXA or aminocaproic acid [3].

The rate of blood transfusion in total joint replacements is quite high, ranging from 20 % to as high as 45 % in some studies [4]. The frequency of blood transfusion was higher in patients with preoperative anemia [4, 5]. This rather anemic lady has a realistic chance of needing blood transfusion with her hip replacement.

I called one of my regional anesthesia colleagues to ask about the use of TXA in their practice. "So, is TXA a miracle drug?"

PRO: As a major orthopedic surgery center, we routinely use TXA for total joint replacements in the absence of contraindications. But, this is not necessarily the practice elsewhere. The evidence is rather clear that TXA reduces blood loss and reduces the need for blood transfusion in both total knee and total hip replacements [1–3]. The surgeons certainly seem to believe that it does reduce bleeding during the surgery.

CON: Respecting the importance of reducing blood loss and the implications of avoiding blood transfusions, TXA sounds like a good idea. But what evidence is there for improved outcomes really? The studies seem to have small sample sizes and are based on single institution data. How confidently can we tell patients that this will work for them so that they would not require a blood transfusion, and more importantly, not suffer any side effects or thromboembolic complications from the TXA?

PRO: Blood conservation is particularly important in orthopedic surgeries because extensive blood loss occurs from surgical manipulation and nailing of bones. Perioperative blood transfusion is frequent in total joint replacement, sometimes even more so for revisions. Besides that, anemia is prevalent in hip replacement patients, even before the surgery [4, 5]. We know that anemia is associated with higher rates of complications, infections, and a longer hospital stay [6]. About half of the patients may end up receiving blood transfusions. So reducing blood loss means

S. Suzuki (✉)
Department of Anesthesiology, New York University Langone Medical Center/Hospital for Joint Diseases, 301 17th Street, New York, NY 10003, USA
e-mail: Suzuko.suzuki@nyumc.org

C.S. Scher et al. (eds.), *You're Wrong, I'm Right*, DOI 10.1007/978-3-319-43169-7_12

better outcomes and avoiding some complications. The use of TXA is probably also cost-effective.

CON: There is some evidence that the risk of thromboembolism with TXA is probably higher for those with risk factors [7]. It is our job to form a risk versus benefit assessment as we always do when we use any medications.

CON: There is a long list of potential risk factors for thromboembolism. Besides the prior history of pulmonary embolism (PE), deep vein thrombosis (DVT), myocardial infarction (MI), and coronary artery disease (CAD), any of the factors for hypercoagulable state are also risk factors such as malignancy, chemotherapy, hormone replacement therapy, use of oral contraceptives and steroids, chronic inflammatory diseases, and anti-lupus antibodies among others. Having surgery itself is a risk factor for DVT. Orthopedic surgery patients are typically obese, sedentary, are relatively immobilized, and often have rheumatological or immunological conditions that led them to have their joint problems. These people are the perfect setup for thromboembolism. If you consider all of these factors, we should not be using TXA in quite a large number of patients.

PRO: To date, no studies have shown an association between the use of TXA and increased rate of thrombotic complication, which include MI, PE, DVT, and stroke [1, 2, 8].

CON: That is hard to believe. And, again, I return to the earlier point that those data are based on a relatively small number of patients. The Cochrane Review did say that the data were sparse. Are you comfortable relying on those small numbers?

PRO: A more recent large database analysis, representing more than 800,000 patients for total hip and knee replacements, agreed with these findings about the benefit of TXA as well as the lack of evidence of increased thromboembolic complications [8].

CON: What about using TXA in this patient with a history of breast cancer who had chemotherapy 5 years ago? She is deemed being in remission from her cancer. Now she is sedentary because of her hip pain. She is at an increased risk of clot formation.

PRO: But she has a history of anemia and has antibodies, making cross-matching challenging, and is having a total hip replacement revision. She is thin, and her risk of needing blood transfusion is significant. Does she continue to take any antineoplastic medications? Looking at just the cancer-related thromboembolism risk, the degree of risk depends on the type of malignancy, extent of disease, and whether the patient is on chemotherapy and combination treatments [9]. Therefore, the risk may be quite different for someone who is actively receiving chemotherapy for recent malignancy and for an otherwise healthy person with history of lumpectomy for low-grade cancer in remission. If she is not on any such medications and has not had any prior history of thromboembolism, and it has been 5 years, I would consider using it, especially since she is also at high risk of needing blood transfusions.

CON: She no longer takes antineoplastic medications. But one fatal PE may be too many while anemia is easier to detect and treat.

PRO: Another interesting and emerging concept in using TXA is the topical or intra-articular application rather than giving it intravenously. There is some evidence of non-inferiority results [10, 11]. For those who are at risk of thromboembolism, the local use of TXA may be a good compromise that avoids much of the systemic complications, but there is not enough evidence to support it and it will also require the surgeons to agree.

Summary

Evidence supports that TXA reduces blood loss and the rate of perioperative blood transfusions in total joint replacements. However, although not yet clearly defined, the risk of thromboembolism exists while the risk factors vary. The risks and benefits of TXA administration should be assessed by clinicians on an individual basis.

References

1. Alshryda S, Sukeik M, Sarda P, Blenkinsopp J, Haddad FS, Mason JM. A systematic review and meta-analysis of the topical administration of tranexamic acid in total hip and knee replacement. Bone Joint J. 2014;96-B(8):10005–15.
2. Yang ZG, Chen WP, Wu LD. Effectiveness and safety of tranexamic acid in reducing blood loss in total knee arthroplasty: a meta-analysis. JBJS. 2012;94:1143-11.
3. Henry DA, Carless PA, Moxey AJ, O'Connell D, Stokes BJ, Fergusson DA, Ker K. Anti-fibrinolytic use for minimising perioperative allogeneic blood transfusion. Cochrane Database Syst Rev. 2011;1, Jan 19. Art. No.: CD001886.
4. Spahn DR. Anemia and patient blood management in hip and knee surgery: a systematic review of the literature. Anesthesiology. 2010;113(2):482–95.
5. Lasocki S, Krauspe R, von Heymann C, Mezzacasa A, Chainey S, Spahn DR. PREPARE: the prevalence of perioperative anaemia and need for patient blood management in elective orthopaedic surgery: a multicenter, observational study. Eur J Anaesthesiol. 2015;32(3):160–7.

6. Saleh A, Small T, ChandranPillai AL, Schiltz NK, Klika AK, Barsoum WK. Allogenic blood transfusion following total hip arthroplasty: results from the national inpatient sample, 2000 to 2009. J Bone Joint Surg Am. 2014;96(18):e155.
7. Whiting DR, Gillette BP, Duncan C, Smith H, Pagnano MW, Sierra RJ. Preliminary results suggest tranexamic acid is safe and effective in arthroplasty patients with severe comorbidities. Clin Orthop Relat Res. 2014;472(1):66–72.
8. Poeran J, Rasul R, Suzuki S, Danninger T, Mazumdar M, Opperer M, et al. Tranexamic acid use and postoperative outcomes in patients undergoing total hip or knee arthroplasty in the united states: retrospective analysis of effectiveness and safety. BMJ. 2014;349:g4829.
9. Lee AY, Levine MN. Venous thromboembolism and cancer: risks and outcomes. Circulation. 2003;107(Suppl 1):I17–21.
10. Gomez-Barrena E, Ortega-Andreu M, Padilla-Eguiluz NG, Perez-Chrzanowska H, Fugueredo-Zalve R. Topical intra-articular compared with intravenous tranexamic acid to reduce blood loss in primary total knee replacement: a double-blind, randomized, controlled, non-inferiority clinical trial. J Bone Joint Surg Am. 2014;96(23):1937–44.
11. Wang C, Xu GJ, Han Z, Ma JX, Ma XL. Topical application of tranexamic acid in primary total hip arthroplasty: a systemic review and meta-analysis. Int J Surg. 2015;S1743–9191(15):00007-2.

Will Operating Rooms Run More Efficiently When Anesthesiologists Get Involved in Their Management?

13

Steven D. Boggs, Mitchell H. Tsai, and Mohan Tanniru

Case

An operating room that has grown continuously has encountered managerial problems. Just a few years ago, there were 7 operating rooms performing annually about 3400 cases. The hospital has built 5 additional operating rooms with a staff of 11, and around 6000 cases will be performed by the end of this fiscal year.

Problems have arisen and these include increased surgical patient cancelation rate, progressively lower Press-Ganey® scores [1] for the perioperative suite, surgeon complaints of lack of instrumentation, staffing difficulties, lower than projected utilization rates and "holds" in the post-anesthetic care unit (PACU) due to insufficient intensive care unit (ICU) beds.

The nurse manager of the OR has been in this position for 20 years. She had been an OR nurse prior to assuming her current position. When the OR caseload was stable and revenue and expenditures were predictable, there had been few complaints. However, even her strongest defenders are now questioning the way the OR is managed.

CON: It seems to me that we need a complete reassessment of the perioperative process [2]. First, we need to look at the perioperative management of patients and we need to optimize patient flows in order to minimize cancelations. Second, it appears that OR resources are not being utilized efficiently, as reflected by lack of instrumentation availability to perform scheduled procedures. Finally, an analysis of the throughput of a patient for the entire perioperative period, from preoperative assessment through intraoperative management to postoperative care to discharge, needs to be undertaken. Roadblocks that occur—such as PACU holds—have to be evaluated and we must correct any systemic problems.

PRO: Actually, what you propose sounds good on paper, but it really will not improve things. In the past, every few years the hospital has hired a consulting company to review its operations. They have interviewed people from each department, collated their ideas, and come up with solutions to improve perceived problems. Then, the consultants have presented these plans to management as if they were their own ideas and nothing has ever changed [3].

CON: I don't dispute what you say about consultants. Even if the management agrees to do what the consultants have suggested, without proper implementation, follow-through, and monitoring, no solution will improve OR productivity. There is a large body of research on OR management, and some issues can be addressed using quantitative metrics [4]. Fundamentally, the management of an OR is no different than any other managerial function. Without leadership committed to change and the creation of the necessary ecosystem to encourage staff to make the changes, no change can be effectively implemented [5]. Also, if the personnel in the OR department don't feel empowered or enfranchised, then the solutions and workflows that are implemented cannot be sustained.

PRO: What you are saying sounds like leadership training for the military. However, we are in the civilian sector and you can't just "order" people around. One can know what needs to be done and one can threaten people, even by telling them that you will fire them if orders are not followed. Ultimately, organizational inertia [6] makes change

S.D. Boggs (✉)
Department of Anesthesiology, James J. Peters VA Medical Center and the Mount Sinai Hospital, 130 West Kingsbridge Road, Bronx, NY 10468, USA
e-mail: Steven.Boggs@va.gov; stevendaleboggs@gmail.com

M.H. Tsai
Department of Anesthesiology, University of Vermont Medical Center, 111 Colchester Avenue, Burlington, VT 05403, USA
e-mail: mitchell.tsai@uvmhealth.org

M. Tanniru
MIS, School of Business Administration Oakland University, 200 I Elliott Hall, 2200 N. Squirrel Road, Rochester, MI 48309, USA
e-mail: Tanniru@oakland.edu

C.S. Scher et al. (eds.), *You're Wrong, I'm Right*, DOI 10.1007/978-3-319-43169-7_13

very difficult and most workers just do only as much as needed to get by.

CON: That is a rather pessimistic and, truthfully, not an accurate reflection of the workplace. You are right. It would be unwise for a leader simply to order people to do what needs to be done. Also, providing incentives for doing the job you are hired to do will likely fail [7]. Rather, one has to look at human factors in the OR and create an atmosphere or ecosystem where every individual member feels that they are contributing to the overall mission of the team.

From the person who cleans the room after a case to the scrub nurse, from the anesthesia healthcare service to the surgical staff members, they all have to recognize the important contributions they each make to patient care. They all need to understand what OR metrics are critical for patient care and how each of them can play a role in addressing these metrics [8]. Such a transparent communication addresses both the tactical (short term) and strategic (long term) needs of an OR. In this way, all members of the team (nurses, physicians, technicians, and ancillary personnel) can address core values of their mission—providing service to the patient. If such a sense of mission does not carry through the entire organization, then people will start seeing discrepancies in what is said and what is done, resulting in status quo and no change.

PRO: So, what do you do about our OR management structure? It has worked for more than 20 years.

CON: Well, you could argue that it has worked for 20 years. But, you could just as effectively argue that it didn't have to work too well for these 20 years. In the past, OR management was relatively easy and painless because the reimbursement was generous. But competition in the healthcare sector has accelerated, insurance and the government have ratcheted down payments, and profit margins have shrunk. We know that operating rooms are at the center of hospitals' business operations [9]. They are pivotal in the sense that they can either generate revenues for the hospital or contribute to significant financial losses [10]. But, the complexity of equipment and pharmaceuticals used in the OR has grown exponentially. Examples include specialized equipment (e.g., video towers for laparoscopic surgery), robotic systems, complicated physiological monitoring systems [e.g., somatosensory evoked potential (SSEP) for cardiovascular medicine], and completely novel treatments that were unheard of not so long ago [e.g., left ventricular assist device (LVAD)]. For all of these reasons, either one person or a group of people in the OR need to have more than "on the job" training in management to make decisions related to costs and benefits. [11].

PRO: I appreciate the growing complexity of medical technology and the collaboration necessary to create a viable, energetic workplace. For the past 20 years, the nurses at this institution have served as the primary gatekeepers, managers, and resource personnel to manage all the clinical workflows demanded by the physicians. Who would you suggest could manage the workload and possess the social skills?

CON: I think that anesthesiologists are in a perfect position to become leaders of any OR in this country. Think about it. Unlike surgeons, we are here in the operating room 24 h a day, every day of the week, much like nurses. Our training gives us the breadth of experience needed to act as consultants for the entire perioperative period. Also, anesthesiologists understand at an intimate level the need for collaboration that is necessary between the surgical and nursing staff in order to care for a patient. We do this every day, probably unwittingly at the beginning. Anesthesiology residents rotate through the ORs, ICU, sedation sites, labor, and delivery, and we are on the floors as hospitalists and acute pain specialists. At a systems level, anesthesiologists understand the operational and tactical needs of a smooth running OR [12]. In fact, many training programs in the country have intuitively anticipated the need for anesthesiologists to play such a leadership role in the OR and created OR management programs for their residents.

PRO: I will accept the argument that anesthesiologists are present in the OR every day. But how would you make the value proposition that they should transition to take on such a leadership role? We have anesthesiologists who show up late every day, who cancel patients on the day of surgery who have already received preoperative clearance, and who at times demonstrate a complete lack of awareness or initiative to take on this new role? They do not seem to be team players.

CON: Let's back up a little bit. You point out a very pertinent, poignant, and painful truth. First, not all anesthesiologists (or surgeons or nurses, for that matter) have the temperament for cardiac anesthesia, for obstetrical anesthesia, or for outpatient anesthesia. Likewise, out of any given residency class, one can only expect a few individuals would be ideal candidates for OR management. Yet, all anesthesiologists should have some exposure to what is involved in this process because—like all other specialties, perhaps more than many—it will affect all of them in their practice throughout their career.

OR management should be divided into different levels of management, just as businesses do such as operational and strategic, depending on the metrics used [13]. Operational management can use efficiency metrics to improve OR processes, as they call for scientific inquiry and measurement for continual improvement. For instance, in order to understand the reason for patient cancelations on the day of surgery, we need to analyze the current work flow used for patient assignment to the OR and data on what contributed to their cancelation. We know that anesthesiologist-driven evaluation of preoperative processes can decrease patient cancelation rates, reduce laboratory expenditures, and improve patient and surgeon satisfaction. In the 1990s, Fischer [14] demonstrated that a preoperative evaluation clinic can be successful in reducing unnecessary preoperative consultations, reduce diagnostic studies by 55 %, and reduce day-of-surgery cancelations by 87.9 %. Establishing such a model has resulted in a savings of $112 per patient.

On the strategic level, we need to address the cultural issues. Lack of physician interest and participation demonstrates the need for an awareness that operational processes have to be coordinated and effectively managed if patient care is the paramount mission of the OR. Until organizational leadership connects operational improvements to strategic mission (patient care) to costs and resources management (e.g., equipment availability) and start to influence the culture of the OR team, success is not feasible.

PRO: Let's say that I agree that some anesthesiologists, who are interested and willing, are right candidates for taking on perioperative leadership. Then, what does the governance structure of a well-managed OR suite look like? The traditional lines of power dictate that nurses have control over physicians, and physicians have influence over nurses and resources of the OR.

CON: I agree that the traditional culture and organizational governance of the OR is set up to create conflicts, frequently falling into disputes between physicians and nurses. We need to change the relationship between nurses and physicians. In fact, we need a level playing field. Dr. Pronovost was able to advance his protocols to prevent central-line infections because he empowered the nurses to stop the process when they saw a breach in precautionary measures [15]. This is not dissimilar to the kaizen method in Toyota manufacturing: Line workers are empowered to stop the assembly line of a multi-billion industry without the prior approval of management when they detect a defect in the line [16]. From the outside looking in, it may seem that Dr. Pronovost created a checklist of things that have to be followed and managed. In actuality, he changed the culture of the ICU by empowering the nurses.

I propose that future OR leadership structures have to bring about such a cultural change. At some institutions, there is a triad that governs the OR: Charge Nurse, Charge Anesthesiologist, and Charge Surgeon. Each day, the Charge Team handles all the operational issues: add-on cases, deals with bumps in schedules, emergencies, and patient needs. A team will be formed using a representative from nurse, anesthesiology, and the surgical staff, and they will have the authority on the decisions made in the OR to address exceptions as they arise.

PRO: What happens when a disgruntled surgeon, with an elective skin tag removal, disagrees with a decision to bump his case for an emergent AAA? Who oversees the Charge Team?

CON: Here, I will borrow from businesses that use matrix organizational structure [17]. Let each Charge representative know that they are in direct communication with the superior officer (or senior management). The Charge Anesthesiologist reports to the Anesthesiology Chair, the Charge Surgeon reports to the Surgery Chair, and the Charge Nurse reports to the Perioperative Services Director. Using your previous example, if the surgeon disagrees with the Charge Team's decision, then he/she would bring the concerns directly up the chain of command. I would love to be a fly on the wall when the surgeon explains to the Surgery Chair on the importance of a skin tag compared to the bleeding, life-threatening AAA.

PRO: I think you are forgetting one major player in this equation: the hospital administration. Even if they are not directly making tactical decisions on the day of surgery, the administration has a vested interest in the successful collaboration of the OR team. They have to structure the OR governance so that decisions lead to optimal performance, both financially and in terms of care delivery. For this reason, effective OR managers (or superior officers as stated earlier) need a transparent system and credible organizational structure to not only help support decisions when conflicts arise, but also to take advantage of opportunities for innovations in care delivery [18]. Also, everyone needs to understand the metrics (e.g., contribution margin per surgeon or per service), so leadership at every level can use these metrics to guide all tactical or strategic decisions regarding which services to provide and where.

CON: So, you are saying that all services are not equal when it comes to receiving block time? That seems like a very politically unsavory position.

PRO: From a long-term perspective, the hospital will not be able to deliver care to every patient if it wants to remain financially viable. As I mentioned before, today's environment is very different from the healthcare delivery systems that existed 10–20 years ago. While all cases will receive time, certain services will receive favorable treatment because they contribute more financially to the hospital. It must be noted that a service may have a lower priority in a hospital, but can have a higher priority (greater contribution margin) in an ambulatory surgical setting. Businesses have used matrix organizational structure to address such trade-offs as well—superior officers of each of the Charge team members can reconcile any differences among themselves or work with the organizational leadership based on the strategic vision of the hospital.

CON: This seems like a tremendous change from the way medicine was practiced just a few decades ago.

PRO: It is. As I mentioned before, this environment is very different from the healthcare delivery systems that existed 10–20 years ago. We have to think more in terms of "systems" now, instead of sole providers advocating care individually for their patients. In the 1970s, 2.5 clinical staff members were involved in the care of each hospitalized patients. In the 1990s, more than 15 clinical staff members were involved in the care of each hospitalized patient. Currently, the number of clinical staff members involved in the care of a hospitalized patient must be even higher. Therefore, when it comes to operational processes, healthcare workers who decry that a patient is "mine" or "yours" completely misunderstand the concept of patient-centered care. Every person involved in the care of a patient in a hospital has a stake in both the patient's clinical outcome and how efficiently they transition through the hospital. Please don't misinterpret what I am saying. There must be accountability and responsibility, but we must also start thinking in terms of teams, cooperation, and "game plans" for our patients. No one provider can provide all of the care that a patient requires in today's complex healthcare environment.

CON: Again, we are back to where we have started this conversation. Teams, collaboration, and process change require leadership. We know that management consultants merely advise but don't help execute. So, how can we create the necessary changes to run an effective OR?

PRO: The challenge today is not simply managing change but supporting change creation, as organizations are asked to continually change as the demands in the environment call for such change. If one were to go through managing change, with cycles of change occurring frequently, managers have to spend too much time managing each change. The goal is to create an innovative and learning environment in organizations so people are driven to change without significant managerial intervention [19, 20]. This is where there a lot of work is going on—creating learning organizations that can create an echo system to support innovation and change creation or be ready to change as the need arises [21]. Healthcare staff must be educated and aware of what is needed for effective care delivery and support profitability (awareness), and empower staff to challenge decisions. Everyone in the organization must be in sync on how conflicts are being resolved in a risk-free or low-risk environment (ability), and create explicit or implicit incentives to work as a team and share in the rewards (intent). Awareness, ability, and intent are key factors for any hospital interested in creating an organizational ecosystem to support learning.

CON: Now, I think we are all on the same page.

References

1. http://www.pressganey.com/. Accessed 29 Oct 2015.
2. Hall R. Patient flow: reducing delay in healthcare delivery. International series in operations research and management science. 2nd ed. New York: Springer; 2013. p. 553.
3. Arfman D, Barbe FGT. The value of lean in the service sector: a critique of theory & practice. Int J Bus Soc Sci. 2014;5(2):18–24.
4. Guerriero F, Guido R. Operational research in the management of the operating theatre: a survey. Health Care Manage Sci. 2011;14 (1):89–114.
5. Hersey P, Blanchard KH, Johnson DE. Management of organizational behavior. 10th edn. Englewood: Prentice-Hall; 2012. p. 360.
6. Pentland BT, Feldman MS, Becker MC, Liu P. Dynamics of organizational routines: a generative model. J Manage Stud. 2012;49(8):1484–508.
7. Kohn A. Why incentive plans cannot work. Harv Bus Rev. 1993 (September-October):54–63.
8. Gawande A. Cowboys and pit crews, New Yorker. 26 May 2011.
9. Herman B. Seven strategies to help hospitals break even on Medicare. Becker's Hospital Review. 2 April 2012.
10. Randa K, Heiser R, Gill R. Strategic investments in the operating room: information technology to generate rapid return on investment and long-term competitive advantage. http://healthleadersmedia.com/content/242938.pdf.
11. http://www.franklindexter.net/education.htm. Accessed 29 Oct 2015.
12. Boggs SD, Frost E, Marn R, Feinleib J. Anesthesiologists as operating room directors. 13–14 Dec 2014. The New York State Society of Anesthesiologists Post-Graduate Assembly.
13. McIntosh C, Dexter F, Epstein RH. The impact of service-specific staffing, case scheduling, turnovers, and first-case starts on anesthesia group and operating room productivity: a tutorial using data from an Australian Hospital. Anesth Analg. 2006;103(6):1499–516.
14. Fischer SP. Development and effectiveness of an anesthesia preoperative evaluation clinic in a teaching hospital. Anesthesiology. 1996;85:196–206.
15. Pronovost P, Needham D, Berenholtz S, Sinopoli D, Chu H, Cosgrove S, et al. An intervention to decrease catheter-related bloodstream infections in the ICU. N Engl J Med. 2006;355:2725–32.
16. Spear SJ. Learning to lead at Toyota. Harv Bus Rev. May 2004. https://hbr.org/2004/05/learning-to-lead-at-toyota.

17. Milgrom P, Roberts J. Complementarities and fit strategy, structure, and organizational change in manufacturing. J Acc Econ. 1995;19 (2–3) March-May:179–208.
18. Stavros JM, Cooperrider D, Kelley L. SOAR: a new approach to strategic planning. In: Homan P, Devane T, Cady S, editors. The Change handbook: the definitive resource on today's best methods for engaging whole systems. 2nd ed. San Francisco: Berrett-Koehler Publishers, Inc.; 2007. p. 375–80.
19. Agarwal R, Krudys G, Tanniru M. Infusing learning into an information systems organization. Eur J Inf Syst. 1997;6 (25):40.
20. Gilley JW, Maycunich A, Gilley AM. Organizational learning, performance, and change: an introduction to strategic human resource development. Cambridge: Perseus; 2000.
21. Weiner BJ. A theory of organizational readiness for change. Weiner; Licensee BioMed Central Ltd; 2009.

Are Outcomes Better for Trauma Patients Who Are Treated Early with Clotting Factors?

14

Steven D. Boggs and Ian H. Black

Case

A 72-year-old male with known coronary artery disease presents to his community hospital's emergency department (ED) with multiple long-bone fractures and a blood pressure of 65/40 following a severe motor vehicle accident. It is also noted that the patient has a widened mediastinum.

You are the anesthesiologist on call. On arrival, you find that the ED physician has already administered 2 l of crystalloid and is instructing the nurse to hang 2 more.

Question

Are outcomes better for patients who are treated with a massive transfusion protocol for hemorrhage?

You begin the dialogue:

PRO: Excuse me, have you started any blood products on this patient?

CON: No, we are treating the patient's blood pressure with crystalloid as a volume expander. The initial hematocrit was 33, and we will be following this patient's hematocrit sequentially with the point-of-care testing instrument that we just purchased for the ED. Then, depending on the results of testing we will order components as indicated.

PRO: This is really a case where we should activate the massive transfusion protocol (MTP). I say that because while only a small percentage of civilian trauma patients require such treatment, approximately 3–6 %, this patient has the potential to require more than 10 units of blood, especially if in addition to his long-bone fractures, he also has an aortic dissection. Massive transfusion can be predicted in cases such as aortic dissection, obstetric catastrophy, and liver transplant. In cases of massive transfusion, it is appropriate to use damage control resuscitation, which involves the 1:1:1 transfusion of packed red blood cells/fresh frozen plasma/platelets [1–10].

While the definitions of massive transfusion have evolved over time, it is important to note that newer definitions include the rapidity of blood loss and not simply a total amount [11]. You will find that this patient's clinical situation highly suggests that he will meet more than one definition of a patient who will require a major transfusion. In case you are not familiar, these would include:

1. 20 units in 24 h (1 blood volume in a 70-kg patient).
2. >10 units in 24 h.
3. >50 % of a patient's blood volume in 3 h.
4. 50 units of blood components in 24 h.
5. >6 units of PRBCs (packed red blood cells) in 12 h.
6. >4 units/1 h.
7. >150 ml/min loss with associated hemodynamic instability.

CON: The difficulty with what you are stating is that we are not a trauma center, we are an isolated medical facility. Our blood bank cannot afford to keep fresh frozen plasma (FFP) unthawed 24/7 for the rare case like this which comes here. Our wastage rate would be unacceptable. We could start the administration of PRBCs now, but you are suggesting that we start infusing

S.D. Boggs (✉)
Department of Anesthesiology, The Icahn School of Medicine at Mount Sinai, Manhattan, NY, USA
e-mail: Steven.Boggs@va.gov; stevendaleboggs@gmail.com

S.D. Boggs
Department of Anesthesiology, James J. Peters VA Medical Center and the Mount Sinai Hospital, 130 West Kingsbridge Road, Bronx, NY 10468, USA

S.D. Boggs
1133 Midland Avenue, Apt. 3G, Bronxville, NY 10708-6472, USA

I.H. Black
Department of Surgery, Cheyenne VA Medical Center, 2360 East Pershing Blvd., Cheyenne, WY 82001, USA
e-mail: ian.black@va.gov; ihb101@hotmail.com

C.S. Scher et al. (eds.), *You're Wrong, I'm Right*, DOI 10.1007/978-3-319-43169-7_14

this patient—who has an acceptable hematocrit—with platelets and FFP. Without evidence of a low hemoglobin, let alone a coagulopathy, it is hard to see the indication.

PRO: Actually, since this patient presented in shock, it is not a bad assumption that he has lost a significant percentage of his blood volume, possibly up to 40 %. If you continue to administer only crystalloid, his hematocrit will be substantially lower than what you are currently measuring. While this may temporarily improve his volume status, we will already be behind the curve in terms of his oxygen-carrying capacity. Admittedly, we do not transfuse to a fixed hematocrit in all patients, but in this patient with known coronary disease and significant blood loss, it is reasonable to maintain a slightly higher hemoglobin. A slightly higher hemoglobin may also make platelets more effective by pushing them against the endothelium [12].

Furthermore, if he has sequestered significant blood internally and then looses additional blood in surgical procedures, not only will he require red cells but there will be significant dilution of his coagulation factors. Substantial evidence exists that it is better in these situations to be proactive in the administration of platelets and coagulation factors [13]. Once you have an established coagulopathy, it is much more difficult to treat. Consequently, a ratio of PRBCs/platelets/FFP of 1:1:1 is usually administered.

CON: The problem with the studies that support your argument is that survivor bias confounds the data. Patients who survive long enough to receive plasma and platelets have already survived a very lethal period—the first few hours in which the more severely injured patients die. So, the data you cite in favor of 1:1:1 or other ratios is not as compelling as you suggest. This is exactly the situation we are in here. If we do order platelets and FFP for this patient, those units may not be available for at least an hour.

PRO: Your point is well-taken. However, Ho and others looked at precisely this issue [5]. While some studies did have a survivor bias (11/26 studies), 10 studies demonstrated the benefit of high plasma to PRBC ratios and a survivor bias was not thought likely when before and after cohorts were used or times were analyzed as time-dependant covariates. Therefore, the best data that we have at present suggest that we should administer blood component therapy early in massive blood loss situations [13–16]. For that reason, this patient is precisely the one in whom the massive transfusion protocol should be activated early. This is even more true in a facility in which these cases are infrequent. In addition, there is some benchtop work that suggests that early administration of FFP makes the endothelium less leaky [14].

CON: Even if I were to concede that blood products should be administered early in resuscitation, what ratio should we select? I have seen everything from 1:1:1 to much higher ratios of platelets and plasma in relationship to red blood cells. Some studies suggest that FFP/RBC ratios of 1:3 are superior [13] and we have to remember that a unit of FFP only contains 80 % of the coagulation factors found in a unit of whole blood.

PRO: You are right, there definitely is controversy in this area. In fact, the original study by Borgman et al. [1] had a 1:1:4 ratio with an interquartile range of 1:1.7–1:1.2 of PRBCs to FFP. To some degree, it depends on the endpoint that you are measuring: 24-h mortality, 30-day mortality, lung injury, or multiple organ failure. Similarly, with the administration of platelets, mortality is improved. The largest, most recent, and best study to date, the PROPPR study shows no 24-h or 30-day mortality difference between 1:1 and 1:2 of PRBCs to FFP [3], but there seemed to be better hemostasis with the 1:1 ratio.

CON: So, should we just toss out our point of care testing (POC)? If you are going to transfuse fixed ratios of red cells, platelets, and plasma, why test?

PRO: No, POC testing is incredibly valuable for managing these patients. You have to recognize where the idea of fixed ratios came from. In wartime situations in the last century, whole blood was administered [17]. However, with the evolution of blood banking and storage of components separately, the idea was that components should be administered in a ratio that more closely approximated that seen in whole blood [13].

In the initial phases of a massive bleeding situation, there is not usually time to measure and treat. Consequently, as a first approach, a fixed ratio is used in MTPs. The coagulopathy seen in these circumstances is also a lagging indicator—by the time you have evidence of the coagulopathy, you should have already started treating. Therefore, it is preferable to order the massive transfusion protocol on the basis of the clinical picture, initiate treatment, and then measure PT/PTT, INR, platelets, fibrinogen, and other parameters (i.e., D-dimer) sequentially. If the patient survives long enough for the hemorrhage to stop, then treatment can be tailored to the patient's measured parameters.

CON: I have heard that some centers utilize thromboelastography (TEG). That would not work here in our ED because we just don't have that capability or volume.

PRO: I don't think a compelling argument can be made for utilization of TEG in a hospital that occasionally receives trauma patients. Traffic highway survival data from the US Department of Transportation show that, for motor vehicular accidents, being close to a Level I or II trauma center improves survival. For centers that receive patients but are not trauma centers, a protocol should be in place and a fixed transfusion ratio might be simplest and easiest to execute.

Ben Taub Hospital, however, has used TEG to guide MTP for over a decade in those expected to receive over 10 units of PRBCs [18]. They found that the addition of TEG to the fixed ratio transfusion schema revealed lower-than-expected coagulation activity. This permitted more precise treatment of coagulopathy. Some centers also use the TEG to guide tranexamic acid (TXA) administration.

CON: Well, if we are going to be really aggressive and want to increase coagulation factors, why shouldn't we just administer Factor VIIa?

PRO: Factor VIIa is not yet licensed in the USA for trauma, and it can only be used on a "compassionate" basis. In general its off-label use in trauma has been waning. It is very costly and unless the patient's temperature and especially pH are optimized, the effect of Factor VII is not significant [19]. Therefore, the best way to treat massive hemorrhage is to administer appropriate doses of platelets, cryoprecipitate, and FFP, and to normalize the patient's temperature and pH. Additionally, Factor VII is no substitute for lack of surgical control of bleeding. That said, if your institution has a protocol that includes Factor VII, and it is appropriate in your clinical judgment, it should be administered. The most recent trauma trial used an initial dose of 200 μg/kg IV with repeated doses of 100 μg/kg at 1 and 3 h [9]. Other trials have used doses of 90 μg/kg with repeated doses every 1–3 h.

CON: It seems to me that your considerations extend beyond the exclusive administration of blood products. If that is the case, it seems to me that the administration of TXA should also be considered in trauma cases. If you look at the CRASH-2 trial, it is very cost-effective and has minimal adverse sequelae [4].

PRO: Tranexamic acid was shown to be useful in the CRASH-2 trial. It was the only study to show an improvement in all-cause mortality. Secondary analysis showed it is most beneficial when administered in the first 3 h and may even be harmful after that window. So, if the patient has a significant risk of bleeding, it would be appropriate to administer 1 g of TXA over 10 min and then continue an infusion of 1 g over 8 h. In fact, TXA has even been administered in air medical transport prior to arrival at hospital to try to decrease blood loss [20].

However, if we are going to look at TXA and Factor VII, then we should also consider the very important and neglected aspects of how to implement an MTP. Even with all blood components and medications available, the choreography of an MTP requires excellent coordination between physicians, nurses, technicians, and the blood bank. This means that the communication systems between the ED (for example) and the blood bank (BB) must be immediate and reliable, and, likewise, the method for transporting the appropriate products to the patient must be similarly reliable.

A recent study on the issues of human factors in the implementation of the MTP showed that in some cases, a dedicated phone line had to be established between the BB and the ED. Also, in a hospital where a pneumatic tube system was utilized, this sped sample delivery from the ED to the BB [2]. One hospital had a "one click" notification in the electronic medical record to notify the BB that the MTP would be used [2]. One study showed that mortality improved after initiation of an MTP even though the ratio of products remained the same. Ultimately, an MTP's overall impact is to change the paradigm to provide blood products earlier and in higher quantities, limit crystalloid, and have a system in place for a relatively rare event. All of those pieces are probably important.

CON: Certainly, some changes in infrastructure are necessary if you want improvements as you suggest. It would be ideal to start the MTP with a single phone call. However, I would argue that training and familiarity with the MTP is even more important than any of the preceding interventions. Not only do everyone need to know what the MTP is and how it is activated, but mock runs with the MTP would be the best way to maintain competency. Furthermore, and this is something that you have not mentioned, it also needs to be clarified when the MTP will be stopped.

Summary

In conclusion, the MTP is a valuable tool, which can be complemented with the use of TXA, point-of-care tests such as TEG, and rehearsal of the protocol with special attention paid to human factors issues. Future research will determine ideal ratios as well as the best way to implement the MTP at low-volume trauma facilities.

References

1. Borgman MA, Spinella PC, Perkins JG, Grathwohl KW, Repine T, Beekley AC, et al. The ratio of blood products transfused affects mortality in patients receiving massive transfusions at a combat support hospital. J Trauma. 2007;63:805–13.
2. Enticott JC, Jeffcott S, Ibrahim JE, Wood EM, Cole-Sincalire M, Fitzgerald M, et al. A review on decision support for massive transfusion: understanding human factors to support the implementation of complex interventions in trauma. Transfusion. 2012;52:2692–705.
3. Holcomb JB, Tilley BC, Baraniuk S, Fox EE, Wade CE, Podbielski JM, et al. Transfusion of plasma, platelets, and red blood cells in a 1:1:1 vs a 1:1:2 ratio and mortality in patients with severe trauma: the PROPPR randomized clinical trial. JAMA. 2015;313:471–82.
4. Shakur H, Roberts I, Bautista R, Caballero J, Coats T, Dewan Y, et al. CRASH-2 trial collaborators. Effects of tranexamic acid on death, vascular occlusive events, and blood transfusion in trauma patients with significant haemorrhage (CRASH-2): a randomised, placebo-controlled trial. Lancet. 2010;376:23–32.
5. Ho AM, Dion PW, Yeung JH, Holcomb JB, Critchley LA, Ng CS, et al. Prevalence of survivor bias in observational studies on fresh frozen plasma: erythrocyte ratios in trauma requiring massive transfusion. Anesthesiology. 2012;56:215–6.
6. Mitra B, O'Reilly G, Cameron PA, Zatta A, Gruen RL. Effectiveness of massive transfusion protocols on mortality in trauma: a systematic review and meta-analysis. ANZ J Surg. 2013;83(12):918–23.
7. Levi M, Levy JH, Andersen HF, Truloff D. Safety of recombinant activated factor VII in randomized clinical trials. N Engl J Med. 2010;363(19):1791–800.
8. Roberts I, Shakur H, Afolabi A, Brohi K, Coats T, Dewan Y, Crash-2 Collaborators, et al. The importance of early treatment with tranexamic acid in bleeding trauma patients: an exploratory analysis of the CRASH-2 randomised controlled trial. Lancet. 2011;377(9771):1096–101.
9. Hauser CJ, Boffard K, Dutton R, Bernard GR, Croce MA, Holcomb JB, CONTROL Study Group, et al. Results of the CONTROL trial: efficacy and safety of recombinant activated Factor VII in the management of refractory traumatic hemorrhage. J Trauma. 2010;69(3):489–500.
10. Mitra B, Gabbe BJ, Kaukonen KM, Olaussen A, Cooper DJ, Cameron PA. Long-term outcomes of patients receiving a massive transfusion after trauma. Shock. 2014;42(4):307–12.
11. McDaniel LM, Etchill EW, Raval JS, Neal MD. State of the art: massive transfusion. Transfus Med. 2014;24:138–44.
12. Escolar G, Mazzara R, Castillo R, Ordinas A. The role of the Baumgartner technique in transfusion medicine: research and clinical applications. Transfusion. 1994;34(6):542–9.
13. Zink KA, Sambasivan CN, Holcomb JB, Chisholm G, Schreiber MA. A high ratio of plasma and platelets to packed red blood cells in the first 6 hours of massive transfusion improves outcomes in a large multicenter study. Am J Surg. 2009;197(5):565–70.
14. Pati S, Matijevic N, Doursout MF, Ko T, Cao Y, Deng X, et al. Protective effects of fresh frozen plasma on vascular endothelial permeability, coagulation, and resuscitation after hemorrhagic shock are time dependent and diminish between days 0 and 5 after thaw. J Trauma. 2010;69(Suppl 1):S55–63.
15. Chapman MP, Moore EE, Ramos CR, Ghasabyan A, Harr JN, Chin TL, et al. Fibrinolysis greater than 3 % is the critical value for initiation of antifibrinolytic therapy. J Trauma Acute Care Surg. 2013;75(6):961–7 (discussion 967).
16. Kutcher ME, Kornblith LZ, Narayan R, Curd V, Daley AT, Redick BJ, et al. A paradigm shift in trauma resuscitation: evaluation of evolving massive transfusion practices. JAMA Surg. 2013;148(9):834–40.
17. Hess JR, Thomas MJG. Blood use in war and disaster: lessons from the past century. Transfusion. 2003;43(11):1622–33.
18. Tapia NM, Chang A, Norman M, Welsh F, Scott B, Wall MJ Jr, et al. TEG-guided resuscitation is superior to standardized MTP resuscitation in massively transfused penetrating trauma patients. J Trauma Acute Care Surg. 2013;74(2):378–86.
19. Meng ZH, Wolberg AS, Monroe DM III, Hoffman M. The effect of temperature and pH on the activity of factor VIIa: implications for the efficacy of high-dose factor VIIa in hypothermic and acidotic patients. J Trauma. 2003;55(5):886–91.
20. Vu EN, Schlamp RS, Wand RT, Kleine-Deters GA, Vu MP, Tallon JM. Prehospital use of tranexamic acid for hemorrhagic shock in primary and secondary air medical evacuation. Air Med J. 2013;32(5):289–92.

Should Cerebral Oximetry Be Employed in Morbidly Obese Patients Undergoing Bariatric Surgery?

15

David Porbunderwala

CASE

A 40-year-old morbidly obese male, body mass index (BMI) 60, with complications including obstructive sleep apnea, hyperlipidemia, hypertension, and type II diabetes mellitus, is undergoing Roux-en-Y gastric bypass weight loss surgery. He has a large neck circumference and a Mallampati score of 3. Difficult intubation is anticipated, so the plan is to proceed with fiberoptic laryngoscopy. A near-infrared spectrometry (NIRS) cerebral oximeter is placed on the patient's forehead to monitor cerebral venous saturation ($rScO_2$); his baseline is 73 %. Peripheral intravenous lines are placed under ultrasound guidance.

The patient is induced with propofol and intubated without difficulty. As the surgeons begin, the patient remains supine as pneumoperitoneum is established, with the blood pressure steady at 100/65 and cerebral venous oxygen saturation at 72 %. Ten minutes into the procedure, the surgeons call for 25° reverse Trendelenburg. One minute following positioning, his $rScO_2$ drops to 64 % and his blood pressure to 98/65. Over the next several minutes, the $rScO_2$ begins to decline steadily to 55 % and the next BP measurement is 64/43.

PRO: Cerebral oximetry allows for continuous monitoring of the patient's circulatory status. Since no arterial line is present, if I'm not proactive, I must wait for the blood pressure cuff to cycle, which may be after a considerable delay. As it stands, I will increase the LR infusion rate and give a bolus of phenylephrine.

CON: In this instance, the course of action was not effectively altered by the $rScO_2$ measurement; rather the change was eclipsed by the marked drop in mean arterial pressure (MAP), prompting immediate intervention. The 64 % reading represents a 10 % change in saturation, certainly not enough for me to emergently reach for a pressor.

PRO: While marked cerebral desaturation might not be common in other abdominal surgeries, obese patients undergoing bariatric procedures are the ones to watch. In 2006, a cohort study by Gipson et al. [1] demonstrated that while significant decreases in $rScO_2$ are not particularly common in abdominal surgery, they were significantly more likely to occur in heavier patients undergoing gastric bypass and in those with longer operations.

CON: The drop in blood pressure or saturation should undoubtedly be anticipated in these patients with so much potential intravascular space undergoing massive sympatholysis. If I am doing my job, I will expect the decrease in blood pressure as the patient is repositioned and I will check the head and tubing, increase FiO_2, and open the IVs, and then I'll be able to react to any drops in BP with less urgency knowing my bases are covered.

PRO: The benefit of the cerebral oximeter transcends surrogate monitoring of systemic perfusion in surgery that is not vascular, cardiac, or neurological. A prospective, randomized trial demonstrated that monitoring cerebral venous saturation in elderly patients undergoing abdominal surgery has additive benefits [2]. Using $rScO_2$ as an indicator for intervention, not only were cerebral venous saturations maintained at a higher level, but in those patients who had desaturations—defined as <75 % of baseline—both length and extent of desaturation correlated with a decrease in the Mini Mental State Examination (MMSE) score at 7 days post-op, implying that postoperative cognitive dysfunction may very well be attributed to desaturation [2]. Another recent meta-analysis supported these findings and found that a prompt reaction to cerebral desaturation reduces hospital stay [3].

CON: Much of these data are derived from elderly patients and those who are considerably sicker; e.g., undergoing liver transplantation. Though this patient may have multiple

D. Porbunderwala (✉)
Department of Anesthesiology, New York University Langone Medical Center, 550 First Avenue, New York, NY 10016, USA
e-mail: davidporbunderwala@gmail.com

C.S. Scher et al. (eds.), *You're Wrong, I'm Right*, DOI 10.1007/978-3-319-43169-7_15

comorbidities, at the end of the day his heart is still good and he is relatively young, and he is putatively more able to recover from this surgery or any minor cerebral injury. MMSE score in these cases was measured at 7 days; barring complications, this patient will have been at home for several days by that point. Furthermore, the second-line therapy in the aforementioned trial was a bolus of propofol to decrease cerebral oxygen demand [2], which I would not be thrilled to give a hypotensive patient.

PRO: While I would not readily give propofol either, it still stands that there is no harm in monitoring cerebral oximetry. Rather, I could have caught the patient on the downslope of his saturation and, ideally, he would never have dropped his MAP or his $rScO_2$ to the extent that he did, regardless of what harm might be done.

Summary

Intraoperative cerebral desaturation and a massive decrease in blood pressure are to be expected in morbidly obese patients when they are placed in reverse Trendelenburg position. The literature suggests that prompt response to desaturation can reduce postoperative cognitive dysfunction, but this phenomenon has not been closely examined in the bariatric population. As the etiology of postoperative cognitive dysfunction continues to be elucidated, monitoring of $rScO_2$ with NIRS provides a simple, noninvasive, and inexpensive means of measuring cerebral perfusion and potentially staying one step ahead of intraoperative hypotension.

References

1. Gipson CL, Johnson GA, Fisher R, Stewart A, Giles G, Johnson JO, et al. Changes in cerebral oximetry during peritoneal insufflation for laparoscopic procedures. J Minim Access Surg. 2006;2(2):67–72.
2. Cavati A, Fanelli G, Pietropaoli P, Proietti R, Tufano R, Danelli G, Fierro G, De Cosmo G, Servillo G. Continuous monitoring of cerebral oxygen saturation in elderly patients undergoing major abdominal surgery minimizes brain exposure to potential hypoxia. Anesth Analg. 2005;101:740–7.
3. Sørensen H, Grocott HP, Secher NH. Near infrared spectroscopy for frontal lobe oxygenation during non-vascular abdominal surgery. Clin Physiol Funct Imaging. 2015; p. 1–6. doi:10.1111/cpf.12244.

16 Is Normal Saline Solution the Best Crystalloid for Intravascular Volume Resuscitation?

Saad Rasheed

Case

A 30-year-old male with no significant past medical history presents to the emergency room with complaints of severe abdominal pain. The patient reports that the pain began 2 days ago. It has since migrated to the right lower quadrant. Associated symptoms include nausea without vomiting, anorexia, and a subjective fever. Significant vital signs include a temperature of 103.4 °F, a heart rate of 110 beats per minute, and a blood pressure of 80/50. Physical examination reveals a diffusely tender abdomen with guarding and rebound tenderness. Pertinent preoperative laboratories include a WBC of 22,000 cells/μ(mu)L and a lactate level of 5.8 mmol/L. An abdominal computed tomography (CT) scan confirms the suspected diagnosis of perforated appendicitis. The general surgery service is consulted and the chief resident recommends IV antibiotics and emergent laparotomy for appendectomy and irrigation and drainage of the peritoneal cavity.

You place 2 large-bore IVs in the emergency room and begin an infusion of lactated Ringer's solution. Once in the operating room you place standard ASA monitors prior to a rapid sequence induction. Postinduction, you place an arterial line. Considering the clinical presentation of severe sepsis, you infuse a total of 30 mL/kg of lactated Ringers. After the infusion, the patient's hemodynamic vital signs have improved; his heart rate is now 95 beats per minute, and blood pressure has improved to 110/65. ABG shows that the lactate is trending downward. The appendectomy and irrigation and drainage are completed successfully, and the patient is extubated without incident. You transport the patient to the postanesthesia care unit (PACU) and give a report to the anesthesiologist covering the recovery room. He tells the nurse taking care of the patient to disconnect the lactated Ringer's and hang a bag of normal saline solution, scolding you and asking, "Don't you know that normal saline solution is the best fluid to resuscitate a patient with?"

Question

Is normal saline solution the best crystalloid for intravascular volume resuscitation?

PRO: The recovery room anesthesiologist notes that sodium chloride is the most commonly used crystalloid solution globally, with more than 200 million liters of normal saline infused each year in the United States. He leans on a common argument of seasoned clinicians who favor normal saline, "I have been practicing anesthesia for more than 20 years and have never encountered a problem using normal saline. Why try and fix it if it isn't broken?"

CON: "Although normal saline was the original crystalloid of choice, there is nothing 'normal' about it. It's composition is based on studies of red cell lysis from the late 1800s that indicated that 0.9 % was the concentration of salt in the human blood, when the actual concentration is actually 0.6 %. Newer crystalloids such as lactated Ringer's approximate extracellular fluid more accurately—intuitively a more physiologically correct fluid should improve patient outcomes and I'm sure there is research to support this common sense assertion."

A quick literature search proves your suspicions: There is an abundance of new research showing the pitfalls of using normal saline for fluid resuscitation. Myburgh and Mythen's article in the *New England Journal of Medicine* summarizes some of the concerns regarding normal saline [1]. The article notes that the "administration of large volumes of saline results in hyperchloremic metabolic acidosis." This makes sense as normal saline has a chloride concentration of 154 mmol/L—much higher than the serum chloride concentration. Further, the article points out that this acidosis is associated with immune and renal dysfunction [1]. The

S. Rasheed (✉)
Department of Anesthesiology, New York University, 545 First Avenue, Apt 10J, New York, NY 10016, USA
e-mail: Saad.w.rasheed@gmail.com; Saad.Rasheed@nyumc.org

C.S. Scher et al. (eds.), *You're Wrong, I'm Right*, DOI 10.1007/978-3-319-43169-7_16

review cites a study by Shaw et al. [2] comparing the use of normal saline versus PlasmaLyte, a balanced fluid similar to lactated Ringer's, which found that in patients undergoing surgery, PlasmaLyte administration was associated with a decrease in major complications such as postoperative infection, the need for renal-replacement therapy, and blood transfusion when compared to normal saline. In light of these findings, the article asserts that physiologically balanced solutions are increasingly recommended in surgical patients [2].

PRO: Your colleague remains unimpressed. He too reads the NEJM article, finding what he believes are key flaws. "You mention that hyperchloremic metabolic acidosis causes an increased incidence of immune and renal dysfunction, but Myburgh and Mythen themselves admit that 'the clinical consequences of these effects are unclear.' Further, the results are for PlasmaLyte, not lactated Ringer's. That study excluded lactated Ringer's because calcium-containing solutions are not used in patients requiring blood transfusion due to the risk of microthrombi. How can you be certain that the results are transferrable? Finally, the results of that study are from a database review! Without the gold standard of a randomized control trial, are you really comfortable changing your clinical practice?"

CON: "You make some fair points. Although Myburgh and Mythen allude to the equivocal results regarding the clinical significance of hyperchloremia in the past, there is growing evidence of its deleterious effects. McCluskey et al. [3] performed a retrospective cohort trial that showed that hyperchloremia was associated with increased morbidity and mortality after noncardiac surgery, specifically showing that hyperchloremia (serum chloride >110 mEq/L) was associated with increased mortality at 30 days postop, a longer hospital stay, and a higher likelihood of postoperative renal dysfunction.

"Although Shaw et al's [2] results were only for PlasmaLyte, I believe the findings are likely transferrable. The results were attributed to a hyperchloremic acidosis caused by normal saline's chloride concentration of 154 mmol/L. PlasmaLyte has a chloride concentration of 98 mmol/L, right in the normal range, and lactated Ringer's has a chloride concentration of 109 mmol/L, only slightly higher than the upper normal limit of plasma chloride concentration. And Noritomi et al's [4] study of crystalloid administration during hemorrhagic shock noted that resuscitation with normal saline solution caused hyperchloremic acidosis while resuscitation with both lactated Ringer's and Plasma-Lyte did not. Thus, it stands to reason that patients would derive similar benefits from lactated Ringer's and PlasmaLyte.

Lastly, your point regarding a randomized control trial is a legitimate one. Although the evidence is growing that normal saline leads to harmful metabolic states, and in turn negatively influences patient outcomes, without large-scale randomized controlled trials making definitive guidelines may prove difficult. This does not, however, mean that your clinical practice shouldn't change. There is no evidence that normal saline is a superior solution, and to continue to use it blindly does your patients a disservice."

PRO: "So are you saying that there is no place for normal saline?"

CON: "My default resuscitation fluid has been lactated Ringer's, and based on these recent studies, I see no reason to change this. In patients who have a hypochloremic metabolic alkalosis, such as those with persistent severe vomiting, the normally harmful physiologic effects of normal saline solution may actually serve some benefit. Outside of this narrow subset of cases, however, there really is no place for normal saline as a resuscitation fluid."

Summary

Normal saline is the most commonly used intravenous fluid globally and in the USA. This is largely due to its place as the original fluid used to treat dehydration and its cost. With the advent of more balanced, physiologically correct solutions, that are only marginally more expensive, these reasons for the use of normal saline no longer hold weight. We recommend the use of normal saline only in patients who have a hypochloremic metabolic alkalosis that would benefit from a high chloride solution such as normal saline. Considering numerous recent studies indicating the advantages of lactated Ringer's over of normal saline, we look forward to a randomized control trial that will definitively prove the superiority of physiologically balanced solutions such as lactated Ringer's.

References

1. Myburgh JA, Mythen MG. Resuscitation fluids. N Engl J Med. 2013;369:1243–51.
2. Shaw AD, Bagshaw SM, Goldstein SL, Scherer LA, Duan M, Schermer CR, et al. Major complications, mortality, and resource utilization after open abdominal surgery: 0.9 % saline compared to Plasma-Lyte. Ann Surg. 2012;255:821–9.
3. McCluskey SA, Karkouti K, Wijeysundera D, Minkovich L, Tait G, Beattie WS. Hyperchloremia after noncardiac surgery is independently associated with increased morbidity and mortality: a propensity-matched cohort study. Anesth Analg. 2013;117:412–21.
4. Noritomi DT, Pereira AJ, Bugano DD, Rehder PS, Silva E. Impact of Plasma-Lyte pH 7.4 on acid-base status and hemodynamics in a model of controlled hemorrhagic shock. Clinics. 2011;66 (11):1969–74.

Part II
Cardiac

17 Should Local Anesthesia with Conscious Sedation Be Considered the Standard of Care Over General Anesthesia for Transcatheter Aortic Valve Replacement via the Transfemoral Approach?

Glen D. Quigley and Jennie Y. Ngai

Case

A new cardiac surgeon, Dr. Jones, has just been hired by the hospital to begin a transcatheter aortic valve replacement (TAVR) program. Prior to his start date, Dr. Jones requested to meet with the cardiac anesthesia attendings to discuss the feasibility of doing all of the transfemoral TAVR cases using only local anesthesia with conscious sedation (LACS). He mentioned that he was at a conference in Europe recently and learned that the majority of transfemoral TAVR cases performed there were done using LACS. Additionally, he stated that he had seen several studies that showed that TAVR procedures done with LACS are just as safe as those done with the patient under general anesthesia (GA) and that they require much less time in the operating room (OR).

"I've been doing cardiac anesthesia for a long time and I have a lot of concerns with trying to do a complicated cardiac procedure like this on a patient who is basically awake," replied one of the senior cardiac anesthesiologists. "One of my biggest concerns is what would happen if the patient moves while the valve is being deployed. Not just because the valve could be malpositioned, but because it could also tear the aorta or block off one of the coronaries and cause a myocardial infarction. I'm not sure it's worth that risk just to save a few minutes of OR time."

G.D. Quigley (✉)
Department of Anesthesiology, Lankenau Medical Center, 100 Lancaster Avenue, Wynnewood, PA 19096, USA
e-mail: Glen.quigley@gmail.com

J.Y. Ngai
Department of Anesthesiology, Perioperative Care and Pain Medicine, New York University School of Medicine, NYU Anesthesia Associates, 560 First Avenue, New York, NY 10016, USA
e-mail: Jennie.Ngai@nyumc.org

Dr. Jones countered, "It's not just about the time savings. I'm also worried that some of these frail elderly patients will have to stay intubated for a long time after the procedure—especially patients coming in with severe lung disease. Is it worth it for a patient to get their valve fixed but then end up needing to get trached because of a prolonged intubation?"

As one of the younger cardiac anesthesia attendings, I was also uneasy about the thought of doing these cases under LACS. However, I wasn't sure that unease alone was reason enough to say these cases shouldn't be done under LACS, especially if studies from other major cardiac centers showed it could be done safely. The hospital had invested a lot of resources into getting this TAVR program started, and it was important for the cardiac anesthesiologists and Dr. Jones to come to some consensus on this issue.

Question

Should local anesthesia with conscious sedation be considered the standard of care over general anesthesia for transcatheter aortic valve replacement via the transfemoral approach?

Transcatheter aortic valve replacement (TAVR) is a procedure that was first performed in 2002 as a less invasive alternative to surgical aortic valve replacement (AVR) and is being increasingly used in very high-risk patients with severe aortic stenoses who are ineligible for open surgical AVR. TAVR uses a stent-valve technology in which a bioprosthetic tissue valve is mounted inside an expandable stent device, which can be deployed inside a patient's native, diseased aortic valve. Although there are numerous approaches through which the device can be introduced (retrograde transfemoral, antegrade transapical, retrograde transaxillary, etc.), most TAVR procedures worldwide are performed via the retrograde transfemoral approach [1, 2]. In the retrograde transfemoral approach (hereafter referred to as

C.S. Scher et al. (eds.), *You're Wrong, I'm Right*, DOI 10.1007/978-3-319-43169-7_17

just the "transfemoral approach"), the stent-valve device is introduced through a percutaneous puncture of the femoral artery and delivered retrograde up the aorta using an over-the-wire technique with fluoroscopic guidance similar to that used to perform coronary angiography and stenting. Thus, in many ways, this procedure is much more similar to procedures typically performed by cardiologists in the catheterization laboratory than it is to the classic open surgical AVR done by cardiac surgeons in the operating room. Since much of the setup and procedural aspects of transfemoral TAVR match those of catheterization laboratory procedures, there has been increasing interest over the past several years in looking at whether transfemoral TAVR can be safely performed under the same type of LACS used for catheterization laboratory procedures. Despite the many similarities though, transfemoral TAVR is still very different from coronary angioplasty in terms of both the *types* and *severity* of complications that can occur. The 30-day mortality rate of TAVR performed in the typical high-risk surgical patient is approximately 10 %, which is much higher than that typically reported for coronary angioplasty with stenting (<1 %) [1].

PRO: My senior anesthesia colleague continued to voice his concerns with this plan. "General anesthesia is the only safe way to do these procedures. It is the only way to guarantee an immobile patient during critical parts of the procedure. It provides a secure airway from the start of the case and it avoids having to worry about rapidly converting to general anesthesia after a surgical catastrophe has occurred. The possible surgical complications of this procedure include injury to the femoral arteries with accompanying retroperitoneal hemorrhage, dissection of the aorta, stroke from embolization of calcific aortic plaques, myocardial infarction from obstruction of coronary ostia, pericardial tamponade, and ventricular fibrillation following rapid ventricular pacing. All of these complications can occur suddenly and can be life-threatening; it would be best to not have to also worry about securing a patient's airway *after* one of these complications occurs."

CON: Dr. Jones countered, "I agree that this procedure can potentially cause life-threatening complications. However, I don't think that just the possibility for serious surgical complications should rule out doing these procedures under LACS. As I mentioned earlier, there are multiple studies that have demonstrated that LACS is equal to general anesthesia in terms of safety and allows for faster recovery after the procedure."

PRO: "Well, I haven't seen these studies yet so I guess I'll have to reserve judgment," remarked my senior anesthesia colleague. "But my feeling is that doing these cases with just local anesthesia and sedation seems to put the patient at increased risk, especially if surgical complications occur. Also, doing these cases under sedation alone means that a transesophageal echocardiography (TEE) probe cannot be used. TEE is critically important as it enables immediate verification of correct valve placement and allows for rapid detection and grading of paravalvular and central leaks. Significant paravalvular leaks are relatively common after TAVR, about 8–10 % from studies that I've seen, which is much more common than after conventional open AVR [3]. This problem can be somewhat alleviated with intraoperative TEE use by allowing for a determination to be made just after deployment regarding whether an additional balloon valvuloplasty should be done or even a valve-in-valve if the paravalvular leak is very severe (i.e., deploying a second TAVR device *inside* the first one)."

CON: "I agree that TEE can be tremendously helpful during these procedures, especially for detecting post-deployment valvular leaks. However, I don't think that TEE is an absolute requirement," replied Dr. Jones. "For starters, we already perform a preoperative TEE prior to coming to the OR to get all the information we need regarding annulus size, annulus area, and aortic root measurements. We can also use transthoracic echocardiography (TTE) in the OR for any cases done with LACS. While imaging of the aorta with TTE is not always as good as TEE, in most cases it would probably give you enough information to determine whether a severe paravalvular leak was present. And we can always perform contrast aortography using fluoroscopy to further determine the severity of regurgitation. How about we take a short break and continue this discussion when we return. I'll see if I can bring some copies of those studies back for us to look at more closely before we make any decisions."

During the break, I returned to my office to review the studies to which Dr. Jones had referred. After a quick search of the literature, I found five clinical trials published in the past 3 years that compared outcomes between TAVR performed under general anesthesia and local anesthesia plus conscious sedation (LACS). I jotted down a few notes, printed out copies of the articles for everyone, and returned to the conference room to share the information I found.

Before the meeting restarted, I compared articles with Dr. Jones and found the ones that I downloaded to be the same articles to which he had referred. As everyone returned to the meeting, we handed out copies of the articles to review as a group. I decided to begin by sharing some of the insights I had taken away from the studies.

"I understand that there are some very strong opinions regarding this topic and that there's probably no one-size-fits-all answer to this question. In front of you are copies of five clinical studies, done within the past 3 years, that compared TAVR performed under either GA or LACS in terms of safety and efficacy."

"In aggregate, these studies looked at 617 patients undergoing transfemoral TAVR—346 under LACS and 276 under GA," I continued [4–8]. "As Dr. Jones had previously mentioned, all five studies showed that there was no difference in terms of mortality, morbidity, or procedure success rate between TAVR done under LACS or GA [4–8]. Four out of the five studies showed that TAVR performed under LACS significantly reduced time in OR when compared with GA, sometimes by as much as 30–45 min [5–8]. Also, three out of the five studies showed that total perioperative and postoperative inotrope/vasopressor requirements were significantly reduced when LACS was used instead of GA [4–6]. So overall, the literature to date seems to support that transfemoral TAVR can be performed under LACS or GA with equal safety and efficacy. LACS also appears to allow for significant time savings in the OR and reduced inotrope/vasopressor requirements."

PRO: "These are definitely interesting studies and I'm impressed at how good some of these results are," stated my senior colleague. "However, I'm not so sure that I'm ready to go ahead and say that all transfemoral TAVR procedures here should be done under LACS. For starters, two of these studies that you provided to us showed a relatively high rate of urgent conversion from LACS to GA. Yamamoto et al. had a 5 % conversion rate and Bergmann et al. reported almost a 17 % conversion rate! [4, 7]. These are very high rates and if almost 17 % of these LACS cases have to be urgently converted to GA, well that's unacceptably high in my opinion. Furthermore, 1 of those studies mentioned that two of those conversions were required because the patients became uncooperative and started moving. Now, it looks like no complications occurred as a result of their movement, but it seems very possible that serious damage could have been done. I'm still not convinced that LACS is appropriate for all transfemoral TAVR patients."

CON: Dr. Jones responded, "I agree that a 17 % conversion rate would be very high. However, this only occurred in 1 study; the other reported conversion rate was 5 % and the three other studies said that zero conversions to GA were needed. Furthermore, it looks like most of those conversions were due to vascular access complications at the femoral sites and occurred during the early part of the study period (2006–2009). Over the past several years, the size of the deployment devices has gotten dramatically smaller (previously 22F–25F, now 16F–19F) leading to much lower rates of femoral vessel injury, especially when combined with improved techniques for percutaneous vessel closure following removal of the device [1]. Given these facts, I would argue that the rate of LACS failure and need to convert to GA due to vascular complications would be much <17 % nowadays."

Concession from PRO: "Fair enough, I know that 17 % was just 1 study," conceded my senior colleague. "But I think it's important to keep in mind that some percentage of cases done under LACS will definitely need to be converted to GA urgently and that instead of just saying all transfemoral cases should be done under LACS, some thought should be given to trying to predict which patients might benefit from doing GA from the start of the case. How about this: Let's try to come up with some criteria regarding which patients would be poor candidates for LACS. Then using these as a guideline, we will evaluate each patient on the day of surgery to see whether they can be done under LACS. Our goal will be to do at least 50 % of our patients under LACS during the first year and as our group gains more experience with it, maybe we can increase from there. Sound reasonable?"

Concession from CON: "Although I would prefer to do most cases using LACS," responded Dr. Jones, "I think that a goal of 50 % of cases done under LACS in the first year and aiming to increase that rate with experience seems very reasonable. Let's come up with some guidelines for LACS suitability and go from there."

Summary

TAVR is being performed with increasing frequency throughout the world as both the number of elderly individuals *needing the procedure* and the number of interventionalists *trained to perform the procedure* increases. Furthermore, TAVR is currently being evaluated as an option in moderate risk patients with severe aortic stenosis who would be able to choose between the less invasive (but less well-studied) TAVR or the current gold standard, open surgical AVR; if approved in this population, the number of TAVR procedures performed annually would likely increase dramatically. As such, it is important for anesthesiologists to continue to evaluate the contribution that anesthetic type makes to patient outcomes for this increasingly important procedure.

As mentioned in the previous discussion, local anesthesia with conscious sedation (LACS), while still controversial, offers many benefits over general anesthesia (GA) including avoidance of airway manipulation and possible prolonged intubation, reduced utilization of OR time, and reduced need for inotrope/vasopressor support—while maintaining similar rates of mortality, morbidity, and procedural success.

However, certain patients would likely be poor candidates for LACS due to a high risk that they would require urgent or emergent conversion intraoperatively from LACS to GA. Identifying these risk factors and using these data to develop guidelines to help with proper patient selection would probably lead to decreases in the rate of LACS failure. Contraindications to LACS for TAVR would likely include: (1) severe obstructive sleep apnea; (2) difficult airway by history or exam; (3) inability to lie flat due to musculoskeletal disease or otherwise; (4) severe GERD; (5) altered mental status, severe dementia, or other barriers to communication; and (6) anatomic considerations in which a TEE may be required (i.e., uncertain annulus size, poor TTE windows, high-risk features such as concern for annular rupture or coronary occlusion). With continued research, anesthesia for TAVR will continue to be refined with the goal of providing each patient with an anesthetic plan that maximizes both safety and comfort.

References

1. Alfirevic A, Mehta AR, Svensson LG. Transcatheter aortic valve replacement. Anesthesiol Clin. 2013;31:355–81.
2. Bufton KA, Augoustides JG, Cobey FC. Anesthesia for transfemoral aortic valve replacement in North America and Europe. J Cardiothorac Vasc Anesth. 2013;27:46–9.
3. Bleiziffer S, Mazzitelli D, Opitz A, Hettich I, Ruge H, Piazza N, et al. Beyond the short-term: clinical outcome and valve performance 2 years after transcatheter aortic valve implantation in 227 patients. J Thorac Cardiovasc Surg. 2012;143:310–7.
4. Bergmann L, Kahlert P, Eggebrecht H, Frey U, Peters J, Kottenberg E. Transfemoral aortic valve implantation under sedation and monitored anaesthetic care—a feasibility study. Anaesthesia. 2011;66:977–82.
5. Dehédin B, Guinot PG, Ibrahim H, Allou N, Provenchère S, Dilly MP, et al. Anesthesia and perioperative management of patients who undergo transfemoral transcatheter aortic valve implantation: an observational study of general versus local/regional anesthesia in 125 consecutive patients. J Cardiothorac Vasc Anesth. 2011;25:1036–43.
6. Motloch LJ, Rottlaender D, Reda S, Larbig R, Bruns M, Müller--Ehmsen J, et al. Local versus general anesthesia for transfemoral aortic valve implantation. Clin Res Cardiol. 2012;101:45–53.
7. Yamamoto M, Meguro K, Mouillet G, Bergoend E, Monin JL, Lim P, et al. Effect of local anesthetic management with conscious sedation in patients undergoing transcatheter aortic valve implantation. Am J Cardiol. 2013;111:94–9.
8. Balanika M, Smyrli A, Samanidis G, Spargias K, Stavridis G, Karavolias G, et al. Anesthetic management of patients undergoing transcatheter aortic valve implantation. J Cardiothorac Vasc Anesth. 2014;28:285–9.

Should Antiplatelet Therapy Be Stopped Preoperatively in a Patient with Coronary Artery Stents?

18

Caitlin J. Guo and Katherine Chuy

Case

A 55-year-old man with hypertension, diabetes, and coronary artery disease (CAD) with 2 drug-eluting stents (DES) placed 3 months ago has been maintained on dual antiplatelet therapy (DAPT) with aspirin and clopidogrel. He is now scheduled for a colectomy for newly diagnosed colon cancer.

The patient arrives at the presurgical testing clinic for his preoperative evaluation. The anesthesiologist is asked for advice on perioperative management regarding his antiplatelet therapy. The cardiologist has already performed a preoperative assessment and determined his cardiac function is optimized to proceed. Given the recent timing of his stent placement, both aspirin and clopidogrel should be continued throughout surgery. However, the surgeon expresses concerns about continuing the dual therapy because of the increased bleeding risk.

Background

An estimated 600,000–900,000 coronary stents are placed every year in the USA for management of acute and chronic coronary artery disease [1, 2]. At least 10 % of these patients undergo surgery within the first year while on antiplatelet therapy [1]. This is an increasingly common scenario that anesthesiologists encounter in the perioperative setting—how to balance the risks of surgical bleeding with major adverse cardiovascular events. Aspirin combined with 1 of the P2Y12 inhibitors (clopidogrel, prasugrel, or ticagrelor) is the current standard of care for oral DAPT after cardiac stent placement to prevent stent thrombosis.

Currently, there are two types of cardiac stents: the bare metal stent (BMS) and drug-eluting stent (DES). Development of the BMS in the 1980s was a major advance over balloon angioplasty, which was associated with a high rate of acute vessel closure and restenosis [3]. BMS attempts to prevent restenosis by reducing arterial recoil and contraction, thus becoming an effective treatment for symptomatic coronary artery disease. By 1999, approximately 84 % of percutaneous coronary interventional (PCI) procedures were done with BMS [3]. However, vascular smooth cell proliferation and migration from stent implantation led to neointimal hyperplasia over time, resulting in restenosis rates as high as 20–30 % [3].

DES, a metallic stent coated with an antiproliferative drug, was developed to reduce neointimal hyperplasia. The dramatic reduction in restenosis (58–70 % [3]) with DES led to an exponential growth of their use. By 2005, 80–90 % of all PCI were performed with DES [3]. Since then, newer and safer DES have been developed, with current usage estimated to be 75 % of all PCI [3]. The downside of a DES is that it requires a much longer duration of DAPT to prevent stent thrombosis, a serious complication that occurs when a previously patent stent undergoes an acute thrombotic occlusion. It almost always leads to complete occlusion of the stent, thus myocardial infarction with ST segment elevation and has an associated mortality of 40–60 % [2]. Patients are at highest risk early after stent placement, prior to vessel re-endothelialization, which takes 4–6 weeks for a BMS and 6–12 months for a DES. Premature cessation of DAPT has been highly associated with stent thrombosis.

C.J. Guo (✉) · K. Chuy
Department of Anesthesiology, Perioperative Care and Pain Medicine, New York University Langone Medical Center, 550 First Avenue, New York, NY 10016, USA
e-mail: Caitlin.Guo@nyumc.org

K. Chuy
e-mail: Katherine.chuy@nyumc.org

K. Chuy
320 Center Street, Englewood Cliffs, NJ 07632, USA

C.S. Scher et al. (eds.), *You're Wrong, I'm Right*, DOI 10.1007/978-3-319-43169-7_18

Questions

What should the patient do regarding surgery and his DAPT? Should this patient proceed with noncardiac surgery 3 months after DES placement? If not, how long should surgery be delayed?

PRO: This surgery is for cancer removal and a possible cure. Any delay could lead to metastases and decrease his chance of a successful complete tumor resection. Surely, the surgeon and the cardiologist can agree on an anticoagulation regimen to minimize the chance of both stent thrombosis and excessive surgical bleeding.

CON: After noncardiac surgery, patients with stents face an 8–10 % risk of developing major adverse cardiac events because of inflammation, stress, and prolonged immobility, compared to a 1–5 % risk in those without stents [2]. The duration between stent placement and timing of the procedure correlates with the risk of these complications. Although his oncologist and surgeon would have to weigh in on this, many types of colon cancer are slow growing. It doesn't help to cure his cancer if he dies perioperatively of a heart attack. Thus, the longer the surgery can wait, the lower the likelihood that the patient will develop stent thrombosis and adverse cardiac events.

According to the 2014 American College of Cardiology (ACC) and American Heart Association (AHA) "Guideline on Perioperative Cardiovascular Evaluation and Management of Patients Undergoing Noncardiac Surgery," [4] the minimal recommendation for DAPT is 1 month after BMS and 12 months for DES (class 1 evidence). Elective surgical procedures, therefore, should be delayed until DAPT is completed.

PRO: Yes, but I would argue that this surgery should not be delayed much longer, which the guidelines address. For emergent surgeries, the recommendation is to continue DAPT (class 1 evidence) [4] unless risk of bleeding is greater than risk of stent thrombosis.

Is a colectomy for colon cancer really a life or death emergency? Or is it urgent? The ACC/AHA suggests waiting at least 6 months (class 2b evidence) for urgent surgeries where risk of delaying the procedure outweighs risks of ischemia and stent thrombosis [4]. In our patient who is 3 months out from stent placement with newly diagnosed colon cancer, the assessment goes beyond simply evaluating the case from a cardiovascular standpoint. We must also consider risk of bleeding while operating with DAPT and oncological consequences of delaying surgery.

Colorectal cancer is the third most common cause of cancer death in the USA, with an estimated 132,700 newly diagnosed cases and 49,700 deaths in 2015 [5]. National Cancer Institute database statistics for 2004–2010 reported that an early diagnosis of a localized colon cancer imparts a 5-year relative survival rate of 90 % [6]. It also allows possibility of a curative therapy with complete resection. In contrast, more advanced cancer has only a 5-year relative survival rate in 71 % if spread regionally versus 13 % if spread systemically [6]. Thus, while colon resection for a localized cancer is not considered an emergency, delaying early treatment and resection for up to a year may lower this patient's long-term survival rate if his cancer spreads.

Consensus

Ultimately the decision process for this patient requires an in-depth discussion with the patient and his or her surgeon, cardiologist, and anesthesiologist, weighing the perceived risk for major adverse cardiac events and stent thrombosis from perioperative discontinuation of DAPT versus bleeding with continuation of DAPT. In this patient, one can argue that surgery should proceed without delay and DAPT should be continued. Uncomplicated colon resection is typically considered low risk for bleeding; in this patient, the benefit of continuing DAPT outweighs the risk of bleeding. However, one can never predict intraoperative complications. For example, if the cancer has invaded major vascular supply, then the risk for bleeding significantly increases. So if DAPT is continued, it is important that the anesthesiologist is familiar with diagnostic and therapeutic options.

Question

Which antiplatelet agents should be continued or discontinued preoperatively and how should they be managed?

For elective surgeries, the majority of American and European guidelines advise patients with cardiac stents to continue ASA therapy perioperatively when possible [2]. This recommendation is based on meta-analyses in which continuation of aspirin did not lead to major adverse outcomes from bleeding, but the discontinuation of aspirin was associated with significantly more adverse cardiac events. For procedures that are deemed high bleeding risk, where even minimal bleeding has severe consequences, such as spinal, intracranial, extraocular, urologic, or major reconstructive procedures, both aspirin and PY2 inhibitor should be held.

If the surgery is urgent and cannot be postponed, depending on when the DES was placed, most agreed that DAPT should be continued unless the consequences of bleeding are extreme. However, many controversies surround perioperative management. Some propose obtaining platelet function assays to determine optimal timing for surgery. However, there are no suggestions for which platelet assays to use or what the bleeding cut-off should be.

For high-risk cardiac patients undergoing high-bleeding-risk surgeries, bridging with intravenous reversible glycoprotein inhibitors such as eptifibatide or tirofiban are reasonable alternatives and should be managed by the patient's cardiologist. Bridging with low-molecular-weight heparin (LMWH) is not advised because of a different mechanism of action.

For our patient undergoing colonic resection, many would suggest he remain on aspirin and, given the recent timing of DES, he should also remain on clopidogrel. If significant bleeding is encountered during or after the surgery, studies that evaluate platelet function or the efficiency of the coagulation cascade, such as thromboelastography, can be used to guide transfusion. The reversal of antiplatelet therapy is platelet transfusion.

Question

When should antiplatelet therapy be stopped and resumed before and after surgery?

If discontinuation of DAPT were deemed necessary within this critical period because of bleeding risk, practice guidelines are variable. While some recommend 5 days, some recommend 7–10 days, and others such as ACC/AHA do not make any statement [2]. For practical purposes, most American hospitals have adopted policies of stopping therapy 7 days before surgery. In terms of resuming DAPT postoperative, the generous consensus appears to be that DAPT should be resumed as soon as possible if there are no surgical contraindications, most recommend within 24–48 h. It is important to note, however, these guideline recommendations are published mostly as narrative commentary. They are based on a level of evidence not stated or not necessarily backed by high quality evidence or are based on either consensus opinions by experts, case studies or a current standard of care [2].

Summary

Managing patients who have coronary stents who are undergoing noncardiac surgeries is challenging and complex. While current guidelines recommend delaying elective surgery for a year in patients who have DES, there are many circumstances in which urgent surgeries are required. The clinicians must weigh the risk of delaying surgery versus the risk of adverse cardiovascular complications.

Furthermore, patients on DAPT are at an increased risk for bleeding if continued, but there is also an increased risk for stent thrombosis and major adverse cardiovascular events if DAPT is discontinued. The US registry showed that in more than 4000 patients who had noncardiac surgery within a year of stent placement, regardless of stent type, there was a 1.9 % event rate for myocardial infarction, death, and stent thrombosis [7]. The perioperative rate for major adverse cardiovascular events was also significantly higher in patients who had surgery within 42 days after stent implantation compared to those who have surgery after 42 days [8].

Guidelines have been helpful; however, level of evidence for most could be stronger. Recent studies show lack of adherence to even the most respected guideline, the ACC/AHA. A 2010 national survey of 295 Veterans Administration physicians showed that 100 % of anesthesiologists and cardiologists were aware of the current ACC/AHA guidelines at that time for perioperative cardiovascular evaluation and care for noncardiac surgery, while only 78 % of surgeons were aware of them. Additionally, only 87 % of anesthesiologists, 90 % of cardiologists, and 64 % of surgeons agreed with published guidelines [9]. The perception of risk of coronary stent thrombosis versus bleeding also varied among these providers. Anesthesiologists and cardiologists focused more on stent thrombosis risk and continuing antiplatelet therapy, and the surgeons focused more on bleeding [9]. Thus, consistent implementation of these guidelines has been difficult.

While existing guidelines have been incredibly useful in guiding perioperative DAPT management before noncardiac surgery, most institutions have adopted their own recommendations based on the current guidelines. Blind adherence to policy without clinical consideration can lead to adverse outcomes. It is important that appropriate specialists evaluate high-risk patients that risks and benefits are discussed among all clinicians taking care of the patient and with the patient himself or herself and those individual hospital policies allow for exceptions.

References

1. Vetter TR, Hunter JM, Boudreaux AM. Preoperative management of antiplatelet drugs for a coronary artery stent: how can we hit a moving target? BMC Anesthesiol. 2014;23(14):73.
2. Darvish-Kazem S, Gandi M, Marcucci M, Douketis J. Perioperative management of antiplatelet therapy in patients with a coronary stent who need noncardiac surgery: a systematic review of clinical practice guidelines. Chest. 2013;144(6):1848–56.
3. Garg S, Serruys PW. Coronary stents: current status. J Am Coll Cardiol. 2010;56(10 Suppl):S1–42.
4. Fleisher LA, Fleischmann KE, Auerbach AD, Barnason SA, Beckman JA, Bozkurt B, et al. 2014 ACC/AHA guideline on perioperative cardiovascular evaluation and management of patients undergoing noncardiac surgery: executive summary. J Am Coll Cardiol. 2014;64(22):2373–405.
5. Siegel R, Miller K, Jemel A. Cancer statistics. CA Cancer J Clin. 2015;65:5–29.
6. American Cancer Society: Cancer Facts and Figures 2015. Atlanta: American Cancer Society. 2015. http://www.cancer.org/

acs/groups/content/@editorial/documents/document/acspc-044552. pdf. Accessed 28 Apr 2015.

7. Berger PB, Kleiman NS, Pencina MJ, Hsieh WH, Steinhubl SR, Jeremias A, et al. Frequency of major noncardiac surgery and subsequent adverse events in the year after drug-eluting stent placement results from the EVENT (Evaluation of Drug-eluting Stents and Ischemic Events) Registry. JACC Cardiovasc Interv. 2010;3(9):920–7.
8. Bell AD, Roussin A, Cartier R, Chan WS, Douketis JD, Gupta A, et al. The use of antiplatelet therapy in the outpatient setting: Canadian Cardiovascular Society guidelines. Can J Cardiol. 2011;27 (Suppl A):S1–59.
9. Graham LA, Maddox TM, Itani KM, Hawn MT. Coronary stents and subsequent surgery: reported provider attitudes and practice patterns. Am Surg. 2013;79(5):514–23.

Is Extubating My Cardiac Surgery Patient Postoperatively in the Operating Room a Good Idea?

19

Joseph Kimmel and Peter J. Neuburger

Case

Following multiple episodes of shortness of breath at home, a 66-year-old man with severe mitral regurgitation undergoes an elective mitral valve repair via mini-thoracotomy. His past medical history is significant for diabetes controlled with metformin and hypertension treated with metoprolol. In the past, he was a casual tennis player, but lately he has been feeling short of breath going up the flight of stairs in his house. It is the first case of the day. Induction, intubation, and line placement are uneventful, and the surgery proceeds without incident. At the end of the case, the surgeon jokes to his assistant, "This gas man over here has the easiest job; he just hits every patient over the head with his cookbook and hopes they wake up some point later in the day."

Question

Should I tailor my anesthetic emergence to extubate the patient in the operating room at the end of the case?

CON: Cardiopulmonary bypass (CPB) induces a stress response in the body evidenced by a sympathetic surge that can persist for hours postoperatively. Despite this, patients typically experience some level of stunned and hibernating myocardium post-CPB, resulting in both systolic and diastolic dysfunction. Additionally, myocardial ischemia is known to peak postoperatively 18–24 h postbypass and to improve with intensive analgesia [1]. Positive pressure ventilation "off-loads" the heart by decreasing afterload and left ventricular end diastolic pressure (LVEDP) and thus may increase coronary perfusion pressure (CPP). Additionally, metabolism is increased postoperatively, leading to increased production of CO_2 and higher work of breathing. Therefore, mechanical ventilation can shift the myocardial oxygen supply and demand curves in favor of promoting optimal healing and favorable myocardial remodeling.

PRO: First of all, the other half of the equation for coronary perfusion pressure is the aortic diastolic pressure, which can be decreased when a postbypass patient with diastolic dysfunction is exposed to positive pressure ventilation, reducing preload, and potentially stroke volume by shifting the Starling curve. Perhaps this is why the studies that showed decreased ischemia with intensive analgesia with positive pressure ventilation never showed a significant benefit in overall patient outcomes in terms of long-term ventricular function, morbidity, or mortality. In fact, the prospective randomized trials that confirmed the safety of fast-track (FT) post-CBP recovery (within 4–6 h of surgery vs. the convention of leaving patients intubated and sedated in the ICU for 18–24 h postoperatively) showed an increase in myocardial ischemic time in the fast-track population, but only with regard to the area under the curve (AUC) of ST segment elevation/depression, and not with regard to blood markers or, more importantly, ventricular dysfunction [2].

In addition, the argument against FT extubation may have been valid 2 decades ago when fast tracking was newly proposed; however, that debate has already run its course. In a prospective randomized trial by Cheng et al. [2], patients were randomized to a fast-track extubation protocol versus conventional therapy. In the fast-track group, the average time to extubation was 4.1 h compared to 18.9 h in the conventional group. Despite extubating during the so-called ischemic period, there was no difference between the 2 groups in cardiac morbidity or mortality. We know it is safe to extubate postbypass cardiac patients within the period of

J. Kimmel
Department of Anesthesiology, Perioperative Care and Pain Medicine, New York University Langone Medical Center, 550 First Avenue, New York, NY 10016, USA
e-mail: Joseph.kimmel@nyumc.org

P.J. Neuburger (✉)
Department of Anesthesiology, Perioperative Care and Pain Medicine, New York University School of Medicine, New York University Langone Medical Center, 550 First Avenue, New York, NY 10016, USA
e-mail: Peter.Neuburger@gmail.com

C.S. Scher et al. (eds.), *You're Wrong, I'm Right*, DOI 10.1007/978-3-319-43169-7_19

postoperative myocardial ischemia, and more recently, this concept was taken even further. In the years since we have switched from the narcotic-heavy "cookbook" protocol to a balanced anesthetic involving inhalational agents, we have found that extubating within 15 min of chest closure is no longer far-fetched. Although there are no randomized prospective trials, there are numerous large retrospective reviews showing both the feasibility and safety of immediate extubation, or ultra-fast-track (UFT) anesthesia.

CON: What about the concern that our patient population is aging? Patients are not just accumulating comorbidities, but they are being medically managed for longer and longer before presenting for surgical correction. With these sicker patients, perioperative complications are on the rise and we need to be more judicious with our aggressive techniques. While fast track was shown to be appropriate for our patient population 10 years ago, our current population may be more liable to the morbidities and complications I just mentioned. The selection bias in these studies might mean that they are not generalizable to our current more debilitated patient population.

PRO: Every 10 years or so an anesthesia journal publishes an article about how our patient population is aging and getting sicker, increasing our risks for perioperative surgical and anesthetic complications. But as our patients have matured, so too has our experience and ability to manage them safely perioperatively. Much as it did with fast-track (and if you look at the first papers published on fast-track anesthesia, they all start with statements about how our population is aging), creating UFT merely requires that we define an eligible population. Some common exclusion criteria in the studies mentioned are patients requiring significant vasopressor or inotropic support, or an IABP; those with morbid obesity; those with severe pulmonary hypertension; and those who are having reoperations [3]. As there are few prospective analyses, a known difficult airway is not typically listed as an exclusion criteria, but I would be more conservative with those patients as well.

CON: Just because something might be safe does not mean it is worth doing. Early extubation clearly exposes the patient to further risk whether it is from ischemia or potential reintubation following respiratory failure; why take an added risk with minimal reward? Granted, our wallets are getting tighter but UFT does not necessarily reduce hospital costs. In fact, the operating room is minute-by-minute the most expensive place in the hospital, and waiting for a patient to meet extubation criteria can increase costs. If our patient is going to stay in the cardiac surgery ICU overnight anyway, why rush to extubate in the OR? Why not allow him to wake up slowly with more intensive pain control?

PRO: Whenever a new protocol is implemented, there is always a learning curve. When fast track was implemented, some initial studies showed that ICU time and costs were not improved. However, in those studies, the patients were eligible for ICU discharge long before they actually left the unit, creating a very expensive financial gap. As institutions became more comfortable with handling these postbypass patients outside the ICU, the financial rewards became more evident. With regard to ultra-fast track, there is literature showing that patients can safely bypass the ICU entirely and be managed in a special cardiac post-op unit providing a step-down level of care. Even with patients recovering in the ICU postoperatively, the Society of Thoracic Surgeons (STS) data from 2010 showed that patients who were extubated in the OR spent 23 fewer hours in the ICU and most were discharged from the ICU within 6 h [4].

Additionally, there are benefits to the patient by reducing the potential for ventilator-associated pneumonia and lung injury and there are also mental health benefits that should not be dismissed. Numerous studies have shown that the development of post-traumatic stress disorder or depression after a surgical ICU stay is a real phenomenon. In fact, some studies in patients 6 months following surgery show decreases in health-related quality of life directly proportional to the duration of their postoperative ICU stay. What's more, it appears that the younger population of patients is more vulnerable to the psychological consequences of an ICU admission, and this is exactly the population that would be the most successful with UFT care. Clearly more research needs to be done in this area, but immediate extubation in the OR might be one method to relieve preoperative anxiety and potentially improve postoperative quality of life.

Concession from CON: I will concede to you that UFT anesthesia may have a place in our future model of cardiac surgery care as we start to move away from required postoperative ICU admissions, especially in the younger patients having minimally invasive surgery. I guess since our surgeons are becoming less invasive, why can't we?

References

1. Siliciano D. Early extubation is not preferable to late extubation in patients undergoing coronary artery surgery. J Cardiothorac Vasc Anesth. 1992;6:494–8.
2. Cheng DC, Karski J, Peniston C, Asokumar B, Raveendran G, Carroll J, Nierenberg H, Roger S, Mickle D, Tong J, Zelovitsky J, David T, Sandler A. Morbidity outcome in early versus conventional tracheal extubation after coronary artery bypass grafting: a prospective randomized controlled trial. J Thorac Cardiovasc Surg. 1996;112:755–64.
3. Singh K, Baum V. Pro: Early extubation in the operating room following cardiac surgery in adults. Semin Cardiothorac Vasc Anesth. 2012;16:182–6.
4. Straka Z, Brucek P, Vanek T, Votava J, Widimsky P. Routine immediate extubation for off-pump coronary artery bypass grafting without thoracic epidural analgesia. Ann Thorac Surg. 2002;74:1544–7.

Is a Pulmonary Artery Catheter Needed If You Have Transesophageal Echocardiography in a Routine Coronary Artery Bypass Grafting?

20

Christopher Y. Tanaka and John Hui

Case

The new anesthesiologist at the hospital, Dr. Pro, is assigned to relieve Dr. Con for the evening from a coronary artery bypass grafting (CABG) surgery. As Dr. Pro enters the room, he sees the case is well underway but not yet on cardiopulmonary bypass (CPB). Dr. Con, obviously anxious to leave, quickly begins to give sign out, "Pretty routine CABG: 67-year-old guy, 3-vessel disease, normal ejection fraction, normal valves, otherwise healthy, easy intubation…"

Dr. Pro scans the monitor and furrows his eyebrows and asks, "Where's the pulmonary artery catheter (PAC)? Where I trained, we put a PAC in all of our cardiac cases."

Dr. Con replies, "So, at this hospital, we only place PACs in patients with specific issues such as poor ventricular function or valvular abnormalities. We should be fine with the central venous catheter (CVC) and transesophageal echocardiography (TEE)" [1].

Question

Is a pulmonary artery catheter needed if you have TEE in a routine CABG?

PRO: Of course, every CABG should have a PAC. Let's review how much useful information you can get from a PAC. First, you get direct measurements of the pulmonary artery pressures (PAP). Second, by wedging the PAC, you can measure the pulmonary capillary wedge pressure (PCWP). Third, you can measure cardiac output (CO) using thermodilution. From these numbers, you can calculate multiple parameters: systemic vascular resistance (SVR), pulmonary vascular resistance (PVR), stroke volume, etc. Finally, you can draw a mixed venous oxygen saturation (SvO_2) to calculate cardiac output using Fick's equation to assess adequacy of oxygen delivery [2].

CON: Yes, we can get a lot of numbers from a PAC, but some of them have potential issues. Accurate measurement of PCWP assumes the catheter tip is in West lung zone 3 [3], and positive pressure ventilation can cause overestimation of left ventricular end diastolic pressure [4]. Thermodilution is inaccurate if performed incorrectly or if there is significant tricuspid or pulmonic regurgitation. TEE can estimate all of the same numbers a PAC gives you, except SvO_2 [2]. For instance, systolic PAP is easily estimated using Doppler measurements of tricuspid regurgitation. You can easily calculate SVR, PVR, CO, and PCWP. You can also assess valvular function, diastolic function, wall motion, and ejection fraction.

PRO: You make it sounds like I am trying to argue that a PAC is better than TEE. The PAC should be a *complement* to TEE. A CABG patient is at high risk of many catastrophic events that are accompanied by acute increases in PAP, including left ventricular dysfunction, mitral regurgitation, and pulmonary arterial vasoconstriction [5]. The PAC's strength is that it continuously displays PAPs and can aid in rapid diagnosis of these complications.

Detecting acute changes in PAPs with TEE requires constant probe manipulation and Doppler measurement. And, if you want to talk about inaccuracies, the TEE has plenty. Measuring cardiac output with TEE is highly operator dependent and is considered less accurate compared to thermodilution [2]. More so, only 53 % of patients have sufficient tricuspid regurgitation to estimate systolic PAP [6].

C.Y. Tanaka (✉) · J. Hui
Department of Anesthesiology, Montefiore Medical Center, Albert Einstein College of Medicine, 111 East 210th Street, Bronx, NY 10467, USA
e-mail: ctanaka@montefiore.org

J. Hui
e-mail: Hui.John@mayo.edu

J. Hui
Department of Anesthesiology, Mayo Clinic, 200 First Street SW, Rochester, MN 55905, USA

C.S. Scher et al. (eds.), *You're Wrong, I'm Right*, DOI 10.1007/978-3-319-43169-7_20

Some of the other calculations you mention are quite sophisticated and difficult to perform quickly in the operating room.

CON: But, you have to consider the financial costs and potential complications of placing PACs. An on-pump primary CABG that takes 4 h bills a total 34 base and time units [7, 8]. Anesthesiologists can bill an additional 10 units for placing a PAC, which adds an additional 29 % to a patient's anesthesia bill [9]. For the average commercial insurance patient, this translates to an additional $700 [10]! That will add up pretty quickly if you place a PAC in every CABG.

Inserting a PAC is an additional invasive procedure with significant risks: arrhythmia, thrombosis, pulmonary artery rupture, infection, myocardial injury, valvular injury, and surgical entrapment [11]. Some of these risks are not uncommon. For instance, bacteremia occurs in 1.3–2.3 % and arrhythmias in up to 70 % of patients with PACs [12].

PRO: Most of these so-called "complications" associated with PACs are arrhythmias that occur transiently during placement and resolve with repositioning the catheter; less than 1 % of patients have significant ventricular arrhythmias that require treatment [12]. The rate of severe complications is actually quite low. In a study of more than 3700 cardiac surgery patients, only 4 had serious mechanical complications [13].

CON: Why should we expose patients to any additional risks or costs when there is no evidence that PACs improve patient outcomes? In fact, a prospective observational trial by Schwann et al. [14] found that PAC use was associated with *worse* outcomes in CABG patients. Analyzing 2500 patients, the study found that PACs were associated with significantly increased cardiac events, cerebral events, renal failure, ICU length of stay, and mortality. Another study found that only 61 % of cardiac anesthesiologists were able to accurately identify and interpret PCWP data [15]. If clinicians are misusing PACs, patient outcomes may suffer.

PRO: That Schwann et al. [14] study is flawed, though. First, it is not a randomized control trial so the decision to place a PAC was up to the anesthesiologist. Second, there was no standardized management using the PAC data. Finally, the study excluded patients with intraoperative TEE monitoring! Again, I am saying PACs should be used in conjunction with TEE.

We also have to consider how this patient will be monitored postoperatively in the ICU. They would not have TEE continuously available to monitor the patient.

CON: Well, a Cochrane Review clearly concluded that the use of PACs in the ICU setting did not improve mortality and length of ICU or hospital stays [16]. Also, we have alternative technologies; we can use in the intensive care unit. We can perform focused transthoracic echocardiography (TTE) in the ICU. More and more critical care physicians and anesthesiologists are using bedside TTE to guide postoperative management [17].

There are also multiple emerging technologies that can quantify cardiac output such as CO_2 rebreathing, esophageal Doppler, pulse contour analysis, lithium dilution, transpulmonary thermodilution, thoracic bioimpedance, and bioreactance [18]. Most can provide continuous monitoring in the OR and ICU, and some do not require additional invasive catheters.

PRO: I can use the same arguments you made a moment ago: Where is the proof these new noninvasive CO monitors improve patient outcomes? There is no evidence they improve morbidity or mortality in cardiac surgery [18]. Also, there is a lack of familiarity and comfort with incorporating these newer technologies into patient management decisions. In a 2015 survey, only 26 % of anesthesiologists reported using noninvasive CO monitors instead of PACs [19]. In the same survey, the majority of cardiac surgeons did not support the use of alternative hemodynamic monitors versus the PAC.

There are no guidelines for the use of these newer technologies, while PACs are addressed by the American Society of Anesthesiologists (ASA) practice guidelines [11]. They state, "PAC is both appropriate and necessary in selected surgical patients undergoing procedures associated with complications from hemodynamic changes (e.g., cardiac surgery…)". This is a pretty clear endorsement for PAC use in a routine CABG.

CON: The ASA recommendations are vague, at best. They do not define "selected patients" and do not specify in which type of cardiac surgeries PACs should be used. Remember, these recommendations were published in 2003 and are outdated. The mortality from CABG surgery decreased nearly 25 % during 2000–2009 [20]. The routine CABG is now a safer procedure and may no longer warrant a PAC.

Additionally, the PAC guidelines do not address concurrent use with TEE. They were written at a time when TEE was not as widely available and utilized. Intraoperative TEE has since proliferated so that now more than 90 % of anesthesiologists use TEE during cardiac surgeries [19].

More recently, in 2011, the American College of Cardiology Foundation (ACCF) and American Heart Association (AHA) Task Force made three recommendations regarding use of PACs in CABG operations [21]:

- Class I: Placement of a PAC is indicated, preferably before the induction of anesthesia or surgical incision, in patients in cardiogenic shock undergoing CABG. (Level of Evidence: C)

- Class IIa: Placement of a PAC can be useful in the intraoperative or early postoperative period in patients with acute hemodynamic instability. (Level of Evidence: B)
- Class IIb: Placement of a PAC may be reasonable in clinically stable patients undergoing CABG after consideration of baseline patient risk, the planned surgical procedure, and the practice setting. (Level of Evidence: B)

So, in our routine CABG patient, use of a PAC is only a class IIb recommendation, and "may be considered." This is only backed by level B evidence, which is only data derived from a single randomized trial or nonrandomized studies. This is a far cry from a strong endorsement for a PAC in our patient, especially considering we use intraoperative TEE in our practice setting.

PRO: But, the ACCF/AHA guidelines do say a PAC is reasonable in a stable CABG, and I think many anesthesiologists would still agree. PACs are still widely utilized in many cardiac anesthesiology practices. A 2015 survey found that 35 % of anesthesiologists use PAC in *all* of their CPB cases, and 45 % of anesthesiologists use a PAC in all off-pump CABGs [19]. The survey also found that 68 % of anesthesiologists use a PAC in at least 75 % of CPB cases.

CON: That means 32 % of anesthesiologists use a PAC in less than 75 % of their cases [22]. I think I will find one of those guys to relieve me instead. It was nice to meet you, though.

Summary

There is still no clear consensus in the literature whether PACs are necessary in routine CABG when TEE is used. The guidelines are vague, although PAC use is considered at least reasonable in a routine CABG.

Until more conclusive evidence is available, decisions to place PACs should be made at the individual clinician and institutional levels on a case-by-case basis. Surgeons and critical care physicians should be included in discussions that review patient and surgical risk factors. The anesthesiologist's skill level with TEE and familiarity with PACs should also be considered.

References

1. Lang RM, Bierig M, Devereux RB, Flachskampf FA, Foster E, Pellikka PA, et al. Recommendations for chamber quantification: a report from the American Society of Echocardiography's Guidelines and Standards Committee and the Chamber Quantification Writing Group, developed in conjunction with the European Association of Echocardiography, a branch of the European Society of Cardiology. J Am Soc Echocardiogr. 2005;18 (12):1440–63.
2. Ranucci M. Which cardiac surgical patients can benefit from placement of a pulmonary artery catheter? Crit Care. 2006;10 (Suppl 3):S6.
3. Summerhill EM, Baram M. Principles of pulmonary artery catheterization in the critically ill. Lung. 2005;183(3):209–19.
4. Brandstetter RD, Grant GR, Estilo M, Rahim F, Singh K, Gitler B. Swan-Ganz catheter: misconceptions, pitfalls, and incomplete user knowledge—an identified trilogy in need of correction. Heart Lung. 1998;27(4):218–22.
5. Denault A, Deschamps A, Tardif JC, Lambert J, Perrault L. Pulmonary hypertension in cardiac surgery. Curr Cardiol Rev. 2010;6(1):1–14.
6. Abramson SV, Burke JB, Pauletto FJ, Kelly JJ Jr. Use of multiple views in the echocardiographic assessment of pulmonary artery systolic pressure. J Am Soc Echocardiogr. 1995;8(1):55–60.
7. Centers for Medicare and Medicaid Services. 2014 base units by CPT code [Microsoft Excel File on Internet]. 2014. [Cited 2015 Oct 11]. Available from: https://www.cms.gov/Medicare/Medicare-Fee-for-Service-Payment/PhysicianFeeSched/Downloads/2014-Anesthesia-BaseUnits-CPT.zip.
8. Centers for Medicare and Medicaid Services. Chapter 12-Physicians/Nonphysician practitioner. Medicare claims processing manual, Rev. 3096. [PDF File on Internet] 2014 Oct. [Cited 2015 Oct 11]. Available from: https://www.cms.gov/Regulations-and-Guidance/Guidance/Manuals/Downloads/clm104c12.pdf.
9. Troianos C. Making dollars and sense from a cardiac anesthesia practice. [Online Meeting Syllabus PDF from Internet] Society of Cardiovascular Anesthesiologist 33rd Annual Meeting and Workshops; 2011 Apr.; Savannah, GA. [Cited 2015 Oct 11]. Available from: http://www.scahq.org/sca3/events/2011/annual/syllabus/annual/submissions/sat/The%20Dollars%20and%20Sense%20of%20Providing%20a%20Cardiac%20Anesthesia%20Service%20-%20Troianos.pdf.
10. Stead SW, Merrick SK. Payment and practice management: ASA 2014 survey results for commercial fees paid for anesthesia services. Am Soc Anesthesiol Newsl. 2014;78(10):64–9.
11. American Society of Anesthesiologists Task Force on Pulmonary Artery C. Practice guidelines for pulmonary artery catheterization: an updated report by the American Society of Anesthesiologists Task Force on Pulmonary Artery Catheterization. Anesthesiology. 2003;99(4):988–1014.
12. Evans DC, Doraiswamy VA, Prosciak MP, Silviera M, Seamon MJ, Rodriguez Funes V, et al. Complications associated with pulmonary artery catheters: a comprehensive clinical review. Scand J Surg. 2009;98(4):199–208.
13. Bossert T, Gummert JF, Bittner HB, Barten M, Walther T, Falk V, et al. Swan-Ganz catheter-induced severe complications in cardiac surgery: right ventricular perforation, knotting, and rupture of a pulmonary artery. J Cardiol Surg. 2006;21(3):292–5.
14. Schwann NM, Hillel Z, Hoeft A, Barash P, Mohnle P, Miao Y, et al. Lack of effectiveness of the pulmonary artery catheter in cardiac surgery. Anesth Analg. 2011;113(5):994–1002.
15. Jacka MJ, Cohen MM, To T, Devitt JH, Byrick R. Pulmonary artery occlusion pressure estimation: how confident are anesthesiologists? Crit Care Med. 2002;30(6):1197–203.
16. Rajaram SS, Desai NK, Kalra A, Gajera M, Cavanaugh SK, Brampton W, et al. Pulmonary artery catheters for adult patients in intensive care. Cochrane Database Syst Rev. 2013;2:CD003408.
17. Royse CF, Canty DJ, Faris J, Haji DL, Veltman M, Royse A. Core review: physician-performed ultrasound: the time has come for routine use in acute care medicine. Anesth Analg. 2012;115 (5):1007–28.

18. Marik PE. Noninvasive cardiac output monitors: a state-of the-art review. J Cardiothorac Vasc Anesth. 2013;27(1):121–34.
19. Judge O, Ji F, Fleming N, Liu H. Current use of the pulmonary artery catheter in cardiac surgery: a survey study. J Cardiothorac Vasc Anesth. 2015;29(1):69–75.
20. ElBardissi AW, Aranki SF, Sheng S, O'Brien SM, Greenberg CC, Gammie JS. Trends in isolated coronary artery bypass grafting: an analysis of the Society of Thoracic Surgeons adult cardiac surgery database. J Thorac Cardiovasc Surg. 2012;143(2):273–81.
21. Hillis LD, Smith PK, Anderson JL, Bittl JA, Bridges CR, Byrne JG, et al. 2011 ACCF/AHA Guideline for Coronary Artery Bypass Graft Surgery. A report of the American College of Cardiology Foundation/American Heart Association Task Force on Practice Guidelines. Developed in collaboration with the American Association for Thoracic Surgery, Society of Cardiovascular Anesthesiologists, and Society of Thoracic Surgeons. J Am Coll Cardiol. 2011;58(24):e123–210.
22. Armstrong WF, Ryan T. Physics and instrumentation. Feigenbaum's echocardiography. 7th ed. Philadelphia: Lippincott, Williams and Wilkins; 2010.

21 When Should You Transfuse a Patient Who Is Bleeding After Cardiopulmonary Bypass?

Cindy J. Wang

Case

A 68-year-old man with hypertension, hyperlipidemia, diabetes mellitus, and coronary artery disease (with a drug-eluting stent placed in the circumflex artery 2 years ago) presents with worsening angina over the past several months. Coronary catheterization reveals multi-vessel coronary artery disease with significant stenosis noted in the right coronary artery (RCA), left anterior descending artery (LAD), and circumflex artery (Cx). A coronary artery bypass graft (CABG) is scheduled, and you are the anesthesiologist. The patient tells you that he stopped taking clopidogrel 5 days ago, but took his aspirin and metoprolol that morning.

Induction, intubation, and placement of lines and monitors proceed smoothly. An arterial blood gas (ABG) taken at the beginning of the case reveals a starting hematocrit of 32 %. After harvesting of the left internal mammary artery (LIMA) and saphenous vein (SV) for bypass grafts, cardiopulmonary bypass (CPB) is initiated and the surgeon proceeds to bypass the stenotic LAD, Cx, and RCA with left internal mammary artery and saphenous vein grafts. Hematocrit coming off CPB is 24 % with no blood products given before or during CPB. The patient is successfully weaned off CPB after spontaneous return to sinus rhythm. Good biventricular function and no regional wall motion abnormalities are noted with transesophageal echocardiography (TEE). After CPB, the blood pressure remains stable with a low-dose infusion of norepinephrine. At this time, the surgeon requests that protamine be given. After a slow infusion of protamine, the blood pressure remains stable and contractility remains unchanged. Activated clotting time (ACT) drawn at this point reveals a return to baseline ACT value, indicating that heparin has been adequately reversed.

C.J. Wang (✉)
Department of Anesthesiology, New York-Presbyterian Hospital/Weill Cornell Medicine, 525 East 68th Street, Box 124, New York, NY 10065, USA
e-mail: ciw9003@med.cornell.edu

This information is relayed to the surgeon who states that he does not see any clot formation and that the patient is "oozy" and bleeding. He asks you to transfuse blood products immediately to help stop the bleeding.

Questions

What is the cause of bleeding? Should you transfuse at this time? If yes, what blood products should you transfuse?

PRO: There are numerous causes of bleeding following CPB in cardiac surgery. These include surgical bleeding, residual heparinization, fibrinolysis, and coagulopathy. Numerous factors may influence platelet function and coagulation including preoperative antiplatelet or anticoagulant therapy, hypothermia, hypocalcemia, dilution of coagulation factors and platelets, renal dysfunction, and more. An ACT that has returned to baseline following protamine administration may rule out residual heparinization. Standard antifibrinolytic therapy (tranexamic acid or aminocaproic acid) helps to minimize fibrinolysis in CPB cases. Standard strategies to decrease hemodilution (i.e., minimizing fluids pre-CPB, decreasing CPB prime volume), repletion of calcium, and rewarming the patient aim to further decrease the risk of bleeding in cardiac surgery. Once surgical bleeding is ruled out, routine laboratory and point-of-care (POC) tests can help to identify causes of bleeding and coagulopathy. Routine laboratory tests such as prothrombin time (PT), partial thromboplastin time (PTT), international normalized ratio (INR), and fibrinogen can help to identify abnormalities in coagulation but can take more than 30 min to obtain results, which is impractical in the setting of rapid and significant bleeding. POC tests include ABG, INR, and visco-elastic tests [thromboelastography (TEG) and thromboelastometry (ROTEM)] that can be run in the operating room with faster results (some obtained within a few minutes).

C.S. Scher et al. (eds.), *You're Wrong, I'm Right*, DOI 10.1007/978-3-319-43169-7_21

If a specific abnormality in coagulation has been identified in the setting of bleeding, the transfusion of blood products that address the specific abnormality can take place. Blood products (red blood cells, platelets, fresh frozen plasma, cryoprecipitate) should not be transfused until the cause of bleeding is identified. This helps to minimize transfusion of unnecessary blood products, which is costly and carries risks. An exception where it may be necessary to give blood products before identifying specific abnormalities is in the setting of brisk, profuse bleeding where the patient requires escalating vasopressor requirements, displays signs of end organ damage, and/or becomes hemodynamically unstable.

CON: The surgeon states that he has checked all of the anastomoses, graft harvest sites, and cannula sites and ruled out surgical bleeding. Despite measures made to decrease hemodilution, the addition of fluids is often necessary to maintain an adequate blood volume on CPB. Therefore, there is always a dilution of red blood cells (RBCs) and coagulation factors resulting in some degree of coagulopathy in all patients after CPB. In addition, this patient was on antiplatelet therapy for his drug-eluting stent prior to surgery and likely has residual platelet inhibition. The surgeon states that the ongoing bleeding is caused by residual platelet inhibition and dilutional coagulopathy and that the patient requires immediate transfusion of platelets and fresh frozen plasma (FFP) to correct these abnormalities. Transfusion of RBCs may also be necessary before the hematocrit reaches a critical level that compromises oxygen delivery.

The surgeon goes on to say that all cardiac surgical patients should routinely receive a transfusion of platelets and FFP after CPB since there is always a degree of dilutional coagulopathy.

Question

Are there any risks to blood product transfusion of cardiac surgical patients on a routine basis?

PRO: Yes. The literature continues to demonstrate many risks related to blood product transfusions. Therefore, it is best to try and avoid transfusion in any patient. Unless the patient is actively exsanguinating and losing a large volume of blood over a short period of time, it is best to identify the cause of bleeding first. Data (usually in the form of routine laboratory or POC testing) can help to identify abnormalities in coagulation and causes of bleeding. This can help guide transfusion of specific blood components to facilitate treatment and hopefully minimize the number of products that are given to each patient. Blood transfusions in and of themselves have been shown to carry numerous risks including transmission of infection, transfusion-related acute lung injury (TRALI), transfusion reactions, and more. Numerous studies have also demonstrated that blood transfusions in cardiac surgical procedures are associated with increased mortality and complications including sternal wound infections, postoperative atrial fibrillation, respiratory issues, renal failure, and neurologic events [1–3].

CON: Although transfusions may have risks, anemia is also an independent risk factor for mortality, with adverse effects seen from poor oxygen delivery to tissues. This is especially true for patients with coronary artery disease who already have decreased oxygen delivery to the myocardium that is further exacerbated by anemia. Multiple large studies have demonstrated that both perioperative and postoperative anemia in cardiac surgery are associated with worse renal function, increased myocardial injury, longer ventilator support, and increased risk of postoperative stroke [1]. To maintain adequate oxygen delivery and improve outcomes in cardiac surgery patients, anemia should be avoided and an adequate hemoglobin level maintained throughout the case, which may require transfusion of RBCs. The risk of anemia in cardiac patients may very well outweigh the risks of transfusion.

Rebuttal from PRO: While it is true that anemia in cardiac surgical patients carries increased risks and morbidity in itself, no definite threshold of hemoglobin has been defined. Transfusion to higher hemoglobin thresholds to avoid anemia have not shown any added benefit. A couple of large randomized trials (TRACS and TITRe2) have demonstrated no advantage to liberal transfusion versus restrictive transfusion in patients undergoing cardiac surgery [2, 3]. A liberal versus restrictive transfusion threshold has not been shown to decrease mortality or morbidity, nor has it been shown to benefit patients. Since no critical hemoglobin or anemia threshold has been defined where risks of anemia clearly outweigh the risks of transfusion, there is no evidence to support routine transfusion of cardiac surgical patients. This further supports limiting transfusions to situations when absolutely indicated.

Question

Do blood conservation strategies minimize transfusion of blood products in cardiac surgery?

PRO: Yes. The risks of both anemia and blood transfusion in cardiac surgical patients are well established and have prompted multimodal approaches to blood conservation strategies. In 2007, the Society of Thoracic Surgeons (STS) and the Society of Cardiovascular Anesthesiologists (SCA) published clinical practice guidelines for perioperative blood transfusion and blood conservation in cardiac surgery, with an update in 2011. Based on evidence from randomized trials, observational studies, and case reports; recommendations for blood conservation include preoperative interventions, intraoperative blood management, blood salvage interventions, perfusion interventions, POC testing, and management of blood resources. These guidelines emphasize a multimodality approach (Class I recommendation) that includes transfusion algorithms with POC testing to optimize blood conservation in cardiac surgery [4, 5].

Several studies comparing blood management pre- and post-implementation of POC testing-guided transfusion algorithms have demonstrated decreased transfusion of blood components and better outcomes including decreased incidence of acute kidney injury, length of postoperative ventilation, length of stay, and cost [6–8].

CON: Despite the release of guidelines in 2007 with recommendations for a multimodal approach to blood conservation in cardiac surgery, the rate of transfusion in cardiac surgery has not changed. A large retrospective study of cardiac surgical patients in the USA by Robich et al. [9] in 2014 actually revealed an increase in overall blood product utilization. Despite the release of the 2007 blood conservation guidelines, blood transfusion in cardiac surgery has not declined. This may be due to a delay or lack of implementation of guidelines by institutions, lack of awareness of the guidelines, higher risk patients undergoing cardiac surgery, and/or other factors. There is also a large discrepancy that remains among institutions performing cardiac surgery and their transfusion practices. This suggests that the majority of cardiac surgeons and anesthesiologists have not adopted blood conservation strategies for one reason or another.

Question

Should we routinely use point-of-care testing as a guide for blood transfusion in cardiac surgery?

PRO: POC testing incorporates visco-elastic tests such as thromboelastography (TEG) or thromboelastometry (ROTEM) in comparison with routine laboratory tests such as PT, PTT, and fibrinogen. Routine laboratory tests have a long turnaround time, often requiring empiric transfusion of blood products prior to receiving results in the setting of ongoing bleeding. POC testing has a much shorter turnaround time (initial information about clotting dysfunction can be obtained within 10–15 min). TEG and ROTEM can provide information on specific dysfunction in clot dynamics including clot formation, clot strength, and clot breakdown (fibrinolysis). This allows for directed transfusion of appropriate blood components to address the identified dysfunction(s) as opposed to empirically transfusing numerous blood components. This has been shown to decrease the amount of transfusion and decrease overall patient exposure to the risks of transfusion.

Additional POC tests such as ACT can help to exclude residual heparin as a cause of bleeding. Prolonged ACT after administration of protamine is often an indication of inadequate reversal of heparin and can be addressed by giving additional protamine.

CON: While POC testing may be useful in identifying specific disturbances in coagulation, it also has numerous limitations. While visco-elastic tests provide results in a shorter time frame than conventional lab tests, they still require at least 10–15 min for preliminary results on clot formation, which may not be an acceptable time to wait in the setting of brisk and vigorous bleeding. These tests also require adequate training and education for performing the test, maintaining quality management, and interpreting the results.

In addition, visco-elastic tests may not be able to identify all causes of bleeding and in certain scenarios may produce normal results when bleeding and coagulation abnormalities are present. In the setting of bleeding with normal POC test results, the usual assumption is that the cause of bleeding is surgical. This assumption may not always be correct. Blood samples for TEG and ROTEM are prepared by heating to a normal body temperature of 37 °C with the addition of calcium and platelet activation factors. Therefore, normal results do not rule out clinically significant platelet dysfunction caused by antiplatelet therapy (i.e., aspirin or clopidogrel), hypothermia, or hypocalcemia. In a study by Welsh and colleagues in 2014, TEG was compared to conventional laboratory tests and was not independently predictive of postoperative bleeding in cardiac surgery with CPB. Conventional laboratory results were always abnormal in patients with coagulopathy, while 15 patients with active bleeding had TEG results in the normal range [10]. Patients with normal TEG results and ongoing bleeding may not have an identifiable cause of surgical bleeding, further demonstrating scenarios where POC tests are not revealing the presence of an underlying coagulopathy. POC tests may not always be reliable in the setting of bleeding and may not serve as an accurate guide to blood component transfusion. Therefore, in the setting of acute bleeding in cardiac surgery with normal POC tests, blood product transfusion may still be necessary.

Summary

Overall blood product usage in cardiac surgery remains significant despite the publication of guidelines for blood conservation in cardiac surgery. Literature supports numerous risks associated with transfusion of blood products in cardiac surgical patients. While anemia is also associated with risks, a critical hemoglobin or hematocrit level where the risks of anemia clearly outweigh the risks of transfusion has not been well established. Numerous studies have shown decreased transfusion requirements and improved outcomes when implementing blood conservation strategies and POC-guided transfusion algorithms in cardiac surgery. Therefore, it is unclear why overall transfusion rates have increased in cardiac surgical patients in the USA over the past years and why there remains a high discrepancy in transfusion rates among institutions. Some potential reasons may be lack of awareness or implementation of STS/SCA guidelines, increasing proportion of patients with a higher risk of anemia or bleeding, and lack of understanding or implementation of POC tests.

Blood conservation in cardiac surgical patients is a multi-disciplinary approach that begins preoperatively and continues postoperatively. Cardiologists, cardiac surgeons, perfusionists, anesthesiologists, and intensivists should all be educated on current guidelines and work together to minimize both anemia and transfusions of blood products in their patients. Multiple strategies should be utilized including guidance from POC testing. Further developments are underway to improve the speed, accuracy, and spectrum of POC tests, which will make them more valuable for real-time decisions during ongoing bleeding in cardiac surgery. For example, more specific platelet function tests may be required to identify medication-induced platelet inhibition that is missed by visco-elastic testing [11]. Implementation of guidelines, education, improvements in POC testing, and multidisciplinary approaches are crucial to improving blood conservation and limiting transfusion in cardiac surgical patients.

References

1. Kilic A, Whitman GJR. Blood transfusions in cardiac surgery: indications, risks, and conservation strategies. Ann Thorac Surg. 2014;97:726–34.
2. Hajjar LA, Vincent JL, Galas FRBG, Nakamura RE, Silva CMP, Santos MH, et al. Transfusion requirements after cardiac surgery: the TRACS randomized controlled trial. JAMA. 2010;304 (14):1559–67.
3. Murphy GJ, Pike K, Rogers CA, Wordsworth S, Stokes EA, Angelini GD, et al. Liberal or restrictive transfusion after cardiac surgery. N Engl J Med. 2015;372:997–1008.
4. Ferraris VA, Ferraris SP, Saha SP, Hessel EA II, Haan CK, Royston BD, et al. Perioperative blood transfusion and blood conservation in cardiac surgery: The Society of Thoracic Surgeons and The Society of Cardiovascular Anesthesiologists clinical practice guideline. Ann Thorac Surg. 2007;83:S27–86.
5. Ferraris VA, Brown JR, Despotis GJ, Hammon JW, Brett Reece T, Saha SP, et al. Update to the Society of Thoracic Surgeons and the Society of Cardiovascular Anesthesiologists blood conservation clinical practice guidelines. Ann Thorac Surg. 2011;2011 (91):944–82.
6. Gross I, Seifert B, Hofmann A, Spahn DR. Patient blood management in cardiac surgery results in fewer transfusions and better outcome. Transfusion. 2015. Epub 2015 Jan 6.
7. Karkouti K, McCluskey SA, Callum J, Freedman J, Selby R, Timoumi T, et al. Evaluation of a novel transfusion algorithm employing point-of-care coagulation assays in cardiac surgery: a retrospective cohort study with interrupted time-series analysis. Anesthesiology. 2015;122:560–70.
8. Weber CF, Görlinger K, Meininger D, Herrmann E, Bingold T, Moritz A, et al. Point-of-care testing: a prospective, randomized clinical trial of efficacy in coagulopathic cardiac surgery patients. Anesthesiology. 2012;117:531–47.
9. Robich MP, Koch CG, Johnston DR, Schiltz N, Pillai AC, Hussain ST, et al. Trends in blood utilization in United States cardiac surgical patients. Transfusion. 2015;55(4):805–14.
10. Welsh KJ, Padilla A, Dasgupta A, Nguyen AND, Wahed A. Thromboelastography is a suboptimal test for determination of the underlying cause of bleeding associated with cardiopulmonary bypass and may not predict a hypercoagulable state. Am J Clin Pathol. 2014;142(4):492–7.
11. Tanaka KA, Szlam F, Kelly AB, Vega JD, Levy JH. Clopidogrel (Plavix) and cardiac surgical patients: implications for platelet function monitoring and postoperative bleeding. Platelets. 2004;15 (5):325–32.

Neuraxial Versus General Anesthesia in a Patient with Asymptomatic Severe Aortic Stenosis

22

Patrick B. Smollen and Arthur Atchabahian

Case

A 72-year-old gentleman with asymptomatic severe aortic stenosis (AS) presents for right hip replacement after a fall at home. He was diagnosed with severe AS months before due to a murmur on physical examination, leading to an echocardiogram showing an aortic valve area of 0.9 cm^2 with a mean gradient of 40 mm Hg and a left ventricular ejection fraction of 55 %. He is fully functional in his activities of daily living and denies dyspnea on exertion, angina, or syncopal episodes. He has no risk factors for a difficult airway on physical examination. You are asked to devise a safe anesthetic plan for his hip replacement, weighing the risks and benefits of neuraxial versus general anesthesia in light of his cardiac condition.

Pro General

In a patient with severe aortic stenosis, two important anesthetic goals are to maintain adequate preload and afterload [1]. Neuraxial anesthesia, both spinal and epidural, produces vasodilation and thus decreases both venous return and peripheral resistance. Failure to maintain these parameters may result in inadequate compensation for a fixed obstruction, hypotension, and reduced coronary perfusion. This creates a vicious cycle in which cardiac output drops, further reducing coronary perfusion and can easily lead to cardiac arrest [2].

P.B. Smollen (✉)
Department of Anesthesiology, Perioperative Care, and Pain Medicine, New York University Langone Medical Center, 550 First Avenue, New York, NY 10016, USA
e-mail: Patrick.Smollen@nyumc.org

A. Atchabahian
Department of Anesthesiology, New York University School of Medicine, 301 East 17th St. Room C2-222, New York, NY 10003, USA
e-mail: arthur.atchabahian@gmail.com; Arthur.Atchabahian@nyumc.org

Pro Neuraxial

When titrated slowly in a patient who has been volume loaded, intrathecal and epidural medications can maintain hemodynamic stability, particularly when a catheter is used in the epidural or intrathecal space [3]. Spinal anesthesia, however, results in a denser block and is less likely to spare certain segments. While there is little evidence comparing the hemodynamics of neuraxial anesthesia to general anesthesia in patients with AS, the stimuli of direct laryngoscopy, intubation, and extubation involved with general anesthesia will result in hemodynamic lability [3].

Pro General

There are only anecdotal case reports of neuraxial anesthesia in the presence of AS, and while successful, they cannot be applied to a large general population. According to the American College of Cardiology, asymptomatic individuals like this patient, who have an aortic valve area >0.8 cm^2, a mean gradient <50 mm Hg, and preserved left ventricular systolic function, are not high risk for non-cardiac surgery [1]. With a reassuring airway exam, an opioid-based anesthetic and induction with etomidate should result in a hemodynamically stable anesthetic appropriate for patients with severe AS.

Pro Neuraxial

Volatile anesthetics have important hemodynamic consequences for patients with AS. In addition to the maintenance of preload and afterload, avoidance of tachycardia and arrhythmias is a key component of the management of patients with severe AS. For example, atrial fibrillation is poorly tolerated in patients with severe AS due to loss of the atrial kick and the poor filling of the left ventricle that results [2].

C.S. Scher et al. (eds.), *You're Wrong, I'm Right*, DOI 10.1007/978-3-319-43169-7_22

Isoflurane and desflurane decrease systemic vascular resistance (SVR), but maintain cardiac output by compensating with an increased heart rate. Though these agents are unlikely to produce extreme tachycardia, higher heart rates increase myocardial oxygen consumption and decrease the filling time needed to maintain left ventricular end-diastolic volume and coronary perfusion. Sevoflurane decreases contractility and SVR with little to no rise in heart rate, dropping the cardiac output and reducing coronary perfusion pressure. Using a neuraxial technique would eliminate the potential harmful hemodynamic effects of these agents [2].

Pro General

Transesophageal echocardiography (TEE), which cannot be used with neuraxial anesthesia alone, may give more insight into the cardiac function in real time. TEE is less invasive and has a lower complication rate than other hemodynamic monitors. With an experienced echocardiographer, a TEE can provide rapid and accurate information to help maintain or restore hemodynamic stability [2]. Using neuraxial anesthesia alone would not allow for TEE as an option.

Consensus

Although there have been no randomized controlled clinical trials comparing general and neuraxial anesthesia in patients with severe AS, expert opinion is that general anesthesia is preferred. There are case reports of neuraxial anesthesia being successfully performed in a select group of patients with AS, so it is not necessarily contraindicated. Each case should be evaluated on its own unique circumstances, with special attention being given to avoiding decreases in preload and afterload, raising the heart rate, and causing arrhythmias.

Regardless of the anesthetic chosen, the patient should be well hydrated and have an invasive blood pressure monitor (an arterial line), as well as a central venous catheter to distinguish between inadequate preload versus decreased systemic vascular resistance. Pulmonary artery catheters can be considered, but they carry a high risk of causing arrhythmias that may not be tolerated. Also, with general anesthesia, a TEE may be considered [1].

Of course, any patient for elective noncardiac surgery with symptomatic AS or systolic dysfunction should be evaluated by a cardiologist and optimized. Further, those categorized as high risk of a poor outcome by the American College of Cardiology (AVA <0.8 cm^2, mean gradient >50 mm Hg) should be evaluated as well [2].

References

1. McDonald S. Is neuraxial blockade contraindicated in the patient with aortic stenosis? Reg Anesth Pain Med. 2004;29:496–502.
2. Samarendra P, Mangione M. Aortic stenosis and perioperative risk with noncardiac surgery. J Am Coll Cardiol. 2015;65:295–302.
3. Kim YS, Park JH, Lee SY, Lim BG, Kim H, Lee IO, Kong MH. Combined spinal-epidural anesthesia for lumbar discectomy in a patient with asymptomatic severe aortic stenosis: a case report. Korean J Anesthesiol. 2014;67:129–32.

Should High-Risk Cardiac Patients Receive Perioperative Statins?

23

Himani V. Bhatt

Case

An 86-year-old woman with an abdominal aortic aneurysm presents for endovascular repair. She has no history of myocardial infarction (MI) or angina symptoms. Her electrocardiogram (ECG) shows no ST changes, q-waves, or T-wave abnormalities, and her echocardiogram is unremarkable. She takes no medications. You decide to administer 20 mg of rosuvastatin to the patient in the holding area since vascular surgery patients are at a high risk of perioperative MI [1]. Shortly, thereafter you proceed to the operating room where a spinal anesthetic is placed and the vascular surgeon begins the procedure.

CON: A colleague later comes into the operating room to chat saying, "I hear you are quitting the field of anesthesiology to go treat high cholesterol instead. An admirable choice, but I heard this patient already has normal cholesterol and has never had a myocardial infarction."

PRO: This patient is not aware of having any cardiac pathology. Most vascular surgery patients, however, likely have coronary artery disease even if it hasn't been detected or become symptomatic yet, and these procedures are often complicated by myocardial necrosis in the perioperative period. While the mechanism of action of statins in the treatment and prevention of cardiovascular disease is primarily from lowering of cholesterol, they also have been shown to have anti-inflammatory and plaque stabilization effects that would be beneficial to this patient in the perioperative period [2].

CON: Alright, I will grant that vascular surgery patients have a high rate of infarction, and statins are useful in patients with coronary artery disease, but aren't you just exposing this patient to the risks of a statin without really knowing if there is a benefit?

PRO: A recent meta-analysis of patients undergoing vascular surgery demonstrated better outcomes for patients who were taking statins. Compared to patients who were not on statin therapy, patients on statin therapy had lower rates of stroke and myocardial infarction, and lower mortality from all causes [2].

CON: In Dr. Antoniou's meta-analysis, most of the patients were in observational trials [1]. In this setting, you can only say that there is a correlation between better outcomes and taking statins, not that the statin was the cause of the difference. The fact that vascular surgery patients who did better were on statins is likely just because these were the patients who saw a doctor regularly and received better preoperative optimization [2].

PRO: Statins could just as easily be a marker for patients who had a more significant overall disease burden. In fact, when statin-taking patients received an extra dose prior to surgery they had fewer cardiovascular and cerebrovascular events compared to placebo.

CON: A prospective study is certainly welcome, but our patient here is not on a statin, so this is not applicable in this case. Can you really say that there is a benefit of giving statins to patients who are not already on them?

PRO: Another review looked only at patients who were statin naive and received a statin prior to surgery. These patients had statistically significant lower rates of death, myocardial infection, stroke, and atrial fibrillation compared to placebo [3].

H.V. Bhatt (✉)
Cardiothoracic Division, Department of Anesthesiology, Mount Sinai Medical Center, One Gustave L. Levy Pl, Box 1010
New York, NY 07093, USA
e-mail: himani.bhatt@mountsinai.org

C.S. Scher et al. (eds.), *You're Wrong, I'm Right*, DOI 10.1007/978-3-319-43169-7_23

CON: Most of those things you mentioned only apply to patients undergoing cardiac surgery. Let us hope that we are not going onto cardiopulmonary bypass for an endovascular repair!

PRO: True, the confirmed benefit for statin-naïve vascular surgery patients given statins prior to surgery was limited to a lower risk of myocardial infarction and death. Although there were not enough patients in the study to demonstrate a benefit in other areas, neither was it shown that there was no improvement in stroke or atrial fibrillation.

CON: While all this talk of heartbreak and death is very stimulating, haven't you put this nice lady at risk of rhabdomyolysis?

PRO: You are correct that statins cause myotoxicity, which is a common barrier to patients remaining on statins long-term. The most common issue is muscle discomfort, although the range of myotoxicity can be anything from an asymptomatic rise in creatine kinase to rhabdomyolysis; the latter being extremely rare. Myotoxicity was not addressed to a significant degree in the studies reviewed, likely because it was not a significant problem compared to the greater issues being addressed [4].

CON: Studies where patients did have significant symptoms from statins probably had a substantial drop-out of the participants and thus simply were not published. Are you planning on keeping her on rosuvastatin until she too develops symptoms and decides to stop on her own accord? Perhaps this will be another item on her medication reconciliation list that no one bothers to stop even if she doesn't need it anymore?

PRO: Ideally, the patient should have started the statin more than 1 week before surgery for maximal value. It is not clear, and however, how long after surgery patients should continue taking statins for optimal benefit. More studies are likely to be needed. On the other hand, patients with coronary artery disease who are statin naïve are a dwindling population, and such studies may not be feasible in the future.

CON: The longer patients stay on these drugs, the more likely they will have complications. Hepatotoxicity, for example, is uncommon, but becomes more likely when the patient is on the medication [5]. Any study of perioperative outcomes will likely be significantly underpowered to adequately address these issues, but hepatotoxicity and rhabdomyolysis are severe and life-threatening issues.

PRO: While I do not want to diminish the risk of taking statin medications, a large study population would likely be needed to adequately evaluate these risks precisely because they are so rare. Myocardial infarction and death, unfortunately, are not rare occurrences.

At this point, our long-forgotten patient decides to interject, "While I appreciate the lively debate the 2 of you have been having on my behalf, I'm wide awake here and would appreciate either some peace and quiet or some effective anesthesia!"

Summary

Statins are highly effective drugs at primary and secondary prevention of myocardial ischemia in the general population. There are good data to support their effects in the perioperative period as well for patients with coronary artery disease undergoing both cardiac and non-cardiac surgery [1–3]. While statins have their risks [4, 5], the potential adverse events associated with them occur at a far lower rate than the events that they help to prevent.

References

1. Antoniou GA, Hajibandeh S, Hajibandeh S, Vallabhaneni SR, Brennan JA, Torella F. Meta-analysis of the effects of statins on perioperative outcomes in vascular and endovascular surgery. J Vasc Surg. 2015;61:519–32.
2. Xia J, Qu Y, Yin C, Xu D. Preoperative rosuvastatin protects patients with coronary artery disease undergoing noncardiac surgery. Cardiology. 2015;131:30–7.
3. de Waal BA, Buise MP, van Zundert AA. Perioperative statin therapy in patients at high risk for cardiovascular morbidity undergoing surgery: a review. Br J Anaesth. 2015;114:44–52.
4. Sathasivam S. Statin induced myotoxicity. Eur J Intern Med. 2012;23:317–24.
5. Björnsson E, Jacobsen EI, Kalaitzakis E. Hepatotoxicity associated with statins: reports of idiosyncratic liver injury post-marketing. J Hepatol. 2012;56:374–80.

Cardiopulmonary Bypass Cases: To Hemodilute or Not?

24

Nicole R. Guinn

Case

As we dropped our patient off in the intensive care unit (ICU), I took a look at the chest tubes: bone dry. We had just finished a Bentall (aortic root plus valve replacement) in a middle-aged patient with a stenotic, bicuspid aortic valve and aortic root dilation. The patient had few other significant comorbidities and an excellent starting hemoglobin value of 14 g/dL, so I had opted to perform acute normovolemic hemodilution (ANH) in addition to our standard blood conservation techniques. We managed to get through the case without blood transfusion and were coming to the unit with a hemoglobin level >11 g/dL. Furthermore, the patient seemed euvolemic, on no vasopressors, and had excellent urine output. "So why don't we do this for all our patients?" queried the resident. He asked a good question.

When we had discussed our case that morning, after reviewing the history and labs, I suggested to the resident that we might perform ANH—something the resident had never heard of before. I explained, "Acute normovolemic hemodilution is the removal of whole blood prior to surgery, with replacement of an appropriate volume of crystalloids and/or colloids to maintain euvolemia. The theory is that by performing hemodilution prior to the expected blood loss, the volume of blood lost has proportionately fewer RBCs per mL. Once the blood loss is complete, at the end of the case, the patient's whole blood is returned to them."

Question

Should acute normovolemic hemodilution (ANH) be used for all patients undergoing surgery with a large expected blood loss?

N.R. Guinn (✉)
Department of Anesthesiology, Duke University Medical Center, DUMC, 2301 Erwin Road, Box 3094, Durham, NC 27710, USA
e-mail: Nicole.guinn@dm.duke.edu; nrguinn@gmail.com

PRO ANH has long been used as a technique to reduce allogeneic blood transfusion. It is safer and cheaper than either allogeneic blood transfusion or pre-autologous donation (PAD), where patients donate their own blood prior to surgery. Unlike PAD, ANH does not have to be done weeks in advance of surgery, necessitating lost days of work for many patients, and there is a reduced risk of infectious exposure and administration errors since there is no need for testing or storage. A quick review of the literature shows multiple studies where ANH reduces intraoperative blood loss and decreases the use of allogeneic blood, although results are equivocal in regard to reducing exposure to transfusion [1, 2]. This may be because hemodilution is only effective in cases with significant blood loss, and we aren't always great at predicting which cases those may be. ANH is especially useful in cases involving cardiopulmonary bypass, because the blood can be removed prior to heparinization, allowing the ability to infuse whole blood post-bypass that has not been cooled, heparinized, or run through a CPB circuit, thus providing improved coagulation. Aortic cases, which undergo a more significant cooling during CPB (cooling impairs platelet function), will particularly benefit from the whole blood and use of ANH may decrease the need for, or amount of, platelet transfusion.

CON That is all well and good for your healthy middle-aged patient with a high starting hemoglobin. But ANH can't be safely performed on all patients. An adequate starting hemoglobin level is necessary to be able to tolerate the anemia associated with hemodilution. We typically target a post-hemodilution hemoglobin level of 9 g/dL, expecting it may drop to 8 g/dL once we initiate CPB. It is also unreasonable to perform ANH in a patient who is already suffering from significant hypovolemia. Furthermore, caution must be used in patients with critical aortic stenosis or left main (or equivalent) coronary disease, as these patients often do not tolerate an acute drop in preload.

C.S. Scher et al. (eds.), *You're Wrong, I'm Right*, DOI 10.1007/978-3-319-43169-7_24

CON As the resident and I discussed the virtues and risks of the technique at the patient's bedside, the ICU attending, a colleague of mine who also practices in the operating room chimed in. "I understand when you do ANH for patients who refuse transfusion, you have few other options then. But why waste your time on it for this patient? It's so labor-intensive, and besides, blood is really safe these days."

Concession from PRO She had a point. When we perform the harvest of autologous blood, we have one provider dedicated to the task, while another monitors and cares for the patient. We perform ANH by connecting tubing from the large bore central venous line to collection bags containing citrate for anticoagulation. Harvest is done by gravity, and it takes great care to ensure that speed of drainage is sufficient to prevent clot formation, as the blood is not anti-coagulated until is reaches the storage bag. Volume of blood is determined using a scale. Overfilling the bags also puts the blood at risk of clotting, as each collection bag is dosed with citrate for an expected total volume of 450 mL. Replacement fluid is given between harvest bags, after the central line has been flushed, with use of vasopressors as needed to maintain adequate mean arterial pressure. Besides ensuring adequate flow during the harvest, the patient must be closely monitored for any signs of ischemia, and the procedure halted if needed. The goal is to complete the harvest prior to heparinization, which can be a busy time for the anesthesia provider, especially if they are trying to perform an echocardiography exam at the same time. With an efficient surgeon, it can be a very short amount of time. Thankfully, we have the benefit of having available highly skilled perfusionists who have been trained on this technique and can assist in performing it with a safe and aseptic technique. But if you don't have someone trained in the technique available to help, and the blood ends up clotting or the patient develops ischemia, you can easily end up doing more harm than good.

PRO Continues But I argued with her about the other comment. "True, risk of contracting an infectious disease from allogeneic blood transfusion is really low these days with advanced testing, <1 in 100,000 for both hepatitis B and hepatitis C, and <1 in 1,000,000 for HIV. But there are new infectious risks constantly emerging, including prion disease, viral severe acute respiratory syndrome (SARS), dengue, and chikungunya just to name a few" [3].

"Not to mention the more common risks of TRALI (transfusion related acute lung injury) and TACO (transfusion related circulatory overload)," my resident chimed in.

But perhaps an even stronger argument is cost. In this age of affordable healthcare, when acquisition and administration of blood averages more than $750 per unit of PRBCs [4], other ways to decrease usage may become more popular.

Summary

So we continue to take it on a case-by-case basis. We perform ANH for all of our blood refusal patients having surgery with cardiopulmonary bypass, who are predominately of the Jehovah's Witness faith. Jehovah's Witnesses refuse blood transfusion based on interpretation of several verses of the Bible. Based on doctrine from the *Watchtower*, the publication for Witnesses, they refuse whole blood, red blood cells, plasma, and platelets, but may accept the "minor fractions" of blood, including immunoglobulins, albumin, and clotting factors, based on an individual's own conscience. Most will accept procedures involving their own blood, as long as it is kept in a closed circuit without storage, such as cell salvage and ANH. For these patients who refuse allogeneic blood transfusion even in life-threatening hemorrhage, ANH is an established and potentially life-saving procedure when undergoing major cardiac surgery [5]. But what about for everybody else? For those patients, it will continue to depend on their particular surgical team, including the anesthesiologist, surgeon, and perfusionists, and their own comfort, experience, and availability on any given day.

References

1. Segal JB, Blaso-Colmenares E, Norris EJ, Guallar E. Preoperative acute normovolemic hemodilution: a meta-analysis. Transfusion. 2004;44(5):632–44.
2. Jamnicki M, Kocian R, Van der Linden P, Zaugg M, Spahn DR. Acute normovolemic hemodilution physiology, limitations, and clinical use. J Cardiothorac Vasc Anesth. 2003;17(6):747–54.
3. Perkins HA, Busch MP. Transfusion-associated infections: 50 years of relentless challenges and remarkable progress. Transfusion. 2010;50:2080–99.
4. Shander A, Hofmann A, Ozawa S, Theusinger OM, Gombotz H, Spahn DR. Activity-based costs of blood transfusion in surgical patients at four hospitals. Transfusion. 2010;50:753–65.
5. McCartney S, Guinn NR, Roberson R, Broomer BW, White W, Hill SE. Jehovah's Witnesses and cardiac surgery: a single institution's experience. Transfusion. 2014;54(10 Pt 2):2745–52.

Are Seizures Really a Problem After the Use of Antifibrinolytics? 25

Dmitry Rozin and Madelyn Kahana

Case

A seven-day-old infant with a hypoplastic aortic arch and membranous ventricular septal defect underwent an aortic arch reconstruction and patch closure of the ventricular septal defect. Total cardiopulmonary bypass (CPB) time was 181 min; aortic cross clamp time was 66 min. There was deep hypothermic circulatory arrest (DHCA) at 18° for 26 min, and regional cerebral perfusion for 11 min. There were no significant problems in the conduct of the CPB. Excellent hemostasis was achieved with meticulous surgical technique, tranexamic acid (TXA) infusion, and balanced blood product transfusion. On post-op day one, the patient was noted to have new onset generalized seizures. The pediatric intensivist phones you to say that your patient is now having seizures secondary to the use of TXA [1–16].

Questions

What are the potential causes of this infant's seizures? Does TXA cause seizures?

CON: Neurologic injury is very common after extensive cardiac surgery with cardiopulmonary bypass, especially when utilizing DHCA. Depending on the length of DHCA, perioperative seizures may be a common complication. If a patient, such as the one described above, suffers a postoperative seizure, it is important to make a prompt diagnosis and to manage accordingly. This includes testing the patient for a number of abnormalities associated with seizures, including blood chemistries and imaging studies as the differential diagnosis is long: hypoglycemia, hypocalcemia, hyponatremia, intracranial bleeding, acute hypoxic ischemic injury, and stroke, to name a few.

PRO: So all of the chemistries and the computed tomography (CT) scan are normal. And, some of the medications used routinely in the operating room have been shown to have epileptogenic potential. Why did you choose the antifibrinolytic that is associated with increased risk of seizures, TXA, and not the available agent that is just as effective and not associated with seizures, ε(epsilon)-aminocaproic acid? Chauhan [14] concluded that ε(epsilon)-aminocaproic acid and TXA are equally effective in reducing postoperative blood loss and transfusion requirements in children with cyanotic heart disease undergoing corrective surgery compared to a control group. Eaton [15] reviewed 22 randomized controlled trials and concluded that there were no significant differences between TXA and ε(epsilon)-aminocaproic acid in reduction of bleeding and transfusion requirement.

CON: The mechanism of action of both lysine analogs, TXA and ε(epsilon)-aminocaproic acid, is similar, but there are several key differences. They both reversibly bind to plasminogen, causing the lysine analog-plasminogen complex to be displaced from the fibrin clot, preventing the conversion of plasminogen to plasmin, ultimately delaying fibrinolysis [1]. At higher concentrations, TXA also has direct plasmin inhibiting action [2, 3], so it may well be superior. Additionally, TXA is approximately 6–10 times more potent than ε(epsilon)-aminocaproic acid. And a recent publication from the Boston group characterized the pharmacokinetics of TXA in infants and children undergoing CPB and found no incidence of perioperative seizures associated with the use of TXA [16].

PRO: TXA has been shown to cause convulsions by GABA antagonism when introduced into the central nervous system [5]. There are a number of studies that have identified seizures as a risk following the administration of TXA in the

D. Rozin · M. Kahana (✉)
Department of Anesthesiology, Montefiore Medical Center, 111 East 210th Street, 4th Floor, Silver Zone, Bronx, NY 10467, USA
e-mail: mkahana@montefiore.org

D. Rozin
e-mail: Rozindmi@gmail.com

C.S. Scher et al. (eds.), *You're Wrong, I'm Right*, DOI 10.1007/978-3-319-43169-7_25

bypass patient [6, 8–10], and at least one study [10] that identified a fourfold risk of seizures following TXA acid than with ε(epsilon)-aminocaproic acid.

Achieving hemostasis after cardiopulmonary bypass, for which extensive anticoagulation is used, is a complex issue. When deciding which agent to select, one must weigh the risks and benefits of both available medications. So at the end of the conversation, it is possible that the seizures could be associated with the use of TXA or with DHCA or both. And perhaps ε(epsilon)-aminocaproic acid would have been a better choice for antifibrinolysis, so that the issue of etiology would not be clouded by a reasonably equivalent drug with a better side effect profile.

Summary

Antifibrinolytic therapy is important in hemostatic control during modern pediatric cardiac surgery. There continues to be controversy regarding which of the available agents, ε(epsilon)-aminocaproic acid and TXA, to utilize. There are data that support TXA as being the more effective of these medications, while other studies suggest they are equally beneficial. Additionally, there are some data that demonstrate a clinically significant increase in risk of seizures with TXA, while other studies do not. The debate continues. One thing is not debated: recommendations regarding optimal dosage as well as timing and duration of administration of the antifibrinolytics need to be specified for infants and children. Until the recent Boston pharmacokinetic data looking at TXA [16] there was almost no pediatric dosing information grounded in solid science. We continue to extrapolate from adult studies. More data addressing optimal pediatric pharmacokinetics and pharmacodynamics, including risk of harm, are clearly needed.

References

1. Hoylaerts M, Lijen HR, Collen D. Studies on the mechanism of antifibrinolytic action of tranexamic acid. Biochim Biophys Acta. 1981;673:75–85.
2. Verstraete M. Clinical application of inhibitors of fibrinolysis. Drugs. 1985;29:236–61.
3. Ogston D. Current status of antifibrinolytic drugs. Blood Rev. 1989;3:1–4.
4. Koster A, Schirmer U. Re-evaluation of the role of antifibrinoltyic therapy with lysine analogs during cardiac surgery in the post aprotinin era. Curr Opin Anesthesiol. 2011;24:92–7.
5. Furtmuller R, Schlag MG, Berger M, Hopf R, Huck S, Sieghart W, Redl H. Tranexamic acid, a widely used antifibrinolytic agent, causes convulsions by a gamma-aminobutyric acid(A) receptor antagonistic effect. J Pharmacol Exp Ther. 2002;301:168–73.
6. Martin K, Wiesner G, Breuer T, Lange R, Tassani P. The risk of aprotinin and tranexamic acid in cardiac surgery: a one year follow-up of 1188 consecutive patients. Anesth Analg. 2008;107:1783–90.
7. Murkin JM, Falter F, Granton J, Granton J, Young B, Burt C, Chu M. High dose tranexamic acid is associated with nonischemic clinical seizures in cardiac surgical patients. Anesth Analg. 2010;110:350–3.
8. Ender J, Brüning J, Mukherjee C, Mohr W. Tranexamic acid increases the risk of postoperative seizures in adults undergoing on-pump cardiac surgery. Abstract presented at the EACT meeting 2010. J Cardiothorac Vasc Anesth 2010; 24:Supplement P-78.
9. Sander M, Spies CD, Martiny V, Rosenthal C, Wernecke KD, von Heymann C. Mortality associated with administration of high-dose tranexamic acid and aprotinin in primary open-heart procedures: a retrospective analysis. Crit Care. 2010;14(4):R148.
10. Martin K, Breuer T, Gertler R, Hapfelmeier A, Schreiber C, Lange R, et al. Tranexamic acid versus e-aminocaproic acid: efficacy and safety in paediatric cardiac surgery. Eur J Cardiothorac Surg. 2011;39(6):892–7.
11. Arnold DM, Fergusson DA, Chan AK, Cook RJ, Fraser GA, Lim W, et al. Avoiding transfusions in children undergoing cardiac surgery: a meta-analysis of randomized trials of aprotinin. Anesth Analg. 2006;102:731–7.
12. Schouten ES, van de Pol AC, Schouten AN, Turner NM, Jansen NJ, Bollen CW. The effect of aprotinin, tranexamic acid, and aminocaproic acid on blood loss and use of blood products in major pediatric surgery: a meta-analysis. Pediatr Crit Care Med. 2009;10(2):182–90.
13. Pasquali SK, Li JS, He X, Jacobs ML, O'Brien SM, Hall M, et al. Comparative analysis of antifibrinolytic medications in pediatric heart surgery. J Thorac Cardiovasc Surg. 2012;143(3):550–7.
14. Chauhan S, Das SN, Bisoi A, Kale S, Kiran U. Comparison of epsilon aminocaproic acid and tranexamic acid in pediatric cardiac surgery. J Cardiothorac Vasc Anesth. 2004;18:141–3.
15. Eaton PM. Antifibrinolytic therapy in surgery for congenital heart disease. Anesth Analg. 2008;106:1087–100.
16. Wesley MC, Pereira LM, Scharp LA, Emani SM, McGowan FX Jr, DiNardo JA. Pharmacokinetics of tranexamic acid in neonates, infants, and children undergoing cardiac surgery with cardiopulmonary bypass. Anesthesiology. 2015;122:746–58.

Is Regional Anesthesia for Cardiac Surgery a Good Idea?

26

M. Megan Chacon

Case

A 47-year-old female with a history of severe mitral regurgitation secondary to posterior leaflet prolapse presents for mitral valve repair/replacement surgery. Her past medical history is significant for hypertension, a remote smoking history, and mild asthma. The cardiac surgeon plans a minimally invasive repair of the valve through a right anterior thoracotomy. The patient is anxious about waking up in the intensive care unit (ICU) while still intubated and concerned about postoperative pain control. You have discussed the anesthetic and placement of access lines, and obtained consent for intraoperative transesophageal echocardiogram. She asks if thoracic epidural anesthesia is an option for her.

High thoracic epidural anesthesia (HTEA) has been used successfully and has many potential advantages. However, its safety and practicality have been called into question because of the need for full heparinization prior to cardiopulmonary bypass, the risks associated with heparin use and neuraxial anesthesia, and the need to delay cardiac surgery in the event of a traumatic epidural placement. You consult your colleagues who have mixed feelings about the risk/benefit ratio of thoracic epidurals for cardiac surgery.

Questions

Is the rate of epidural hematoma higher when HTEA is placed prior to cardiac surgery? What are the benefits of thoracic epidural anesthesia for this patient population? Is paravertebral blockade a reasonable alternative?

PRO: High thoracic epidural anesthesia provides superior postoperative pain control than general anesthesia alone. There is evidence of additional benefits including a reduction in postoperative pulmonary complications, a lower incidence of postoperative supraventricular arrhythmias and acute kidney injury, and improvement in glycemic control. Several studies have demonstrated that the cardiac sympathetic blockade from HTEA has a direct anti-ischemic effect by vasodilation of stenotic coronary arteries and attenuates stress-induced myocardial ischemia [1]. A randomized study revealed HTEA was associated with improved perioperative cardiac index in patients undergoing cardiac surgery [2]. And while it is still debatable whether use of HTEA facilitates fast-track potential and early extubation; it certainly is a useful technique to avoid large doses of intravenous opioids that may delay awakening and extubation.

CON: HTEA may have benefits, but the complications can be catastrophic. The greatest limitation to its widespread acceptance and use is the presumed increased risk of epidural hematoma associated with high-dose heparin administration prior to initiating cardiopulmonary bypass. With the increasing frequency of same-day hospital admissions prior to cardiac surgery, epidural catheters are placed on the morning of surgery. While the American Society of Regional Anesthesia and Pain Medicine considers it safe to place an epidural 1 h prior to heparinization, many clinicians would prefer a longer interval [1]. And of course, if there is a traumatic epidural, it is likely the case will need to be postponed for at least 24 h to decrease the likelihood of epidural hematoma. Few surgeons would be willing to accept both the neurologic risk to their patients and the unexpected delays it would create in the cardiac surgery schedule.

PRO: I can understand the reservations due to the theoretical hazards; however, there have not been any studies that demonstrate an increased risk of epidural hematoma in cardiac surgery. In fact, in the last two published meta-analyses, no estimates of the risk of HTEA in cardiac surgery could be made due to the lack of events [1, 3, 4]. There is no evidence

M.M. Chacon (✉)
Department of Anesthesiology, University of Nebraska Medical Center, 984455 Nebraska Medical Center, Omaha, NE 68198-4455, USA
e-mail: mchacon@unmc.edu; m.meganchacon@gmail.com

C.S. Scher et al. (eds.), *You're Wrong, I'm Right*, DOI 10.1007/978-3-319-43169-7_26

that anticoagulation during cardiac surgery contributes to an increased incidence of hematoma.

CON: What about paravertebral blockade (PVB) as an alternative technique? Multiple prospective, randomized studies have proven PVB to be as efficacious as HTEA for thoracic surgery, yet the side effects and complication profile appear superior to HTEA. It is associated with fewer dural punctures and a smaller risk of epidural hematoma. A single injection may be effective for as long as 23 h. A prospective randomized study by Neuburger et al. [5] demonstrated decreased postoperative pain and narcotic usage in patients who received PVB in addition to general anesthesia compared to general anesthesia alone when undergoing minimally invasive cardiac surgery. A retrospective study by Rodrigues et al. [6] suggests the addition of PVB to general anesthesia may be associated with lower intraoperative narcotic requirements and a greater likelihood of successful immediate extubation.

PRO: HTEA has been shown to improve more than just postoperative pain control; there are fewer arrhythmias, pulmonary complications, and acute kidney injuries. However, the more acceptable side-effect profile may favor the routine use of PVB for cardiac surgery [5], particularly as minimally invasive techniques become more common. PVB has a well-documented role in pain control after thoracoscopic surgery.

Summary

HTEA is excellent for postoperative pain control, and there is evidence HTEA can have a positive impact on short-term mortality. The benefits probably outweigh any risk of epidural hematoma. However, potential delays due to traumatic epidural placement may not be tolerated by the surgery team, the anesthesia team, perioperative services, or the hospital administration. Paravertebral blockade is a safe and equally efficacious alternative to improving pain control, early extubation, and patient satisfaction. More studies are needed on bilateral PVB for median sternotomy incisions, but there certainly is a role for PVB during minimally invasive cardiac surgery with benefits that far outweigh the risks.

References

1. Jakobsen CJ. High thoracic epidural in cardiac anesthesia: a review. Semin Cardiothorac Vasc Anesth. 2015;19:38–48.
2. Jakobsen CJ, Bhavsar R, Nielsen DV, Ryhammer PK, Sloth E, Greisen J. High thoracic epidural analgesia in cardiac surgery: part 1—high thoracic epidural analgesia improves cardiac performance in cardiac surgery patients. J Cardiothorac Vasc Anesth. 2012;26(6):1039–47.
3. Svircevic V, van Dijk D, Nierich A, Passier M, Kalkman C, van der Heijden G, Bax L. Meta-analysis of thoracic epidural anesthesia versus general anesthesia for cardiac surgery. Anesthesiology. 2011;114:271–82.
4. Bignami E, Landoni G, Biondi-Zoccai G, Boroli F, Messina M, Dedola E, Nobile L, Buratti L, Sheiban I, Zangrillo A. Epidural analgesia improves outcome in cardiac surgery: a meta-analysis of randomized controlled trials. J Cardiothorac Vasc Anesth. 2010;24(4):586–97.
5. Neuburger PJ, Ngai JY, Chacon MM, Luria B, Manrique-Espinel AM, Kline RP, Grossi EA, Loulmet DF. A prospective randomized study of paravertebral blockade in patients undergoing robotic mitral valve repair. J Cardiothorac Vasc Anesth. 2015.
6. Rodrigues ES, Lunch JJ, Suri RM, Burkhard HM, Li Z, Mauermann WJ, Rehfeldt KH, Nuttall GA. Robotic mitral valve repair: a review of anesthetic management of the first 200 patients. J Cardiothorac Vasc Anesth. 2014;28:64–8.

Are Surgical and Anesthesia Medical Missions in Low- and Middle-Income Countries Helping or Hurting? The Evolving Fields of Global Anesthesia and Global Surgery

27

Jamey Jermaine Snell

Case

A pediatric surgeon volunteering for a charitable, international, non-governmental organization contacts you to solicit your help for an upcoming surgical mission to Guatemala to perform cleft palate repairs. She is a world-renowned expert in oral and facial surgery in need of a skilled pediatric anesthesiologist to assist, so you join her along with her team of nurses and surgical assistants.

Upon arrival at a small city hospital, you find meager resources, but a local anesthesia technician is there to show you around. You are shown their outdated, but functional anesthesia machines fitted only with halothane vaporizers, a poorly stocked supply cabinet, and medications consisting of thiopental, "suxamethonium," morphine, diazepam, "lignocaine," and bupivacaine. Fortunately you have brought supplies and medications with you, so you feel confident in being able to care for patients safely here.

By the end of an exhausting week, you and the team are proud to have completed more than 120 cases, including an impromptu case for resection of an obstructing congenital airway mass in a neonate, without a single intraoperative complication.

A few weeks after returning home, you email the anesthesia technician back in Guatemala for an update on how things are back at the hospital. He replies with some discouraging news. The infant with the airway mass who required postoperative intubation and ICU care did not survive. She could not receive the appropriate mechanical ventilation or parenteral nutrition she required because the hospital rarely cares for neonates. Now, the family is upset with the hospital staff because the patient's protracted and expensive course drained them of all their resources and they are struggling to feed their remaining children. He then tells you about a 5-year-old patient who had a successful cleft palate repair on the last day of the trip, but returned days later with a significant wound infection and has yet to improve. The patient is only being treated with antibiotics since the sole local surgeon capable of managing the case left town when the mission team arrived and has yet to return. Apparently, the reason being that in the weeks leading up to the mission team's arrival, the small hospital was emptied of all other patients in order to make room for the cleft palate patients and the local surgeon had no work during that time and no reason to stay. The technician laments about the dismal state of surgery and anesthesia in his hospital and of all healthcare in his country and hopes your team will return soon to help them again.

J.J. Snell (✉)
Department of Anesthesiology, Perioperative and Pain Medicine, Boston Children's Hospital/Harvard Medical School, 300 Longwood Ave, Bader 3, Boston, MA 02120, USA
e-mail: jamey.snell@gmail.com

Questions

Are international endeavors in surgery and anesthesia in low- and middle-income countries (LMICs) helpful or harmful? Does the successful treatment of 120 patients justify the harm done to 2 families? How can efforts in global anesthesia and global surgery be done better?

PRO: Classically the field of global health has focused on conditions that have the ability to cross borders and therefore affect the entire globe—namely infectious diseases. Increasingly, however, as initiatives aimed at reducing the burden of communicable diseases in LMICs have recognized that scaling up healthcare systems is the ultimate solution, a more comprehensive definition of global health has come to take into account non-communicable diseases as well. This includes chronic and surgically treatable diseases. It is estimated that surgically treatable diseases make up 28 % of the global burden of illness and contribute to 30 % of deaths in some countries. Nearly 2 billion people lack access to safe surgical care worldwide. And though LMICs make up 70 % of the world's population, they receive only 4–25 % of the more than 230 million surgical procedures

C.S. Scher et al. (eds.), *You're Wrong, I'm Right*, DOI 10.1007/978-3-319-43169-7_27

performed annually. If access to safe medical care is considered a human right and moral imperative, so too should access to safe surgery and the compulsory provision of safe anesthesia and perioperative care [1, 2].

CON: Taking an even further step back, global health is one of many forms of global aid or foreign aid that Western countries have been providing to spur development in LMICs since the end of World War II. If we take Sub-Saharan Africa as an example, which has received more than 300 billion dollars in global aid since 1970, the statistics unequivocally prove the ineffectiveness of aid. Not only do poverty, disease, and corruption continue unabated in most of these countries, but also those with the highest dependence on foreign aid actually saw a negative economic growth rate of −0.2 % and increase in poverty from 11 to 66 %, during this time frame. It's estimated that at most, only half of the funds donated ever actually make it to their intended target [3]. The explanation for this failure, and perhaps harm, is complex and varies with the geographic, cultural, and political setting. However, one observation seems to be universal: conditions do not improve when foreigners try to impose their solution to fix a poor country's problems with aid, and they may actually be making it worse. Fixing someone else's problem for them only removes the pressure and impetus for them to fix the problem themselves. To be motivated based upon the assumption that they are incapable of finding their own solutions is not altruism but paternalism. This platitude in global aid and economics can also be seen in transnational military-led democratization campaigns, and is analogous to endeavors in global health. The conclusion of the aforementioned Guatemalan story—the technician expressing the need for the foreign surgical team to return—illustrates the indefinitely dependent relationships that these types of well-meaning projects can engender.

PRO: Well, if one does take the all-encompassing point-of-view, then we must also recognize that we as citizens and physicians in Western countries are the executives of geopolitical decisions and recipients of commercial wealth that has exploited many LMICs and are at least partially responsible for the dismal state of their economies and healthcare systems. Are we to sit by idly and watch people die when there is something we can and *should* do about it?

CON: There are some scenarios where the risk benefit ratio is unarguably in favor of global health aid. Humanitarian aid and medical care provided in the context of natural disasters, armed conflict, and infectious disease outbreaks are a necessity due to the absence or debilitation of preexisting healthcare systems. If the field of global anesthesia does require those with experience and training, let it be for these situations where there are no systems in place to cause unintended harm. The focus is appropriately on the patients first and the system second. But for planned, non-emergency, medical and surgical missions, the priorities should be reversed. The holy grail of any endeavor in global health aid should be sustainability. Surgical missions by their very nature of relying on volunteered time, charitable donations, and importing the human and technical resources needed—in this case the entire surgical staff and necessary medical supplies—are by no means sustainable. And though this story gives an optimistic example of only 2 complications out of 120, the actual statistics of perioperative morbidity or mortality are largely unknown, but are likely higher when one considers the frequent circumstance illustrated above. Practitioners on surgical missions, like our anesthesiologist, must often provide care in a new, often austere, setting with unfamiliar drugs, antiquated equipment, limited additional hands to help, and often a language barrier. Poorer outcomes are also more likely due to limitations to comprehensive preoperative screening and testing as well as inadequate follow-up and post-op care. But these statistics may be unknown for a reason. Just as is the case with global aid in economic development, the stakeholders involved in these medical missions want to see good outcomes resulting from their financial contributions. Neither the volunteer organizations nor the recipients want to keep track of data that may demonstrate that the emperor indeed has on no clothes, or that behind the Potemkin Village is shambles. Along with external funding also comes external priorities. What dictates the type of surgery and perioperative care provided is not a question of what a resource-limited population needs, but what the resource-rich mission team wants to provide. The power dynamic, often complicated by a culture of hospitality, is not in favor of the hosts being anything but agreeable to what the visiting team wants to do and how they want to do it. This inequality of priorities can also be responsible for disrupting preexisting operations in a hospital, displacing local healthcare professionals, and even interfering with educational activities and the appropriate care of other patients to make room for the surgical missions team [4].

PRO: So if sustainability is the ultimate goal, then the solution should be focusing on building up local human resources through education. In fact, the dearth of human resources in LMICs is cited as the ultimate bottleneck to scaling up healthcare systems. The focus of efforts in global anesthesia and surgery, when not in the emergency/humanitarian context, should be through mutually beneficial, international education collaboratives. Ideally these would be twinning collaboratives between academic medical institutions where both organizations have something to gain—unique training and research opportunities for the residents and faculty in the donor program in exchange for clinical and educational support for the host program. Sustainability can further be enhanced by going beyond the single surgeon-led model to a collaborative reinforced with multi-disciplinary (anesthesia, surgery, medicine, etc.) and inter-professional (physicians, nurses, technicians, etc.) relationships. The leadership structure would include high-ranking local officials to provide context-specific goals and objectives. In terms of duration, it should be long enough to transfer the necessary educational knowledge and clinical skills, but with a predetermined endpoint so that plans and expectations are that the local hosts will gradually assume full responsibility for building up their human resources in healthcare [5].

CON: Perhaps a program of that design would work in theory, however, the reality still falls far short. From personal first-hand experiences with global health collaboratives in Tanzania, Uganda, Ethiopia, Rwanda, Costa Rica, and Italy, I have seen with surprising consistency the magnitude of destruction cultural disharmony can have on even the most well-intentioned, well-designed programs. Anecdotes are numerous and include an assumption that patients in LMICs do not need to provide informed consent before receiving interventions with risk, the use of a "sterilized" zip-lock bag used to cover an open wound, assuming a double-standard or overall lower standard-of-care, the question of if a practitioner could "experiment" with different anesthetic techniques on patients, the use of a chlorhexidine and tap water mixture used to irrigate the peritoneal cavity, research protocols that would never pass one's institutional review board at home, working beyond the boundaries of one's own scope-of-practice or training experience, local healthcare workers being fired by their superiors when a foreign physician made even a benign complaint, and many, many more. Although these cultural faux pas are more often the exception and not the norm, few can disagree with the common sentiment of frustration Westerners often experience when they work in the resource-poor context—"the locals just aren't doing enough!" This is not apathy being observed, but a cultural misunderstanding. A Western point-of-view superimposed on the LMICs' context. For this reason, the long-term international physician may be better served by a supplemental degree in anthropology or sociology than in education or even public health. Cultural misunderstandings are not only responsible for making twinning partnerships less effective but can even pose a risk of unintended harm for those they wish to serve.

With regard to unintended harm to the local profession, examples are also numerous and include local doctors being uncooperative with foreign doctors because they were not consulted in the decision to have them there, being offended because foreign doctors are younger and less experienced but consider themselves equal or superior due to their credentials, local doctors physically interrupting foreign doctors teaching physician-extenders because they fear the empowerment of a competing profession and job insecurity, leaving their job posts or being fired indirectly due to the presence of foreign doctors, foreign doctors damaging the respect and stature of local doctors by professionally disagreeing with or demeaning them in public in a manner considered acceptable back at home, and, at its worst, the medico-legal fallout and damage to the trust of local physicians in the community that can follow a patient's death or complication suffered at the hands of a foreign doctor.

With regard to unintended harm to the patients, the classic example is of the heroic surgeon (and accompanying anesthesiologist) who go *around* the system—doing uncommon procedures, requiring uncommon resources—in order to save the life of a single patient in desperate need of a procedure that could not and would not be done if the foreign team was not there. It is not uncommon to see physicians go so far as to donate their own money or take drastic measures to build a micro-healthcare system around the patient. This, at first glance, seems to the foreign physician like a laudable response to a moral imperative that cannot be ignored. His or her short-sighted goal fails to ask the questions:

- "Can the family afford the care this child will need postoperatively or long-term?"
- "Am I consuming local resources that will now be unavailable for other patients?"
- "Will the surgeons who I'm teaching this procedure to be willing and able to do this procedure after I leave?"
- "Just because I can, does that mean I should?"

These questions are challenging ethical conundrums that do not have simple or easy answers. Nevertheless, they should be asked and considered.

The sustainable approach is from the long-term point-of-view that aims to work *through* the system—broken as it may be—instead of around it. A real-life example that illustrates this point was a recent experience while working as an anesthesiologist in a resource-stricken, academic referral hospital of a Sub-Saharan African country. There was an observation that the incidence of hypoxia was significantly high following routine inductions of general anesthesia. A fact-finding survey found one of many contributing factors to be only 4 laryngoscopes that existed for 6 operating theaters. Practitioners were often leaving to search for equipment or attempting to proceed without the appropriate laryngoscope. The results of the survey proved that the lack of laryngoscopes was directly associated with compromising patient safety and was used as objective data and leverage to convince the hospital's director general to allocate funds and procure more laryngoscopes. About a month later, additional laryngoscopes were provided. In this case, we as the foreign physicians had to intentionally work within the broken system, resist the urge to bring our own or donate resources, and facilitate the growth and evolution of the system. This approach takes much more time, much less ego, is less under our control, is not nearly as impressive as quoting the number of operations done, and may even require watching patients suffer the tragic consequences that their hospital's lack of resources subjects them to all the time when we are not around. But this system-centered approach has the potential to help thousands of patients while the patient-centered approach can help only one at a time.

Summary

It can be safely assumed that regardless of its efficacy, the practice of international aid—whether in the context of economic or healthcare development—is not going away any time soon. We must therefore accept the fact that endeavors in global surgery and global anesthesia will continue as well. But we should never lose sight of the fact that the ultimate goal is to not be needed—to equip a system to sustain itself autonomously. All of our efforts should be screened and assessed with regard to this system-centered criterion, in addition to placing leadership and prioritization in local hands, and giving deference to ethical and cultural considerations. Let us hope that as this field evolves, each new iteration of a particular collaborative builds upon lessons learned from its predecessor. Then, one day we may achieve the goal of realizing a sustainable model for improving healthcare in resource-limited settings and ensuring quality and access for patients regardless of the country in which they reside.

References

1. Schecter WP. Academic global surgery: a moral imperative. JAMA Surg. EPub 2015 May 6.
2. Steffner KR, McQueen KA, Gelb AW. Patient safety challenges in low-income and middle-income countries. Curr Opin Anesthesiol. 2014;27:623–30.
3. Moyo D. Dead aid. New York: Farrar, Straus and Giroux; 2009.
4. Ginwalla R, Rickard J. Surgical missions: the view from the other side. JAMA Surg. 2015;150(4):289–90.
5. Binagwaho A, Kyamanywa P, Farmer PE, Nuthulaganti T, Umubyeyi B, Nyemazi JP, et al. The human resources for health program in Rwanda—new partnership. N Engl J Med. 2013;369 (21):2054–9.

Part III

Thoracic

Can Oxygenation in Single-Lung Thoracic Surgery Be Affected by Inhibition of Hypoxic Pulmonary Vasoconstriction?

28

Rebekah Nam

Case

A 60-year-old male is undergoing video-assisted thoracoscopic surgery (VATS) for the resection of a lung mass. We induce general anesthesia, and endotracheal intubation is performed with a double-lumen tube. The appropriate lung is isolated, and correct tube placement is confirmed with fiberoptic guidance. Single-lung ventilation is established with an FiO_2 of 1.0, which the patient tolerates without desaturation or hemodynamic disturbance. As the surgeons get to work, the cardiothoracic fellow who is feeling gregarious today turns to us and initiates a discussion on the topic of hypoxic pulmonary vasoconstriction (HPV).

Questions

What exactly is hypoxic pulmonary vasoconstriction? Are there scenarios where this phenomenon could be harmful rather than advantageous? What are some of the mediators of this reflex under the anesthesiologist's control?

PRO: Hypoxic pulmonary vasoconstriction is a highly conserved reflex. Pulmonary blood flow is diverted away from gravity-dependent, poorly ventilated, relatively hypoxic areas of the lungs and toward better-ventilated regions. This effectively optimizes ventilation and perfusion (V/Q) matching throughout the lungs and maximizes oxygenation under hypoxic conditions. The major stimulus for this reflex is alveolar as well as pulmonary capillary oxygen tension. HPV is described with 2 distinct phases. Phase 1 takes effect within just a few seconds and peaks at 15 min. With sustained hypoxia (30–60 min), Phase 2 begins and pulmonary vascular resistance (PVR) continues to steadily increase over 2 h. Vascular tone and PVR decrease slowly to baseline over a period of hours following a return to normoxia [1].

HPV plays an essential role in compensating for hypoxia associated with asthma, chronic obstructive pulmonary disease, pneumonia, adult respiratory distress syndrome, and atelectasis. It especially plays a significant role during anesthesia and single-lung ventilation surgical cases.

CON: Although HPV has evolved for the purpose of improving oxygenation through V/Q matching, there are also conditions in which long-standing hypoxia leads to increased pulmonary vascular resistance resulting in pulmonary hypertension and even cor pulmonale. There exists the fascinating entity of high-altitude pulmonary edema (HAPE), which is a form of noncardiogenic pulmonary edema affecting mountaineers as they ascend to areas of low FiO_2.

PRO: There are many additional factors that contribute to the attenuation or augmentation of HPV including oxygen levels, carbon dioxide, acid–base status, temperature, and coexisting medical conditions. The strength of HPV is also responsive to many of our anesthetic decisions. Volatile inhalational agents (isoflurane, sevoflurane, desflurane), for example, all impair HPV whereas fentanyl and propofol seem to have no significant effects. The pulmonary vasculature contains alpha, beta, and dopamine receptors, which may respond inconsistently to pressors as different receptors are stimulated at varying doses of medication. In studies, phenylephrine has been shown to increase oxygenation in certain populations. Furthermore, vasoactive drugs and many classes of medications such as calcium channel blockers, beta-blockers, ACE inhibitors, prostacyclins, phosphodiesterase inhibitors, and inhaled nitric oxide (iNO) all affect the degree of pulmonary vasoconstriction [1].

CON: There appear to be too many variables that ultimately determine the degree of pulmonary vasoconstriction present. Patients come in with complex medical histories and complicated medication lists. Anesthesia and surgical conditions

R. Nam (✉)
Department of Anesthesiology, New York University Langone Medical Center, 550 First Avenue, New York, NY 10016, USA
e-mail: Rebekah.nam@gmail.com; Rebekah.Nam@nyumc.org

C.S. Scher et al. (eds.), *You're Wrong, I'm Right*, DOI 10.1007/978-3-319-43169-7_28

induce a myriad of physiological changes many of which affect HPV from both the patient internally (physiologic parameters) and from iatrogenesis (anesthesiologist-administered drugs and mechanical ventilation parameters, for example). Furthermore, many of the studies on hypoxic pulmonary vasoconstriction were performed on laboratory animals and findings may not strictly pertain to human subjects [2].

Summary

In the event of severe hypoxemia during one-lung ventilation, the anesthesiologist must be prepared with maneuvers to restore adequate oxygen delivery. FiO_2 should be increased, and proper double-lumen tube positioning confirmed. The delivery of volatile anesthetic may be decreased to <1 MAC to reduce HPV inhibition, and PEEP (5 cm H_2O) can be applied to the ventilated lung following a recruitment maneuver. More advanced interventions include adding CPAP (1–2 cm H_2O) to the nonventilated lung following a recruitment maneuver, intermittently inflating the nonventilated lung, or introducing a bronchial blocker for targeted isolation of the operative lobar bronchus. In the event of critical desaturation under OLV, timely communication with the surgeon is key. Two-lung ventilation should be resumed if possible and the surgeon may be able to assist by occluding or compressing the blood flow to the operative lung [3].

Hypoxic pulmonary vasoconstriction is an extremely critical and adaptive reflex that allows for compensation in conditions of hypoxemia. Known mediators of HPV may be employed by the anesthesiologists to optimize oxygenation. However, it must be realized that HPV is profoundly responsive to numerous stimuli. The best anesthetic strategy may be to aim for normal physiological parameters and be mindful how deviation and medications may affect HPV in critical situations with dangerous hypoxia.

References

1. Lumb AB, Slinger P. Hypoxic pulmonary vasoconstriction physiology and anesthetic implications. Anesthesiology. 2015;122:932–46.
2. Nagendran J, Stewart K, Hoskinson M, Archer SL. An anesthesiologist's guide to hypoxic pulmonary vasoconstriction: implications for managing single-lung anesthesia and atelectasis. Curr Opin Anaesthesiol. 2006;19(1):34–43.
3. Miller RD. Miller's anesthesia. 8th ed. Philadelphia: Elsevier; 2015.

Is a Bronchial Blocker Just as Good as a Double-Lumen Tube for Achieving Adequate Lung Isolation?

29

Alexandra Lewis and David Amar

Case

A 48-year-old female (height 155 cm; weight 64 kg) with a history of moderate chronic obstructive pulmonary disease (COPD) was scheduled for right video-assisted thoracoscopic surgery (VATS) and segmentectomy for a lower lobe mass measuring 2.5 × 2.4 cm. On examination, she had a Mallampati Class II airway, a high-arched palate, a mouth opening >3 cm, and full range of neck motion. Anesthesia was induced with propofol and vecuronium. Direct laryngoscopy revealed a grade 3 view of the larynx with visualization only of the tip of the epiglottis. After 3 failed attempts with a Mac #3, a Miller #3, and a video laryngoscope, a supraglottic airway (SGA) was inserted and her oxygen saturation was maintained at >95 %. The anesthesia team called for help due to increasing airway edema, concerned that this could lead to a "can't ventilate, can't intubate" situation.

An 8.0 endotracheal tube was loaded onto the fiberoptic scope and successfully advanced into the trachea through the supraglottic airway. The thoracic surgeon now requested placement of a double-lumen tube (DLT) for optimal lung isolation. The anesthesiologist responded, "Taking into account this patient's airway anatomy and increased edema from intubation, we were planning on using a bronchial blocker (BB)."

A. Lewis
Department of Anesthesiology and Critical Care Medicine,
Memorial Sloan Kettering Cancer Center,
1275 York Avenue, R, M-330, New York, NY 10065, USA
e-mail: lewisa1@mskcc.org

D. Amar (✉)
Department of Anesthesiology and Critical Care Medicine,
Memorial Sloan Kettering Cancer Center, 1275 York Avenue,
M-304, New York, NY 10065, USA
e-mail: amard@mskcc.org

Question

Do you really think it is wise to exchange a single-lumen tube for a DLT in this setting?

PRO (Surgeon): Why can't we use an airway exchange catheter? I've seen many anesthesiologists use it to place DLTs. My greatest concern is poor surgical exposure with the use of a bronchial blocker (BB). I have never had a good experience with those devices.

CON (Anesthesiologist): We should be able to achieve adequate lung isolation with a BB. Given this patient's known history of difficult intubation, the exchange of a single-lumen tube for a DLT is fraught with the risk of airway trauma and loss of the airway. In our practice, we use a video laryngoscope during the tube exchange to guide the DLT under direct vision and minimize these risks. In this particular situation, we had an unexpected difficult airway and worsening airway edema from multiple intubation attempts. We had a poor view with the video laryngoscope, which would make direct visualization for the exchange virtually impossible. Under these circumstances, it is dangerous to use an exchange catheter and I am not willing to take that risk.

PRO: Isn't there evidence of better lung isolation with a DLT compared to a BB?

CON: I agree, the time to adequate lung isolation was significantly less for 1 type of DLT (~93 s) when compared to 3 types of BBs (~203 s) in 1 randomized trial [1]. While repositioning was also needed more frequently using a BB, good surgical exposure was achieved with BB in this study. Although using the BB may require more patience on your part, I believe that it will be much safer for the patient to not exchange the endotracheal tube in this case.

PRO: Well, a BB is not ideal in a patient with obstructive lung disease. The narrow lumen of a BB produces increased airway resistance to flow compared to a DLT. This patient has moderate COPD with hyperinflation on her CXR. The

C.S. Scher et al. (eds.), *You're Wrong, I'm Right*, DOI 10.1007/978-3-319-43169-7_29

speed of lung collapse in this patient will likely be slower than in a patient with normal lung parenchyma due to hyperinflation and severe gas trapping. How would you expedite lung collapse with a BB under these circumstances?

CON: Several procedures can accelerate lung collapse, including the apnea disconnection technique or the bronchial suction technique. With the apnea technique, the patient is disconnected from the circuit and the BB is inflated after end-expiration when the $EtCO_2$ falls to zero [2]. If the lung is still slightly inflated after the chest is open, a second period of apnea is implemented; the circuit is disconnected and the BB is deflated coupled with gentle pressure from your surgical instruments to collapse the lung further. However, this technique is not recommended in patients with limited pulmonary reserve, such as the morbidly obese and patients with severe parenchymal disease. Alternatively, with the bronchial suction technique, gentle, intermittent suction can be applied incrementally to the suction port of the BB to a pressure of −30 cmH_20 [3].

PRO: Even if you achieve lung isolation, I was under the impression that BBs have a higher incidence of malposition. The BB can easily be dislodged with surgical manipulation of the lung. It is not just inconvenient but potentially dangerous if we are dissecting around the pulmonary artery. How do you reduce the risk of malposition?

CON: Although there may be a higher incidence of malposition with a BB versus DLT, this is still uncommon. There are different types of BBs available on the market. A new device is a single-lumen tube with a camera at the tip, which can be used in combination with the BB to continuously visualize the BB and immediately identify impending herniation or malposition, which can then easily be corrected.

PRO: The major benefit of a DLT is the ease of freely alternating ventilation between the lungs and the ability to suction and irrigate as needed. This advantage is irrefutable, and I am not sure whether the BB offers any additional benefits, except for difficult or prolonged intubations. If there is tumor in the mainstem bronchus, a BB can lead to serious bleeding in the airway, and the BB will be in the way of the surgery. A DLT on the contralateral side could avoid disruption of the bronchial tree.

CON: You make a compelling argument, and I agree with some of your points, especially in the presence of an intraluminal tumor. I am not convinced, however, that the DLT has any advantage over the BB for ventilation or suctioning. If necessary, the BB may simply be deflated to facilitate suctioning and ventilation with short periods of apnea.

Summary

The use of BBs versus DLTs continues to remain a subject of much debate among thoracic anesthesiologists and surgeons. A growing number of studies demonstrate no difference in the degree of lung collapse between the 2 devices. BBs are often selected in clinical scenarios when a double-lumen tube is contraindicated. In cases with restricted mouth opening from trismus, airway swelling, or facial trauma, a nasal fiberoptic intubation with a single-lumen tube is the only option and precludes the use of a DLT. Alternatively, a BB can be used in such a way to minimize the degree of intrapulmonary shunt by selective lobar blockade in patients with severe pulmonary disease [4–6]. Considering these scenarios, BBs are among the most versatile airway devices for lung isolation and have clear advantages over DLTs.

Among the reasons that BBs are not widely accepted is that positioning may be challenging in patients with unusual anatomic variations, and there is a risk of malposition in these situations. Thus, placement requires a skilled anesthesiologist familiar with airway anatomy and comfortable with the use of fiberoptic bronchoscopy to position a BB. The use of BBs should be in every anesthesiologist's armamentarium for lung isolation. Their use should be encouraged in training programs to ensure that the anesthesiologist can adapt to situations where a BB is necessary. With the introduction of single-lumen tubes with integrated cameras, BBs may gain wider acceptance for purposes of training and monitoring. The VivaSight single lumen tube has been successfully used to provide visualization and continuous monitoring of endobronchial blockers [7]. Thus far, limited research exists on the use of these newer airway devices compared to traditional BBs among less experienced anesthesiologists, but close attention to this area of research is warranted in the future.

Disclosures Dr. Lewis—None. Dr. Amar—Member, Scientific Advisory Board of ETView Medical.

References

1. Narayanaswamy M, McRae K, Slinger P, Dugas G, Kanellakos GW, Roscoe A, Lacroix M. Choosing a lung isolation device for thoracic surgery: a randomized trial of three bronchial blockers versus double-lumen tubes. Anesth Analg. 2009;108:1097–101.
2. Yoo JY, Kim DH, Choi H, Kim K, Chae YJ, Park SY. Disconnection technique with a bronchial blocker for improving lung deflation: a comparison with a double-lumen tube and bronchial blocker without disconnection. J Cardiothorac Vasc Anesth. 2014;28:916–9.

3. El-Tahan MR. A comparison of the disconnection technique with continuous bronchial suction for lung deflation when using the Arndt endobronchial blocker during video-assisted thoracoscopy: a randomized trial. Eur J Anaesthesiol. 2015;32:411–7.
4. Karzai W, Schwarzkopf K. Hypoxemia during one-lung ventilation: prediction, prevention, and treatment. Anesthesiology. 2009; 110:1402–11.
5. Slinger P, Suissa S, Triolet W. Predicting arterial oxygenation during one-lung anaesthesia. Can J Anaesth. 1992;39:1030–5.
6. Campos J. Effects on oxygenation during selective lobar versus total lung collapse with or without continuous positive airway pressure. Anesth Analg. 1997;85:583–6.
7. Gaitini L, Yanovski B, Mustafa S. A feasibility study using the VivaSight Single Lumen™ to intubate the trachea through the fastrach laryngeal mask airway: a preliminary report of 50 cases. Anesth Analg. 2013;116:604–8.

Your Thoracic Epidural is Not Working: How Do You Provide Analgesia Post-thoracotomy?

30

Angela Renee Ingram and Anuj Malhotra

Case

You are carrying the pain pager and are paged to the floor for a patient who is 2 days following (POD#2) a thoracotomy for a pulmonary lobectomy. When moving the patient from a chair to her bed, her epidural catheter was inadvertently pulled out and now the patient is in severe pain. Should you replace her epidural or seek alternative techniques for adequate pain control?

Question

Are thoracic epidurals the gold standard for managing post-thoracotomy pain? What alternative regional techniques and systemic medications are available to provide adequate pain control post-thoracotomy? Do these different techniques have equianalgesic effects and similar side-effect profiles?

PRO: Epidural blockade has provided reliable pain management in postoperative patients since the 1980s and has become the "gold standard" in the management of post-thoracotomy pain. In general, epidural anesthesia has been shown to attenuate the surgical stress response, which causes a pro-inflammatory state with catecholamine surges and potential cardiovascular consequences. Epidural analgesia after surgery helps to prevent the contribution of severe pain to this inflammatory state. Multiple factors contribute to post-thoracotomy pain including the skin incision, intraoperative retraction of intercostal muscles and ligaments, direct intercostal nerve damage, and pleural irritation. Post-surgical pain is also related to the presence of chest tubes as well as pleural irritation from residual pleural fluid and blood [1]. Well-controlled pain with an epidural facilitates deep breathing, coughing, and earlier mobilization to prevent atelectasis while reducing overall opioid consumption. In a meta-analysis of the effectiveness of postoperative epidural analgesia, Block et al showed improved pain scores for epidural versus parenteral opioids at all time points, including postoperative days 2–4 [2]. In this post-thoracotomy patient with reduced pulmonary reserve, replacing the epidural and getting her comfortable quickly is the way to go, provided there are no absolute contraindications for a neuraxial block.

CON: Well, that's great that epidurals are considered the gold standard from 20+ years ago for post-thoracotomy pain; however, they are not without morbidity. Complications related to the epidural include hypotension, urinary retention, delayed gastric emptying, and potentially devastating epidural hematoma. Although epidurals do demonstrate better short-term outcomes in terms of acute pain, including earlier mobilization and earlier return of intestinal function, there is no conclusive evidence of a mortality benefit of epidural over other modes of analgesia, including systemic opioids, after thoracic surgery. Furthermore, the success of thoracic epidurals in treating acute postoperative pain has not been shown to translate definitively into the prevention of chronic post-thoracotomy pain syndrome. Additionally, thoracic epidural placement can be more technically challenging than the lumbar route because of the steep angle of the thoracic vertebrae, leading to difficulty with placement, which may delay treatment of the acute pain. Failure of thoracic epidurals is not uncommon and depends on both patient anatomy and the level of experience of the person performing the procedure. Systemic opioids in conjunction with other adjuvant medications such as NSAIDs, acetaminophen, and gabapentin would still be able to control

A.R. Ingram (✉)
Department of Anesthesiology, Children's Hospital of Pittsburgh of UPMC, Pittsburgh, PA 15244, USA
e-mail: ingrama2@upmc.edu

A. Malhotra
Department of Anesthesiology, Pain Management, Icahn School of Medicine at Mount Sinai, 5 East 98th St, 6th Floor, Box 1192New York, NY 10029, USA
e-mail: anuj.malhotra@mountsinai.org

C.S. Scher et al. (eds.), *You're Wrong, I'm Right*, DOI 10.1007/978-3-319-43169-7_30

post-thoracotomy pain. Using multimodal analgesia should help to minimize the side-effect profiles of each individual drug.

PRO: There are no data specifically showing survival benefit in post-thoracotomy patients with thoracic epidurals because prospective, randomized clinical trials have been underpowered for this relatively rare endpoint. However, a recent meta-analysis does suggest decreased mortality [3]. Additionally, there may be contraindications to using individual systemic medications, thus making multimodal analgesia using only these agents difficult to achieve. Systemic opioids can contribute greatly to postoperative nausea and vomiting as well as decreased intestinal motility, leading to postoperative ileus and its sequelae. Opioid-induced respiratory depression may lead to aspiration or hypercarbic respiratory failure. Acetaminophen may be contraindicated in patients with liver dysfunction. NSAIDs could be challenging to use in the setting of postoperative bleeding or in patients with significant renal dysfunction. Gabapentin has been shown to decrease postoperative pain scores within the first 24 h but has not demonstrated an opioid-sparing effect past this time point [1], and can itself cause increased sedation.

CON: It's POD #2, a time when many patients begin to have their anticoagulation restarted and therefore placing a new thoracic epidural would be contraindicated. If a thoracic epidural is of concern due to an increased risk of hematoma or hypotension (e.g., planned anticoagulation, hypovolemia), an alternative to a neuraxial blockade could be a single-shot regional technique, or if there is no absolute contraindication, a paravertebral catheter. A meta-analysis by Davies, Miles, and Graham showed that when paravertebral catheters were directly compared to thoracic epidural catheters for thoracotomy, there was no significant difference in pain control, and that paravertebral catheters had a more favorable side-effect profile than epidurals, with decreased failure rates and a reduction in pulmonary complications [4]. If this patient were in severe pain, even a single-shot paravertebral block done at the bedside would be able to decrease acute pain in conjunction with systemic medications. Intercostal blocks would be another regional technique that could be performed post-thoracotomy, but they may require multiple injections to cover pain adequately. Other research into using liposomal bupivacaine in single-shot paravertebral and intercostal blocks is ongoing and may prove to be yet another alternative to managing post-thoracotomy pain.

PRO: I agree that if a thoracic epidural is contraindicated, it should not be replaced and that a regional technique, if possible, plus systemic medications is the way to go; however, I would also point out that the majority of the paravertebral catheters in the meta-analysis quoted earlier were placed under direct visualization by the surgeon at the end of the procedure. Direct visualization intraoperatively increases the chances of the paravertebral catheter working beyond its initial insertion and also decreases the chances of a complication. More research must be done that directly compares ultrasound-guided paravertebral catheter placement versus thoracic epidural in thoracotomy patients before I am convinced about paravertebral catheters replacing epidurals as a rescue therapy in post-thoracotomy patients. Additionally, paravertebral injections and blocks are still considered "deep blocks" or non-compressible in the event of vascular puncture. Although anticoagulation and hypotension are not considered absolute contraindications to this block, alternative regional techniques such as intercostal nerve blocks may be a better option.

Summary

When treating severe acute post-thoracotomy pain, one must weigh the risks and benefits of treating the individual patient with neuraxial blocks, other regional techniques, or parenteral medications. Although thoracic epidurals are the gold standard for managing post-thoracotomy pain, there are multiple alternative techniques to provide good pain relief. In general, a multimodal technique using regional anesthesia plus parenteral medications will create adequate analgesia to synergistically relieve pain. Research directly comparing ultrasound-guided regional techniques with thoracic epidurals as well as longer acting liposomal bupivacaine in regional techniques is ongoing [5] and may yield alternate options for treating post-thoracotomy pain.

References

1. Pennefather SH, McKevith J. Pain management after thoracic surgery. In: Slinger PD, editor. Principles and practice of anesthesia for thoracic surgery. New York: Springer; 2011. p. 675–707.
2. Block BM, Liu SS, Rowlingson AJ, Cowan AR, Cowan JA Jr, Wu CL. Efficacy of postoperative epidural analgesia: a meta-analysis. JAMA. 2003;290:2455–63.
3. Pöpping DM, Elia N, Van Aken HK, Marret E, Schug SA, Kranke P, Wenk M, Tramèr MR. Impact of epidural analgesia on mortality and morbidity after surgery: systematic review and meta-analysis of randomized controlled trials. Ann Surg. 2014;259:1056–67.
4. Davies RG, Myles PS, Graham JM. A comparison of the analgesic efficacy and side-effects of paravertebral vs epidural blockade for thoracotomy—a systematic review and meta-analysis of randomized trials. Br J Anaesth. 2006;96:418–26.
5. Rice DC, Cata JP, Mena GE, Rodriguez-Restrepo A, Correa AM, Mehran RJ. Posterior intercostal nerve block with liposomal bupivacaine: an alternative to thoracic epidural analgesia. Ann Thorac Surg. 2015;99:1953–60.

Part IV
Pediatric

Pediatric Upper Respiratory Infection: You Cancelled the Case and Told the Parents to Reschedule, Right?

31

Brian Blasiole

Case

After travelling 3 h early one morning in September, a young family registers their 4-year-old son at the preoperative desk for a tonsillectomy and adenoidectomy (T&A) with Dr. Rhino. The child is placed in a pre-op evaluation room, and the nurse obtains vital signs and assesses the patient. The newly minted pediatric anesthesiology fellow reviews the chart outside the room and notes an otherwise healthy 4-year-old with sleep disordered breathing and obstructive sleep apnea (OSA) diagnosed by a formal sleep study presenting for T&A.

The fellow knocks on the door and almost recoils upon entry with the odor of stale cigarette smoke saturating the room. The nurse in the room reports that the child had a cold with a fever "to touch" last week and asks the fellow if the case will be cancelled. The parents quickly interrupt the nurse and state that the child has been on antibiotics for 3 days from their local pediatrician who also cleared him for surgery. They also state that he always has a cough and runny nose, and their pediatrician told them the frequency of colds would decrease after the T&A.

The fellow obtained more history and ascertained that the child has been afebrile and behaving normally after starting antibiotics. His symptoms consist of non-purulent rhinorrhea and occasional non-productive cough. On auscultation, coarse breath sounds are heard, which clear after the child coughs.

The fellow explains to the parents the risk of anesthesia in a child with a recent upper respiratory infection (URI) and intimates that the case may be cancelled. The parents become visibly upset and start to argue with the fellow, stating that they were told by their pediatrician the kid will be fine for surgery and that they both took the day off from work, drove 3 h to get to the hospital, and coordinated child care and school transportation for their other children. The fellow quickly retreats stating that he will review this case with his attending.

After leaving the room, the fellow consults with a colleague who shows him an article by a preeminent researcher in the field of pediatric URI and anesthesia suggesting that blanket cancellation of kids with URIs "may be a thing of the past" [1].

Question

"You cancelled the case and told the parents to reschedule, right?" asks the veteran anesthesiologist after hearing the fellow's presentation of the patient.

PRO: It is generally felt that elective surgery should be cancelled in children with an active and/or recent URIs because of an increased risk of perioperative respiratory events. URIs lead to the release of inflammatory mediators that are associated with airway hyper-reactivity and can cause perioperative bronchospasm, atelectasis, and hypoxemia with an increased alveolar–arterial oxygen gradient. Additional respiratory complications include breath holding, increased secretions, laryngospasm, and stridor from subglottic edema. URIs are most commonly of viral origin and self-limiting; however, the airway hyper-reactivity can persist from 2 to 6 weeks. Risk factors for respiratory adverse events that can be identified during the pre-anesthetic assessment include an active URI or respiratory symptoms within the past 2 weeks, nasal congestion, parent's statement that child has a "cold" and is not acting normally, tobacco smoke exposure, and a history of prematurity (<37 weeks), reactive airway disease, atopy, and/or snoring [1]. Severe symptoms that typically lead to postponement of a case for at least 4 weeks include mucopurulent secretions (not just clear rhinorrhea), productive cough, fever >38 °C, lethargy,

B. Blasiole (✉)
Department of Anesthesiology, Children's Hospital of Pittsburgh of UPMC, 4401 Penn Avenue, Suite 5643, Pittsburgh, PA 15224, USA
e-mail: balsioleb@upmc.edu

C.S. Scher et al. (eds.), *You're Wrong, I'm Right*, DOI 10.1007/978-3-319-43169-7_31

or signs of pulmonary involvement (lower airway). This child is at a higher risk of a perioperative respiratory event due to his history of URI with moderate respiratory symptoms, fever, and tobacco smoke exposure. The conservative approach would be to postpone this case for at least 2 weeks.

CON: Children in daycare or in nursery school can have up to 6–8 URIs in a year. Postponing surgery for up to 6 weeks between each URI makes it very difficult to schedule a surgery that could possibly ameliorate a cause for the child's frequent colds. Besides, there have been numerous cases of children undergoing major surgery with an URI that did not affect their hospital course. In fact, there have been no cases of serious adverse events in the closed claims database associated with anesthesia and URIs [1]. The adverse events associated with URIs are treatable and can possibly be mitigated by certain anesthetic approaches. Finally, it is important to weigh the risks and benefits of proceeding with this case. The family has arranged time and transportation to get here, which they may not be willing to do again. The optimal time frame to allow for resolution of the URI and symptoms and reschedule surgery is also known. Furthermore, a T&A in this relatively uncomplicated child may decrease the likelihood of another URI. Surgery should proceed as scheduled. Inform the parents about the risks of anesthesia with a URI including the possibility of a hospital admission.

The new pediatric anesthesia fellow pushes his attending to proceed with the case in the light of the seemingly mild, resolving URI and the family's hardship. As the patient is brought into the operating room, the grizzled attending asks the young physician if he plans an intravenous or inhalational induction. The fellow hesitates, as he assumed that the standard inhalational induction and placement of peripheral IV would suffice. The attending quickly becomes impatient, shakes his head and grumbles.

Question

Should this 4-year-old be held down to obtain peripheral IV access prior to administration of an inhalational agent?

PRO: Pre-induction administration of IV anticholinergics agents will block muscarinic receptors, which may help to decrease airway secretions (secretions that may trigger bronchospasm). Additional adjunctive agents that could be administered with an IV include lidocaine and opioids. Most importantly, blunting the airway reflexes with a sufficient depth of anesthesia is paramount in avoiding respiratory events and triggering airway hyper-reactivity. Intravenous induction will provide the fastest way to achieve a deep plane of anesthesia, regardless of which induction agent is used. If given sufficient time to work (15–20 min), premedication such as oral midazolam and distraction techniques should make the patient a satisfactory candidate for IV placement.

CON: Obtaining IV access in an awake 4-year-old child can be difficult, and possibly psychologically damaging to the child if multiple attempts are required. Mask induction of inhalation anesthesia with sevoflurane in oxygen, with or without nitrous oxide, is a common and safe approach to induction in a child of this age. A peripheral IV can reliably be placed in a motionless child once a sufficient plane of anesthesia has been reached. An inhalational induction is also more amenable to parental presence.

The anesthesiology attending, determined to push the fellow further, now demands a decision on airway management. He asks whether the fellow will place a laryngeal mask airway (LMA) or endotracheal tube (ETT)? Or, he sarcastically proposes with an artful smile, would the fellow prefer to mask the patient between cauterizations?

Question

Should an ETT be placed for this procedure?

PRO: An oral right angle endotracheal (RAE) tube is preferred for T&A to allow for placement of the grooved blade tongue retractor for surgical exposure. Ideally, the RAE tube should be cuffed to prevent aspiration of blood and other material as well as gas leaks around the tube. Topical lidocaine spray to the vocal cords prior to placement of the tube may reduce the incidence of laryngospasm and/or bronchospasm. Using a LMA for this case would make it technically more difficult for the surgeon secondary to inadequate positioning and surgical exposure. This could potentially prolong the surgery, increase the risk of surgical complications, and lead to more pain. The LMA does not provide the protection from aspiration or laryngospasm that an ETT would confer. Finally, the ETT would allow the provision of higher airway pressures and more direct application of aerosolized beta-bronchodilator therapy in the event of bronchospasm in the child with a URI.

CON: Use of an ETT in a child with a URI is associated with an increased risk of airway complications [1]. Although the lowest risk of airway complications is associated with use of a face mask, it would be impractical and possibly dangerous to manage the airway with a face mask for a T&A. The LMA is a safe alternative since it does not require the instrumentation of the airway and is associated with the lower incidence of perioperative complications compared to the ETT [1].

Following an uneventful inhalation induction, intravenous line, and oral RAE tube placement, the surgery is conducted uneventfully. The surgeon finishes and returns the head of the bed to the anesthesiology fellow who dutifully calls his attending to report that he is ready extubate the patient "deep." The attending sighs and asks for the fellow to wait for him to get to the room before he does anything.

Question

Should the patient with a recent URI be extubated under deep anesthesia after a T&A for obstructive sleep apnea?

PRO: There is no evidence for increased respiratory complications after deep extubation following T&A, even in children with a URI [2, 3]. Removal of the tracheal tube under deep anesthesia removes the stimulus for coughing and bronchospasm. Coughing and bucking on the endotracheal tube during emergence also increases the risk for postsurgical bleeding and the possibility of wound dehiscence. If the airway and stomach are appropriately suctioned while the child is asleep, the risk of laryngospasm and aspiration can be decreased. Upper airway obstruction can be avoided by gentle placement of adjunctive devices such as a nasal trumpet or oral airway. Proper head, neck, and body positioning of the child and vigilant monitoring for airway obstruction will allow the child to awaken safely from anesthesia.

CON: A deep extubation requires that the child emerge from anesthesia with an unprotected airway, leading to the possibility of laryngospasm or bronchospasm. If the child is brought to the postanesthesia care unit while still in stage 2 or 3 anesthesia, these events could occur in the hallway, a truly dangerous situation. This child also has an increased risk for upper airway obstruction after his T&A due to his diagnosis of obstructive sleep apnea. Extubating the trachea completely awake after return of the laryngeal and pharyngeal reflexes prevents the occurrence of airway obstruction and aspiration.

The endotracheal tube is removed while the patient is still deeply anesthetized in the operating suite. The patient is transported to the postanesthesia care unit (PACU) on oxygen via simple face mask. On arrival, the fellow notes that the child is cyanotic, tachypneic, and has audible wheezing. Pulse oximetry shows low oxygen saturation. The fellow quickly applies positive pressure via face mask while simultaneously handing his attending atropine and epinephrine. The bronchospasm breaks and the oxygen saturation returns to baseline. The attending orders nebulized albuterol, and the fellow gives a dose of intravenous methylprednisolone. Once the patient is stable, the parents are allowed to see the child in the PACU and are informed of the bronchospasm event. By this time, the attending has long since vanished, and the fellow explains to the family that he believes the child should be admitted overnight for observation. The upset parents ask, "Why?"

Question

Should this child be admitted for overnight observation after treatment for bronchospasm?

PRO: This child should be admitted to the hospital for observation in light of his T&A, URI, and subsequent bronchospasm on emergence in the PACU. Discharging this child on the same day could be deadly if he undergoes another event in the car or at home when the effect of the beta-2 agonists and steroids wane. Overnight monitoring of the patient allows for rapid detection and treatment of any additional respiratory events. In addition, postoperative bleeding after a T&A could conceivably be worse in a child with intermittent coughing from a URI.

CON: The family's social situation has again come into play. An overnight admission would require them to take another day off work and arrange for care of their other children.

Summary

URIs are the most common cause of procedure cancellation in pediatric anesthesia and present a unique challenge to the pediatric anesthesiologist. The anesthesia risks for a child with a URI are laryngospasm, bronchospasm, increased secretions, coughing, and resultant decreased oxygen saturations. These risks are increased in the setting of exposure to second-hand smoke, sleep disordered breathing, a more invasive type of airway instrumentation (ETT>LMA>mask), presence of an underlying RAD, and prematurity. High-risk symptoms are parental report of a URI, nasal congestion, copious secretions, sleep disordered breathing, passive smoking, family history of atopy/asthma, and airway surgery.

The risks and benefits of proceeding with anesthesia in a child with a URI must be considered and include the urgency and nature of the surgery, the anesthetic management required, the severity of the URI, and the social situation. Airway risks can be mitigated by tailoring the anesthetic to safely perform certain surgeries in the presence of a mild URI. The dilemma for the anesthesiologist is to decide when to proceed or postpone elective cases in children with a moderately severe URI. If the decision is made to continue with the case, the increased risk and dangers of an adverse respiratory event including the possibility of an overnight admission must be made clear.

References

1. Tait AR, Malviya S. Anesthesia for the child with an upper respiratory tract infection: Still a dilemma? Anesth Analg. 2005;100:59–65.
2. Baijal RG, Bidani SA, Minard CG, Watcha MF. Perioperative respiratory complications following awake and deep extubation in children undergoing adenotonsillectomy. Paediatr Anaesth. 2015;25:392–9.
3. Von Ungern-Sterberg BS, Davies K, Hegarty M, Erb TO, Habre W. The effect of deep vs. awake extubation on respiratory complications in high-risk children undergoing adenotonsillectomy: a randomized-controlled trial. Eur J Anaesthesiol. 2013;30:529–36.

Does a Low Mean Blood Pressure in the Neonate Under Anesthesia Lead to Cognitive Deficits?

32

Anna Clebone and Corey S. Scher

Case

A 3-day-old presents for surgery to deal with a tethered cord. This congenital disorder is characterized by a membrane (the filum terminale) abnormally anchored to the spinal cord at the L2 level or lower. If untreated, there may be progressive lower extremity weakness and incontinence, due to stretching on the spinal cord from the child's movements. Early surgery yields better outcomes.

The "untethering" surgery involves a careful dissection to free the spinal cord. Neuromonitoring and nerve testing intraoperatively are essential to preserve motor function in the lower extremities and avoid incontinence later in life. The need for intraoperative nerve monitoring prohibits the use of muscle relaxants. The neurosurgeon rightly insists that the infant stay completely still while she is dissecting out the spinal cord. Sevoflurane is kept at 3.6 atm%, slightly above the MAC of 3.3 atm% for neonates. In addition, an infusion of remifentanil is added. You realize the blood pressure will be lower than ideal, but you don't want the patient to move, which would be catastrophic. Your colleague comes in the room to give you a lunch break, and starts to harangue you about the persistent blood pressure of 50/28 (35)…

"You may not know it, but you are probably not perfusing the brain and above all the spinal cord," your colleague says derisively.

A. Clebone (✉)
Department of Anesthesia and Critical Care, The University of Chicago, 5841 S. Maryland Ave. MC-4028, Chicago, IL 60637, USA
e-mail: aclebone@gmail.com

C.S. Scher
Department of Anesthesiology, Perioperative Care and Pain Medicine, New York University School of Medicine, New York, NY 10016, USA
e-mail: coreyscher@gmail.com

Questions

Is autoregulation present at birth? If not, is a mild level of hypotension a threat to the central nervous system at a critical mean arterial blood pressure (MAP)?

PRO: "As you know, the variables involved are cerebral perfusion pressure (CPP), MAP, intracranial pressure (ICP), and central venous pressure (CVP). CPP = MAP − ICP (or CVP, whichever is higher)." Your colleague continues with a smug look on his face, "In this case we cannot calculate CPP. We do not know the CVP. The ICP is almost impossible to measure noninvasively, although the wide-open diamond-shaped posterior fontanelle and square-shaped anterior fontanelle will be bulging if it is high. Having said that, MAP is what we can control related to brain perfusion. The normal MAP in a full-term 3-day-old is 40 mmHg! Talk about a narrow window for error!!!"

CON: "Three days ago the infant went through labor and delivery, during which the umbilical cord was periodically being compressed during contractions—with presumed decreased oxygen to the brain. What's different now? General anesthesia most likely decreases the amount of oxygen that the brain needs by decreasing the cerebral metabolic rate. If you are really worried about perfusing the brain, employ near-infrared spectroscopy (NIRS), which in my opinion, is greatly underutilized. Jöbsis first reported in 1977 that the relatively high degree of transparency of myocardial and brain tissue in the near-infrared (NIR) range enabled real-time non-invasive detection of tissue oxygen saturation using transillumination spectroscopy [1]. By 1985, Ferrari and colleagues reported some of the first human cerebral oximetry studies using near-infrared spectroscopy (NIRS in patients with subarachnoid haemorrhage) [2]. According to Bhatia et al, 'Episodes of angiographic cerebral vasospasm were strongly associated with a reduction in the trend of the ipsilateral NIRS signal. Furthermore, the degree of spasm (especially more than a 75 % vessel diameter reduction) were associated with a greater reduction in the same-sided

C.S. Scher et al. (eds.), *You're Wrong, I'm Right*, DOI 10.1007/978-3-319-43169-7_32

NIRS signal demonstrating real-time detection of intracerebral ischaemia' [3]."

PRO: "The NIRS is constantly changing with the $EtCO_2$. Not to mention the variation if the surgery becomes bloody and the hematocrit drops. There are no defined trigger points to tell me when the infant's brain is becoming ischemic, whether the interference with the signal be anemia or pH status."

CON: "Well, fine, even if you don't look at the NIRS, the MAP estimates cerebral blood flow pretty well. If there's nothing else bad going on in the brain, a MAP over 45 mmHg is great, between 35 and 45 mmHg is probably OK, and only when you get under 35 you are getting into trouble. Rhondali et al. [4] looked at this in children under 6 months old, with the $EtCO_2$ level held relatively constant. If you want the transcranial Doppler to show good perfusion, aim for a MAP of 45 mmHg. The NIRS still looks decent and shows increased oxygenation versus an awake infant with MAPs between 35 and 45 mmHg, probably because sevoflurane decreases the cerebral metabolic rate. With a MAP below 35 mmHg, cerebral perfusion is likely poor, but you are stuck between a rock and a hard place because most pressors in babies will compromise splanchnic flow and renal flow [4]."

PRO: "Yeah, but Rhondali's study was done in healthy infants, with an ideal fluid balance. Who is to say that with longer surgeries or sicker kids, those numbers are right? Why not better safe than sorry and keep the blood pressure up? And besides, do those sketchy monitors correlate with long-term outcomes for these kids, our most vulnerable population?"

CON: "Are you not concerned with intraventricular hemorrhage (IVH) as you try to keep the pressure up? It has evolved in the literature from case reports to actual studies. IVH DOES happen."

PRO: "If intraventricular hemorrhage is going to occur, it has likely already happened in utero, during delivery of the infant, or otherwise way before the infant gets to the operating room. This may or may not be applicable to full-term infants, but in one large meta-analysis of preterm low birth weight and very low birth weight infants, over half of IVH occurred in the first 6 h of life [5]."

Summary

The data on safe minimal blood pressures for infants undergoing general anesthesia are still in its, well, infancy. Large database studies correlating intraoperative blood pressures and long-term cognitive outcomes are needed. Close attention is warranted to this area of research in the future.

References

1. Jöbsis FF. Noninvasive, infrared monitoring of cerebral and myocardial oxygen sufficiency and circulatory parameters. Science. 1977;198(4323):1264–7.
2. Ferrari M, Giannini I, Sideri G, Zanette E. Continuous non invasive monitoring of human brain by near infrared spectroscopy. Adv Exp Med Biol. 1985;191:873–82.
3. Bhatia R, Hampton T, Malde S, Kandala NB, Muammar M, Deasy N, et al. The application of near-infrared oximetry to cerebral monitoring during aneurysm embolization: a comparison with intraprocedural angiography. J Neurosurg Anesthesiol. 2007;19 (2):97–104 (Case Reports Comparative Study).
4. Rhondali O, Pouyau A, Mahr A, Juhel S, De Queiroz M, Rhzioual-Berrada K, et al. Sevoflurane anesthesia and brain perfusion. Paediatr Anaesth. 2015;25(2):180–5.
5. Al-Abdi SY, Al-Aamri MA. A systematic review and meta-analysis of the timing of early intraventricular hemorrhage in preterm neonates: clinical and research implications. J Clin Neonatol. 2014;3 (2):76–88.

Does Rapid Sequence Induction Have a Role in Pediatric Anesthesia?

33

Michale Sofer

Case

A 5-year-old male presents to the emergency department (ED) with a right supracondylar fracture after falling from the monkey bars. He has no other injuries, no notable past medical history, and no past surgical history. He ate lunch about an hour prior to his fall and arrived to the ED approximately 30 min later. He has a 22-gauge IV in his left upper extremity and a splint to his right upper extremity. He is noticeably upset and tucked into his mother's arms. The pediatric orthopedic surgeon would like to take him urgently to the operating room (OR) for a closed reduction with percutaneous pinning (CRPP), and possible open reduction with internal fixation if needed. The surgeon anticipates 20–30 min operative time and minimal blood loss for the case.

Just as you are finishing preparing the room for the case, your friend, a pediatric anesthesiologist, peeks into the operating room to offer you a hand. You are not pediatric trained, but often take care of older children when on call. You welcome your friend, along with her professional input, into the room and ask her to peek at your setup and see if there is anything you forgot.

As she looks over your anesthesia machine and cart, she notices the medications you prepared for induction and asks, "Are you planning to do a rapid sequence induction?"

Questions

Does Rapid Sequence Induction (RSI) have a role in pediatric anesthesia? Should we instead consider "modified-RSI?" If we do utilize RSI, which muscle relaxant is most appropriate: succinylcholine or rocuronium?

M. Sofer (✉)
Department of Anesthesiology, Perioperative Care and Pain Medicine, New York University Langone Medical Center, 550 First Avenue, New York, NY 10016, USA
e-mail: soferm@email.chop.edu

PRO: Of course! He's a trauma patient. He is a "full stomach."

I was planning to do a classic RSI. I don't want to ventilate and insufflate his stomach. He ate lunch a measly 2 h ago! Thankfully, he already has an IV from the ED, so that's one less thing to worry about. I was going to place all my monitors and pre-oxygenate for at least 3 min. I've prepared propofol, fentanyl, and rocuronium for induction. With an intubating dose of rocuronium, he should have adequate intubating conditions in about a minute or so. I've done it this way before in older children, it works well.

CON: My main concern is that he won't tolerate apnea, even for that minute. In fact, the younger the child, the less likely they are to tolerate classic RSI. First, he simply may not cooperate. Wrestling a mask on his face for pre-oxygenation is likely to just leave you both out of breath! He is already in tears, and the mask may not do much more than add to his (and your) anxiety, without accomplishing adequate pre-oxygenation. Even if you accomplish pre-oxygenation, he is still much more likely to have hypoxemia between induction and intubation than to have an aspiration event. Aspiration events in children are not only infrequent, but appear low risk [1]. I'd be more concerned about the hypoxemia than aspiration.

PRO: It only takes about a minute for the rocuronium to take effect. That's not a long time for apnea! I can hold my breath longer than that! Why do you think he won't tolerate it?

CON: Compared to an adult, he has a decreased functional reserve capacity to minute ventilation ratio, increased oxygen consumption, and a greater closing capacity after induction of anesthesia and use of muscle relaxant. You may only have seconds until his oxygen saturation starts to drop, while older children do tend to tolerate apnea better.

For example, with adequate pre-oxygenation, a healthy adult can tolerate apnea for at least 8 min before desaturation to less than 90 % SaO_2. On room air, this same adult will

C.S. Scher et al. (eds.), *You're Wrong, I'm Right*, DOI 10.1007/978-3-319-43169-7_33

start to start to desaturate within 45–60 s [2]. In a child who is pre-oxygenated, you may see desaturation in under a minute. Without pre-oxygenation, that time is even less, and the smaller the child, the less time you have [3].

Aspiration just isn't nearly as likely as desaturation in children. It shouldn't be more of a focus than hypoxemia.

PRO: We shouldn't just ignore the possibility of aspiration. It does happen, and it does increase morbidity and mortality. Our goal should still be to minimize its occurrence, utilizing all possible measures. Perhaps it happens so infrequently because we have been doing things right: minimizing ventilation, minimizing time between induction and intubation, and using rapid onset muscle relaxants.

In this case, cricoid pressure may do more harm than good. It will probably distort the airway and make intubation more difficult. Plus, a 5-year-old is unlikely to understand the benefit of pressure on his neck [3].

I would omit cricoid pressure, but I still feel that we should utilize all other measures to minimize his aspiration risk. I don't want him sitting in an intensive care unit because I chose to ignore the hotdog in his stomach.

CON: I agree, but aspiration in pediatric anesthetic practice appears to occur at a rate of 2 per 10,000 cases. It is potentially higher in emergency situations, but not significantly. Aspiration in young children is even rarer, and no pediatrics deaths from aspiration have been appreciated in any recent reviews or studies [1]. There will always be risk factors that we can't control for, such as a difficult airway, gastrointestinal pathology, gastro-esophageal reflux, obesity, and esophageal disease. However, anxiety, increased abdominal pressure, and inadequate or light anesthesia were also found to be risk factors for aspiration and are in some realm of our control.

In his case, regurgitation and vomiting are most likely to result from direct laryngoscopy in the setting of light anesthesia or incomplete paralysis. This is classically what happens when a child starts to desaturate with classic RSI and the anesthesiologist rushes to intubate: the patient can buck and regurgitate, become a more difficult intubation, or experience hypoxemia or bradycardia [1, 4].

How about trying "controlled" RSI, with gentle mask ventilation? Mask ventilation pressures maintained below 10–12 cm H_2O allow oxygenation, limit hypercarbia, and keep small airways open, with a very low likelihood of resulting gastric inflation and regurgitation. Neuhuas et al. reported a retrospective cohort analysis of 1001 children who underwent controlled RSI with less than 4 h NPO after solids or 2 h after clears. This study reports significantly fewer episodes of hypoxemia, bradycardia, and difficult intubations compared to classic RSI, with no observed pulmonary aspiration events. This is in stark comparison to Gencorelli et al. retrospective study of 1070 children who underwent classic RSI, with high incidences of hypoxemia, especially in younger patients, and increased difficult intubations, but also no reported aspiration events [4].

It seems that either way, the risk of aspiration is low in the pediatric population and compromising ventilation to minimize the rare aspiration event may be overzealous. Controlled RSI allows time for adequate muscle relaxation and depth of anesthesia, while maintaining oxygenation. If you are worried about the time to intubation, you can also consider using succinylcholine as an alternative to high-dose rocuronium.

PRO: You would use succinylcholine? What about the side effects? What about the risks of hyperkalemic cardiac arrest, malignant hyperthermia, or rhabdomyolysis? We don't know that he's not susceptible! His lack of medical history doesn't exclude him from the possibilities of an undiagnosed muscular dystrophy or malignant hyperthermia. I'm not sure it's worth the risk. Besides, Mazruek et al. [5] study in 26 pediatric patients found comparable intubating conditions 30 s after RSI with administration of rocuronium 1.2 mg/kg as compared to succinylcholine 1.5 mg/kg. The only significant difference was the time until the return of the first twitch response. If the two drugs are comparable with respect to intubation, rocuronium seems safer to me.

CON: I would consider succinylcholine only because this is expected to be such a short case. Rocuronium isn't going to wear off in a timely fashion, and succinylcholine is another appropriate option, although less popular. The pediatric product labeling was revised and now states that succinylcholine is indicated for "emergency intubation or instances where immediate securing of the airway is necessary, [such as] laryngospasm, difficult airway, full stomach or intramuscular use when a suitable vein is inaccessible." Due to the potential side effects, I would generally agree with your use of rocuronium, but in this case, it may leave you with some waiting time at the end of the procedure.

References

1. Kelly CJ, Walker RWM. Perioperative pulmonary aspiration is infrequent and low risk in pediatric patients. Paediatr Anaesth. 2015;25:36–43.
2. Weingart SD, Levitan RM. Preoxygenation and prevention of desaturation during emergency airway management. Ann Emerg Med. 2012;50(3):165–75.
3. Engelhardt T. Rapid sequence induction has no use in pediatric anesthesia. Paediatr Anaesth. 2015;25:5–8.
4. Walker RWM. Pulmonary aspiration in pediatric anesthetic practice in the UK: a prospective survey of specialist pediatric centers over a one-year period. Paediatr Anaesth. 2013;23:702–11.
5. Mazurek AJ, Rae B, Hann S, Kim JI, Castro B, Coté CJ. Rocuronium versus succinylcholine: are they equally effective during rapid-sequence induction of anesthesia? Anesth Analg. 1998;87:1259–62.

34 Anesthetic Neurotoxicity: Is Anesthesia Toxic to the Developing Brain? Should I Cancel My Baby's Surgery?

Misuzu Kameyama and Corey S. Scher

Case

A 4-month-old boy with congenital sensorineural hearing loss presents for bilateral cochlear implant placement under general anesthesia. The child was born full term with no problems in the perinatal period. The mother did an Internet search for "anesthesia for children" and was shocked at what she found: Papers that claimed that anesthesia in growing children can impact cognitive development. While she was not familiar with the language of scientific reporting, she was more than proficient to determine that anesthesia in the growing neuroplastic brain could be a danger for her child [1]. In addition, her child was already falling behind in reaching developmental milestones due to hearing loss. The mother's concern grew, as her child had multiple anesthetics to evaluate for hearing loss since the child's first month of life. At the pre-surgical testing clinic, the parents asked the anesthesiologist how exposing their child to another anesthetic could affect his future development.

Question

Is anesthesia toxic to the developing brain? Should I cancel my baby's surgery?

PRO The parents certainly have valid concerns. The literature on neurotoxicity is replete with animal models that demonstrate that exposure to inhaled anesthetics is associated with neurotoxicity. The deposition of beta amyloid protein, increased apoptosis, tau phosphorylation, and mitochondrial changes are just a few of the markers that show up in well-designed animal models [1]. Much of the research in pediatric anesthesiology over the past 10 years has been dedicated to determining whether these changes occur in humans. This is very difficult to do prospectively, due to overwhelming ethical concerns. Obviously, we cannot biopsy the brain after a child has had an anesthetic. I have looked at so many papers from infant rats and primates, and the results are the same: apoptosis, beta amyloid protein, and the rest of the markers. I am convinced that anesthesia-induced neurotoxicity has to occur in humans [2].

CON This procedure needs to occur. Even though being deaf is not "life-threatening," it is a major disability that will hinder the child's verbal development. There is strong evidence that when cochlear implants are placed early in a pre-lingual child, there is significant improvement in auditory speech reception and perception skills.

The American Society of Anesthesiologists (ASA) addressed this issue with a consensus statement from an expert examination of the literature. The original statement addressed the intense controversy of giving anesthetics to a child, due to neuroplasticity of the infant brain. In essence, the statement declared that children younger than 3 years old should not have elective surgery. More recently, two trials have brought this into question. In the most definitive study to date, researchers examined 700 infants, up to 60 weeks old, who were undergoing hernia repair in hospitals across 7 countries. Half of the patients were randomly assigned to receive general anesthesia, while the other half received spinal anesthesia and remained awake. The median duration of surgery in both groups was approximately 1 h. The authors assessed the children's neurological development at 2 years of age [3] and found that children in both the general and regional anesthesia groups had similar cognitive scores. Another recent investigation looked at premature infants (on average, born at 26 weeks gestation) who were randomized to receive sevoflurane versus a spinal for inguinal hernia

M. Kameyama (✉)
Department of Anesthesiology, New York University Langone Medical Center, 550 First Avenue, TH530, New York, NY 10016, USA
e-mail: Misuzu.kameyama@nyumc.org

C.S. Scher
Department of Anesthesiology, Perioperative Care and Pain Medicine, New York University Langone Medical Center, New York, NY 10016, USA
e-mail: coreyscher@gmail.com

C.S. Scher et al. (eds.), *You're Wrong, I'm Right*, DOI 10.1007/978-3-319-43169-7_34

repair. The neurodevelopmental outcome did not differ between the two groups. Simply stated, this child can have surgery now.

PRO Yes, while very impressive, there will be constant shifts on the pendulum of this issue. I can assure you that there are ongoing trials that will show the opposite. That is the inherent nature of scientific investigation. The animal studies were initially conducted in immature baby mice and later in rhesus monkeys. The pharmacologic agents that have been identified as potentially harmful are the gamma-aminobutyric acid (GABA) agonists and *N*-methyl-D-aspartate (NMDA) receptor antagonists. And although the studies are inconclusive, opioids and alpha agonists may be neuroprotective.

The design of most of these controlled animal investigations can cover the variables better than a clinical human study. The two prospective studies in human infants are well designed. However, the scale used to measure intelligence—the Wechsler Pre-School and Primary Scale of Intelligence—may not be sensitive enough. It may be years before this issue is definitive.

CON A single brief exposure to anesthesia is unlikely to do harm. With repeated exposures, the risk of learning disabilities, behavioral problems, and cognitive dysfunction in children will probably rise, although not as much as we previously imagined. The only reason why an increase in developmental delay is even on our radar lies in increased surveillance for these disorders. Better diagnostics, not anesthesia is the reason for this trend.

PRO Concession to CON In summary, you are correct. I would recommend that they proceed with the cochlear implant surgery without reservation. The benefit of this life-changing operation far outweighs the risk of a single exposure to anesthesia, provided that this child is otherwise in good health. I would proceed with general anesthesia, which is considered the current standard, since this is not a surgery that can be done with local or regional anesthesia. I am not compelled to do a total intravenous anesthetic as it is unclear which intravenous drugs may be related to neurotoxicity.

Summary

While the best clinical human studies now appear to show that a single, short general anesthetic is not neurotoxic in children, more work must be published to add to that literature. If a small child needs to undergo an invasive procedure, it is not only unethical but also dangerous to withhold anesthesia and analgesia. As with any medical decision, one should weigh the risks and benefits of proceeding with surgery and anesthesia. If a procedure is completely elective, perhaps it should be delayed until the child is older. But urgent and emergent cases, as well as potentially life-changing cases should proceed without altering our current practice.

References

1. Hansen T. Anesthesia-related neurotoxicity and the developing animal brain is not a significant problem in children. Pediatr Anesth. 2015;25:65–72.
2. Miller TL, Park R, Sun L. Report of the fourth PANDA symposium on "Anesthesia and Neurodevelopment in Children". J Neurosurj Anesthesiol. 2014;26:344–8.
3. Davidson AJ, Disma N, de Graaff JC, Withington DE, Dorris L, Bell G, et al. GAS Consortium. Neurodevelopmental outcome at 2 years of age after general anesthesia and awake-regional anesthesia in infancy (GAS): an international multicentre, randomised controlled trial. Lancet. 2016;387(10015):239–50.

Should an Anxious Parent Be Allowed to Be Present for the Induction of Anesthesia in Her Child?

35

Paul A. Tripi and Mark M. Goldfinger

Case

Two attending pediatric anesthesiologists are colleagues in a busy pediatric operating room. Although a departmental policy exists that permits parental presence during induction of anesthesia (PPIA) in a child, they have very differing views on the effectiveness of this intervention for decreasing child anxiety and improving cooperation during induction. Because of these differences in viewpoint, one anesthesiologist, Dr. John Friendly, frequently allows PPIA, while the other, Dr. Michael Firm, avoids it in almost every case.

Dr. Firm is assigned to the urology room for the day and is caring for many children having minor ambulatory procedures. In the preoperative area, he meets Billy Whiner, who is scheduled to undergo an inguinal hernia repair, along with his mother. Both are very anxious about the upcoming surgery, and the mother insists on coming with Billy to the operating room (OR) until he is asleep. Dr. Firm responds that he can sedate Billy to reduce his anxiety and refuses mom's request to go with Billy on the grounds that it will be of no benefit. Mom angrily responds that she would like to have a different anesthesiologist who is willing to allow her to come to the operating room.

P.A. Tripi (✉)
Department of Anesthesiology and Perioperative Medicine, University Hospitals Case Medical Center, Rainbow Babies and Children's Hospital, 11100 Euclid Avenue, LKSD 2500, Cleveland, OH 44106-5007, USA
e-mail: Paul.Tripi@uhhospitals.org

M.M. Goldfinger
Department of Anesthesiology and Perioperative Medicine, University Hospitals Case Medical Center, Rainbow Babies and Children's Hospital, 11100 Euclid Avenue, LKSD 2526, Cleveland, OH 44106-5007, USA
e-mail: Mark.Goldfinger@uhhospitals.org

Question

Should an anxious parent be allowed to be present for the induction of anesthesia in her child?

Pro-Con Discussion

In an attempt to diffuse the situation, Dr. Firm responds to mom by telling her that he will discuss the case with his colleague, Dr. Friendly, who is also working in the surgery center that day. He manages to track down Dr. Friendly, who is between cases in his busy ear, nose, and throat (ENT) room.

Dr. Firm: Hey, John, I've got this anxious mother who is insisting on coming to the OR with her 6-year-old for an inguinal hernia repair. She is incredibly anxious, so I told her, "Absolutely not. I can sedate him to take away his anxiety." She is still insisting!

Dr. Friendly: I'm not surprised, Mike. You know it is natural for a parent to remain close to her child, especially during stressful situations.

Dr. Firm: Yes, John. No doubt that is true. But, the data are clear about anxious parents in the operating room. They are not any help and often can make the child even more anxious. For instance, Kain did a large prospective cohort study that reviewed much data from his prior studies. He showed that children who benefited from PPIA had calm rather than anxious parents [1]. Furthermore, Bevan showed that anxious parents can actually worsen a child's behavior during induction and make the child more upset than if the parent was not present [2].

Dr. Friendly: Just because the parent is anxious does not mean that you should always say "no" to the parent's request to come to the operating room. In that study by Kain you

C.S. Scher et al. (eds.), *You're Wrong, I'm Right*, DOI 10.1007/978-3-319-43169-7_35

mentioned, he showed that there were several factors other than a calmer parent associated with less anxious children during induction. These factors included older age, child temperament characterized by lower activity and impulsivity, and parental motivation to participate. The study also indicated that much of the variation in child anxiety and compliance could not be accounted for by any of these factors [1]. Refusing to allow PPIA can upset the parent, and we have entered the age of consumerism, where the satisfaction of the parent is very important. Parents generally have very positive attitudes about PPIA, and they will usually say "yes" when given a choice to participate [3]. A recent study looking at parental motivation to be present during induction confirmed parents' preference for this option and showed that being sensitive to the family's culture was also important [4]. I think it is imperative to consider how motivated the parent is to participate. In my own practice, I have allowed parents to participate in thousands of cases, and I have never had an adverse event.

Dr. Firm: Well, apparently you did not hear about that case from a couple of years ago. A mother was present during induction of her 7-year-old son for an umbilical herniorrhaphy, and she attempted to remove him from the induction room after he was fully anesthetized [5]! It turns out the OR team had noted that she was anxious, and she subsequently reported that the experience resurfaced traumatic memories. It does not seem worth the risk to ever let an anxious parent go to the OR.

Dr. Friendly: That was an unusual event that was the first of its kind reported in the literature. It just points out that it is important to carefully explain to a parent what she should expect during the induction. An extra person should be available to monitor the parent and escort her from the induction area after the child is anesthetized. Just as important, a departmental or hospital policy should be in place to identify the screening process for determining eligibility of patients, outline the procedures for educating parents, and identify steps in the process to make it as safe as possible.

Dr. Firm: I do not see why we do not just go ahead with sedation and skip parental presence in all cases. The literature is clear that premedication is more effective than parental presence to reduce child anxiety and improve cooperation during induction of anesthesia [6]. Oral midazolam has a long history as a safe and effective preoperative sedative for children, and newer agents such as dexmedetomidine are gaining in popularity and offer additional benefits such as improved analgesia [7].

Dr. Friendly: All drugs have adverse effects, and it would not be practical or economical to sedate every patient. I like to use a balanced approach to providing preoperative anxiolysis in children [8]. I draw on three major strategies to achieve anxiolysis: psychosocial preparation, PPIA, and premedication. Every patient should receive information and preparation based upon his psychological development and social interactions. With the help of the Child Life Service to provide some child-friendly preparation for mask induction, this may be all that is necessary to achieve a smooth induction of anesthesia. If your patient remains anxious, it is certainly reasonable to provide premedication, usually in a noninvasive fashion that avoids placing an IV in the awake child. A lot of times, the parent becomes less insistent on coming to the OR once she sees her child calm down with the sedation.

Dr. Firm: Why bother with parental presence in the OR once your patient is adequately sedated?

Dr. Friendly: There still may be some benefit, more so to the parent than the child. In 2000, Kain showed decreased parental anxiety and improved satisfaction when comparing parents who accompanied sedated children to the OR versus parents who did not [9]. Remember, it is the parent rather than the child who completes the follow-up satisfaction survey! Furthermore, in keeping with practicing family-centered care, I consider the parent to also be my patient.

Dr. Firm: Well, be my guest in taking this parent on as one of your patients. I still do not see any benefit to bringing that anxious parent to the OR.

Dr. Friendly: Mike, if you do not mind, I would be happy to take care of Billy. We can switch assignments for now, and trade back once the case is completed.

Summary

There is no right answer contained within this argument between Dr. Friendly and Dr. Firm. Views concerning parental presence vary widely among anesthesiologists, ranging from complete avoidance to liberal use of the intervention. There is general consensus that it is best avoided in certain situations, such as the anesthesia induction of a young infant or a child with anticipated airway management difficulties. Anesthesiologists should respect colleague's differing opinions and try to work within the framework of the departmental/hospital policy regarding parental presence. The ultimate goal for each patient is to provide adequate anxiolysis to achieve a smooth and safe induction of anesthesia.

References

1. Kain ZN, Mayes LC, Caldwell-Andrews AA, Saadat H, McClain B, Wang SM. Predicting which children benefit most from parental presence during induction of anesthesia. Pediatr Anesth. 2006;16:627–34.
2. Bevan JC, Johnston C, Haig MJ, Tousignant G, Lucy S, Kirnon V, et al. Preoperative parental anxiety predicts behavioural and emotional responses to induction of anaesthesia in children. Can J Anaesth. 1990;37(2):177–82.
3. Kain ZN, Caldwell-Andrews AA, Wang SM, Krivutza DM, Weinberg ME, Mayes LC. Parental intervention choices for children undergoing repeated surgeries. Anesth Analg. 2003;96(4):970–5.
4. Fortier MA, Gomez SH, Kain A. Motivation and parental presence during induction of anesthesia: an examination of the role of ethnicity and language. Pediatr Anaesth. 2012;22(11):1094–9.
5. Johnson YJ, Nickerson M, Quezado Z. An unforeseen peril of parental presence during induction of anesthesia. Anesth Analg. 2012;115(6):1371–2.
6. Kain ZN, Mayes LC, Wang SM, Caramico LA, Hofstadter MB. Parental presence during induction of anesthesia versus sedative premedication: which intervention is more effective? Anesthesiology. 1998;89(5):1147–56.
7. Pasin L, Febres D, Testa V, Frati E, Borghi G, Landoni G, et al. Dexmedetomidine vs midazolam as preanesthetic medication in children: a meta-analysis of randomized controlled trials. Paediatr Anaesth. 2015;25(5):468–76.
8. Tripi PA. Preoperative anxiolysis and sedation. In: Kaye AD, Fox CJ, Diaz JH, editors. Essentials of pediatric anesthesiology. Cambridge: Cambridge University Press; 2015. p. 315–22.
9. Kain ZN, Mayes LC, Wang SM, Caramico LA, Krivutza DM, Hofstadter MB. Parental presence and a sedative premedicant for children undergoing surgery: a hierarchical study. Anesthesiology. 2000;92(4):939–46.

What Is the Role of Premedication in the Pediatric Patient?

36

Elliot S. Schwartz and Anna Clebone

Case

A 5-year-old boy presents for surgery to repair a large inguinal hernia. The inguinal mass is reducible and enlarges when the boy coughs or cries. The boy has no nausea or vomiting and has been having normal bowel movements. The mass is not tender and there are no signs of inflammation.

As the anesthesiologist starts the preoperative evaluation, the child clings to his mother and starts crying. The parents state that they are very anxious as well.

Question

Should this child receive premedication with sedative drugs? If not, what are alternatives to premedication?

PRO: Many pediatric patients show signs of significant preoperative anxiety. Preoperative anxiety is associated with postoperative complications including higher levels of perceived pain, increased incidence of emergence delirium, and higher rates of postoperative maladaptive behaviors [1]. I use premedication with sedative drugs regularly because it reduces anxiety in children and their parents, shortens the time required for induction, and decreases the risk of negative psychological events after the surgery. Pharmacologic intervention is more effective and more cost sensitive than resource-intensive behavioral preparation programs. The ideal premedication has a rapid and reliable onset, a short duration of action, and minimal side effects. There is a range of options, but oral midazolam (0.5–1 mg/kg, 20 mg maximum) should be routinely administered in the pediatric patient as it comes closest to achieving this ideal profile. Maximum effect occurs after 15–20 min.

CON: A classic study in anesthesiology demonstrated that a preoperative visit from an anesthesiologist reduced anxiety to a greater extent than a sedative medication [2]. This study was done in adults, but the lesson here can also be applied to pediatrics in that there is no replacement for a thorough and thoughtful preoperative visit from an empathic anesthesiologist. This preoperative visit can reduce patient and parent anxiety by providing the details of what the patient and parent should expect and how the child's safety will be ensured. The more information and communication the better: videos, literature, and hospital tours can all reduce anxiety without any of the drawbacks of adverse effects from an additional medication. Additionally, many children respond positively to play therapy and parental presence during induction of anesthesia. An empathetic approach with the anxious patient makes the routine use of premedication unnecessary.

PRO: The development of midazolam has reshaped the approach to premedication because of its quick action and minimal effect on respiration. What are your concerns about the administration of midazolam?

CON: An ear tube surgery lasts 10 min; the effects of midazolam are obviously much longer. This likely contributes to increased rates of postoperative delirium and agitation in some premedicated patients, especially those treated during short procedures. In addition, paradoxical reactions have been noted where anxiety is actually increased after the administration of midazolam. Other

E.S. Schwartz
Department of Anesthesiology and Perioperative Medicine, University Hospital, Case Western Reserve University, 11100 Euclid Ave., Cleveland, OH 44106, USA

E.S. Schwartz (✉)
2022 Murray Hill Road, Apt 2, Cleveland, OH 44106, USA
e-mail: elliot.schwartz@case.edu

A. Clebone
Department of Anesthesia and Critical Care, The University of Chicago, 5841 S. Maryland Ave. MC-4028, Chicago, IL 60637, USA
e-mail: aclebone@gmail.com

A. Clebone
60 E Monroe no. 4703, Chicago, IL 60603, USA

C.S. Scher et al. (eds.), *You're Wrong, I'm Right*, DOI 10.1007/978-3-319-43169-7_36

factors that may limit its use include bad taste, burning sensation upon IV or nasal administration, and increased risk of hiccups [3]. What other medications do you use? It is essential to know that a syringe full of a premed may provoke as much anxiety as a mask induction.

PRO: Oral midazolam is the most widely used premedication, but there are many effective regimens. A smaller dose of midazolam, for example, can be used in conjunction with oral ketamine (4-6 mg/kg). Midazolam can also be administered orally, intramuscularly, intravenously, rectally, or nasally. As an alternative to a benzodiazepine, fentanyl (5-15 mcg/kg) can be administered even in the form of a lollipop or nasal sufentanil can be administered at a dose of 2 mcg/kg, although close monitoring is required due to the high risk of respiratory depression. Other alternatives that require more research include the alpha-2 adrenergic receptor agonist clonidine and dexmedetomidine, which may have the potential to reduce the risk of postoperative delirium and pain. Dexmedetomidine can be used both orally and nasally. The delayed onset of action of oral clonidine and the limited oral bioavailability of dexmedetomidine do limit their use (although a higher oral dose has been tried with some success). Unfortunately, a recent randomized controlled study using clonidine administered nasally showed that only about half of the children responded adequately 30 min following its administration [4].

CON: As the pharmacology evolves, so too does research into non-pharmacologic approaches to reduce anxiety. One study has demonstrated that an intensive family-centered preparatory program is as effective as midazolam [5]. The most important elements contributing to this reduction in anxiety in this preparatory program seemed to be prior education and exposure of the child to the anesthesia mask and parental use of distraction [6]. Other creative approaches to reduce anxiety include the use of clown doctors [7], web-based resources [8], and fish aquariums [9]. By whichever method, the goal is to create a family-friendly environment.

PRO: Some of the approaches listed are resource intensive and may not be feasible in a surgical facility that only occasionally has pediatric patients. My other concern is the child who initially responds well to these behavioral preparation programs, but suddenly becomes anxious as you enter the operating room. What are your non-pharmacologic approaches to the children that were calm in the presurgical area, but become terrified as you prepare for induction?

CON: For children that go from calm to terrified tears in the operating room, I first stop what I am doing and, if old enough to communicate with, I ask about their concerns. I provide reassurance that they will see their family after they awake and that they will not feel anything or remember anything from the procedure. I remind them that everything will be done to make sure that they are not in any pain after they wake up. If there is any specific misunderstanding, I clarify the process using concrete language. If the child asks for a parent to be present in the operating room, I honor the request. In some circumstances, having the child or adolescent hold the anesthesia mask provides a degree of control that can relieve anxiety.

PRO: What if after these attempts at relieving the child's anxiety, the patient continues to be hysterical and uncooperative?

CON: In our youngest patients, parental presence is often effective, possibly combined with premedication. If a school-age patient is still hysterical and inconsolable after every other avenue has been attempted, I would have a conversation with the parents about rescheduling the surgery or offering a premedication.

PRO: I am familiar with research showing that parents overwhelmingly want to be present for induction in the operating room [10], but realize this does not happen in the vast majority of cases. Are there any randomized controlled studies describing the usefulness of parental presence during induction?

CON: Parental presence in the operating room during induction remains controversial, especially among anesthesiologists in the USA. However, I have found parental presence provides another opportunity for reassurance during the most anxiety-provoking component of the patient's experience. The child can be reassured through eye contact and touch from the parent resulting in increased cooperation of the child. Randomized controlled studies have mixed results about the benefits of parental presence. For example, parental presence during anesthesia reduces the anxiety of the child compared to the level of anxiety in children without parents present, but this anxiolytic effect is less than the effect of children premedicated with midazolam [11]. Additionally, there may be no benefit to the child if the parent has a significant level of anxiety, and the benefit may vary based on the age of the patient [12].

CON: How would your approach differ based on the age of the patient?

PRO The typical 6-month-old infant will rarely require premedication as separation anxiety is not an issue at this age. However, in an older infant with separation anxiety, premedication should be routinely administered. From ages 2–5, the need for premedication is generally the highest.

Summary

Reducing anxiety in the preoperative period improves postoperative outcomes and parent satisfaction. Whether the goal of anxiety control is best achieved through premedication is still a matter of debate in the literature, and many in the USA regularly use premedication. A challenge in the research on premedication is the external validity of even the most rigorous studies. Expectations can play a crucial role in anxiety, and expectations can vary enormously among patients in different regions, countries, and cultures.

References

1. Kain ZN, Mayes LC, Caldwell-Andrews AA, Karas DE, McClain BC. Preoperative anxiety, postoperative pain, and behavioral recovery in young children undergoing surgery. Pediatrics. 2006;118(2):651–8.
2. Egbert LD, Battit GE, Turndorf H, Beecher HK. The value of the preoperative visit by an anesthetist. A study of doctor-patient rapport. JAMA. 1963;185(7):553–5.
3. Lönnqvist P-A, Habre W. Midazolam as premedication: Is the emperor naked or just half-dressed? Pediatr Anesth. 2005;15 (4):263–5.
4. Larsson P, Eksborg S, Lönnqvist P. Onset time for pharmacologic premedication with clonidine as a nasal aerosol: a double-blind, placebo-controlled, randomized trial. Pediatr Anesth. 2012;22 (9):877–83.
5. Kain ZN, Caldwell-Andrews AA, Mayes LC, Weinberg ME, Wang S-M, MacLaren JE, et al. Family-centered preparation for surgery improves perioperative outcomes in children: a randomized controlled trial. Anesthesiology. 2007;106(1):65–74.
6. Fortier MA, Blount RL, Wang S-M, Mayes LC, Kain ZN. Analysing a family-centred preoperative intervention programme: a dismantling approach. Br J Anaesth. 2011;106(5):713–8.
7. Vagnoli L, Caprilli S, Robiglio A, Messeri A. Clown doctors as a treatment for preoperative anxiety in children: a randomized, prospective study. Pediatrics. 2005;116(4):e563–7.
8. North I. Evaluation of a virtual tour for children undergoing same-day surgery and their parents. Pediatr Nurs. 2011;37 (4):177.
9. Sanchez M, Delpont M, Bachy M, Kabbaj R, Annequin D, Vialle R. How can surgeonfish help pediatric surgeons? A pilot study investigating the antinociceptive effect of fish aquariums in adult volunteers. Pain Res Manag. 2015;20(1):e28–32.
10. McEwen AW, Caldicott LD, Barker I. Parents in the anaesthetic room—parents' and anaesthetists' views. Anaesthesia. 1994;49 (11):987–90.
11. Kain ZN, Mayes LC, Wang SM, Caramico LA, Hofstadter MB. Parental presence during induction of anesthesia versus sedative premedication: which intervention is more effective? Anesthesiology. 1998;89(5):1147–56.
12. Kain ZN, Mayes LC, Caramico LA, Silver D, Spieker M, Nygren MM, et al. Parental presence during induction of anesthesia. A randomized controlled trial. Anesthesiology. 1996;84(5): 1060–7.

Presence of Family Members in the Operating Room: Is This Really Helpful? 37

Michelle N. Gonta and Misuzu Kameyama

Case

A 3-year-old boy presents to the ambulatory surgery unit of a large city hospital for a bilateral tonsillectomy and adenoidectomy for mild sleep apnea and snoring. He was born full term with no other medical history. While discussing the anesthetic plan for inhalational induction using a mask, the child's mother interrupts and states that she heard from friends of hers that she would be able to stay with her child while he went to sleep. The child seems uncomfortable with your presence and clings to his mother's leg. You feel that it would be appropriate for the mother to accompany her child to the operating room given the child's clear discomfort with strangers; however, your supervising anesthesiologist, who comes from an institution that never allows parents in the operating room, does not agree.

Question

Is the presence of family members in the operating room really helpful in easing the child's anxiety?

PRO Given the child's anxiety, there is clearly an advantage to allowing the parent to be present for induction. There is a significant negative correlation [1] between age and anxiety. Children who are younger are much more anxious during induction of anesthesia than older children. In this particular study, the mean age for the most anxiety was 2.6 years old, so this child is of the appropriate age to receive the most benefit.

M.N. Gonta (✉) · M. Kameyama
Department of Anesthesiology, Perioperative Care and Pain Medicine, New York University Langone Medical Center, 550 First Avenue, TH530, New York, NY 10016, USA
e-mail: michelle.gonta@med.nyu.edu

M. Kameyama
e-mail: misuzu.kameyama@med.nyu.edu

CON It's true that younger children experience more anxiety, but often this is a result of the anxiety of their parents. Children of calm parents are less anxious during induction of anesthesia, whether the parent is present or not. Children of anxious parents were more anxious when their parent was present during induction. Another randomized controlled trial [2] found that serum cortisol was decreased in children aged >4 with a parent with a low anxiety level. These were the only children found to benefit strongly from parental presence during induction of anesthesia. Further, this study found that children aged <4 were more anxious when the parent was present during induction of anesthesia.

PRO You concede that the findings of this study strongly argue against bringing the parents of this child into the operating room, especially given that his mother does appear to be quite anxious. However, the child is also very anxious and has now started to cry. You suggest premedicating the child with midazolam 0.5 mg/kg, but the patient's mother says that her presence is all the child needs and she doesn't want her kid to get more medicine.

CON Your attending explains to the parents that a study [3] compared parental presence to midazolam premedication to no intervention and found that while there were no differences in the child's anxiety among the three groups in the preoperative holding area, on separation from the parents it was found that the children in the midazolam group exhibited significantly less anxiety than both the parental presence group and the no intervention group. The group of children that received midazolam was also found to have the least anxiety overall on entry into the operating room and application of the anesthesia mask. The children who were premedicated with midazolam were also found to be more compliant during induction of anesthesia.

PRO The child's parents agree to premedicate the child and not accompany the child to the operating room until the child's uncle bursts into the room and states that he heard

C.S. Scher et al. (eds.), *You're Wrong, I'm Right*, DOI 10.1007/978-3-319-43169-7_37

other parents speaking in the waiting room about the possibility of having clowns accompany their child and thinks that clowns should be considered to ease the child's anxiety. The parents now would like to know if they could once again forgo the midazolam premedication and simply have a clown join them and their child in the operating room.

CON You defer to your attending for a response, as you have never seen clowns in the hospital and certainly not in the operating room. Your attending cites a recently published study [4] that compared the anxiety of children in three unique groups: (1) a clown group, which consisted of two clowns and a parent accompanying the child; (2) a premedication group, which consisted of midazolam premedication as well as a parent accompanying the child to the operating room and through induction; and (3) a control group in which the child was simply accompanied to the operating room by one parent. Your attending states that the results of this study showed that the level of anxiety was significantly lower in the clown group compared to the premedication group at the time of induction of anesthesia, and the level of anxiety in the control group was significantly higher compared to both the premedication and clown group. The level of anxiety in the waiting area showed no significant differences across the three groups. A related study [5] also looked at the effect of clowns versus hand-held video games on children's preoperative anxiety and found that clowns were more effective than video games at reducing the patient's apprehension. While these studies seem to indicate that the distraction component the clowns provide plus the presence of a parent at induction was the most effective at reducing the child's anxiety, it is important to note that this was never compared to midazolam alone, which in prior studies was shown to be more effective than parental presence. Further, these studies looked at children ages 5–12, which represents an older age group than this particular 3-year-old patient. Therefore, applying these results to this patient may end up heightening his anxiety.

PRO The patient's parents agree to proceed without a clown or their presence in the operating room, and with a midazolam premedication following the extensive advice of your attending. The induction is uneventful and the child is cooperative, even holding the mask himself for the inhalational induction. The case proceeds without incident, and the parents happily meet their sleeping child in the recovery room.

Summary

Nearly every child having a surgical procedure experiences some level of anxiety regarding entering the operating room and induction of anesthesia. Whether utilizing midazolam, calm parental presence, or even introducing clowns and other distraction techniques into the mix, it is our opinion that decreasing the patient's anxiety with whatever techniques are currently available at your institution should be the goal of the pediatric anesthesiologist, whenever safe and feasible.

References

1. Kain ZN, Mayes LC, Caldwell-Andrews AA, Saadat H, McClain B, Wang SM. Predicting which children benefit most from parental presence during induction of anesthesia. Paediatr Anaesth. 2006;16:627–34.
2. Kain ZN, Mayes LC, Caramico LA, Silver DM, Spieker M, Nygren MM, Anderson G, Rimar S. Parental presence during induction of anesthesia: a randomized control trial. Anesthesiology. 1996;84:1060–7.
3. Kain ZN, Mayes LC, Wang SM, Caramico LA. Parental presence during induction of anesthesia versus sedative premedication. Anesthesiology. 1998;89:1147–56.
4. Vagnoli L, Caprilli S, Messeri A. Parental presence, clowns, or sedative premedication to treat preoperative anxiety in children: what could be the most promising option? Paediatr Anaesth. 2010;20:937–43.
5. Messina M, Molinaro F, Meucci D, Angotti R, Giuntini L, Cerchia E, Bulotta AL, Brandigi E. Preoperative distraction in children: hand-held videogames vs clown therapy. Pediatr Med Chir. 2014;36:203–6.

Is It Appropriate for Complicated Pediatric Surgical Patients to Receive Care Outside of Specialized Pediatric Centers?

38

Mark M. Goldfinger and Paul Tripi

Case

The annual American Society of Anesthesiologists (ASA) meeting is a great place to assemble with colleagues and reacquaint with friends from the past. Sherry and I hadn't seen each other since we graduated medical school 20 years ago. We walked to the Ether Pub, est. 1846, in the French Quarter, New Orleans, Louisiana, hoping to reminisce over 2 Moscow Mules. They were closed for renovations so we went to Café Du Monde, est. 1862, instead. We then began to chat over café au lait with chicory. Little did I know that she was a practicing anesthesiologist at St. Elsewhere, 60 miles from the Children's Hospital where I practice in Ohio. She elaborated on how she loves living near the Amish countryside. "My son and daughter ride our horses on 10 acres of land," she commented with a smile. Thinking of a quick retort I said, "My kids practice their unicycle riding in the hallway of our penthouse."

After completing an anesthesiology residency program, Sherry went to work at a community hospital in rural Ohio. As a fellowship-trained board-certified pediatric anesthesiologist, I was curious to know if she had done any interesting pediatric cases at her hospital.

"Well, yes," she said with a furrowed brow. "Last month there was a 4-week-old baby born at home and subsequently admitted to our community hospital with a diagnosis of pyloric stenosis. We thought about shipping the baby out, but after adequate rehydration and appropriate electrolyte data he was booked for a pyloromyotomy. I hadn't cared for an infant in a while but when the child's mother said, 'Take care of my baby,' I knew that I was destined to be that child's anesthesiologist. Besides, we have a general surgeon who's really good with his hands," Sherry commented.

M.M. Goldfinger (✉) · P. Tripi
Department of Anesthesiology and Perioperative Medicine, University Hospitals Case Medical Center, Rainbow Babies and Children's Hospital, Euclid Avenue, LKSD 2526, Cleveland, OH 44106-5007, USA
e-mail: Mark.Goldfinger@uhhospitals.org

P. Tripi
e-mail: Paul.Tripi@uhhospitals.org

Question

Should this baby receive care in a community hospital?

PRO (Sherry) It's a question of supply and demand. For many decades, children have been cared for in community hospitals. With more than 5 million operations performed annually on children in the USA, there just aren't enough pediatric-trained anesthesiologists and surgeons to attend to every case. There are an estimated 800 practicing pediatric general surgeons in the USA [1]. The overall ratio of pediatric general surgeons to the pediatric population 0–17 years is 1/108,000. In the year 2000, there were no pediatric general surgeons in the states of Montana, Idaho, Wyoming, and North Dakota.

CON (I) There may be a shortage of specialists, but patient safety must trump other concerns.

"Is it safe to anesthetize children at community hospitals?" I asked.

"Yes. We have a long track record at our hospital in Ohio," Sherry said. "And so do other states." she added. "I know what you're thinking, but the reported anesthetic-related death of a 19-month-old at a California community hospital was the first such death in 16 years at that institution as reported by the *Los Angeles Times*" [2].

"True, it's rare," I said, "but if that's your child, the fact that the devastating event is rare won't make a difference, much less bring back the child."

PRO (Sherry) "Well how about cost? In this country we are experiencing the Patient Protection and Affordable Care Act ('Obamacare'), along with its complexities and myriad ramifications. There is a study that demonstrates that the cost of a pyloromyotomy is lowest at a general hospital ($10,197) as compared to a children's hospital ($11,160) or a children's

C.S. Scher et al. (eds.), *You're Wrong, I'm Right*, DOI 10.1007/978-3-319-43169-7_38

unit within a general hospital ($12,284) [3]. We must also consider convenience. In my experience, families prefer being close to home. When visiting a loved one at a hospital, they don't want to travel long distances, especially through heavy traffic in the big cities. If they forget something at home they can easily retrieve it. If transportation is an issue, it is generally less costly to travel a shorter distance."

CON (I) "That may be true, but again the value of a life is priceless. A group at UCLA reported that infants treated at community hospitals for pyloric stenosis experienced an increased likelihood of surgical complications. Complications include viscous perforation, postoperative infection, and small bowel obstruction. This must drive up costs considerably" [4].

PRO (Sherry) "Well, another complication looked at in that paper includes readmission to the same or a different hospital. As it turns out, hospital type and volume did not impact the 30-day readmission rate (3.4 %). By the way, the most common diagnosis on readmission was electrolyte imbalance/dehydration and respiratory illness. We are prepared to treat both of those."

CON (I) "What we really want to focus on though is safety. Adverse events in younger children are a universal concern. In Japan, critical incidents such as laryngospasm and hypotension are 4 times more common during an anesthetic in infants younger than 1 year [5]. The Hellenic Society of Anesthesiology in Greece recommends that children under 3 years of age undergoing a surgical procedure be transported to specialized centers [6]. Authors in France recommend that a minimum case load of 200 pediatric anesthetics (per group per year) is necessary to reduce the incidence of complications in children [7]. Are you really prepared to treat an infant who has a cardiac arrest from massive hemorrhage (and hypovolemia) or hyperkalemia (related to the transfusion of stored blood)? According to The Pediatric Peri-Operative Cardiac Arrest (POCA) registry, these cardiovascular causes are the most common reasons for cardiac arrest, at least since we got rid of halothane" [8].

PRO (Sherry) "Let me tell you about my case. I proceeded with intravenous administration of atropine, suctioning of the infant's stomach, preoxygenation, and a rapid sequence induction. The circulating nurse's cell phone rang while she was holding cricoid pressure, and the nurse stepped away to answer. At that point in time, the patient vomited his stomach contents. His head was bathed in a soupy mix and my hands were slipping as I attempted laryngoscopy. The last oxygen saturation number I noticed was 58 %. After quickly suctioning the baby's mouth with a yankauer and drying off the baby's face, I intubated the baby with a 3.5 mm microcuff endotracheal tube. The SaO_2 rose to 97 %. The baby was extubated at the end of the case and did just fine. Does this happen at your hospital?"

CON (I) "Yes. But, at an academic center there are more skilled people around to deal with complications. For instance, it's more likely that someone experienced in holding cricoid pressure would be available. There are numerous personnel to intubate if the laryngoscopist fails, or to start a new intravenous line if the existing one infiltrates. Attendings, fellows, residents, and anesthetists to name a few. If the baby requires tertiary level care postoperatively due to aspiration pneumonia, as an example, we have a pediatric intensive care unit (PICU) and level IV neonatal intensive care unit (NICU). Consultants such as pediatric pulmonologists are readily available. We don't have to worry about transporting the baby to another medical facility. Sherry, how would you have transported your patient to a tertiary care facility if needed?"

PRO (Sherry) "By ambulance. The family would have followed by horse and buggy as their driver was ill at the time."

"Let's take a closer look at your world of pediatric anesthesiology. I've been doing some reading on this topic since my soupy mix case. Pediatric anesthesiology has only relatively recently been formalized as a unique specialty. The Society for Pediatric Anesthesia (SPA) formed in 1987. In 1997 the Accreditation Council for Graduate Medical Education (ACGME) recognized pediatric anesthesia as a subspecialty. There are currently 42 accredited fellowship programs. In 2013 the American Board of Anesthesiology (ABA) administered the first examination offering the opportunity for interested candidates to become board certified in pediatric anesthesiology. After the 2013 and 2014 exam administration there are 2214 board certified physicians in this field. Again, there clearly aren't enough specialists to cover the pediatric surgical population in the United States."

CON (I) "Well let's look at the difference in training between *generalists* and *specialists*. The pediatric requirement per the ACGME for anesthesia residents during their training mandates caring for 100 patients younger than 12 years of age. Within this group, 20 children must be younger than 3 years of age, including 5 that are younger than 3 months of age. This means, Sherry, that you may never have taken care of a 1-month-old in training, much less a 1-month-old with a full stomach like the patient with pyloric stenosis. In contrast, Pediatric Anesthesia fellows must care for 75 children between the ages of 3 and 11, 40 children between the ages of 1 and 2, 40 infants between the ages of 1 month and 11 months, and 15 neonates. I would respectfully argue that caring for the minimum of 55 (40 + 15) infants and neonates will prepare a specialist well when presented with the opportunity to care for a 1-month-old with pyloric stenosis. Next time put the neonate in an ambulance and have him transported from St. Elsewhere in Amish country to our tertiary Children's Hospital."

PRO (Sherry) "What about *surgical* training?"

CON (I) "Well, per the ACGME, general surgical residents must perform 750 cases during their training. Pediatric surgery is one of the essential content areas that is emphasized amongst a host of other areas. Pediatric surgical fellows in comparison must document 800 major pediatric surgical procedures during their 24-month program. In addition, Sherry, did you know that the ASA has published a statement on practice recommendations for pediatric anesthesia? This was approved by the ASA House of Delegates on October 19, 2011. Under sections 3, 3.2 it states: '...it is suggested that anesthesiologists providing and/or directly supervising the anesthetic care of patients in the categories designated by the facility's department of anesthesiology as being at increased risk for anesthetic complications should be graduates of pediatric anesthesiology fellowship training programs accredited by the ACGME.'" [9].

PRO (Sherry) "Yes I did. But, did YOU know that the same paragraph you quote continues to state that '...or should be fully credentialed members of the department of anesthesiology who have demonstrated continuous competence in the care of such patients as determined by the department of anesthesiology'? I am one of those members. And I'm not sure that a perfectly healthy full-term baby with pyloric stenosis would even be considered at increased risk for anesthetic complications."

CON (I) "Soupy mix. Soupy mix. The plague of the first-born male. In March 2014, the American College of Surgeons published guidelines that define the resources that surgical facilities need for safe care of infants and children [10]. The upshot is that there are 3 tiers of children's surgical care. Level I is comprehensive care at the highest level, including complex surgical procedures and children with severe illness. This necessitates *pediatric* surgeons and anesthesiologists as well as a level IV NICU. Level II is advanced surgical care in children with moderate risk medical conditions. This level also necessitates a facility staffed with pediatric surgeons and anesthesiologists as well as a Level III NICU. Level III is basic surgical care. This involves low-risk surgical procedures in children older than 1 year who are otherwise healthy. A *general* surgeon and anesthesiologist are adequate at this level. No NICU is necessary, but the facility must have the ability to stabilize and transfer the patient to a Level I or II facility. I think St. Elsewhere would be a Level III facility. This means that performing an inguinal hernia repair on a healthy 2-year-old would be appropriate."

PRO (Sherry) "Now that you mention it, I did read an article in the *Wall Street Journal* that relates a story about a child having surgery and summarizes the 3 levels" [11].

I ordered a beignet drizzled with dark chocolate for Sherry. We left Café Du Monde, hailed a cab back to the convention center and arrived just in time for the inaugural ASA apple bobbing contest. Sherry joined the rural anesthesiologist group while I connected with the urban group.

References

1. American College of Surgeons Health Policy Research Institute. The surgical workforce in the united states: profile and recent trends. Chapel Hill: American College of Surgeons Health Policy Research Institute; April 2010. p 25.
2. Ornstein C. Infant anesthesia problems spark debate. Los Angeles Times. 24 Feb 2003.
3. Raval MV, Cohen ME, Barsness KA, Bentrem DJ, Phillips JD, Reynolds M. Does hospital type affect pyloromyotomy outcomes? Analysis of the Kids' Inpatient Database. Surgery. 2010;148 (2):411–9.
4. Kelley-Quon LI, Tseng CH, Jen HC, Shew SB. Hospital type predicts surgical complications for infants with hypertrophic pyloric stenosis. Am Surg. 2012;78:1079–82.
5. Morita K, Kawashima Y, Irita K, Kobayayashi T, Goto Y, Iwao Y, et al. Committee on Operating Room Safety of Japanese Society of Anesthesiologists. [Perioperative mortality and morbidity in 1999 with a special reference to age in 466 certified training hospitals of Japanese Society of Anesthesiologists—report of Committee on Operating Room Safety of Japanese Society of Anesthesiologists]. Masui. 2001;50(8):909–21 (Japanese).
6. Malissiova A, Papageorgiou-Brousta M, Anagnostidou A, Georgoussi S, Sfira E. Hellenic Society of Anaesthesiology. Guidelines for the perioperative pediatric anesthesia environment. http://anaesthesiology.gr/media/File/pdf/GL22.pdf.
7. Auroy Y, Ecoffey C, Messiah A, Rouvier B. Relationship between complications of pediatric anesthesia and volume of pediatric anesthetics. Anesth Analg. 1997;84:234–5.
8. Bhananker SM, Ramamoorthy C, Geiduschek JM, Posner KL, Domino KB, Haberkern CM, et al. Anesthesia related cardiac arrest in children: update from the Pediatric Perioperative Cardiac Arrest Registry. Anesth Analg. 2007;105(2):344–50.
9. American Society of Anesthesiologists. Committee of Origin: Pediatric Anesthesia. Statement on practice recommendations for pediatric anesthesia. Approved by the ASA House of delegates on October 19, 2011. http://www.asahq.org/quality-and-practice-management/standards-and-guidelines.
10. Task Force for Children's Surgical Care. Optimal resources for children's surgical care in the United States. J Am Coll Surg. 2014 Mar;218(3):479–87.
11. Landro L. Programs aim to standardize surgical care for children. Wall Street J. 2 Sept 2014.

Are the Transfusion Goals for a Premature Infant the Same As for a 7-Year-Old?

39

Olga N. Albert

Case

A 26-week-old ex-28-week premature infant presents for the resection of a congenital pulmonary adenomatous malformation (CPAM). He is intubated and sedated in the Neonatal Intensive Care Unit (NICU). You notice that the patient's hemoglobin is 7 and his hematocrit is 21. The NICU fellow giving you the report informs you that in preparation for the upcoming surgery the patient was transfused with fresh frozen plasma "just to give him volume" (which doesn't seem like a good reason to you) and is ready for the operation. You tell the fellow that this critically ill neonate needs to have hemoglobin of at least 10.

He disagrees, stating, "This infant has physiologic anemia of prematurity, which can be well tolerated. In premature infants, this occurs at an earlier post-conceptual age than in full term neonates. He is no different then a 7-year-old going for surgery."

Question

Should anemia be treated differently in the preemie than in the older child?

CON Until recently, transfusion guidelines for children were based on experiences with adults. In a 2007 Canadian study, investigators found that stable critically ill children can tolerate hemoglobin of 7 and a hematocrit of 21 without any sequelae [1]. These findings were similar to results published in an earlier adult Intensive Care Unit study [2]. The PINT (Premature Infants in Need for a Transfusion) study determined that a restrictive transfusion policy did not result in a higher incidence of death, neurodevelopmental impairment, or significant visual or hearing deficits in preemies [3]. "So your patient does not need to be transfused, he is ready," the fellow insists.

PRO "I would disagree," you say. "In the PINT study, if ventilatory support needed to be escalated to provide adequate oxygenation, then a transfusion was given [3]. In patients needing an increasing level of ventilator support, some centers have adopted guidelines to transfuse to a hemoglobin of 10 and hematocrit of 30. And why not?! The risks of transfusion today are very low across all age groups."

CON "But there is more to consider," the fellow replies. "Risks of transfusion can be much higher in the premature neonate, including developing a CMV infection; transfusion-associated graft-versus-host disease, necrotizing enterocolitis, and even severe intraventricular hemorrhage (from the solute load in the blood-product preservative). Transfusion-related hyperkalemia and resulting cardiac arrest is well documented in the infant and child. In addition, several retrospective studies show that transfusion of PRBCs carries an increased risk of neurocognitive abnormalities in preemies and is linked to chronic lung disease and retinopathy of prematurity [4]."

PRO "You aren't considering the risks of inadequate oxygen delivery," you point out to the fellow. "The major reason for the PRBC transfusion is to increase oxygen delivery to the tissues (DO_2). As you may recall if you paid any attention in med school physiology, this is defined as the product of cardiac output (CO) and arterial oxygen content (CaO_2). So,

$$DO_2 = CO \times CaO_2.$$

The arterial oxygen content is dependent upon the hemoglobin concentration, arterial oxygen saturation (SaO_2), oxygen-carrying capacity of hemoglobin (1.34 mL/gm

O.N. Albert (✉)
Department of Anesthesiology, Perioperative and Pain Medicine, Stanford University Medical Center, 300 Pasteuer Drive, Suite H3689, Stanford, CA 94305, USA
e-mail: olabert@stanford.edu

C.S. Scher et al. (eds.), *You're Wrong, I'm Right*, DOI 10.1007/978-3-319-43169-7_39

hemoglobin), and to a minor extent, the partial pressure of oxygen (PaO_2). So,

$$CaO_2 = (Hb \times 1.34 \times SaO_2) + (PaO_2 \times 0.003).$$

Oxygen supply can be increased by increasing cardiac output, arterial oxygen saturation, or hemoglobin concentration. Hemoglobin concentration is the major player in this equation. I agree that currently there are not any good biomarkers for measuring oxygen delivery to the tissue. However, I still think this preterm infant should be transfused."

CON "Well, to really improve quality of life in premature neonates, one must consider treatment with erythropoietin or darbepoetin, not a transfusion. In a prospective, randomized, blinded, multicenter study evaluating the effect of erythropoietin versus darbepoetin on neurodevelopmental outcomes of preterm infants, Ohls et al. showed that treated patients had significantly higher composite cognitive scores and higher language scores, with results approaching statistical significance. The patients in the treatment group were exposed to fewer transfusions, which could have been the reason for their better neurodevelopmental outcome [5]."

PRO "I agree that erythropoietin is a great idea, but one can't always wait for 4–6 weeks before surgery for this medication to work. Furthermore, I am worried that this preterm is ill equipped to handle blood loss during surgery. In healthy adult volunteers, Weiskopf et al. [6] showed that reduction of hemoglobin to 6 g/dl leads to reversible intellectual impairment: both increases in reaction time and impairments in early and late memory. This trend also held true in premature neonates. In a study by van Hoften et al. improved cerebral oxygen saturation occurred with transfusion at or below a hemoglobin level of 6 g/dl [7]. The implication is that overly restrictive transfusion guidelines may impair adequate cerebral oxygenation in patients regardless of age."

Summary

Although many transfusion principles are similar for premature infants and older children, there are multiple differences as well. Premature neonates need CMV-negative, leukocyte-reduced, and irradiated blood. Premature infants with respiratory insufficiency may also require transfusion. Unique risks with transfusion certainly exist for the premature infant, and these must be weighed against the benefits on a case-by-case basis.

References

1. Lacroix J, Hébert PC, Hutchison JS, Hume HA, Tucci M, Ducruet T, TRIPICU Investigators, Canadian Critical Care Trials Group, Pediatric Acute Lung Injury and Sepsis Investigators Network, et al. Transfusion strategies for patients in pediatric intensive care units. N Engl J Med. 2007;356:1609–19.
2. Hébert PC, Wells G, Blajchman MA, Marshall J, Martin C, Pagliarello G, Transfusion Requirements in Critical Care Investigators, Canadian Critical Care Trials Group, et al. A multicenter, randomized, controlled clinical trial of transfusion requirements in critical care. N Engl J Med. 1999;340(6):409–17.
3. Kirpalani H, Whyte RK, Andersen C, Asztalos EV, Heddle N, Blajchman MA, et al. The premature infants in need of transfusion (PINT) study: a randomized, controlled trial of restrictive (low) versus liberal (high) transfusion threshold for extremely low birth weight infants. J Pediatr. 2006;149:301–7.
4. Aher SM, Ohlsson A. Late erythropoetin for preventing red blood cell transfusion in preterm and/or low birth weight infants. Cochrane Database Syst Rev. 2014;4:CD004868.
5. Ohls RK, Kamath-Rayne BD, Christensen RD, Wiedmeier SE, Rosenberg A, Fuller J, et al. Cognitive outcomes of preterm infants randomized to darbepoetin, erythropoietin or placebo. Pediatrics. 2014;133:1023–30.
6. Weiskopf RB, Kramer JH, Viele M, Neumann M, Feiner JR, Watson JJ, Hopf HW, Toy P. Acute severe isovolemic anemia impairs cognitive function and memory in humans. Anesthesiology. 2000;92(6):1646–52.
7. van Hoften JCR, Verhagen EA, Keating P. Cerebral tissue oxygen saturation and extraction in preterm infants before and after blood transfusion. Arch Dis Child Fetal Neonatat. 2010;95:F352–8.

How Should You Get the Autistic Child into the Operating Room When the Mother Objects to Intramuscular Ketamine?

40

Glenn E. Mann and Jerry Y. Chao

Case

Freddy is a 15-year-old autistic obese teenager who presents for elective circumcision due to phimosis. His mother is present in the preoperative area and is quite concerned about the induction of anesthesia. Her friend, who also has an autistic child, told her that Freddy will have to have an intramuscular injection of medicine in order to "go to sleep" for surgery. Based on prior experiences at the dentist's office the mother explains that as soon as someone comes near him with a needle he becomes agitated; using a needle for induction of anesthesia would be challenging. When you go to see Freddy he is sitting in a chair with his mother and sister at his side. As you approach him, Freddy gets up and tries to walk out, but his mother tells him to sit down again. He seems to listen to her directions well.

Your colleague says to you, "Better go get the ketamine dart ready!"

Question

You are now considering the various options for anesthetic management of a patient with autism. How can one safely induce general anesthesia for this patient while being mindful and sensitive to the needs of Freddy's family?

Autism spectrum disorder (ASD) is characterized by a wide range of social and communication disabilities that can encompass repetitive behaviors and interests, sensory issues, phobias, and in some cases severe cognitive delay. The ability of these patients to perform activities of daily living may be severely impaired. Patients with ASD can be hypersensitive to situations or activities that bring them discomfort and provoke fearful and sometimes aggressive behavior. Fortunately, there are often simple interventions that evoke more calming reactions. While cognitively impaired, patients with ASD are aware of unfamiliar surroundings and can be shy and fearful of strangers, especially if they have had prior traumatic encounters. It will be important to have a discussion with the family about options for thoughtful care in the perioperative setting.

PRO Freddy is very aware of his surroundings and appears quite afraid of the medical staff. If he is approached with a needle, he will likely become aggressive and combative. We will need to enlist the help of his mother, his sister, and our child life specialist. They will be important in assessing Freddy's needs and can help determine alternative techniques we can employ to desensitize Freddy to the perioperative environment. Hopefully, during this time of non-threatening interaction we can gain some insight into what he will tolerate. Perhaps he will eventually accept brief periods of mask placement.

CON This is going to take a lot of time to assess and may delay other scheduled cases. It also seems like an excessive effort given how safe a ketamine injection is as a first-line sedative. It has favorable properties of sedation, analgesia, and amnesia. In high enough doses it can be used to induce general anesthesia. Ketamine has a rapid onset and a predictable duration of action, generally preserves airway patency and spontaneous breathing with little impact on functional residual capacity, and avoids cardiovascular compromise [1]. Why would you want to try any other strategy with this patient?

PRO While these are positive pharmacologic features, ketamine also has adverse properties such as increased salivation, hallucinations, hyperventilation, random limb movements, and emergence reactions, especially after short surgical procedures [1]. Not to mention that traumatizing

G.E. Mann (✉) · J.Y. Chao
Department of Anesthesiology, Montefiore Medical Center, The University Hospital for Albert Einstein College of Medicine, 111 East 210th Street, Bronx, NY 10467, USA
e-mail: gmann@montefiore.org

J.Y. Chao
e-mail: jechao@montefiore.org

C.S. Scher et al. (eds.), *You're Wrong, I'm Right*, DOI 10.1007/978-3-319-43169-7_40

Freddy with a needle also may have consequences. He could have behavioral disturbances that last for days or weeks after today's procedure as a result of our interaction. And all future encounters with medical professionals could be negatively impacted as well. Using desensitization techniques can greatly benefit our patient and his family. The benefits of involving a skilled child life specialist cannot be overstated, and close participation and investment of the primary caretaker(s) are crucial in this endeavor.

Early engagement by the child life specialist and demonstration of the use of medical equipment such as the pulse oximeter probe, blood pressure cuff, and anesthesia mask in a non-threatening, playful setting have been shown to be of real benefit [2]. Role playing and distraction with electronic media (tablet computer, video game console, etc.) have also been shown to decrease anxiety and ease induction [3]. These strategies have also been shown to reduce emergence delirium, decrease analgesic requirements, and improve parental satisfaction with the perioperative experience [4].

Of course, I acknowledge that for patients with developmental delay, behavioral interventions may be of variable benefit. But, surprising Freddy with a ketamine "dart" likely will make him more mistrustful of healthcare workers in the future and could lead postoperatively to the development of post-traumatic stress disorder symptoms such as nightmares, increased aggression, increased anxiety, eating problems, and withdrawal [5]. Anesthetic management can have far-reaching consequences beyond the immediate perioperative period.

CON Are you not concerned that Freddy could put himself and the providers taking care of him in danger by becoming aggressive with everyone?

PRO I am very concerned about self-injurious behavior as well as risk to nurses, physicians, and support staff. If behavioral interventions alone are ineffective, we can give him oral midazolam, which has been shown to be a highly effective anxiolytic. After oral premedication, Freddy may allow examination of his arms for candidate veins with the participation and engagement of his primary caretaker and the child life staff. Application of a eutectic mixture of local anesthesia (EMLA) cream may also be possible before or after oral midazolam. Freddy may tolerate venipuncture with oral premedication, distraction, and/or EMLA cream. This approach allows for the possibility of an intravenous induction of anesthesia as opposed to intramuscular injection or inhalational induction. There is also evidence supporting the use of intranasal dexmedetomidine for sedation [6]. Only after we have exhausted these possibilities and Freddy remains a risk to himself and the staff would I agree to intramuscular ketamine. I view this induction technique as a strategy of last resort.

Summary

Successful anesthetic induction of the developmentally delayed and potentially combative child requires a true multidisciplinary effort and the foresight and leadership of the anesthesiologist and allied staff. Educated primary caretakers should be empowered to take on a significant role in the induction of their child as well. Early desensitization, observing what the patient will allow, well-timed distraction, and pharmacologic interventions may all be of benefit in contributing to a safe and smooth induction. Indeed, there are many alternative approaches to the induction of anesthesia in these challenging situations. The "ketamine dart" is but one of those alternatives and in our view should be the anesthesiologist's last resort.

References

1. Haas DA, Harper DG. Ketamine: a review of its pharmacologic properties and use in ambulatory anesthesia. Anesth Prog. 1992;39:61–8.
2. Brewer S, Gleditsch SL, Syblik D, Tietjens ME, Vacik HW. Pediatric anxiety: child life intervention in day surgery. J Pediatr Nurs. 2006;21:13–22.
3. Patel A, Schieble T, Davidson M, Tran MC, Schoenberg C, Delphin E, Bennett H. Distraction with a hand-held video game reduces pediatric preoperative anxiety. Paediatr Anaesth. 2006;16:1019–27.
4. Kain ZN, Caldwell-Andrews AA. Preoperative psychological preparation of the child for surgery: an update. Anesthesiol Clin N Am. 2005;23:597–614.
5. Kain ZN, Caldwell-Andrews AA, Maranets I, McClain B, Gaal D, Mayes LC, Feng R, Zhang H. Preoperative anxiety and emergence delirium and postoperative maladaptive behaviors. Anesth Analg. 2004;99:1648–54.
6. Jia JE, Chen JY, Hu X, Li WX. A randomised study of intranasal dexmedetomidine and oral ketamine for premedication in children. Anaesthesia. 2013;68:944–9. doi:10.1111/anae.12312.

Is "Deep" Extubation Preferable in Patients at Risk for Bronchospasm?

41

Manoj Dalmia

Case

You walk up to your next patient, a slim 10-year-old boy, as his clubbed fingernails rapidly pound away at a keyboard, his eyes fixated on the screen. You sigh, recognizing this physical examination sign of chronic hypoxia (the fingers, not the video game addiction). As you suspect, he has cystic fibrosis complicated by recurrent lung infections and failure to thrive. He is scheduled for a soft tissue mass excision of the lower back. The parents are unsurprisingly nervous though the child is relatively calm. You introduce yourself to the child who shakes your hand but then immediately goes back to his game, pausing briefly first to cough up a tissue full of phlegm. The parents explain to you that he had a recent bronchial infection (on day 5 of 7 of antibiotics) that is now just resolving but is, unfortunately, par for the course. The patient is very compliant with his inhaler use. The parents are just as concerned as you about the increased pulmonary risks associated with general endotracheal anesthesia and recent lower respiratory infection, especially in light of his cystic fibrosis; however, this surgery has been cancelled twice already, and their son never seems to have a clear window to have the procedure done. In addition, the mass is deep and painful to lie on, and the surgeon states it cannot be done under local anesthesia. After a detailed discussion involving the parents and surgeon, you decide to proceed with the surgery. The parents accept the risks and appreciate your help.

The patient arrives in the operating room and you proceed to put in an intravenous line under nitrous oxide—you'd rather not risk a mask induction without intravenous access considering the risk of a severe bronchospasm or laryngospasm on induction. After pre-oxygenating the patient for 3 min, you proceed to induce the patient with a combination of fentanyl, lidocaine, propofol, and rocuronium. The patient is easy to mask, and intubation is uneventful. Anesthesia is maintained with sevoflurane at a minimum alveolar concentration (MAC) of 0.8 plus intermittent boluses of fentanyl and rocuronium (both of which are unlikely to cause clinically significant histamine release). You keep the total gas flow to a minimum to help warm/humidify the gas and minimize the chances of further drying up this patient's already thick secretions. The patient is turned prone and you have caught up on your charting when your pediatric anesthesia colleague comes in to relieve you for the day. You give report to your colleague and explain your plan to extubate the patient during stage 3 anesthesia—"deep" to minimize the chance of airway reactivity. His eyes narrow and, thinking that he does not understand, you explain that this involves deepening the level of anesthesia at the end of the case, tracheal suctioning, recruitment maneuvers, and neuromuscular blockade reversal prior to having the patient breathe spontaneously with 6–10 mL/kg tidal volumes and a regular respiratory rate prior to extubation.

On this suggestion, your pediatric colleague looks at you quizzically, saying, "Why would you ever WILLINGLY remove a definitive airway from a patient irrespective of their underlying disease? Wake them up and if they bronchospasm during stage 2, you can treat it while knowing you have a secure airway!"

Question

Does evidence demonstrate that "deep" extubation of pediatric patients at risk for bronchospasm (e.g., from asthma, cystic fibrosis, recent upper respiratory infection, or bronchopulmonary dysplasia) is safe, or even preferred?

PRO: You retort with all of the calm you can manage, "I don't think it's crazy at all. We know that cystic fibrosis is an autosomal recessive disorder that leads to a defect in the cystic fibrosis transmembrane conductance regulator (CFTR)

M. Dalmia (✉)
Department of Anesthesiology, Perioperative Care and Pain Management, New York Langone Medical Center, 550 First Avenue, TH530, New York, NY 10016, USA
e-mail: Manoj.Dalmia@nyumc.org

M. Dalmia
New York, NY 10026, USA

C.S. Scher et al. (eds.), *You're Wrong, I'm Right*, DOI 10.1007/978-3-319-43169-7_41

gene affecting multiple organs, including the lungs, pancreas, hepatobiliary tract, and intestine. Specifically in the lungs, it leads to hyperviscous mucus, which is difficult to clear, serving as a perfect petri dish for chronic infections including Staph and *Pseudomonas*. Consequently, there is a cycle of chronic inflammation both from the infectious processes and the disease itself leading to progressive lung injury/destruction [1]. Add to this the fact that this child has a resolving lower respiratory tract infection (LRI), which significantly increases ANY patient's airway reactivity plus the introduction of a foreign object into his trachea (the endotracheal tube!), and this patient is a clear set-up for bronchospasm, severe coughing, and other possible respiratory complications. It would seem irresponsible NOT to extubate him deep!"

CON: "Where is your evidence that demonstrates that deep extubation in a high-risk patient actually DECREASES the risk of perioperative complications? Are there are any studies that show superiority to awake extubation? Think of this logically: If a child bronchospasms without a secure airway and you're unable to ventilate him, what would you do? Intubate. If a child laryngospasms without a secure airway and you're unable to break it with positive pressure ventilation, what would you do? Intubate. If a patient vomits without a secure airway, you think he might have aspirated, and he starts desaturating, what would you do? You get the idea. You're removing the answer to the problem. And with modern-day anesthetics and how quickly they are removed from our bodies, the patient should wake up very quickly."

PRO: "Your initial point is logical, but I don't think it's necessary to prove that deep extubations decrease perioperative complications as long as they don't INCREASE them. von Ungern-Sternberg et al. initially performed a prospective cohort study looking to identify any associations between family history, anesthesia management, and occurrence of perioperative respiratory events by assessing children in the preoperative period with an adapted version of the International Study Group for Asthma and Allergies in Childhood (ISAAC) questionnaire. They evaluated 9297 completed questionnaires and found the following groups were all associated with a statistically significant increase in perioperative respiratory events (i.e., bronchospasm, laryngospasm, perioperative persistent cough, desaturation <95 %, or airway obstruction) (see Table 41.1 [2])."

"Recently, von Ungern-Sternberg et al. also performed a prospective, randomized controlled trial comparing deep versus awake extubations in 100 high-risk patients for adenotonsillectomy using the risk factors as laid out in their prior study. Although a small sample, this study found NO increase in the overall incidence of complications. Persistent coughing occurred more in the awake extubation group and mild airway obstruction (relieved with simple airway maneuvers) occurred more in the deep extubation group [3]. This is consistent with more recent studies demonstrating no overall difference in the incidence of perioperative respiratory complications in children undergoing T&A in high-risk children (albeit with different criteria defining 'high risk') (see Table 41.1 [4])."

Table 41.1 Pediatric patients considered to be at high risk for perioperative respiratory events [2, 4]

Study	Considered "high risk" for perioperative respiratory events
von Ungern-Sternberg et al. [2]	Positive respiratory history (i.e., nocturnal dry cough, wheezing during exercise, wheezing more than 3 times in the past 12 months, history of eczema)
	Recent upper respiratory infection (<2 weeks before procedure)
	History of ≥ 2 family members with asthma, atopy, or smoking
	Inhalation induction (vs. intravenous)
	Intravenous maintenance of anesthesia (vs. inhalational)
	Airway management by general anesthesiologist (vs. pediatric specialist)
	Endotracheal intubation (vs. facemask)
Baijal et al. [4]	<3 years old
	Craniofacial abnormalities
	Down syndrome
	Obstructive sleep apnea
	Morbid obesity
	Failure to thrive
	Recent upper respiratory infection (<2 weeks before procedure)
	History of reactive airway disease

"*Primum non nocere*: First do no harm, which is supported by the most recent evidence. And if I can decrease postoperative coughing fits, then that also improves the quality of the postoperative period for the child and family!"

CON: "You're still helping to prove my point. If there is no overall BENEFIT to extubating deep, then there is no reason to deviate from the 'gold standard' of an awake extubation. Sure, bucking or coughing could damage the surgical suture line—but the incidence is low. Persistent coughing in the postoperative period is easily treated with some blow-by humidified oxygen or an albuterol nebulizer. Patient satisfaction is important, but just because I can do it, doesn't mean I should. Call me conservative. And here you're not simply dealing with a patient with asthma or a simple cold. Cystic fibrosis patients have a greater degree of underlying pulmonary disease, and general anesthesia leads to numerous impairments in pulmonary mechanics: decreased functional residual capacity, increased atelectasis, increased airway resistance (due to obstruction), just to get started."

PRO: "Again, great point. Pandit et al. looked at a cohort of 19 cystic fibrosis patients from 8 to 18 years old who were admitted for intravenous (IV) antibiotic treatment for pulmonary exacerbation and required general anesthesia (GA) for peripheral intravenous central catheter (PICC) line placement—a decent comparison for our current patient! Seventeen underwent GA with a supraglottic airway (e.g., an LMA) and 2 underwent GA with endotracheal intubation. Their study compared spirometry results, cystic fibrosis clinical scores (CFCS), and forced oscillation technique (FOT) results for the cohort in the preoperative period, as well as 24 and 48 h postoperatively after GA. He found no statistically significant differences in spirometry, CFCS, or FOT besides a statistically significant DECREASE at 48 h in respiratory system resistance in the CF group! [5]."

CON: "This is clearly a very debatable topic, and honestly, I am still not comfortable with the idea of a deep extubation in this patient. I see where you're coming from, but I am not going to change my practice until I see evidence that deep extubation is superior to what I've always done."

PRO: "No problem. I understand your viewpoint and don't want to put you in an uncomfortable position. I'll stay and finish the case since I have no plans tonight. See if there's another one of our peds colleagues who needs relief!"

Summary

Both sides make great points, and there is no clear answer yet to strongly support one method over the other. Until there is, each anesthesia provider should make this decision based on the individual patient, the risks and benefits, as well as their own clinical skills—unfamiliarity with a technique is likely to lead to perioperative complications. Obviously, certain patient and surgical factors can lean a practitioner toward one technique versus another. In a patient with a difficult airway, an awake extubation is appropriate. If the surgical suture line is fragile, deep extubation (and backup from a colleague familiar with this technique) should be considered.

References

1. Gregory GA, Andropoulos DB, editors. Gregory's pediatric anesthesia. 5th ed. Hoboken: Wiley-Blackwell; 2012.
2. von Ungern-Sternberg BS, Boda K, Chambers NA, Rebmann C, Johnson C, Sly PD, Habre W. Risk assessment for respiratory complications in paediatric anaesthesia: a prospective cohort study. Lancet. 2010;376(9743):773–83.
3. von Ungern-Sternberg BS, Davies K, Hegarty M, Erb TO, Habre W. The effect of deep vs. awake extubation on respiratory complications in high-risk children undergoing adenotonsillectomy. Eur J Anaesthesiol. 2013;30(9):529–36.
4. Baijal RG, Bidani SA, Minard CG, Watcha MF. Perioperative respiratory complications following awake and deep extubation in children undergoing adenotonsillectomy. Paediatr Anaesth. 2015;25(4):392–9.
5. Pandit C, Valentin R, De Lima J, Robinson P, Fitzgerald D, van Asperen P, et al. Effect of general anesthesia on pulmonary function and clinical status on children with cystic fibrosis. Paediatr Anaesth. 2014;24(2):164–9.

What Is the Best Approach to a Pediatric Patient with an Unexplained Intraoperative Cardiac Arrest?

42

Sherryl Adamic and Anna Clebone

Case

Still bleary-eyed from a long night on call doing a liver transplant, you stumble into the local coffee shop looking for a jolt of caffeine before the drive home. One of your new colleagues, fresh out of fellowship, bounces in the front door.

You attempt to duck out of the shop through a side door, but unfortunately she spots you and starts talking at a rapid pace, "Hi, Doctor! Boy, you look tired! I have to tell you, I did the craziest case yesterday."

You sigh and look up at her through half-closed eyelids.

"This kid suddenly lost end-tidal carbon dioxide ($EtCO_2$) and became pulseless during the middle of the surgery!" Dr. Sprightly squeaks.

Realizing that you DID go into academics to mentor residents and younger faculty, you shift into professor mode and ask her about the case.

She replies, "The patient was a healthy 4-year-old who presented for resection of a renal tumor that extended into the inferior vena cava."

"Healthy patients tend to do well," you muse. "Was there anything else in the medical history? What about the labs?"

"We checked a chemistry, complete blood count, and coagulation studies. All the lab values were within normal limits. Besides the tumor, the only abnormal finding was a tumor thrombus that was located in the inferior vena cava."

S. Adamic
Department of Anesthesiology, University Hospitals of Cleveland, 11100 Euclid Ave, Cleveland, OH 44106, USA

S. Adamic (✉)
7752 Debonaire Dr., Mentor, OH 44060, USA
e-mail: sgadamic@gmail.com

A. Clebone
Department of Anesthesia and Critical Care, The University of Chicago, 5841 S. Maryland Ave. MC-4028, Chicago, IL 60637, USA
e-mail: aclebone@gmail.com

A. Clebone
60 E Monroe no. 4703, Chicago, IL 60603, USA

"Interesting," you state. "I can guess how this story ends. The patient arrests secondary to a massive pulmonary embolus, correct?"

"That would be the most obvious reason, but the short answer is no."

"You have now peaked my curiosity. Can we talk over coffee and you can tell me what happened?"

"Sure!" she exclaims, excited to have a mentor hear her story.

You now wonder what you have started.

Question

What is the best approach to a pediatric patient with an unexplained intraoperative cardiac arrest?

PRO: You tell her, "I would follow the Pediatric Advanced Life Support (PALS) guidelines and consult the pulmonary embolus algorithm."

She continues, "We initiated the PALS guidelines. Chest compressions were started immediately and we called for help and the automated external defibrillator (AED). The rhythm was checked, and it was shockable ventricular fibrillation. The patient weighed 17 kg, so we gave 170 μg of epinephrine (10 μg/kg) and planned on defibrillating the patient at 40 J ($\sim$2 J/kg). Once the defibrillator was available, we attempted to place the 'fast patches' (self-adhesive defibrillation electrodes), but there wasn't enough area available on the chest due to the sterile surgical field. We lost time trying to figure out how to defibrillate the patient. Fortunately one of our team members suggested using the external paddles. More time was lost because our surgeon objected that the paddles would contaminate the sterile field because there was no way to make them sterile. We were able to convince the surgeon to accept contamination, as defibrillation could be life-saving, and we defibrillated at 40 J without success."

C.S. Scher et al. (eds.), *You're Wrong, I'm Right*, DOI 10.1007/978-3-319-43169-7_42

You reply sagely, "That doesn't surprise me. Unanticipated cardiac arrests are very rare. Adding the sterile field to a stressful situation only makes matters worse. Going to the external paddles when the fast patched aren't available or when they can't be quickly placed due to a draped surgical field is a good idea. Plus, it may be difficult to resuscitate a patient with a massive pulmonary embolus anyway. What happened next?"

CON: Your colleague looks down and sighs, "Kept following the PALS guidelines without success."

"That's unfortunate. The PALS guidelines should be successful, as long as you treat the underlying cause. Did you perform a TEE?" you ask.

"We did and no thrombus was identified."

Now alert, you say, "I am intrigued. There has to be more to this story. What events led up to the arrest?"

She goes on, "The patient had been losing blood throughout the case. It was more oozing than massive bleeding. We treated it with lactated Ringers and 5 % albumin boluses. When the patient became hypotensive and anemic, we initiated a blood transfusion. After starting the second unit of blood the patient suddenly arrested."

PRO: "So it sounds like a hypovolemic arrest—one of the most common causes of unanticipated cardiac arrests in children," you muse. "I would have continued to transfuse the blood while continuing the PALS resuscitation."

"That's exactly what we did and the patient did not respond. We continued to give epinephrine and defibrillated the patient at 80 J (~4 J/kg) with no conversion of the ventricular fibrillation. It had been over 15 min since the arrest and I was sweating bullets. I couldn't figure out why the patient wasn't responding to treatment."

"Hmmmm. Did you check labs?" you reply.

"I tried but wasn't able to get blood from the arterial line. I felt all was lost, and then a team member suggested giving calcium. I thought that it wouldn't hurt the patient and it might help even though there wasn't a clear indication. I gave 340 mg of calcium intravenously while chest compressions were continued. At the next rhythm check (and 20 min into the arrest), the patient was still in v-fib. We defibrillated at 80 J, and this time there was conversion of the rhythm to normal sinus with a perfusing blood pressure."

CON: You now state definitively, "Sounds like while following the PALS guidelines, you concentrated on one possible underlying cause to the exclusion of other possibilities. Due to the successful resuscitation after giving calcium, I'm now changing my guess to a hyperkalemic cardiac arrest. Of course this now makes sense since the arrest happened during a blood transfusion, with the high potassium concentration in a unit of packed red blood cells. Hyperkalemia is one of the most common causes of pediatric cardiovascular arrest under anesthesia according to the Pediatric Perioperative Cardiac Arrest (POCA) Registry [1]. This registry encompassed 80 hospitals reporting all cardiac arrests in children 18 years old and younger. Over a 6-year period, ~400 arrests were reported, half connected to an anesthesia cause."

She looks at you knowingly and says, "Your second guess is correct. We ran a full panel arterial blood gas once the line was functional. The potassium was 9.1 mEq/L."

"There are some great teaching points here," you muse.

"Such as?"

"This is a great reminder for me as well. What you think is obvious may not be so obvious. Going down the pulmonary embolus algorithm would never have gotten you to the correct answer. Also, strictly adhering to PALS guidelines wouldn't have gotten you quickly to the correct answer either. I think that it is very easy to get stuck on what seems to be the obvious pathway and become blinded to other possibilities (e.g., the use of the external paddles instead of the fast patches). Back in the day, the paddles were all we had, but now 'fast patches' are usually the best choice. But what happens when you don't have them or can't use them? Most medical professionals wouldn't even think to use the external paddles since they may not have had experience with them."

"It's amazing how obvious it becomes once the answer is staring at you," she states.

You answer, "Even though I'm more experienced than you, I would have thought it was a PE from the tumor thrombus too. I do have to say that I'm glad that you shared this experience with me. It has certainly educated me to many points that I would not have thought about."

Summary

Intraoperative cardiac arrest in children is a rare event, especially in children without cardiac disease; 34 % of children with an intraoperative cardiac arrest had cardiac disease, either acquired or congenital [2]. When intraoperative cardiac arrest occurs, the PALS guidelines are a good starting point, but the PALS algorithm itself only begins to consider the treatment of underlying causes (Hs and Ts). Fixation error, which occurred in this case, can lead to focusing on one cause of cardiac arrest and ignoring all other possibilities [3]. Frequent simulation training, as well as specific training on avoiding cognitive errors, may be a solution, but more research is needed to determine the best means of implementation.

References

1. Bhananker SM, Ramamoorthy C, Geiduschek JM, Posner KL, Domino KB, Haberkern CM, et al. Anesthesia-related cardiac arrest in children: update from the Pediatric Perioperative Cardiac Arrest Registry. Anesth Analg. 2007;105(2):344–50.
2. Ramamoorthy C, Haberkern CM, Bhananker SM, Domino KB, Posner KL, Campos JS, et al. Anesthesia-related cardiac arrest in children with heart disease: data from the Pediatric Perioperative Cardiac Arrest (POCA) registry. Anesth Analg. 2010;110(5):1376–82.
3. Stiegler MP, Neelankavil JP, Canales C, Dhillon A. Cognitive errors detected in anaesthesiology: a literature review and pilot study. Br J Anaesth. 2012;108(2):229–35.

Malignant Hyperthermia: "It Certainly Is" Versus "It Certainly Is Not!"

43

Corey S. Scher

Case

The first case of the day in room 12 is a 4-year-old boy who is scheduled for a bilateral inguinal hernia repair. Three days before the procedure, the child had presented to pre-surgical testing for evaluation. Pertinent history includes birth at 31-week gestation, and predictably, the common morbidities of a premature infant, including lack of lung surfactant requiring a week of intubation and ventilation, apnea of prematurity, bronchopulmonary dysplasia (BPD), hyperbilirubinemia, a grade 2 intraventricular hemorrhage, and 2 seizures. Luckily, all of these problems have resolved. The child did receive an ill-defined anesthetic for a peripherally inserted central catheter (PICC) line during his initial hospitalization in the neonatal intensive care unit (NICU). The Mandarin-speaking father reported that the child needed 3 days of postoperative mechanical ventilation due to lung problems related to prematurity. He did not recall any other problems.

You proceed with induction. With the father in the room, an inhalational induction is performed with oxygen and 70 % nitrous oxide with 8 atm% sevoflurane quickly added. When the child appeared to be asleep, the father was escorted out of the room and an intravenous line was placed without incident. Intubation without muscle relaxation was smooth. Activation of the underbody heat transfer device was activated. A minute after beginning the inhalational induction the end tidal CO_2 ($EtCO_2$) immediately rose to 62 mm Hg. After stage 2 anesthesia had passed, the anesthesia attending turned the sevoflurane down to 3 atm% and assisted ventilation by squeezing the bag with every breath. The $EtCO_2$ was 70 at the time of intubation. The CO_2 increased with each breath on pressure-controlled mechanical ventilation. Ventilation settings were set to hyperventilate the child, but the CO_2 continued to climb to the mid-80s. Vital signs after a minute of mechanical ventilation were a pulse of 156, BP of 110/70, and a temperature of 38.1. Breath sounds were equal bilaterally, and heart tones were normal.

PRO: It seems that the more we ventilate, the worse the CO_2 becomes. I have never had a case of malignant hyperthermia, but the increasing CO_2 with ventilation is very worrisome. Please bring in the malignant hyperthermia cart now!!!

CON: All you have is an elevated CO_2. Nothing else fits MH. The temperature and vital signs are not very different than they would be after an inhalational induction in a normal 4 year old. Call a tech to check out the machine, and in the meantime, hand ventilate rapidly to lower the CO_2.

PRO: We have enough information to give dantrolene at this point. Nothing else fits!

CON: This could be any lung problem ranging from atelectasis to mucous plugging to mainstem intubation to pneumothorax, not to mention air embolus or cardiac shunt. Breath sounds in a child are transmitted across the chest to both lung fields, and it is very common to hear bilateral breath sounds in an infant or child when you are only ventilating one lung (e.g., with a mainstem intubation, large mucous plug blocking 1 bronchus, or from a pneumothorax). The child had or has residual BPD. The lung remodels to correct BPD, and it is very possible that you now have a pneumothorax from your overzealous ventilation. So far, you have very little to label him for life as a patient who has MH. Actually, you have almost nothing.

PRO: You are clueless as you probably have no idea what is actually going on. If you did understand MH, giving dantrolene now is essential!! The normal state of events must be understood before the MH state is understood. During excitation–contraction coupling, acetylcholine is liberated from muscles and binds to the nerves at the neuromuscular

C.S. Scher (✉)
Department of Anesthesiology, Perioperative Care and Pain Medicine, New York University School of Medicine, New York, NY 10016, USA
e-mail: coreyscher@gmail.com

C.S. Scher et al. (eds.), *You're Wrong, I'm Right*, DOI 10.1007/978-3-319-43169-7_43

receptors. This causes an action potential at the neuromuscular endplate. This action potential is propagated to the transverse tubule, causing a voltage change at the dihydropyridine receptor. A conformational change at the voltage-gated dihydropyridine receptor is directly transmitted to the ryanodine receptor subtype (RYR1), which is located at the sarcoplasmic reticulum [1]. The ryanodine receptor then opens and facilitates release of calcium from the sarcoplasmic reticulum into the cytosol. This leads to muscle contraction by initiating cross-linking of myofilaments. Active reuptake of calcium back into the sarcoplasmic reticulum via an adenosine triphosphate-dependent calcium pump terminates the muscle contraction [2]. It is no surprise that there are so many clinical expressions of MH as there are more than 400 variants in the RYR! gene. With the administration of triggering agents such as inhaled anesthetics and/or succinylcholine, the huge storage bin of calcium in the sarcoplasmic reticulum is released through the RYR1 channels causing a relative overdose of cytosolic calcium. This leads to intense muscle contraction, the destruction of vital cell functions including the loss of the integrity of the cell membrane. Upon the cell's death, CO_2 and heat are released. I am sure that is going on in our patient. What else does this?

CON: With the use of succinylcholine, an abrupt rise in CO_2 is common. You did not use sux! Now that the routine use of succinylcholine has been abandoned, the rise in CO_2 is much more gradual. In this case, the rise is more than abrupt. The mildly elevated body temperature and the relative increase in heart rate also argue against that.

PRO: The operating room is freezing, which would conceal the early signs of hyperthermia. I would get an early arterial blood gas. If I have a mixed respiratory and metabolic acidosis, I would initiate dantrolene and follow the remainder of the Malignant Hyperthermia Hotline algorithm, which is available on any cell phone or operating room computer. Delay would add to significant rhabdomyolysis. Then I would have to deal with renal dysfunction with myoglobin deposits in the kidney.

CON: Larach et al. [2] determined that hyperthermia was one of the first signs of hyperthermia, and in the very aggressive presentation of this case, the room temperature is never at a point to suppress the temperature elevation of MH.

PRO: I cannot believe that you can take a con position against giving dantrolene. The old Dantrium is being replaced by Ryanodex. It is available in 250 mg ampoules and on need 5 cc of sterile water to constitute. One amp will cover the initial presentation of MH.

CON: I now know why you are so eager to call the MH. Are you not the doctor who gave anesthetic for a tonsillectomy and the patient, 7 h after arriving at home, returned to the hospital with a temperature of 40° and then had a cardiac arrest!! Malignant hyperthermia does not present itself that far out after an anesthetic. It was taught back in the day that any elevation of temperature in the first 24 h after anesthesia could be MH, but it is no longer considered to be true. You feel like you have been burned, but the facts are that whatever caused the child to present back to the hospital, had nothing to do with the anesthetic.

PRO: The ABG is back! pH 7.17, CO_2 81, O_2 250 (with FiO_2 of 50 %), and a base excess of −15. At this point, you must admit that this is MH!! Stop the anesthetic. Hook up an Ambu bag and hook it up to wall oxygen. Start a propofol infusion to provide a non-triggering anesthetic. I am calling for help and getting both excellent IV access and an arterial line for both hemodynamics and blood sampling. Let us start out with 1 meq of sodium bicarbonate and 2.5 mg/kg of dantrolene. I do hope we have the Ryanodex as classic dantrolene takes a few minutes to mix with sterile water. Every second counts, and once the arterial line goes in, we will get a gas to see the response to dantrolene and have a CK (creatinine kinase) level to determine the relative muscle breakdown at this point. I do not think that alkalizing the urine has safety issues.

CON: How does the dantrolene work and are you dosing by ideal body weight or actual weight?

PRO: Dosing should be based on real weight to make sure that the dantrolene works on all of the muscle mass. Muscle contraction is hindered directly by dantrolene; the calcium in the muscle cell is diminished. Rigidity from muscle relaxation wanes. Dantrolene halts the ongoing release of calcium from the storage sites in muscle (the sarcoplasmic reticulum). There is no block of neuromuscular transmission from dantrolene itself. A decrease occurs in the physical response to nerve stimulation. It potentiates non-depolarizing neuromuscular blockade. When dantrolene is used with non-depolarizing muscle relaxants, care should be taken to ensure muscle strength has returned prior to extubation.

CON: Was he at risk for all of this? While the genetics support an autosomal dominant predisposition, most cases involve a mutation and the ryanodine receptor. Forty-four different mutations at the ryanodine receptor have been documented. There are some rare muscle diseases that are markers for MH, but I have never seen one of them. Central core disease is clearly a case where triggering agents should be avoided. King-Denborough [3] D′, centronuclear myopathy, and myotonic muscular dystrophy have a strong relationship with MH. I have not seen one of these diseases.

PRO: The ABG after 1 dose of dantrolene is completely normal, and the child is now breathing on his own. Let's repeat the gas in 10 min and re-evaluate further dosing of dantrolene. In days back, dantrolene was given on a schedule for 24 h with a maximum dose of 10 mg/kg. Patients were kept intubated for the first day. The dosing has changed. Give one dose and re-evaluate. If there remains a mixed metabolic and respiratory acidosis, give another dose. Remember to get a CK with each dose. There are rare cases when you need to exceed more than 10–30 mg/kg has been described but it is rare.

CON: It seems that there are so many variable clinical pictures of this disorder, I now know if the possibility exists, no real harm in treatment. Your instincts were correct.

PRO: While we are waiting for the next gas, get the father in the PACU. I need to talk to him.

FATHER: What is going on with my son?

PRO: Your son looks like he had a reaction to the anesthetic that is called malignant hyperthermia. (A detailed dissertation follows)

FATHER: I was married to a woman 10 years ago. We had a child who also had a reaction to anesthesia. He was sick and kept on life support for a day and discharged after 5 days. Your description of this case is similar to the one that was in the past. Now I am married to another woman, and it happened again. I have never had anesthesia, but it sounds like I passed it on.

PRO: Incredible. I need to go back to the operating room to take care of your son.

CON: The ABG is normal again. Let's call the Pediatric ICU, keep him on a propofol drip and re-evaluation.

PRO: While the return to the full MH signs and symptoms is 25 %, I want to stop the propofol, get him ready for extubation! I think he is fine now.

CON: You are out of your mind. In no way are you out of the woods.

PRO: If the blood gases are stable, the dantrolene worked and there is no reason he needs to be intubated and sedated. The patient will be in the pediatric ICU, and if signs and symptoms return, we can give another dose of dantrolene.

CON: Don't you need to see the CK to make sure that we do not end up with a renal issue?

PRO: He does not need to be intubated and sedated for that. I have had 8 cases over 30 years, which is more than most clinicians have had. Each one is different than any other one. The signs and symptoms vary in each one. In this case, the temperature was barely elevated and the underbody could account for it. I think that the elevated temperature was a clear signal that something was not right as it was elevated only moments after the tachycardia and end tidal CO_2 shot up.

CON: I think you are out there alone in your perspective of such an early extubation. MH can kill.

PRO: If diagnosed early and treated with dantrolene early, MH cannot kill.

Summary

It is essential that every anesthetizing location that includes the use of inhaled anesthetics must have an adequate quantity of dantrolene in a cart that includes ACLS meds, cooling systems, ice, NG tubes, central line kits to cover the possibility of poor venous access, and any other supportive materials. MH is a disease of high variability and requires flexibility on anesthesiologists as it rarely fits in the box that contains all the signs and symptoms. While there remain several gaps in a comprehensive understanding of this disorder, the treatment is highly effective. While the incidence of this disorder is rare, the mortality of this disorder should be also rare.

References

1. Chamley D, Pollock NA, Stowell KM, Brown RL. Malignant hyperthermia in infancy and identification of novel RYR1 mutation. Br J Anaesth. 2000;84(4):500–4.
2. Larach MG, Allen GC, Brandom BW, Lehman EB. Temperature changes are not late signs of malignant hyperthermia: a NMAH registry of NHAUS study. Anesthesiology. 2008;109:A374.
3. D'Arcy CE, Bjorksten A, Yiu EM, Bankier A, Gilles R, McLean CA, et al. King-Denborough syndrome caused by a novel mutation in the ryanodine receptor gene. Neurology. 2008;71 (10):776–7.

Is There a "Right" Drug to Choose When the Blood Pressure Is Low and More Volume Is not the Answer in a Pediatric Patient?

44

Jennifer L. Liedel and Madelyn Kahana

Case

A 5-month-old presents for urgent drainage of a suspected empyema associated with a community-acquired pneumonia. The infant was a full-term product of an uncomplicated pregnancy and delivery and was healthy until developing an upper respiratory tract infection (URI) 10 days ago. She was admitted to the hospital 2 days prior to the procedure with continued fever and increased work of breathing and is on a high-flow nasal cannula. Her respiratory viral panel is positive for respiratory syncytial virus (RSV), and her blood culture is positive for *Staph aureus*. She was treated with vancomycin for 36 h. Her temperature is 39 °C, she is tachycardic to 190, her respiratory rate is 58, and her blood pressure is 85/38. Her oxygen saturation is 94 on 100 % oxygen at 8 L per minute. Your colleague is helping you prepare and suggests having a dopamine infusion available in case the child becomes hemodynamically unstable and is poorly responsive to volume resuscitation. You tell him that you do not want to manipulate the anterior pituitary output with dopamine, you want to support the blood pressure, and epinephrine would be a better choice [1]. He is skeptical that it matters.

Question

Does it matter if you choose epinephrine or dopamine for small children and neonates who are septic and require inotropic support?

J.L. Liedel
Division of Pediatric Critical Care, Department of Pediatrics, Albert Einstein College of Medicine, Children's Hospital at Montefiore, 3415 Bainbridge Avenue, Bronx, NY 10467, USA
e-mail: jliedel@montefiore.org

M. Kahana (✉)
Department of Anesthesiology, Montefiore Medical Center, 111 East 210th Street, 4th Floor, Silver Zone, Bronx, NY 10467, USA
e-mail: mkahana@montefiore.org

M. Kahana
50 Murray St Apt 2101, New York, NY 10007, USA

PRO A fluid bolus is obviously the first choice to treat hypotension from sepsis or systemic inflammation. When this isn't enough, dopamine has historically been the inotrope of choice [2]. More recently, the use of dopamine has been questioned, especially in the young child.

In this 5-month-old, several organ systems are maturing at a rapid pace. Dopamine reduces the anterior pituitary output, impacting thyroid hormones. Potential long-term neurodevelopmental consequences include a negative impact on brain development, which is dependent on normal thyroid function [3, 4]. There is no advantage, and only detriment to using dopamine. Epinephrine is a clear alternative.

CON Dopamine is still on the recommended treatment list for pediatric sepsis [1].

PRO Dopamine has a long history of being used for pediatric sepsis and as such is listed as a therapy for hypotension. However, it functions not only as a catecholamine (after being converted in the body to norepinephrine), but also as a central nervous system neurotransmitter and a peripheral paracrine hormone.

Dopamine acts via D2 receptors to maintain hypothalamic pituitary homeostasis. Two important anterior pituitary hormones are affected by changes in dopamine—thyroid stimulating hormone and prolactin [3–5]. The effect of dopamine on TSH is particularly important in the neonate and infant for whom brain maturation is occurring at a rapid rate. Dopamine has been shown to prolong the sick euthyroid state in critically ill patients. Increasingly, evidence suggests that even a short period of relative hypothyroidism has lasting effects on development [3, 4].

Epinephrine is also on the recommended treatment list for pediatric sepsis. Although no data prove that dopamine-induced reductions in thyroid hormone impact brain development, why risk it when there is a good, if not better, alternative? And dopamine reduces prolactin levels as well, and that could be problematic [5].

C.S. Scher et al. (eds.), *You're Wrong, I'm Right*, DOI 10.1007/978-3-319-43169-7_44

CON I know you could not be worried about lactation in this setting.

PRO You're right. I do not care about lactation, but I do care about the immune system, and prolactin is a key hormone involved in regulating lymphocyte number and function. Exogenous dopamine causes a marked reduction in prolactin secretion via the hypothalamic pituitary axis. Receptors for prolactin are present on many tissues in the body. The absence of stimulation is thought to put patients at risk of immunosuppression and infection [5].

CON Well, dopamine can be used to protect renal function. I am sure you have heard of "renal dose dopamine." Epinephrine may increase the likelihood of acute kidney injury.

PRO The notion of "renally dosed" dopamine has been disproven [6]. Dopaminergic activation (D1) in the kidney is in part responsible for the natriuresis observed with lower doses of dopamine in the setting of normotension. Renal tubule cells also produce dopamine, which activates a Na–K ATPase and enhances natriuresis. This is augmented by local vasodilation. So while I admit that dopamine may increase urine flow, there is no evidence that administration of dopamine in the setting of renal failure or insufficiency will prevent progression or reverse the ongoing acute kidney injury [6].

With regard to epinephrine and the induction of renal injury, the best protection for the kidney is adequate cardiac output. Epinephrine does not and should not replace adequate volume replacement, but should additional inotropy be needed to maintain sufficient cardiac output, epinephrine does not produce direct renal injury.

CON With dopamine, you can still titrate the effect you want based on the dose you choose. At doses <10 mcg/kg/min the drug is primarily a beta adrenergic agonist and at doses above that it becomes an alpha-adrenergic agent. That is convenient. You only need one drug.

PRO Although that is true, I would argue it is true for both agents. With the administration of either exogenous dopamine or epinephrine, adrenergic receptors are activated. Importantly, for both catecholamines, beta responses predominate at lower doses and alpha at higher doses (dopamine >10 ug/kg/min, epinephrine >0.05 ug/kg/min). As doses increase and alpha responses predominate, organ perfusion is diminished.

In fact, epinephrine is a downstream product of the metabolism of dopamine. In the adrenal medulla and with peripheral secretion, dopamine is converted to norepinephrine. A portion of that norepinephrine is further modified to create epinephrine. In the past, epinephrine has been utilized as a second-line agent for the treatment of hypotension in sepsis. Both epinephrine and dopamine act via beta-1 receptors to increase cAMP. The increase in cAMP leads to increased intracellular availability of calcium, resulting in positive inotropy and chronotropy.

Loss of vasomotor tone can occur in sepsis, requiring the use of an intravenous vasoconstricting agent. Although high-dose dopamine is effective, new evidence shows low-dose vasopressin would be a better choice [1]. Vasopressin does not cause tachycardia and can result in the ability to decrease the dose of other medications, such as epinephrine.

CON Isn't dopamine less injurious to cardiac muscle cells? That would be an important reason to choose it over epinephrine.

PRO At doses that produce an equivalent pharmacologic effect, all adrenergic agonists are cardiotoxic. All of them. Dopamine is no better than epinephrine and no worse [7].

CON OK. What if the infusion extravasates? Dopamine will not cause as much tissue damage as will epinephrine. That is a real advantage [8].

PRO It would be an advantage if it were true. Extravasation of dopamine and epinephrine are both bad. Both can cause extensive soft tissue injury and both should ideally be infused in a central line, but in an emergency, both can be infused peripherally until a central access is established. Care should be taken to directly visualize and frequently check the peripheral infusion site for any signs of extravasation or infiltration [8]. Good try.

Summary

The choice of vasoactive medications in the setting of sepsis or systemic inflammation is an important one. Although there is no real "right" answer, the neuroendocrine impact of dopamine administration is an important consideration. Although outcomes are not well established in randomized controlled trials, the preclinical science is powerful. When making this decision, one should consider the potential negative impact of dopamine on neurocognitive development in the infant through thyroid hormone suppression and on the immune system in all ages through depression of prolactin levels.

References

1. Dellinger RP, Levy MM, Rhodes A, Annane D, Gerlach H, Opal SM, et al. Surviving sepsis campaign: international guidelines for management of severe sepsis and septic shock: 2012. Crit Care Med. 2013;41(2):580–635.
2. Ventura A, Góes P, Fernandes IC, Hsin SH, Souza DC, Gaiga L, Bousso A, Gilio AE. Randomized double blind trial of dopamine or epinephrine as first line vasoactives in fluid refractory pediatric septic shock. Pediatr Crit Care Med 2014;15(4_ Suppl): 5.
3. de Zegher F, Van den Bershe G, Dumoulin M, Gewillig M, Daenen W, Devlieger H. Dopamine suppresses thyroid-stimulating hormone secretion in neonatal hypothyroidism. Acta Paediatr. 1995;84(2):213–4.
4. Filippi L, Pezzati M, Cecchi A, Poggi C. Dopamine infusion: a possible cause of undiagnosed congenital hypothyroidism in preterm infants. Pediatr Crit Care Med. 2006;7(3):249–51.
5. Freeman ME, Kanyicska B, Lerant A, Gyorgy N. Prolactin: structure, function, and regulation of secretion. Physiol Rev. 2000;80(4):1524–83.
6. Friedrich JO, Adhikari N, Herridge MS, Beyene J. Meta-analysis: low-dose dopamine increases urine output but does not prevent renal dysfunction or death. Ann Intern Med. 2005;142:510–24.
7. Liaudet L, Calderari B, Pacher P. Pathophysiological mechanisms of catecholamine and cocaine mediated cardiotoxicity. Heart Fail Rev. 2014;19:815–24.
8. Loubani OM, Green RS. A systematic review of extravasation and local tissue injury from administration of vasopressors through peripheral intravenous catheters and central venous catheters. J Crit Care. 2015;30(3):653e9–17.

Part V
Obstetric

45 Which Is Safer: A Traditional Epidural or a Combined Spinal Epidural?

Juan Davila-Velazquez and Jeffrey Bernstein

Case

A 32-year-old primigravida at 5-cm dilatation, with regular contractions and intact membranes, is admitted to the labor floor in active labor. She is obese [body mass index (BMI) 41] and has a Mallampati Class III airway. The rest of her medical history is unremarkable. After addressing her questions and concerns and signing consent, you perform a traditional epidural with loss of resistance to air, 6 cm from the skin. Aspiration and test dose are negative. The epidural catheter is loaded with 10 ml bupivacaine, 0.125 %, and fentanyl, 50 μ(mu)g. Patient-controlled epidural analgesia with both continuous and demand dosing is initiated before you leave the room.

Thirty minutes later, the nurse calls and informs you that the patient is still reporting moderate to severe pain during her contractions. You decide to load the epidural catheter with an additional 5 ml of a stronger concentration of bupivacaine (0.25 %). Fifteen minutes after the top-up, you return to the labor room. As per the nurse, cervical dilatation is unchanged. The patient still looks uncomfortable, and after your assessment, you realize there is no discernible sensory or motor block. You explain to the patient that the epidural catheter appears not to be working and should be replaced. The patient agrees.

It is 6 p.m., and the overnight resident is here to relieve you. After excusing yourself, you meet the senior night float resident in the on-call room. Explaining what has just happened; the resident interrupts you and says, "This has just taken too long. Poor lady! You should have done a combined spinal epidural (CSE) from the beginning."

J. Davila-Velazquez (✉) · J. Bernstein
Department of Anesthesiology, Montefiore Medical Center—Weiler Division, 1825 Eastchester Road, Bronx, NY 10461, USA
e-mail: Judavila@montefiore.org

J. Bernstein
e-mail: jbernste@montefiore.org

Question

Compared to a traditional epidural, is a combined spinal epidural technique more reliable and safer?

PRO Acceptance of the CSE technique among certain practitioners has been slow because of the concern that an epidural catheter placed after administration of an intrathecal anesthetic is untested and unreliable. This is especially evident if the epidural needs to be activated soon after placement (~1 h) for an emergent cesarean section. When a catheter is placed utilizing the traditional technique, we must wait 20 min after the loading dose to assess whether it is working. If the patient remains uncomfortable and the initial sensory block is not what was anticipated, most practitioners will err on the side of manipulating or redosing the catheter with a higher concentration and reassessing 20 min later. By the time the patient agrees to a replacement and a new catheter is placed and loaded, an hour has elapsed. This is no difference in the time it takes the initial sensory block achieved with a standard subarachnoid CSE dose [2.5 mg bupivacaine and 10–15 μ(mu)g fentanyl] to resolve or wear off. Thus, the time during which the catheters remain untested is similar, regardless of the technique utilized for placement. Ultimately, it is our vigilance and clinical suspicion that will help us identify which catheters are likely to fail.

CON If a CSE technique is used and the patient requires an emergency cesarean delivery, the untested epidural anesthetic can be patchy, one-sided, or not work at all. This puts the patient, newborn, and anesthesiologist at risk should a general anesthetic be required for a true emergency. If a CSE is performed with 2.5 mg of bupivacaine and 10–15 μ(mu)g of fentanyl, the patient will be comfortable for an hour, and at best you can reliably test for intravascular placement without truly knowing the risk of dosing an inadvertent intrathecal catheter. After placement of a pure epidural catheter, it should not take more than 20 min to determine whether your catheter is properly placed.

C.S. Scher et al. (eds.), *You're Wrong, I'm Right*, DOI 10.1007/978-3-319-43169-7_45

By performing a dural puncture with a 25-, 26-, or 27-gauge needle you increase the risk of a headache, which is of primary concern because of patient dissatisfaction and lawsuits. By penetrating the dura, which serves as a protective barrier, you create a channel through which infectious agents can reach the CNS, increasing the possibility of meningitis. I agree that a CSE provides more reliable initial analgesia than an epidural. But I feel safer knowing I have a reliable working catheter should an emergency arise.

PRO I agree that albeit small, there is increased morbidity when a CSE is performed. Nonetheless, if passing a 27-G pencil-point needle with its 1 % chance of spinal headache helps an anesthesiologist confirm location of the epidural space, such a risk is justifiable. A 1 % incidence of post-dural puncture headache (PDPH) is smaller than that incurred if you continue to advance and pierce the dura unintentionally with the epidural needle. Furthermore, the consequences of a spinal headache are far less detrimental than those that may complicate the replacement of an epidural catheter (bleeding, infection, nerve damage). Thus, when faced with the predicament of passing a spinal needle and confirming it with the visualization of CSF, or threading a catheter after a "suspicious" loss of resistance, it is preferable to pass the spinal needle. In fact, seeing CSF removes some of the subjectivity from the procedure. It is not surprising that a growing amount of evidence shows that there is a lower rate of catheter replacement and a higher rate of successful catheter activation for cesarean sections after a CSE [1, 2]. Safety is not compromised but rather enhanced with a CSE technique.

CON What if it is a dry tap (you are really in the epidural space but there is no CSF)?

When placing an epidural, if I encounter a loss of resistance but I am not sure that I have entered the epidural space, I pull it out and start again rather than advancing my needle or puncturing the dura unnecessarily with a spinal needle. Even if you have CSF confirmation, it does not guarantee that the epidural catheter will function appropriately should the need arise. The advantage of a CSE is that in some patients, it is hypothesized that the communication channel created allows for the diffusion of local anesthetic from the epidural into the spinal canal, thus providing better sacral analgesia.

Summary

The advantages of the combined spinal epidural technique are that it provides faster analgesia and better sacral coverage. The disadvantages are that it comes at the expense of a small increase in the risk of PDPH and meningitis. Which catheter is more reliable, one placed during a CSE or during a traditional epidural, is a subject of much debate. Beside the technique or approach used for catheter placement, there are probably other factors that will ultimately affect catheter safety. How experienced the anesthesiologist is with either technique and his/her ability to detect and replace suboptimal or non-working catheters are difficult to measure, yet critical factors. In other words, the CSE or the epidural is only as good as the anesthesiologist performing and managing it.

References

1. Pan P, Bogard T, Owen M. Incidence and characteristics of failures in obstetrical neuraxial analgesia and anesthesia: a retrospective analysis if 19,259 deliveries. Int J Obstet Anesth. 2004;13:227–33.
2. Gonzalez A, Sachs A, Aaronson J, Smiley R. Catheter replacement rates in labor; combined spinal epidural vs. epidural technique. Abstract presented at 46th Annual Meeting Society of Obstetric Anesthesia and Perinatology; 14–18 May 2014; Toronto.

46 When Should a Patient Undergoing Dilation and Evacuation of Products of Gestation Be Intubated?

Barbara Orlando, Agnes McNamara Lamon, and Migdalia Saloum

Case

A 32-year-old G4P0030 at 22 weeks is seen by her obstetrician for moderate vaginal bleeding that began 2 days ago upon returning from a trip to the Bahamas. She explains that this morning after breakfast, she experienced severe cramping and worsening bleeding. She is worried because "I've already lost 3 babies and I really want a child."

Unfortunately, after examining her, no fetal heart tones are found, and the ultrasound confirms the suspected diagnosis of an incomplete abortion. Because the bleeding is quite heavy, the obstetrician decides to have her emergently admitted to the hospital. He recommends a dilation and evacuation (D & E).

The patient is extremely upset. When the anesthesiology resident arrives, the first thing the patient utters is, "I want to go to sleep! I cannot deal with another dead baby."

Upon examination, she is hemodynamically stable, but pale. Besides the previous spontaneous miscarriages for which workups were negative, the patient is healthy, obese [body mass index (BMI) 30.8], and has no allergies. Her airway is a Mallampati class III and she had a full breakfast at 8 a.m. It is now 3:15 p.m. The anesthesiology attending arrives as the patient is signing the consent for general anesthesia only. She refuses neuraxial or regional blocks, even though the resident explained the risks of general anesthesia in a patient considered to have a "full stomach."

B. Orlando
Department of Anesthesiology, Mount-Sinai West Hospital, 1000 10th Avenue, New York, NY 10019, USA

B. Orlando (✉)
145 Old Army Rd, Scarsdale, NY 10583, USA
e-mail: borlando@chpnet.org

A.M. Lamon
Department of Anesthesiology, Mt. Sinai Roosevelt Hospital, 1111 Amsterdam Ave, New York, NY 10025, USA
e-mail: Agnesmlamon@gmail.com; alamon@chpnet.org

A.M. Lamon
300 Blackwell Street Apt 410, Durham, NC 27701, USA

M. Saloum
Department of Anesthesiology, Mt. Sinai West/Mt. Sinai St. Luke's, 1000 Tenth Avenue, New York, NY 10019, USA
e-mail: msaloum@chpnet.org

M. Saloum
299 16th St., Brooklyn, NY 11215, USA

Question

Should all patients undergoing a D & E be intubated?

PRO: As the anesthesiology attending introduces himself to the patient, he realizes how upset she is. Anxiety and stress in the context of 3 previous miscarriages seem to be an adequate reason to choose general anesthesia.

CON: The resident does not agree and expresses her concerns about a potential difficult airway. She recently read a retrospective study from the UK, finding that failed intubation occurred in 1/224 pregnant patients with Mallampati scores > I [1]. She then suggests to the attending, "Maybe we could just do deep sedation. It should be a short case and the patient is almost 8 h away from her last food intake. To be on the safe side, we could ask the obstetrician to wait 45 more minutes!"

PRO: The attending replies, "Well, I am familiar with this study and it also shows that obstetric patients are at a higher risk for aspiration" [1]. Even if gastric emptying has recently been shown to be normal during pregnancy, this risk is still increased because of decreased pressure at the lower esophageal sphincter [2]. Sedation without protecting her airway would put her at an increased risk for aspiration even if she was NPO, because she is in her second trimester, obese, and very anxious, which further delays gastric emptying. I would not administer deep sedation; I would definitely intubate the trachea. This patient is to be considered "full stomach" regardless of her last intake.

The attending adds that the patient has been crying a lot, and she was throwing up as the resident was setting up the

C.S. Scher et al. (eds.), *You're Wrong, I'm Right*, DOI 10.1007/978-3-319-43169-7_46

room. He continues, as the resident is shaking her head, "Maybe if she was <20 weeks gestation and had a normal BMI, I would consider sedating her."

CON: The resident does not seem convinced by her attending's arguments. For her, the potential difficult airway combined with the aspiration risk seem a relative contraindication to general anesthesia. As for the patient's anxiety, she says, "I would rather do a spinal and comfort her through the whole procedure than having to deal with an aspiration risk or worse! In addition, would it allow closure if she was able to hold the baby? What do you think?"

PRO: "You bring up an interesting point. The *British Journal of Medicine* published an article in 2013 that showed that women who had a vaginal delivery of a stillborn and were able to hold their child had a lower incidence of post-traumatic stress disorder later in life [3]. However, those were cases of intrauterine fetal demise (IUFD) where the mother was hemodynamically stable. I understood from her obstetrician that she has already lost ~800 cc! She might become severely hypotensive when you create a sympathetic block with the spinal! I feel it is really safer to have this patient asleep with a controlled airway from the beginning, especially if we anticipate further bleeding and the need for a transfusion."

CON: The resident thinks for a minute then replies, "We could do an epidural and slowly titrate the level to avoid a sudden sympathectomy?"

PRO: "But what if the patient goes into disseminated intravascular coagulation (DIC) and you need to start a massive transfusion protocol? This patient is actively bleeding! Do you want to have an awake patient who you might have to intubate emergently? It is safer to control the airway when you are in a relatively stable situation as opposed to a crash intubation! You do know that the risk of DIC is increased when the fetus dies at a relative advanced gestational age, and this patient is in her late second trimester" [4, 5].

Summary

The obstetric patient has always been a source of anxiety for anesthesiologists because of the potential for immediate, severe, and sometimes even fatal complications. The increased Mallampati score [6], airway edema and friability, decreased oxygen reserve (lower functional residual capacity), and increased aspiration risk combine to create a recipe for disaster. No anesthesiologist wants to find themselves in the "cannot intubate, cannot ventilate" situation. Deep sedation is clearly not a prudent option in a pregnant patient since the airway may be lost when mild sedation leads to deep sedation or general anesthesia without a protected airway. Additionally, increased gastric contents leading to a higher risk of aspiration ("full stomach") should be presumed in all patients with severe GERD or obesity, and pregnant patients likely after week 12, but certainly after 16 weeks of gestation [3, 7]. The American Society of Anesthesiologists (ASA) recently reviewed, in conjunction with the American Congress of Obstetricians and Gynecologists (ACOG), the statement on non-obstetric surgery during pregnancy, but it did not include any specific recommendations on intubation of pregnant patients.

This leaves the anesthesiologist with the anesthetic options of neuraxial anesthesia vs general anesthesia with an endotracheal tube.

Other complications seen with incomplete abortions and intrauterine fetal demise are blood loss and disseminated intravascular coagulation. Determining the hemodynamic stability of the patient is critical. An otherwise healthy, young patient may be able to compensate for a large blood loss until hemodynamic collapse. Monitoring vital signs, accurately estimating ongoing blood loss, and being thoroughly prepared to resuscitate the patient cannot be overstated. It is essential that a hemodynamically unstable patient or one that is at risk to require aggressive resuscitation should have a definitive protected airway. A parturient with a closed cervix, no blood loss that is experiencing an IUFD or uncomplicated incomplete abortion might be offered regional anesthesia.

References

1. Quinn AC, Milne D, Columb M, Gorton H, Knight M. Failed tracheal intubation in obstetric anaesthesia: 2 yr national case–control study in the UK. Br J Anaesth. 2013 Jan;110(1):74–80.
2. Reitman E, Flood P. Anaesthetic considerations for non-obstetric surgery during pregnancy. Br J Anaesth. 2011;107:i72–8.
3. Gravensteen IK, Helgadóttir LB, Jacobsen EM, Rådestad I, Sandset PM, Ekeberg O. Women's experiences in relation to stillbirth and risk factors for long-term post-traumatic stress symptoms: a retrospective study. BMJ Open. 2013;3(10):e003323.
4. The American College of Obstetricians and Gynecologists. Practice Bulletin No. 135: Second-trimester Abortion. Obstet Gynecol. 2013;121(6):1394–406.
5. Lurie S, Feinstein M, Mamet Y. Disseminated intravascular coagulopathy in pregnancy: thorough comprehension of etiology and management reduces obstetricians' stress. Arch Gynecol Obstet. 2000;263:126–30.
6. Pilkington S, Carli F, Dakin MJ, Romney M, De Witt KA, Doré CJ, Cormack RS. Increase in Mallampati score during pregnancy. Br J Anaesth. 1995;74(6):638–42.
7. Bedson R, Riccoboni A. Physiology of pregnancy: clinical anaesthetic implications. Contin Educ Anaesth Crit Care Pain. 2013. http://ceaccp.oxfordjournals.org/content/early/2013/09/11/bjaceaccp.mkt036.full.

Two Blood Patches Have Failed. Now What?

47

Alexander Sinofsky and Arthur Atchabahian

Case

I was not thrilled when the newest patient requested an epidural at the end of my shift on the obstetrics floor. To put it nicely, her anatomy promised it would be a technically challenging procedure—there were no palpable landmarks to speak of on her back. After my Tuohy needle hit bone for a fifth time, I called the supervising anesthesiologist covering obstetric anesthesia that day to provide assistance and moral support. He struggled for several minutes before his needle seemed to find a promising spot. And as he advanced the needle a touch more, his persistence was rewarded with a steady stream of cerebrospinal fluid. A "wet tap"—the attending and I stared at each other. He quickly removed the epidural catheter from the tray and threaded it through the needle into the intrathecal space.

Ultimately, we left the catheter in place and did not attempt an epidural at another level. The attending stepped into the hallway as I counseled the patient on the strong possibility of developing a headache, reportedly 50–70 % [1].

"Well, what are we going to do now?" I called after my supervising anesthesiologist.

A. Sinofsky (✉)
Department of Anesthesiology, New York University Langone Medical Center, 550 First Avenue, New York, NY 10016, USA
e-mail: asinofsky@gmail.com

A. Sinofsky
946 Goss Avenue, Apartment 1306, Louisville, KY 40217, United States

A. Atchabahian
Department of Anesthesiology, New York University School of Medicine, 301 East 17th St. Room C2-222, New York, NY 10003, USA
e-mail: arthur.atchabahian@gmail.com; Arthur.Atchabahian@nyumc.org

A. Atchabahian
10 W 15th St #414, New York, NY 10011, USA

Looking over his shoulder as I caught up, he answered, "There isn't much to do right now—we just have to wait."

I wasn't convinced this was the best course of action.

Question

What should the initial treatment of a post-dural puncture headache (PDPH) be? Does timing matter?

PRO: The attending explained outside, "One of the most widely used initial treatments for known wet tap is inserting the epidural catheter intrathecally with possible conversion to continuous spinal anesthesia. Previous data were inconclusive, but a recent study demonstrated that insertion of an intrathecal catheter reduced the risk of PDPH compared to placing an epidural catheter elsewhere" [2].

CON: I didn't like the idea of threading anything into the intrathecal space, given the risk of infection and the possibility of someone unwittingly administering a dose of medication intended for an epidural.

I proposed an alternative, "There may be some efficacy in performing a blood patch prior development of symptoms. A recent study concluded that performing a prophylactic blood patch at a different interspace reduced the incidence of post-dural puncture headache" [3].

PRO: "Typically, we wait a day or two after a wet tap when a patient develops a headache to offer a blood patch. Previous literature has shown very little difference between prophylactic blood patches and sham procedures. Additionally, blood patches were known to fail at a much higher rate if given in the first 48 h after dural puncture [1]," the supervising anesthesiologist said.

CON: "Well, using the onset of the headache as a trigger for an epidural blood patch (EBP) can be complicated as well. Although uncommon, the onset of intense headache immediately or on the same day as dural puncture is most likely

C.S. Scher et al. (eds.), *You're Wrong, I'm Right*, DOI 10.1007/978-3-319-43169-7_47

pneumocephalus—the injection of air into the subarachnoid or subdural space. This headache can be almost indistinguishable from PDPH, although it typically resolves within several days. In contrast, PDPH is more often seen 24–48 h after dural puncture and can last much longer than pneumocephalus."

As the on-call supervising anesthesiologist left the obstetrics ward, I took a quick detour to an office to search for articles. I was reminded that a blood patch is believed to work by sealing the dural leak with blood clot, thus increasing both intracranial and intraspinal pressure toward normal, relieving the vasodilation that may cause the headache.

I was surprised by how conflicting the evidence was regarding prophylactic blood patches. Some studies, including meta-analyses, concluded that prophylactic EBP (PEBP) demonstrated a significant reduction in PDPH incidence, while others showed no benefit. According to a focused review by Agerson et al., the available data suggest that PEBP does not reduce PDPH incidence after dural puncture, but may reduce intensity and duration of symptoms [4]. This reinforced what I already had been taught: There just didn't seem to be sufficient evidence to draw reliable conclusions about the benefit of PEBP.

As for the idea that epidural blood patches have higher failure rates if administered early, there were some results to suggest increased failure of therapeutic blood patches given within 24 and 48 h after dural puncture. Yet, these studies seemed to have many confounding variables: needle size and type, the surgical procedure, sex, and age. I also considered a concession: PDPH is known to have a variable course that can last from days to weeks. Some patients may have full resolution of their symptoms within the first 48 h and thus could avoid having to undergo a blood patch if we would just wait.

Two days later, I was back on the obstetrics floor with a different supervising anesthesiologist. The intrathecal catheter had been accidentally removed on the first day, and the patient was complaining of an intense headache while sitting up or standing, which was relieved when she lay flat. She had no other neurologic symptoms. I went to grab the new supervising anesthesiologist on call to offer a therapeutic epidural blood patch (TEBP). The attending seemed hesitant to offer the blood patch at that time.

Question

Should all patients with a post-dural puncture headache receive an epidural blood patch?

PRO: Surprised by his reluctance, I said, "An epidural blood patch is the only treatment for post-dural puncture headache supported by evidence. It is as close to a sure thing as we have."

CON: "That's questionable at best," he continued, not sounding very impressed. "Most recent studies have shown that complete relief from post-dural puncture headaches is actually much less common after blood patch than we think. One study of accidental dural puncture in 100 obstetric patients found complete headache relief after EBP in only 50 % of patients; a different study by Paech et al. showed permanent cure in only 22 % [5]. Furthermore, PDPHs tend to resolve by themselves in days to weeks regardless, so even those patients with resolution of symptoms after TEBP may just have had spontaneous resolution. There have also been case reports of scarring in the epidural space after blood patch, rendering future epidural anesthesia patchy and ineffective [6]. Also, there are case reports of delayed radicular pain from large injections of blood [7]. We should treat most of these patients with expectant, conservative management…."

PRO: "There is almost no evidence at all in support of 'conservative management': hydration, bed rest, and adjuvant medications. A Cochrane review concluded that bed rest and fluid supplementation is not effective in relieving PDPH symptoms [8]. In different studies, gabapentin and hydrocortisone did decrease pain scores over placebo, but only for up to 96 and 48 h after intervention, respectively. Both of these studies were limited by small sample size and short follow-up time [9]. And the role for agents such as sumatriptan and ACTH remains unclear, as studies thus far have not yielded significant results."

I knew that PDPH had a course varying from days to weeks (or even years), but withholding treatment while a patient suffers was unacceptable to me.

CON: "Well, there are studies of caffeine that show it may help lower the incidence of headache, but is not effective at treating symptoms. Analgesics such as NSAIDs, acetaminophen, and opioids may have a role in symptomatic relief, but have not been shown to prevent or reduce the duration of headaches." It didn't sound like this senior attending really wanted conservative management. His point was merely that TEBP was an invasive procedure and its effectiveness was questionable; it was wrong to offer a treatment just for the sake of doing *something*. Transient back pain after the procedure is common [1], meningeal symptoms have been reported, and case reports have associated TEBP with subdural hematomas.

Concession from CON: He concluded, "I'm not opposed to offering TEBPs, but it is not the right treatment for every patient. It may be best suited for the treatment of severe cases where there are signs of traction on the cranial nerves like diplopia and tinnitus, or the severity of the headache has forced the patient to be bedbound. Additionally, a promising alternative to EBPs is sphenopalatine ganglion block (SPGB), a much less invasive intervention. In early data, 69 % of 32 obstetrics patients with PDPH had resolution of their headaches after SPGB without needing an EBP" [10].

Although the patient did not have any other neurologic sequela of dural puncture, the attending soon relented and we performed a therapeutic epidural blood patch at the bedside. I was pleased when I returned an hour later to find the patient smiling and sitting up in bed. I was convinced we were successful, and the patient was discharged home.

Yet, when I called the patient 2 days later, her headache had returned. Now, I was really unsure of what to do. I went to speak with the new on-call supervising anesthesiologist to determine whether we should offer a second blood patch.

Question

After an unsuccessful therapeutic epidural blood patch, should a second blood patch be offered?

PRO: "I think we need to repeat a TEBP today—the patient's symptoms are back and exactly as they were 2 days ago. I'm just not sure what went wrong; we waited 48 h after dural puncture and injected 20 mL of blood," I said.

CON: "The data on performing a second TEBP are almost nonexistent. There are no randomized controlled trials of repeat blood patches. Many patients are discharged and lost to follow-up before we see whether the first blood patch even worked. There are some case reports of patients requiring more than two blood patches for relief of their PDPH [11]—the third blood patch was performed under computed tomography (CT) guidance to direct blood to the site of CSF leakage. Explanations for failure of these blood patches include inadequate volume, patching too early, and presence of CSF in the epidural space. CSF may dilute or have an anticoagulant effect that decreases the success of EBPs" [12].

PRO: "The usefulness of repeat EBPs is not well established. Most practitioners will offer a second patch, but are hesitant to do more than two if that fails. A recent survey of North American practitioners reported that nearly 75 % of responders would perform a second TEBP. If the second one fails, or the patient develops neurologic sequela, nearly 90 % of responders would obtain neurologic consultation and additional imaging" [13].

Summary

Epidural blood patch following inadvertent dural puncture has been considered the "standard of care." A recent survey of North American practices reported that more than 90 % of patients with PDPH are treated with EBP [13]. Before the procedure was performed, physicians quoted success rates of greater than 90 % to their patients [12], although recent investigations have shown the success rate of EBP to be much lower. EBP as it is performed now is likely not the gold standard we need to eliminate PDPHs. We need to investigate more solutions to this complication that can result from any epidural anesthetic. In the meantime, we can continue to use epidural blood patches as a valuable treatment in a very limited armamentarium against post-dural puncture headaches.

References

1. Duffy P, Crosby E. The epidural blood patch: resolving the controversies. Can J Anesth. 1999;46:878–86.
2. Verstraete S, Walters M, Devroe S, Roofthooft E, Van de Velde M. Lower incidence of post-dural puncture headache with spinal catheterization after accidental dural puncture in obstetric patients. Acta Anaesth Scand. 2014;58:1233–9.
3. Boonmak P, Boonmak S. Epidural blood patching for preventing and treating post-dural puncture headache. Cochrane Database Syst Rev. 2010;20(1):CD001791.
4. Agerson AN, Scavone BM. Prophylactic epidural blood patch for unintentional dural puncture for the prevention of postdural puncture headache in parturients. Anesth Analg. 2012;115:133–6.
5. Paech M, Banks S, Gurrin L. An audit of accidental dural puncture during epidural insertion of a Tuohy needle in obstetric patients. Int J Obstet Anesth. 2001;10:162–7.
6. Collier CB. Blood patches may cause scarring in the epidural space: two case reports. Int J Obstet Anesth. 2011;20(4):347–51.
7. Desai MJ, Dave AP, Martin MB. Delayed radicular pain following two large volume epidural blood patches for post dural puncture headache: a case report. Pain Physician. 2010;13:257–62.
8. Arevalo-Rodriguez I, Ciapponi A, Munoz L, Roque I. Bonfill Cosp X. Posture and fluids for preventing post-dural puncture headache. Cochrane Database Syst Rev. 2013;12(7):CD009199.
9. Basurto Ona X, Martinez Garcia L, Sola I, Bonfill X. Drug therapy for treating post-dural puncture headache. Cochrane Database Syst Rev. 2013;28(2):001792.
10. Cohen S, Ramos D, Grubb W, Mellender S, Mohiuddin A, Chiricolo A. Sphenopalatine ganglion block: a safer alternative to epidural blood patch for postdural puncture headache. Reg Anesth Pain Med. 2014;39:563.
11. Ho KY, Gan TJ. Management of persistent post-dural puncture headache after repeated epidural blood patch. Acta Anaesth Scand. 2007;51:633–6.
12. Morley AP, Messer CP. Failure of repeated blood patch in a parturient with spinal headache. Int J Obstet Anest. 1993;2(4):204–6.
13. Baysinger C, Pope E, Lochart E, Mercaldo N. The management of accidental dural puncture and postdural puncture headache: a North American survey. J Clin Anesth. 2011;23:349–60.

Should a Spinal Be Used for Surgical Anesthesia After a Failed Labor Epidural?

48

Antonio Gonzalez Fiol and Suzanne K.W. Mankowitz

Case

The obstetrical team (OB) calls the anesthesia resident to inform him that one of the laboring patients will have a cesarean delivery for failure to progress. The anesthesia resident calls his attending: "I am calling to discuss our 24-year-old G1P0 parturient in labor room 8 who will be having a cesarean delivery for failure to progress. The patient's medical history is significant only for obesity. She denies any surgeries in the past. Her airway examination reveals a Mallampati 3, with good mouth opening, normal thyromental distance, full range of motion, and a short, thick neck. We placed her epidural this morning, and I have been asked to give additional medication (top-up) three times since then.

The patient's epidural catheter is bolused with 15 mL of 2 % lidocaine in divided doses. Fifteen minutes later, the patient has a right-sided blockade to T10 and a left-sided block to L1 by pin prick. The anesthesia resident approaches the two anesthesia attendings on the labor floor and asks them how to proceed. The resident suggests quickly doing a low-dose spinal.

A.G. Fiol (✉)
Department of Anesthesiology, Rutgers, New Jersey Medical School, 185 South Orange Ave., MSB E-538 NJ, Newark, NJ 07103, USA
e-mail: gonzala6@njsm.rutgers.edu

A.G. Fiol
182 County Ave, Secaucus, NJ 07094, USA

S.K.W. Mankowitz
Department of Anesthesiology, Columbia University Medical Center, 3959 Broadway, New York, NY 10032, USA
e-mail: sw397@cumc.columbia.edu

S.K.W. Mankowitz
813 Downing Street, Teaneck, NJ 07666, USA

Question

Should a spinal be used for surgical anesthesia for cesarean delivery after a failed labor epidural?

Attending: I wish that you had informed me that you gave numerous boluses to this patient. An increased number of epidural top-ups are associated with epidural anesthesia block failure at cesarean delivery [1]. Before we commit to a plan, have you manipulated the catheter in an attempt to improve the quality of the block? Simple catheter manipulation, such as pulling the catheter back 1 cm, can lead to successful epidural anesthesia. In fact, this intervention may lead to successful epidural anesthesia in greater than 80 % of cases in which there is an initially inadequate surgical block [2].

Resident: I noticed the level to be one-sided after I gave 10 mL of 2 % lidocaine. I pulled back the catheter 1 cm and gave an additional 5 mL. After 15 min, the block remains one-sided. Perhaps a low-dose spinal might work in this case.

Attending: You seem pretty sure about this "low-dose spinal." Why do you think this is our best anesthetic option?

Resident (PRO): A spinal technique offers a quick onset blockade and a dense block. This avoids the "patchy" or unilateral block that is sometimes associated with an epidural, as we are experiencing here. Spinals are a far more reliable technique for cesarean delivery with fewer intraoperative failures and less intraoperative pain [3]. I have seen other anesthesiologists routinely remove the epidural catheter without even attempting to use it for a cesarean delivery; they prefer to place a single-shot spinal. Kinsella [3] and Visser et al. [4] are two authors who have published the literature in favor of this practice.

C.S. Scher et al. (eds.), *You're Wrong, I'm Right*, DOI 10.1007/978-3-319-43169-7_48

Attending (CON): Simply removing a labor epidural catheter and performing a spinal is different from what you are proposing here. Remember, our case is different because we already bolused the epidural with 15 cc of local anesthetic. I think that it would be a bad idea to place a spinal after an epidural bolus, because this could lead to a high or total spinal [5]. Can you imagine having your birth experience destroyed by apnea and intubation? I absolutely forbid you to do this on my watch. Kinsella et al found that there is a significantly greater likelihood for a high spinal in patients who had this procedure performed after already receiving an epidural bolus for cesarean delivery, 7/71 versus 1/68 [3]. However, be aware that high spinals have also occurred even in the absence of a recent epidural bolus. The Serious Complication Repository project (SCORE) found that spinal anesthesia after failed labor epidural represented 27 % of the total high neuraxial blocks secondary to epidural or spinal techniques (excluding unrecognized intrathecal catheters during labor or at the time of cesarean delivery). Obesity accounted for 41 % of those total high neuraxial techniques [6]. Thus, I prefer not to do a single-shot spinal after epidural.

Questions

What is considered low-dose spinal anesthesia? Is it 10 mg of bupivacaine, 7.5 mg, or even less than that? How can you know how much to use, particularly in this case where we already have quite a lot of local anesthetic in the epidural space?

PRO: You have some excellent questions. We do not really know what dose to use. However, looking here at my iPad, I found one article in which a reduced spinal dose was used, between 7.5 mg and 11.3 mg (median 9.38) of 0.75 % hyperbaric bupivacaine with 15–25 mcg of fentanyl. This dose led to zero high spinals in 115 parturients who had a spinal anesthetic after epidural analgesia. No boluses were administered for 30 min prior to spinal placement and the patients remained sitting for 2 min after the neuraxial block [7]. I also found a second study that reported no increased incidence of high or total spinal after labor analgesia compared to de novo spinals, when spinals are placed after labor analgesia without bolusing the epidural catheter for cesarean delivery. In this second study, 128 women were administered 1.5–3 mL of hyperbaric or isobaric 0.5 % bupivacaine with or without 1–3 mcg of sufentanil [4]. Thus, I concur with these authors that a 20 % reduction in spinal dose is a reasonable plan after a labor epidural that has not been recently bolused [7].

CON: Good luck trying to explain to the surgeon why you are going to delay his case for an additional 2 min after doing your spinal! That is a long time, especially if the baby is already having late decelerations, or worse. I think that we really just do not know what dose to use. You must also take into consideration how much volume is in the epidural space from a continuous infusion or bolus. This volume in the epidural space can lead to extension of a spinal blockade [5, 7]. Complicating the situation, remember that this patient has a Mallampati score of 3, which is associated with an incidence of difficult direct laryngoscopy that is eight times higher [8]. We cannot change the body mass index or airway of our patients, but we can modify our anesthetic technique to provide the safest alternative using evidence-based medicine. Therefore, I would advocate a low-dose spinal only as part of a combined spinal-epidural so that the block could be extended as necessary. This particular patient has two risk factors for a high or total spinal: (1) obesity and (2) a failed labor epidural that was bolused less than 30 min before the cesarean delivery. Hence, I would recommend the placement of an epidural and slow titration of the local anesthetic until a surgical level is obtained. It is important to take into consideration the fact that at this point there is a risk of reaching toxic levels of the local anesthetic in question [9]. The authors recommend the use of chloroprocaine-2, 3 % to obtain a surgical level. This would allow a fast evaluation of the level of anesthesia and avoid reaching toxic levels of lidocaine.

Regional anesthesia (epidural, spinal, or combined spinal-epidural) remains the preferred anesthetic technique for the management of urgent/elective cesarean delivery. General anesthesia (GETA) is usually reserved for emergency cesarean delivery, when there is a contraindication for neuraxial anesthesia or in some instances when neuraxial anesthesia fails. GETA carries risks of pulmonary aspiration, difficult airway, a "can't intubate, can't ventilate" situation, neonatal depression, and/or maternal recall. It is critical to remember that the parturient has particularly friable airway mucosa and an increased incidence of difficult airway, even compared to the same patient when she is not pregnant.

It is important to recognize factors that could possibly lead to a situation in which epidural analgesia cannot be used as an anesthetic for cesarean delivery. Some of those risk factors include: the need for multiple top-ups, an urgent cesarean delivery, and training of the anesthesiologist (non-obstetric anesthesia specialist) [1]. The replacement of a poorly functioning labor epidural is the best way to prevent a failed epidural catheter in the event that the patient should end up needing a cesarean delivery. Although spinal anesthesia after an epidural catheter bolus is an acceptable technique, it should be done with great caution and recognition that a high or total spinal could occur, albeit infrequently. Lowering the spinal dose could adversely impact duration of the spinal blockade or result in block failure. Replacement of the original labor epidural with a combined spinal epidural (CSE) or a de novo epidural is other options. A CSE is a good option because it might be more reliable and have a faster onset with better anesthesia than a standalone epidural. Again, however, the best dose for the spinal component of this technique remains unknown, particularly after a bolus is administered. The decision of which technique to perform when faced with a parturient needing an emergency cesarean delivery, who presents with a failed labor epidural, is a difficult one. The patient's risk factors for a total high spinal (i.e., obesity, bolus <30 min ago) must be taken into consideration. Each option has benefits and risks, and the final plan must be tailored to each patient.

References

1. Bauer ME, Kountanis JA, Tsen LC, Greenfield ML, Mhyre JM. Risk factors for failed conversion of labor epidural analgesia to cesarean delivery anesthesia: a systematic review and meta-analysis of observational trials. Int J Obstet Anesth. 2012;21:1–16.
2. Campbell DC, Tran T. Conversion d'une analgésie péridurale pour travail obstétrical en une anesthésie péridurale pour césarienne. Can J Anaesth. 2008;56:19–26.
3. Kinsella SM. A prospective audit of regional anaesthesia failure in 5080 caesarean sections. Anaesthesia. 2008;63:822–32.
4. Visser WA, Dijkstra A, Albayrak M, Gielen MJM, Boersma E, Vonsée HJ. Spinal anesthesia for intrapartum cesarean delivery following epidural labor analgesia: a retrospective cohort study. Can J Anaesth. 2009;56:577–83.
5. Carvalho B. Failed epidural top-up for cesarean delivery for failure to progress in labor: the case against single-shot spinal anesthesia. Int J Obstet Anesth. 2012;21:357–9.
6. D'Angelo R, Smiley RM, Riley ET, Segal S. Serious complications related to obstetric anesthesia: the serious complication repository project of the Society for Obstetric Anesthesia and Perinatology. Anesthesiology. 2014;120:1505–12.
7. Dadarkar P, Philip J, Weidner C, Perez B, Slaymaker E, Tabaczewska L, Wiley J, Sharma S. Spinal anesthesia for cesarean section following inadequate labor epidural analgesia: a retrospective audit. Int J Obstet Anesth. 2004;13:239–43.
8. Boutonnet M, Faitot V, Katz A, Salomon L, Keita H. Mallampati class changes during pregnancy, labour, and after delivery: can these be predicted? Br J Anaesth. 2010;104:67–70.
9. Riley ET, Papasin J. Epidural catheter function during labor predicts anesthetic efficacy for subsequent cesarean delivery. Int J Obstet Anesth. 2002;11:81–4.

Accidental Dural Puncture: Should an Intrathecal Catheter Be Threaded?

49

Katherine Chuy and Shruthima Thangada

Case

It was a late night on the obstetrics floor. I was the resident on call, overseeing the management of 7 epidurals in laboring patients. Just as I was about to lay my head down in the call room, I received a call from the nurse, who told me that a patient being admitted was asking to speak with me about an epidural. I looked over her chart and saw that she was a healthy 32-year-old female giving birth to her second child. She had 1 uncomplicated pregnancy in the past and no previous miscarriages or abortions. When I met the patient in the labor room, the obstetrics resident informed me she was 6 cm dilated and would likely deliver that evening.

After reviewing the case with my attending and determining that the patient had no contraindications for an epidural placement, I prepared for the procedure while my attending supervised me. Everything was going smoothly as I slowly advanced the 10-cm, 18-G Tuohy epidural needle. Suddenly, however, with the next advancement, a gush of fluid started filling the syringe attached to the needle. With my hands still on the needle and the patient's back, I shook my head in disappointment and looked at my attending. I had accidentally punctured the dura once before, and I felt discouraged with this second blunder during my obstetric anesthesia rotation. Still not used to making quick decisions, I froze as cerebrospinal fluid (CSF) rushed into the syringe.

"Should I take the epidural out and place it at another level?" I whispered to my attending. This is what I did the last time with a different attending.

"You could," he said. "Or you could just thread the epidural catheter."

What? I thought. *I've never heard of such a thing. At the same time, here is a chance to do something new.* Following my attending's step-by-step instructions, I threaded the catheter and injected a small amount of local anesthetic. Within moments, the patient was much more comfortable. I confirmed good bilateral pain relief up to the T7 level and ensured she did not have any signs of a high spinal. I labeled the catheter with a bright red sticker, informing everyone on the medical staff that this was a *spinal catheter*, not an epidural catheter. I hooked the catheter up to a medication pump, slowly infusing the local anesthetic at a low, constant rate. The patient did well, ultimately giving birth several hours later.

I later sat down with my attending to discuss this case. I recognized the accidental dural puncture immediately and understood that we did not want to leave the needle in place with CSF leaking, because that would increase the risk of post-dural puncture headache (PDPH). The harder part for me was quickly making a decision about how to rectify the situation. I suggested doing what I was familiar with: removing the needle and reinserting it at another level. But this was residency. I had to expose myself to different schools of thought as well as critically analyze and determine alternatives when the initial anesthetic plan did not play out as expected.

Question

An accidental dural puncture (ADP) during an epidural placement increases the chance of PDPH. Should we thread the epidural catheter into the intrathecal space when this occurs, or reintroduce the epidural at a new interspace? Does threading the catheter reduce the risk of PDPH?

CON (Resident): I understand that puncturing the dura exposes a patient to the risk of PDPH caused by decreased

K. Chuy (✉)
Department of Anesthesiology, Perioperative Care and Pain Medicine, New York University Langone Medical Center, 550 First Avenue, New York, NY 10016, USA
e-mail: Katherine.chuy@nyumc.org

S. Thangada
Department of Anesthesiology, New York University Langone Medical Center, 309 5th Avenue, Apt. 4C, New York, NY 10016, USA
e-mail: midazgal@gmail.com

C.S. Scher et al. (eds.), *You're Wrong, I'm Right*, DOI 10.1007/978-3-319-43169-7_49

pressure as CSF leaks through the dural tear. This causes CSF volume loss and intracranial hypotension. It can be caused by a spinal or combined spinal/epidural procedure, if we intend for the dura to be punctured. If the dura is punctured during an epidural placement, however, it's referred to as ADP or "wet tap." Epidural needles have larger bores (16 or 18 G) than spinal needles. Because they are larger, ADP would increase the amount of CSF leak, thus increasing the risk of PDPH [1].

If the dura were punctured during an epidural placement, I would immediately recognize this by observing CSF exiting through the needle. My approach, based on my limited experience, would involve immediately taking the needle out and reinserting it at another interspace. Hopefully, my prompt response of removing the needle would prevent too much CSF leakage, which could lead to PDPH. I would keep a close eye on the patient for any symptoms that would suggest PDPH, such as headache presenting in the occipital or frontal regions, which is exacerbated by assuming an upright position and relieved by lying down [2]. Once I established that my newly placed epidural was working well, I would manage it as I normally would. I would load the epidural to establish a good sensory level, and then I would set an appropriate infusion rate to maintain adequate analgesia. I would report to the nurse and team taking care of the patient so they are familiar with the plan of care.

PRO (Attending): You have some good points and a good line of thinking. Although nobody wants to accidentally puncture the dura during an epidural needle placement, it happens to the best of us. According to some published reports, the rate of ADP varies from 0.19 to 6.6 %. Of the patients affected, PDPH can occur in 50–70 %, so it's not insignificant [1]. The question then turns to what you should do when you recognize ADP during an epidural attempt. One option, as you mentioned, is removing the epidural needle and restarting the procedure in a new interspace. The second option is threading the epidural catheter intrathecally to continue with spinal analgesia. You are still giving analgesia as you would with an adequately placed epidural, but studies have suggested that threading the catheter after ADP can help decrease the chances of PDPH. The third and fourth options, both less likely in this case, are to give a single-shot spinal dose through the epidural needle or to abandon the procedure entirely [3]. We won't go into the last 2 options in this discussion.

There are some benefits to immediately threading the epidural catheter intrathecally. For one, this obviates the need to retry the epidural, which can expose the patient to another ADP and place them at even higher risk of PDPH if the needle punctures the dura a second time. Once a catheter is placed intrathecally, it can be dosed appropriately with local anesthetics and opioids to provide rapid and effective labor analgesia, anesthesia for operative delivery, or for other procedures where neuraxial anesthesia is beneficial.

Secondly, some studies have suggested a decreased incidence of PDPH when the spinal catheter is threaded during ADP. One recent meta-analysis showed a risk ratio for PDPH after spinal catheterization of 0.82. The laboring patients in this study with ADP, who had a catheter in place for at least 24 hours, had a reduced incidence of PDPH compared to those who had an epidural attempted at another location (42 vs. 62 %, odds ratio = 2.3) [1]. Another study also showed that the group who had an intrathecal catheter placed for at least 24 hours also had a decreased PDPH incidence of 6.2 % [4]. While these studies seem promising, they also have limitations. Additionally, a recent meta-analysis analyzed 9 studies on parturients and concluded that the incidence of PDPH was reduced, but not significantly, by intrathecal catheters after ADP [5].

So, while recent studies have been conflicting, we ultimately want to do what we can to reduce the chance of PDPH—an unpleasant experience for patients; it can hinder ambulation and prolong the hospital stay [4]. It is at least worth considering the option of threading an intrathecal catheter after ADP, as there seem to be suggestions that it can help decrease the incidence of PDPH and, at least, avoid another epidural attempt.

Question

Does threading a catheter decrease the need for an epidural blood patch (EBP)? What about a prophylactic EBP?

CON (Resident): OK, I understand that some studies suggest that threading the catheter decreases the chance of getting PDPH, but patients who get a spinal catheter can still get PDPH. In the event that they do develop this complication, there are options we can choose to manage it, such as conservative treatment like intravenous hydration and bed rest. Ultimately, if these do not work, I would recommend doing EBP, which has a pretty high success rate. If studies are not conclusive that a spinal catheter will decrease the incidence of PDPH, I don't quite see the benefit of threading the catheter, particularly if I'm quite confident I can insert it successfully the second time around. If it comes to the point where the patient gets PDPH, I will manage it accordingly, even if it means performing an EBP.

PRO (Attending): I understand that you are getting into your comfort zone. I do want to challenge you, though, to at least be able to assess your options, and know why and how you come to your decisions. To be able to perform epidurals quickly, safely, and successfully is great. Remember, though, performing an EBP is also not always benign—it comes with the same risks as performing an epidural. If our goal is to provide a safe way to manage pain and decrease side effects, complications, and risks, I want you to at least consider that a continuous spinal anesthetic is also an option if we do not want to risk another ADP. In addition to what I mentioned earlier about analyses suggesting a decreased incidence of PDPH, studies have also suggested a lower incidence of patients needing a therapeutic EBP with intrathecal catheters compared to patients who received another attempted epidural [4, 5]. However, other studies have suggested no statistical difference in EBP rates when comparing spinal catheters to epidurals reinserted at another location after ADP [1, 6].

Conservative treatment such as hydration and bed rest has not been shown to be very effective at treating PDPH [1]. Thus, if threading the epidural catheter intrathecally at the time of ADP can possibly help prevent PDPH and decrease the chance of needing EBP, my opinion is that this would be an option worth considering. Performing EBP has its own risks, so it seems to me that a spinal catheter may be a better choice than reintroducing the epidural at a new interspace in that it can provide quick, adequate pain relief and possibly prevent a higher risk of PDPH and the need for EBP.

Question

We have to be so careful with the dosing in these catheters. Are they worth the risk if other people taking care of the patient are not familiar with the epidural?

CON (Resident): There appears to be a lot of risk with these catheters, especially on a busy obstetrics floor where there is a lot of turnover among residents and medical staff. Giving a large dose and causing a high spinal despite correctly labeling the catheter and giving adequate turnover instructions would be a devastating error. I would rather not take this chance. I would rather know that if my patient ended up having PDPH, there are several different management options available, even if it means performing a therapeutic EBP.

PRO (Attending): The placement of a spinal catheter indeed poses risks if it is not managed correctly. Thus, only those trained to manage these catheters should be involved in their placement. There must be clear labeling that they are *intrathecal catheters*. I'm glad you recognize the concerns surrounding this procedure and other aspects of its management that might make it risky in the hospital setting. I hope that this discussion at least allows you to broaden your scope of options when ADP occurs. I would encourage you to continue reading literature that comes out on this. While the information I have mentioned points toward certain possible benefits of spinal catheters, remember that much of the literature are meta-analyses, or observational and retrospective studies. We have yet to see a large-scale, prospective, randomized control study on this topic, mainly because the rates of ADP and PDPH are low, and such studies would require a significant length of time, many patients, and many participating medical centers in order to get results that are statistically significant.

Summary

Interestingly, 1 study investigated injecting intrathecal morphine with short-term spinal catheterization (i.e., less than 24 hours), as a means of preventing PDPH in non-obstetric surgery [3]. In their case series, 11 of 686 adult patients undergoing pelvic/lower limb surgery with plans for a combined spinal/epidural procedure received a continuous spinal catheter following an ADP. At the end of surgery, intrathecal morphine and hyperbaric bupivacaine were given. There were no reports of any morphine side effects (nausea, vomiting, pruritus, respiratory depression, or urinary retention), symptoms of PDPH, paresthesias, fever, or signs of infection upon daily follow-up for 7–10 days after surgery. According to this study, it is perhaps the intrathecal opioids that helped decrease the incidence of PDPH and thus the need for EBP after ADP with spinal catheterization [3].

More large, multicenter, prospective randomized control trials have to be done to determine what exactly can help prevent PDPH and decrease the need for therapeutic EBP after ADP. Current studies suggest the benefit of threading an epidural catheter intrathecally to prevent PDPH and decrease the need for EBP, but results vary.

Inserting a spinal catheter after ADP can lead to immediate pain relief and decreases the need to reintroduce the epidural at another site; some studies suggest that it may also help reduce the risk of PDPH and EBP. Ultimately, the decision to thread a spinal catheter depends on the anesthesiologist's comfort and on the team that will be managing the catheter thereafter.

References

1. Verstraete S, Walters MA, Devroe S, Roofthooft E, Van de Velde M. Lower incidence of postdural puncture headache with spinal catheterization after accidental dural puncture in obstetric patients. Acta Anaesth Scand. 2014;58:1233–9.
2. Turnbull DK, Shephard DB. Post-dural puncture headache: pathogenesis, prevention and treatment. Br J Anaesth. 2003;91:718–29.
3. Chaudhary K, Saxena KN, Taneja B, Gaba P, Anand R. Intrathecal catheterisation for accidental dural puncture: a successful strategy for

reducing postdural puncture headache. Indian J Anaesth. 2014;58:473–5.
4. Ayad S, Demian Y, Narouze SN, Tetzlaff JE. Subarachnoid catheter placement after wet tap for analgesia in labor: influence on the risk of headache in obstetric patients. Reg Anesth Pain Med. 2003;28:512–5.
5. Heesen M, Klöhr S, Rossaint R, Walters M, Straube S, van de Velde M. Insertion of an intrathecal catheter following accidental dural puncture: a meta-analysis. Int J Obstet Anesth. 2013;22:26–30.
6. Russell IF. A prospective controlled study of continuous spinal analgesia versus repeat epidural analgesia after accidental dural puncture in labour. Int J Obstet Anesth. 2012;21:7–16.

Should Intraoperative Cell Salvage Be Used During Cesarean Delivery?

50

Alaeldin A. Darwich and Sharon E. Abramovitz

Case

A 32-year-old woman, G3P2, at 38-week gestation presented to triage with vaginal bleeding. She had two previous cesarean sections: the first for breech presentation and the second at her request, both of which were complicated by uterine atony and postpartum hemorrhage. She received a blood transfusion, but did not recall the amount or type of blood products administered.

The patient was scheduled for repeat cesarean section in 8 days. She was hemodynamically stable, but the obstetrician suspected mild placental abruption and he wanted to proceed with cesarean section urgently.

You are the obstetric anesthesiologist covering the labor and delivery unit. With a high risk of bleeding in this case, you contact the blood bank to assure that blood is available before proceeding to the operating room. Your colleague, who came to start his shift and take over labor and delivery, called the anesthesia technician to set up the cell salvage machine. You are in complete disagreement with your colleague about using intraoperative cell salvage (IOCS) during cesarean section.

Obstetric hemorrhage is the leading cause of maternal mortality worldwide. In the USA, hemorrhage was the cause of 11.3 % of all pregnancy-related deaths in 2011 [1]. Pregnancy-related transfusion accounts for up to 6 % of the total quantity of red blood cells transfused in developed countries. In the USA, this is equivalent to approximately 830,000 units of red cells transfused annually secondary to obstetrics-related anemia and hemorrhage [2].

The practice of intraoperative blood salvage has increased substantially during the last two decades during surgeries where large volumes of blood loss are anticipated. Allogeneic blood transfusions are certainly beneficial in specific situations, but this practice is also associated with many risks and side effects including postoperative infection, acute lung injury, perioperative myocardial infarction, and low cardiac output failure. The rate of allogeneic blood transfusion and its associated risks and costs has decreased with the use of IOCS. There is strong evidence for the use of intraoperative cell salvage in cardiac and orthopedic surgery, but there are concerns about its use in obstetrics [3].

A.A. Darwich (✉) · S.E. Abramovitz
Department of Anesthesiology, New York Presbyterian Hospital - Weill Cornell Medicine, 525 East 68th Street, Box 124
New York, NY 10065, USA
e-mail: Aad2004@med.cornell.edu

S.E. Abramovitz
e-mail: Sea2003@med.cornell.edu

Question

Should intraoperative cell salvage be used during cesarean section? If so, what are the safety concerns and economic benefits of IOCS?

Risk of Iatrogenic Amniotic Fluid Embolism

CON: Using IOCS in the obstetrical setting is not a safe practice due to the risk of contamination with amniotic fluid and fetal cells, and re-administration of the shed blood can trigger an iatrogenic amniotic fluid embolism (AFE). Parturients are different from general surgery patients.

PRO: This is a theoretical concern. The presence of fetal cells and amniotic fluid in the maternal blood has been regarded as a marker of AFE, but both components are present in the maternal blood even when AFE does not develop.

Intraoperatively, two suctions can be utilized: one to remove the initial blood that is rich in amniotic fluid and the other for subsequent bleeding. The suctioned maternal blood

C.S. Scher et al. (eds.), *You're Wrong, I'm Right*, DOI 10.1007/978-3-319-43169-7_50

is mixed with anticoagulant and then filtered, washed, centrifuged, suspended in saline, and re-administered to the patient. This process will remove multiple contaminants of shed blood, which include free hemoglobin, anticoagulant, inflammatory mediators, cellular debris, and amniotic fluid. When leukocyte depletion filtration is used after washing, the salvaged blood product will be comparable to the circulating maternal [4].

Clinical experience with about 400 case reports supports the use of IOCS. With this technology, maternal blood contaminated with amniotic fluid has been re-administered to the mother after washing without the development of amniotic fluid embolism.

CON: IOCS has been used in obstetric hemorrhage. But there are no randomized controlled trials that exist to support the safety of blood salvage in obstetrics and the supporting data that do exist are based only on case reports. AFE can be a life-threatening complication.

PRO: AFE is a rare event with an incidence of 1–12 cases per 100,000 deliveries [5]. A study to prove the safety of blood salvage in OB would require a huge sample, which would be impractical and very expensive. The available data show that there is currently no reported case of AFE associated with the use of cell salvage in obstetrics. As anesthesiologists, we use off-label drugs and devices and adopt practices without definite support from data. For example, we add fentanyl and/or morphine to local anesthetics when performing spinal and epidural anesthesia, which is an off-label use of these drugs.

The etiology of AFE is not clear. The pathophysiology of AFE is considered to be similar to anaphylactic- or endotoxin-mediated shock rather than an embolic event. Therefore, AFE could occur regardless of the presence of fetal tissue or blood in the maternal circulation [6].

Rh-Immunization

CON: What about concerns for Rh-immunization? Cell salvage cannot distinguish maternal blood from fetal blood. In a parturient who is Rh-negative, there is a risk of Rh-immunization if the fetus is Rh-positive.

PRO: This should not be of great concern. All Rh-negative parturients receive anti-D immunoglobulin after delivery. A Kleihauer test should be performed in the immediate postpartum period to calculate the appropriate dose of anti-D immunoglobulin.

Risks of Allogenic Blood Transfusion

CON: There is hesitation in using IOCS, particularly since the blood bank is available 24 h per day. In elective cesarean sections with a high risk of postpartum hemorrhage, such as known placenta accreta, there is time to alert the blood bank and prepare for massive hemorrhage. In emergency situations, O-negative blood is available in the labor and delivery unit for immediate use, and the massive transfusion protocol can be activated. Why is cell salvage advantageous over the blood bank supply?

PRO: Allogeneic blood transfusion is not without adverse effects. Traditionally, blood transfusion-related adverse effects have focused on infectious complications. These risks are extremely rare due to pre-donation testing and screening. However, when multiple units are transfused, this risk is increased substantially. The risk of having any type of infection is about 1:30,000 after exposure to 1 unit of blood and is dose-dependent. After ten units of blood, the patient's risk increases to 1:3000 [4].

A more commonly recognized risk is transfusion-related acute lung injury (TRALI), which is indistinguishable from acute respiratory distress syndrome (ARDS) and has an incidence of 1:12,000 transfused units.

Transfusion-associated circulatory overload (TACO) occurs in 1–6 % of transfused patients and may be seen in young patients after transfusion of as little as 1 unit of RBCs [7].

Immunomodulation is a unique concern after blood transfusion, especially in the younger patient. Short- and long-term effects include nosocomial infection, postoperative infection, and cancer recurrence [8].

A systematic review and meta-analysis of health care-associated infections after RBC transfusion found that a restrictive transfusion strategy might lower the incidence of health care-associated serious infection [9].

The aim of cell salvage is to reduce the need for allogeneic blood transfusion and its associated risks. If a patient is a Jehovah's Witness or has a rare blood group or antibodies, this blood saving technique is readily available. Cell salvage is acceptable to some Jehovah's Witnesses who refuse allogenic blood transfusion, provided that blood remains in continuity with their circulation.

Question

Is the use of cell salvage in the obstetric setting cost-effective?

CON: The majority of cases of postpartum hemorrhage have no known risk factors, and predicting who would benefit from cell salvage is difficult. In order for cell salvage to be beneficial, it should be available at all times, especially during emergency situations. Emergency cesarean sections have been shown to be associated with more hemorrhage than scheduled cesarean sections, and utilization of cell salvage is most needed in this situation [10]. A 24-h service with experienced personnel to initiate the cell salvage when needed will mandate additional costs, manpower, and training.

PRO: The cost-effectiveness of cell salvage in obstetrics may depend on the facility's case volume, risks, and the volume of blood loss for each case. Financial and education investments in such technology would be beneficial in high-volume tertiary obstetric units with high-risk parturients. In such settings, cell salvage can be cost-effective compared with allogenic blood transfusion [10].

Postpartum hemorrhage is notorious for unpredictability, and blood loss is usually underestimated. With the increase of uterine blood flow at full term, which may reach 700–900 mL/min, large amounts of blood can be lost in minutes. One way to minimize cost and to be ready for transfusion is to set up the cell salvage machine in "stand-by mode," which is using only the collecting system. When sufficient blood is collected, the processing components can then be utilized [11].

CON: One of the goals of using IOCS in obstetrics is to eliminate or minimize the use of allogeneic blood. The available data show that the median salvaged blood transfused does not exceed two units, and the percentage of women who avoided allogeneic blood transfusion is 28.5 %. However, it is unknown whether these data will support IOCS to reduce the use of blood bank supply [12].

PRO: The available data are based on studies with small sample sizes, and the groups were not homogenous. The starting hemoglobin was not the same, and transfusion guidelines and thresholds were different. A randomized control study to establish the efficacy of IOCS on the blood bank would require about 4500 patients to detect a 33 % reduction in allogeneic blood usage. Despite the lack of data, the American College of Obstetrics and Gynecology recommends the use of IOCS in women when massive hemorrhage is anticipated [12]. Also the American Society of Anesthesiologists recommends its use in cases of intractable hemorrhage when banked blood is not available or the patient refuses [13]. Similarly in the UK, several official scientific bodies recommend the use of IOCS in specific circumstances.

A multicenter randomized controlled trial of IOCS use during cesarean section conducted in the UK was scheduled to end in April 2015. This trial recruited 3050 participants to determine whether routine use of IOCS during cesarean section will reduce the need for blood bank transfusion in comparison with the current practice. Such a large study will hopefully answer questions about efficacy of IOCS usage and concerns about adverse effects [14].

Summary

Intraoperative cell salvage is a blood conservation technique with the main goal of reducing the use of banked blood and its associated risks. The use of IOCS in the obstetrical setting was limited initially by concerns for risks of AFE and Rh-immunization. To date, there are about 400 case reports describing the safe use of IOCS to manage postpartum hemorrhage. There are no proven cases of AFE after IOCS reported in the literature. Medical societies in the USA and UK are endorsing its use to manage postpartum hemorrhage (PPH). Randomized controlled trials are needed to show its effectiveness and the impact on the supply of allogeneic blood.

References

1. Centers for Disease Control and Prevention. Pregnancy mortality surveillance system; 2011. http://www.cdc.gov/reproductivehealth/maternalinfanthealth/pmss.html. Accessed 23 Apr 2015.
2. Blood transfusion safety. World Health Organization; 2006. http://www.who.int/bloodsafety/en/Blood_Transfusion_Safety.pdf?ua=1. Accessed 23 Apr 2015.
3. Herd JM, Joseph JJ, McGarvey M, Tsimbouri P, Bennett A, Meek RMD, Morrison A. Intraoperative cell salvage in revision hip surgery. Ann Med Surg (Lond). 2014;3:8–12.
4. Waters JH. Pro/con debate: is cell salvage a safe technique for the obstetric patient? Soc Obstet Anesthesiol Perinatol Newsl. 2005;7–8.
5. Baldisseri MR, Manaker S, Lockwood CJ, Finaly G. Amniotic fluid embolism syndrome; 2015. http://www.uptodate.com/contents/amniotic-fluid-embolism-syndrome. Accessed 23 Apr 2015.
6. Clark SL. Clinical expert series. Amniotic fluid embolism. Obstet Gynecol. 2014;123:337–48.
7. Scavone BM. Antepartum and postpartum hemorrhage. In: Chestnut DH, Wong CA, Tsen LC, Ngan Kee WD, Beilin Y, Mhyre J, editors. Chestnut's obstetric anesthesia principles and practice. 5th ed. Philadelphia: Mosby; 2014. p. 881–914.
8. Lannan K, Sahler J, Spinelli SL, Phipps RP, Blumberg N. Transfusion immunomodulation—the case for leukoreduced and (perhaps) washed transfusions. Blood Cells Mol Dis. 2013;50:61–8.

9. Rohde JM, Dimcheff DF, Blumberg N, Saint S, Langa KM, Kuhn L, et al. Health care-associated infection after red blood cell transfusion: a systematic review and meta-analysis. JAMA. 2014;311:1317–26.
10. Brearton C, Bhalla A, Mallaiah S, Barclay P. The economic benefits of cell salvage in obstetric haemorrhage. Int J Obstet Anesth. 2012;21:329–33.
11. Esper SA, Waters JH. Intra-operative cell salvage: a fresh look at the indications and contraindications. Blood Transfu. 2011;9:139–47.
12. Liumbruno GM, Meschini A, Liumbruno C, Rafanelli D. The introduction of intra-operative cell salvage in obstetric clinical practice: a review of the available evidence. Eur J Obstet Gynecol Reprod Biol. 2011;159:19–25.
13. American Society of Anesthesiologists Task Force on Obstetric Anesthesia. Practice guidelines for obstetric anesthesia: an updated report by the American Society of Anesthesiologists Task Force on Obstetric Anesthesia. Anesthesiology. 2007;106:843–8.
14. Dhariwal SK, Khan KS, Allard S, Wilson M, Moore P. SALVO study group. Does current evidence support the use of intraoperative cell salvage in reducing the need for blood transfusion in cesarean section? Curr Opin Obstet Gynecol. 2014;26(6):425–30.

Should Damage Control or Traditional Resuscitation Be Used for Abnormal Placentation Cases?

51

Anna Korban, Antonio Gonzalez Fiol, and Stephanie R. Goodman

Case

A healthy 25-year-old G_3P_{2002} patient at 38-week gestation was referred to the high-risk obstetric anesthesia service due to the presence of abnormal placentation. Her past surgical history included 2 previous cesarean deliveries. The ultrasound examination was suspicious for a complete anterior placenta previa with multiple placental lakes, which looked even more likely after magnetic resonance imaging (MRI).

One day prior to the scheduled cesarean delivery, the team discussed the anesthetic plan. The resident told the attending that she read about damage control resuscitation for a presentation, and asked, "Do we have any evidence to support the use of this transfusion strategy for severe obstetric hemorrhage?"

Question

Should damage control or traditional resuscitation be used for abnormal placentation cases (expected or unexpected)?

A. Korban
Department of Anesthesiology, Rutgers, New Jersey Medical School, 48 Veterans Drive, South River, NJ 08882, USA
e-mail: korbanan@njms.rutgers.edu

A. Gonzalez Fiol (✉)
Department of Anesthesiology, Rutgers, New Jersey Medical School, 185 South Orange Ave., MSB E-538 NJ, Newark, NJ 07103, USA
e-mail: gonzala6@njsm.rutgers.edu

A. Gonzalez Fiol
182 County Ave, Secaucus, NJ 07094, USA

S.R. Goodman
Department of Anesthesiology, Columbia University Medical Center, New York Presbyterian – Columbia, 630 West 168th Street, P and S Box 46, New York, NY 10025, USA
e-mail: srg24@cumc.columbia.edu

S.R. Goodman
310 West 99th Street, Apt 106, New York, NY 10025, USA

PRO: Your attending explained, "You are correct that early coagulopathy, specifically enhanced fibrinolysis, is not exclusive to trauma and is also a known problem in obstetrical hemorrhage [1]. Some authors refer to the normal coagulation changes at the end of pregnancy (increase of several clotting factors and anticoagulants, and a decrease in fibrinolytic activity) as a low-grade compensated disseminated intravascular coagulation (DIC). It is not uncommon to see DIC develop in patients with placental abruption, amniotic fluid embolism (AFE), or hemorrhagic shock [1]. That being said, it is important to respond to severe hemorrhage quickly, not only by replacing packed red blood cells (PRBCs) but also considering that a rapid consumption of coagulation factors (i.e., DIC) might follow."

CON: A second attending, known for being more conservative, retorts, "I think that we do not have enough evidence to support the use of damage control resuscitation (PRBCs to fresh frozen plasma [FFP] to platelets 1:1:1) in obstetrical patients compared to traditional resuscitation (PRBCs to FFP to platelets 3:1:1 after 10 U PRBCs). The damage control strategy has been shown to be effective only in trauma patients. Rheologically speaking, parturients are known to be in a hypercoagulable state [2] and obstetric hemorrhage is not necessarily the same as traumatic hemorrhage. Why would parturients need early or aggressive replacement of their coagulation factors?"

PRO: "I would like you to see this review article by Gallos et al. [3]. They cite several studies showing that trauma patients who received a 1:1 PRBC:plasma ratio had less coagulopathy and improved survival. Most importantly, just as I mentioned before, they stress the relationship between the early coagulopathy and DIC associated with severe hemorrhage, which is what we expect in a patient with a placenta accreta. In addition, they shares their positive experience (personal and institutional) with using a 1:1:1 strategy when managing patients with known abnormal placentation."

C.S. Scher et al. (eds.), *You're Wrong, I'm Right*, DOI 10.1007/978-3-319-43169-7_51

CON: "After your explanation of the coagulation changes during pregnancy, this makes sense physiologically, but where is the evidence?! Plenty of ideas in the history of medicine have seemed great on paper, but studies have proven them false."

PRO: "I agree with you that we do not have a lot of literature to support using a 1:1 ratio of PRBCs to FFP in treating postpartum hemorrhage (PPH). What is proven, though, is the importance of fibrinogen and its early replacement during resuscitation. Here, let's quickly review this article I have. Charbit et al. [1] collected blood from 128 parturients the moment administration of prostaglandin E2 was deemed necessary, typically after first-line maneuvers (manual exploration/massage of the uterus and administration of oxytocin) failed to control excessive bleeding. The blood was collected at 0, 1, 2, 4, and 24 h. From all of the many laboratory values measured, (PT, PTT, INR, fibrinogen, Factor II and Factor V, D-dimer, antithrombin, protein C, thrombin-antithrombin [TAT] and plasmin-antiplasmin [PAP] complexes, soluble fibrin, euglobin lysis time and soluble thrombomodulin), multivariate analysis showed that fibrinogen was the only factor independently associated with progression to severe hemorrhage (defined as peripartum decrease of hemoglobin by 4 g/dL or more; transfusion of at least 4 units of PRBCs, the need for hemostatic intervention such as embolization, surgical vascular ligation, or total hysterectomy, or death). Fibrinogen levels of less than 2 g/L at time zero had a 100 % positive predictive value for severe hemorrhage, which strongly suggests that fibrinogen levels should be maintained above 2 g/L during massive hemorrhage. Early administration of FFP (damage control transfusion) is of the utmost importance in order to avoid progression to severe hemorrhage. As you can see, in traditional resuscitation, FFP would not be given until after 10 units of PRBCs, and fibrinogen would not be replaced until much too late!"

CON: "There is no way to tell from this study design if the low fibrinogen levels were the cause or a consequence of the bleeding. FFP isn't a great way to replace fibrinogen anyway—it only contains 2 g/L, which means that large volumes of FFP would be needed to achieve this goal. Cryoprecipitate has a much higher fibrinogen concentration (388 mg/Unit), but also poses higher risks of immune and transfusion reactions [4]. Is the benefit worth the risk of exposing patients to the volume and risk of infection and allergic reaction? Aiming to correct hypofibrinogenemia with FFP might result in transfusion-acquired circulatory-overload (TACO)."

PRO: "How about fibrinogen concentrate? The volume is low, and it is processed to decrease the risk of infection.

"Early administration of fibrinogen concentrate for treatment of PPH was addressed in a recently published randomized controlled trial by Wikkelso et al. [5]. Unfortunately, their liberal use of tranexamic acid in both study groups, inability to include patients with massive and rapid bleeding, and the fact that only 2 % of the enrolled patients had a fibrinogen level <2 g/L limit the generalizability of this study. The majority of their patients would have been categorized as low risk for severe hemorrhage according to Charbit et al. [1] (fibrinogen of >4 g/L). I do admit that I am waiting for better evidence before incorporating fibrinogen concentrate into my practice, though."

CON: "Should we send STAT blood work and direct our management to maintaining a fibrinogen level >2 g/L?"

PRO: "Waiting for blood work results such as a fibrinogen level or coagulation profile could result in delayed administration of blood products. Although clinical judgment is important, in massive hemorrhage, there isn't time to play catch-up. Protocols can assist with 'staying ahead' once a massive hemorrhage situation has been declared, keeping a balance between replacement of oxygen-carrying PRBCs and replenishment of important coagulation factors. In our institution, per our request, cryoprecipitate is in the second box of blood products sent with activation of the obstetric massive transfusion protocol (MTP). In contrast, in the trauma MTP, cryoprecipitate is not transfused until after the fourth box of products.

"Some institutions use point-of-care thromboelastography devices such as the ROTEM®, TEG®, or FIBTEM® for guiding hemorrhage treatment. Although not a 'real-time' result, thromboelastography comes close, detecting the strength of clot formation in approximately 10 min. This test can also help with early detection of abnormal fibrinolysis and its response to therapy [2]."

CON: "It makes sense then to use more yellow products early in a case of obstetrical hemorrhage. But why not also use an anti-fibrinolytic drug such as tranexamic acid, as you mentioned in the study by Wikkelso et al. [5]? I can get it from the cardiac room and we can use it in the case tomorrow."

PRO: "The data, in terms of safety and efficacy of tranexamic acid in cases of PPH, are not clear and more work is needed before making a practice-changing decision. The CRASH-2 trial demonstrated that the use of tranexamic acid reduced mortality in trauma patients with no increase in thromboembolic events [6]. On the other hand, the obstetric literature is inconclusive (mainly as a result of a lack of well-designed studies) in terms of its routine use during elective or urgent cesarean deliveries or for PPH management. There is an ongoing trial looking into the efficiency of tranexamic acid for obstetric hemorrhage (WOMEN trial) [6]."

CON: "OK. I overheard the nursing staff saying that we were going to be using cell salvage during this delivery. I thought that the use of cell salvage was a relative contraindication in patients with obstetric hemorrhage due to the risk of AFE?"

PRO: "The use of cell salvage was restricted out of fear of exposing the maternal circulation to amniotic fluid and fetal material, which were believed to be triggers of AFE. We now understand, however, that AFE is not an embolic phenomenon but a rare, severe anaphylactoid reaction and that the presence of amniotic fluid and fetal material in the maternal circulation is not uncommon. The use of cell salvage has been reported in hundreds of obstetric hemorrhage cases without causing iatrogenic AFE [3]. Caution should be used as there are some case reports in which hypotension has been associated with the use of cell salvage during cesarean delivery. Despite these reports, cell salvage is commonly used in many institutions in patients with known or highly suspected abnormal placentation. In fact, the use of cell salvage is recommended by the American College of Obstetricians and Gynecologists for such patients [7]."

Summary

Postpartum hemorrhage remains one of the leading causes of maternal morbidity and mortality [2]. Recently, we have seen an increase in the literature describing low fibrinogen levels related to severe hemorrhage. Yet it still remains unclear whether this is the cause of, or merely associated with, the bleeding [4]. Given the association between this coagulation factor and PPH, it is not surprising that many obstetric anesthesiologists have adopted the damage control transfusion strategy that has normally been reserved for trauma patients. Not only have we provided early availability and transfusion of FFP, but have we modified this strategy as well in order to better suit our obstetric patients' needs.

In our institution, the obstetric MTP (Table 51.1) uses cryoprecipitate early, which is aimed at restoring fibrinogen levels as aggressively as possible. It is reasonable to consider that in the near future, we might replace fibrinogen with fibrinogen concentrate. Even though the FIB-PPH trial (fibrinogen concentrate) by Wikkelso et al. [5] showed no efficacy from pre-treatment with fibrinogen concentrate in PPH, we still think that the use of this drug and tranexamic acid might become part of our pharmacologic therapy for PPH.

The management of PPH is an enormous task that requires a multidisciplinary approach involving physicians, nurses, and the blood bank, among others. The primary goal of this approach is early recognition and aggressive management of patients at risk of, or suffering from, PPH. There is even a nationwide movement toward the creation and implementation of protocols aimed at decreasing the morbidity and mortality associated with severe PPH. This is exemplified by the creation of the Obstetric Hemorrhage Care Guidelines and Hemorrhage Tool kits by the California Maternal Quality Care Collaborative Task Force (https://www.cmqcc.org) and the recent study by Shields et al. [8]. The key elements of these protocols are the early identification of patients at risk and the creation of algorithms for early and aggressive intervention for patients suffering from antepartum, intrapartum, or postpartum hemorrhage. Recognition of the primary cause of hemorrhage (i.e., atony, laceration of the uterus or vaginal canal, accreta) is of the

Table 51.1 OB massive transfusion protocol (MTP)

Step #1: Activation of OB MTP (packs released 15 min apart) Pack #1	
PRBCs	5 units of type-specific or 5 O neg
Thawed plasma	5 units type-specific, or compatible
SDP	1 unit type- and Rh-specific or RH neg
Step #2: After 15 min retrieve Pack #2	
PRBCs	5 units of type-specific or 5 O neg
Thawed plasma	5 units type-specific, or compatible
Cryoprecipitate	5 units cryo pooled
Step #3: After 15 min retrieve Pack #3 (same as pack #1)	
Step #4: After 15 min retrieve Pack #4 (same as pack #2)	
15 min after step #4: Repeat steps 1 through 4 until MTP is discontinued	

utmost importance because if bleeding persists, replacement of blood products only temporizes and does not fix the true problem.

References

1. Charbit B, Mandelbrot L, Samain E, Baron G, Haddaoui B, Keita H, et al. The decrease of fibrinogen is an early predictor of the severity of postpartum hemorrhage. J Thromb Haemost. 2007;5(2):266–73.
2. Ducloy-Bouthors A-S, Susen S, Butwick A, Vallet B. Medical advances in the treatment of postpartum hemorrhage. Anesth Analg. 2014;119(5):1140–7.
3. Gallos G, Redai I, Smiley RM. The role of the anesthesiologist in management of obstetric hemorrhage. Semin Perinatol. 2009;33 (2):116–23.
4. Butwick AJ. Postpartum hemorrhage and low fibrinogen levels: the past, present and future. Int J Obstet Anesth. 2013;22:87–91.
5. Wikkelsø AJ, Edwards HM, Afshari A, Stensballe J, Langhoff-Roos J, Albrechtsen C, et al. Pre-emptive treatment with fibrinogen concentrate for postpartum haemorrhage: randomized controlled trial. Br J Anaesth. 2015;114:623–33.
6. Sentilhes L, Lasocki S, Ducloy-Bouthors AS, Deruelle P, Dreyfus M, Perrotin F, et al. Tranexamic acid for the prevention and treatment of postpartum haemorrhage. Br J Anaesth. 2015;114:576–87.
7. Rogers WK, Wernimont SA, Kumar GC, Bennett E, Chestnut DH. Acute hypotension associated with intraoperative cell salvage using a leukocyte depletion filter during management of obstetric hemorrhage due to amniotic fluid embolism. Anesth Analg. 2013;117: 449–52.
8. Shields LE, Wiesner S, Fulton J, Pelletreau B. Comprehensive maternal hemorrhage protocols reduce the use of blood products and improve patient safety. Am J Obstet Gynecol. 2015;212:272–80.

52 Managing the Noncompliant HIV-Positive Mother: A PRO/CON Debate

Simon Kim and Corey S. Scher

Case

It was another busy night at the hospital when around 10 p.m., a disheveled, unkempt young woman walked in from the rain. While the patient was oriented to name and place, and was able to tell us that she was pregnant, she also remained confused, somewhat somnolent, and altered, making me question the reliability of her medical history.

With regard to the history, the obstetrics (OB) team had no better luck. On manual examination, the residents noted her amniotic sac was still intact, but she was having active contractions on the monitor.

As the patient was being taken care of by the OB team, I went to go check up on some of the labs that were sent. She had active human immunodeficiency virus (HIV) with a $CD4^+$ count of 20 cells/mm^3 and a large detectable viral load of >1000 copies/mL. My mind raced for an answer to the endless possibilities of what could explain her diminished mental capacity: Primary lymphoma, toxoplasmosis, cerebral abscess? Kaposi's with cerebral involvement? HIV encephalitis or HIV-associated dementia? Other infectious causes [i.e., herpes simplex virus (HSV) encephalitis]? Or could this be substance-related? Did she ever have a workup in the past, and was she ever on antiretroviral (ARV) therapy?

Question

What is the HIV management protocol for a pregnant patient with a CD4 count of 20 and a large detectable viral load (>1000 counts/mm^3) and diminished mental capacity? What drug therapy would be appropriate?

The obstetrics resident, known to cite the American College of Obstetricians and Gynecologists (ACOG) guidelines religiously, reaffirmed the fact that it was imperative to identify and treat pregnant women for HIV and to provide appropriate prophylaxis to the newborn in the first hours of life. "Generally, the same regimen recommended for non-pregnant adults is used in pregnant women, unless known adverse effects outweigh the benefits to the woman, fetus, or infant. While it is unclear whether or not the patient was ever on anti-retroviral therapy in the past, the mother needs to be started on zidovudine (ZDV), given her HIV status, especially since it appears that she is near delivery."

PRO: It is important to prevent further progression of the disease in the mother as well as vertical transmission to the fetus. "A retrospective review of HIV-exposed infants in New York state showed a transmission rate of approximately 10 % when zidovudine (ZDV) prophylaxis was begun intrapartum or given to newborns within 48 hours of life; no significant reduction of neonatal transmission if therapy was started after 3 days of life" [1].

CON: I interposed, "What about resistance testing for HIV? What if she had a similar episode of active HIV in the past, and was previously treated with ZDV? In the setting of potential ZDV resistance, should ZDV still be given?"

I recalled that the National Institutes of Health (NIH) provides detailed recommendations for use of antiretroviral drugs (ARVs) in HIV-infected mothers; their guidelines are reviewed and updated frequently. I decided to take another look to see when resistance testing is warranted—if HIV RNA is above threshold (i.e., >500–1000 copies/mL) [2]. However, while the NIH provides detailed guidelines for HIV pregnant patients

S. Kim (✉)
Department of Anesthesiology, Bellevue Hospital, 462 1st Ave, New York, NY 10016, USA
e-mail: simonkk@uci.edu; Simon.Kim@med.nyu.edu

C.S. Scher
Department of Anesthesiology, Perioperative Care and Pain Medicine, New York University School of Medicine, New York, NY 10016, USA
e-mail: coreyscher@gmail.com

S. Kim
Department of Anesthesiology and Perioperative Care, University of California Irvine, 333 City Blvd W #2150, Orange, CA 92868, USA

C.S. Scher et al. (eds.), *You're Wrong, I'm Right*, DOI 10.1007/978-3-319-43169-7_52

with known ARV status, our patient is unable to provide any reliable history. Hence, for this patient who was likely ARV naïve or who may have lacked compliance if ever treated with ARVs in the past, immediate therapy and prophylaxis should be initiated without waiting for results of resistance testing [2].

Optimal prophylaxis in drug-resistant HIV pregnant patients is unknown; it is important to consult a pediatric acquired immunodeficiency syndrome (AIDS) specialist for optimizing therapy in an infant, especially when weighing the risks of side effects (i.e., risk of teratogenicity with efavirenz). However, the NIH states ZDV should still be given intravenously regardless of ZDV resistance given its demonstrated benefits even in the face of resistance [2].

The patient was given ZDV. The OB team decided to page the AIDS pediatric consult to assist in optimizing ART therapy (i.e., 3 regimen HIV drug therapy).

The next question came up in my mind: given her HIV status, should the infant be delivered via cesarian or vaginal delivery? It seemed logical to me that a cesarean delivery would be the way to go to prevent vertical transmission from exposure to the high viral load in the blood or vaginal fluids.

PRO: I decided to do a quick search on the Internet, which seemed to validate my thoughts. ACOG recommends scheduling cesareans at 39 weeks in patients with a viral load >1000 copies/mm^3; in these patients, cesarean deliveries performed before labor onset and ROM effectively reduce the risk of vertical transmission [3]. On the other hand, when HIV viral load <1000 copies/mL, the benefits of a cesarean delivery are not as clear in decreasing HIV vertical transmission.

Furthermore, ZDV alone reduced risk of vertical transmission from 25 to 5–8 %; in combination with a scheduled cesarean delivery, the risk is further reduced to 2 % [3].

CON: However, while the benefit to the newborn was clear, what of the risk to the mother? I asked the OB attending, Dr. S who was standing nearby, "Is there an increased risk of mortality for the mother with a cesarian delivery?"

Concession from CON: Dr. S took a moment before he replied, "While that is true, complication rates in most studies of HIV-infected women undergoing cesarean deliveries have been shown to be generally similar to HIV-uninfected women [4]."

By repeat ultrasound, the gestational age of the fetus was determined to be around 36 weeks. While scheduled cesarean delivery at 38–39 weeks seemed to be the general consensus, given that the patient was in active labor, it was decided to schedule her for a cesarean within the next few hours.

Dr. S further added, "Even if a pregnant woman with HIV has taken her ARVs throughout her pregnancy but continues to have a viral load above 1000 copies/mL at 34 to 36 weeks, we still advise cesarean over vaginal delivery."

I went to talk with the patient again to see if I had any better luck this time figuring out any relevant history, only to find out she had eaten recently before her C-section. The American Society of Anesthesiologists (ASA) Guidelines for Obstetrical Anesthesia recommend that patients undergo a fasting period of 2 h for clear liquids and 6–8 h for solids (depending on the fat content of the food) [5].

Question

Under the given circumstances regarding the patient's upcoming c-section, is a neuraxial technique or a general anesthetic preferred?

PRO: Pregnant patients are considered to have a full stomach given the physiological and anatomical changes of pregnancy. With an additional oral intake of solids, there may be a potential for an increased risk of aspiration with the loss of airway reflexes associated with the induction of general anesthesia. To minimize aspiration risk, a regional technique may be a better alternative for anesthesia [5].

CON: This patient might not cooperate during a cesarean delivery with a neuraxial anesthetic, due to her altered mental status. A general anesthetic might be necessary to ensure her safety during this surgical procedure. The risk of aspiration pneumonitis may be decreased further with the use of H2-blockers to decrease stomach acid.

As I examined the patient's back, to my horror, I found an old, worn out, flimsy epidural catheter loosely taped in place. How in the world did she end up with this catheter for so long? I attempted to remove it, only to find part of the tip break off (unclear how much was left inside, or if there was anything significant left) from the rest of what I could pull out. Murphy's Law was in full effect.

Great, just great, I thought to myself.

It was hard to tell whether or not the catheter itself was infected. Blood cultures were immediately drawn and sent. The patient was already started on broad-spectrum antibiotics given her immunocompromised status, fever, and tachycardia by the primary OB team when she first presented. We ordered a computed tomography (CT) scan, which did not show any signs of a broken catheter, nor any significant lesions in the brain that may have served a contraindication to a neuraxial. When we finally decided to do another epidural at a different level, Murphy's Law continued to prove resilient as we punctured the epidural membrane, causing the tip of the needle to go intrathecally, also known as a "wet tap."

Awesome job, I thought to myself sarcastically.

We decided to convert to a spinal instead, which went more smoothly. We threaded the catheter intrathecally and achieved an excellent block with spinal dosing through the catheter. With reassurance, the patient did well during the cesarean under neuraxial anesthesia, and luckily her infant was born with Apgar scores of 9 and 9, with no immediately obvious medical issues.

At the end of the case, we gave an intrathecal dose of preservative-free morphine and then removed the intrathecal catheter. Although some authors suggest leaving an accidental intrathecal catheter in situ for 24 h to decrease the risk of post-dural puncture headache (PDPH), we thought that it would be best for the patient to remove it, given the risk of her leaving against medical advice. Unfortunately, 6 h later, the patient began to exhibit classic signs of a PDPH. We decided to start standard management of IV fluids, caffeine, and analgesia, but the patient continued to indicate her headache was not going away following the dural puncture. Epidural saline relieved the headache temporarily, but the effect was transient and patient was found to be experiencing the headaches again.

Question

The question arose, would an autologous epidural blood patch (EBP) be safe given her HIV-positive status?

CON: There is very little literature regarding HIV-positive patients and autologous EBPs after a post-dural puncture. Some major fears with use of autologous EBPs from a HIV-seropositive patient are the potential enhancement of HIV spread through the central nervous system (CNS), masking of neurologic sequelae of the autologous EBP with coexisting neurologic HIV complications, possible epidural infection in the immunocompromised patient, and epidural hematoma and HIV-associated coagulopathy.

PRO: While not many studies exist given the complexity and scarcity of these patients, in 1 longitudinal study, 9 of 218 HIV-seropositive patients undergoing at least 1 diagnostic lumbar puncture (LP) required an EBP, all administered between 5 and 13 days post-LP, for PDPH [6]. Of the 9 patients, 6 underwent serial longitudinal neuropsychological evaluations over varying periods of time from 6 to 24 months. None were found to have declined in neurocognitive performance or any other adverse neurologic or infectious sequelae [6].

CON: However, the sample in the cited study included only patients with no history of prior HIV-related nervous system disease. Our patient may very well have HIV-related CNS involvement. Furthermore, the risk of secondary infection in the CSF as a result of an autologous EBP in an HIV-positive patient seems unknown in the literature.

Concession from CON: Yes, our patient may have CNS involvement, but HIV infection involves the CNS early in the course of the disease regardless. Hence, it is highly unlikely that an autologous EBP would be the initial CNS exposure to HIV. Many HIV-induced neurologic disorders (toxoplasmosis, CNS lymphoma, cryptococcal meningitis) are secondary to the HIV-induced immunocompromised state. It is true, however, that other HIV-induced neurologic diseases such as AIDS dementia complex, HIV aseptic meningitis, and vacuolar myelopathy may be attributable directly to the HIV infection itself [6].

To treat a PDPH, one may also consider epidural saline or dextran, but effects tend to be transient. Homologous EBPs can also be considered, but a donor needs to be present. Stored blood is anti-coagulated and therefore cannot be used for EBP.

The patient continued to have a PDPH 24 h after conservative therapy. She was given an autologous EBP, and her headache soon resolved.

I later overheard one of the nurses rush into the call room the day after delivery with news that the patient was nowhere to be found. The patient seemed to have left against medical advice (AMA) and was never to be heard from again. It was a sad story, one that seemed meant for the books. And the rest is history... or so we thought.

The patient returned a year later, in acute distress, and due to significant blood on her clothing, she was taken immediately to the trauma bay.

After the initial ruckus, the staff got her quickly situated in her room. How long was she like this? Was she actively hemorrhaging? Back to the ABCs: Airway, check. Breathing, check. Circulation? She looked a bit pale overall but pressures remained stable after large bore IVs and fluid boluses were initiated. Type and cross and blood was ordered stat. The staff was doing a great job responding to the acute situation. On examination, the patient was found to have a retained placenta not yet delivered, and it was unknown where her baby was or how long since the delivery.

I began to think about the anesthetic plan for a patient with a retained placenta, assuming most of the delivery occurred outside the hospital. Should we give a regional anesthetic, ketamine or general (inhalational?) anesthesia? The patient was around 91 lb and her height 5 ft 2 in.

Question

Furthermore, might she benefit from intravenous nitroglycerine?

This could be a simple case of an undelivered versus a retained placenta, although on ultrasound the obstetrics team did not see any signs of an invasive placenta. Retained placenta occurs in a very small percentage of vaginal deliveries and necessitates manual exploration. The risk of primary or secondary postpartum hemorrhage (PPH), uterine inversion, and puerperal sepsis all increases with a retained placenta. One also needs to be aware of drugs that may contract the cervix, trapping the placenta.

Nitroglycerin could be used to assist placental delivery, given that it relaxes the uterus and thus assists in manual exploration and delivery of the placenta. However, given the possibility the patient has been hemorrhaging given the unknown details of her delivery, nitroglycerin (and regional techniques) may increase hypotension via vasodilation. Ketamine, on the other hand, may be a better candidate given its rapid onset, sympathomimetic effects and preferred hemodynamic effects in the setting of PPH. Moreover, it is synergistic with opiates in reducing pain. As a dissociative anesthetic, however, it may cause hallucinations. In this patient, who has diminished mental capacity, this combination with a dissociative may make it more difficult to assess her neurologic function, and potentially become a disaster in the case of a bad reaction.

General anesthesia may make manual exploration of her uterus easier, given her neurologic status. In addition, an inhalational anesthetic is rapidly acting with dose-dependent relaxation (of the uterus).

The patient ended up receiving general anesthesia given her altered mental status, along with 50–100 mcg nitroglycerin IV push q 1–2 min initially, with necessary adjustments made as needed for desired clinical effect and maternal hemodynamics. Fortunately, she remained hemodynamically stable without the need to consider ketamine.

I'm happy to say, the placenta was successfully delivered. Finally, I could breathe a sigh of relief.

Summary

In the treatment of the HIV-positive parturient, zidovudine remains an important prophylactic drug regardless of patient resistance. In an HIV-positive parturient, scheduled cesarean delivery is recommended when the viral load is greater than 1000 copies/mm^3. The limited literature so far suggests that in HIV-seropositive patients, an autologous EBP for a PDPH refractory to conservative treatment may be done without worsening of the patient's neurologic symptoms of HIV, although studies are currently limited.

References

1. American College of Obstetricians and Gynecologists, Committee on Obstetrics Practice. Committee opinion 418 prenatal and perinatal human immunodeficiency virus testing: expanded recommendations. ACOG, Washington, DC; 2008.
2. Panel on Treatment of HIV-Infected Pregnant Women and Prevention of Perinatal Transmission. Recommendations for use of antiretroviral drugs in pregnant HIV-1-infected women for maternal health and interventions to reduce perinatal HIV transmission in the United States. http://aidsinfo.nih.gov/guidelines/html/3/perinatal-guidelines/0/. Accessed 25 Apr 2015.
3. Committee on Obstetric Practice. ACOG committee opinion scheduled cesarean delivery and the prevention of vertical transmission of HIV infection. Number 234, May 2000 (replaces number 219, August 1999). Int J Gynaecol Obstet. 2001;73:279.
4. Benton S, Reese A. HIV and the obstetric patient: anesthetic considerations. Int J Anesthesiol 2009;24(1):1–7. http://ispub.com/IJA/24/1/4503.
5. Wong C. Analgesia and anesthesia for labor and delivery. Glob Libr Women's Med 2009; ISSN: 1756-2228. doi: 10.3843/GLOWM.10216. http://www.glowm.com/section_view/heading/Analgesia%20and%20Anesthesia%20for%20Labor%20and%20Delivery/item/216.
6. Tom DJ, Gulevich SJ, Shapiro HM, Heaton RK, Grant I. Epidural blood patch in the HIV-positive patient. Review of clinical experience. San Diego HIV Neurobehavioral Research Center. Anesthesiology. 1992;76:943–7.

Part VI
Neuroanesthesia

At What Hematocrit Should a Patient Who is Undergoing Craniotomy for Tumor be Transfused?

53

Mark Burbridge

Case

A 67-year-old retired operating room nurse is scheduled for craniotomy for tumor resection. The presumptive tissue diagnosis is a renal cell carcinoma metastasis. The lesion measures 3 cm by 2 cm, and imaging shows that the tumor encases a segment of the middle cerebral artery. This will be her third craniotomy in the last 3 years, all on the right side. This unfortunate woman had a right radical nephrectomy, and the left kidney has significant tumor burden. Her preoperative hematocrit is 25. She mentions that she received a blood transfusion after coronary artery bypass graft (CABG) surgery 15 years ago following a ST-segment elevation myocardial infarction (STEMI) and ended up in the intensive care unit (ICU) for 2 weeks with septic shock; she thinks from contaminated blood products. She asks you what the likelihood is of needing a blood transfusion, and she would like to know what your transfusion strategy is because she only wants to receive blood if it is absolutely necessary.

As you are about to tell her that there is an absolute lack of evidence on the subject, she looks you in the eye and states that she trusts you and knows you will do the right thing. Shortly after induction, you call for blood to be brought to the operating room due to the high potential for surgical bleeding. One of the senior neuroanesthesiologists in the department then enters the room and asks whether you will use a liberal or restrictive transfusion strategy for blood transfusion, and why.

Question

At what hematocrit should a patient who is undergoing craniotomy for tumor be transfused?

M. Burbridge (✉)
Department of Anesthesia, Stanford University Medical Center, 300 Pasteur Drive, Stanford, CA 94304, USA
e-mail: markburb@stanford.edu

PRO There are no published guidelines. The decision to transfuse, and at what hematocrit is unknown. Therefore, one must understand the physiology of cerebral bloodflow and the risks and benefits of blood transfusion.

CON I agree that there are no published guidelines, but the incredibly large variation in transfusion practice among anesthesiologists for neurosurgery would indicate that there is more to consider than simply the physiology of cerebral bloodflow [1].

PRO The issue of whether or not to transfuse can be distilled down to cerebral oxygen delivery in the perioperative period. What we know is that the relationship between oxygen delivery and consumption in the human brain exists in a precarious balance. The brain has a high oxygen extraction ratio, and receives 15 % of cardiac output yet consumes 20 % of total body oxygen. The brain has essentially no energy reserve. We must ensure adequate delivery of oxygen to the brain at all times or risk ischemia or infarction. Complicating matters further, it is uncertain at which point oxygen delivery will be compromised as hematocrit falls [2], thereby justifying a higher transfusion trigger. A liberal transfusion strategy is a nebulous term, but would correspond to a hematocrit of approximately 30–33 %. This patient has coronary artery disease, for which a hematocrit above 30 % would be advised [2]. Similar to the brain, the heart requires a constant supply of glucose and oxygen and has limited energy stores, and the flow to this patient's heart is already compromised. Multiple risks of significant and abrupt blood loss exist during this case, including the location of the tumor next to a major blood vessel, the fact that this is her third craniotomy in the same area, and the fact that renal cell carcinoma metastases are notoriously vascular tumors. This tumor has also not been embolized preoperatively. Embolization could significantly reduce intraoperative blood loss if she had been a good candidate. Coupled with her low preoperative hemoglobin and history of coronary artery disease, there are multiple

C.S. Scher et al. (eds.), *You're Wrong, I'm Right*, DOI 10.1007/978-3-319-43169-7_53

reasons to maintain the hematocrit above 30 and to "stay ahead" of the blood loss.

CON While you outlined some factors that must be considered in the decision to transfuse, let us not forget that administration of blood is not a benign event. Blood should only be given when absolutely necessary. In fact, this patient has already suffered from a rare complication of blood transfusion: bacterial contamination leading to septic shock. It is obvious that this patient's cardiac status is poor, and a transfusion-related complication could worsen her cardiac status further and increase the risk of death. Inadvertent over-transfusion could impair oxygen delivery to her brain due to increased blood viscosity [3]. This could actually be more harmful than letting her hematocrit fall too low. Over-transfusion will also lead to circulatory over-load, which will place incredible stress on this woman's heart, which we know is already damaged from her STEMI. This could precipitate an intraoperative MI. When you factor in the additional, although rare, risks of transfusion-related acute lung injury, hemolytic transfusion reactions, febrile reactions, and ABO incompatibility and the risk of infectious disease transmission, it becomes clear that blood must only be given when the clinical scenario necessitates it. The immunosuppression that is caused by any blood transfusion must also be considered [2]. I am choosing to transfuse more conservatively based on my continuous intraoperative evaluation of the patient's physiology, the surgical success, and the ongoing blood loss.

PRO Of course there is risk to transfusion of blood products, but it has never been safer to transfuse. I personally think that the risk associated with blood transfusion takes a back seat to the need to supply enough oxygen to the brain. We cannot let rare complications cloud our assessment of what the patient needs in an operation that carries significant risk. We could extend the argument that what we do can cause rare or even theoretical complications also applies to the choice of anesthetic agents. While some preliminary evidence would suggest that general anesthetics also play an immunosuppressive role [2], we do not eliminate these from our anesthetic practice. The overriding principle is to provide sound perioperative care to patients that gives them the lowest morbidity and mortality.

CON My case is about to start in the other room, so I will have to go in a few moments. One last point of discussion must involve the use of blood conservation strategies. Have any of these been employed in this case?

PRO While we can agree that the practice of permissive hypotension has largely been abandoned, there are several blood conservation strategies that have been investigated. These include: acute normovolemic hemodilution, use of antifibrinolytics such as tranexamic acid and aminocaproic acid, autologous predonation, intraoperative cell salvage, acute normovolemic hemodilution, and erythropoietin. While these are theoretically attractive, the evidence currently does not support their routine use in craniotomy for tumor [1].

Summary

In general, guidelines for blood transfusion practices for anesthesiologists are lacking in neurosurgical patients. Evidence shows that both anemia and blood transfusion are associated with poor clinical outcomes [3]. There is essentially no high-quality evidence to guide transfusion practice for cases of craniotomy for tumor resection. The heterogeneity of patient presentation is the major reason. One study found that the risk of transfusion for all patients having a craniotomy for tumor resection was 1.4 % [2]. There are a number of risk factors, however, that increase the likelihood of transfusion. Meningiomas are the primary tumors with the highest potential for blood loss, while renal cell carcinoma metastases have the highest blood loss when considering secondary tumors. Proximity to major vascular structures must also be considered. Re-operation is, as with other organs, a risk factor for increased potential for blood loss as well. Patient factors that would increase the likelihood for transfusion are numerous and include, but are not limited to, coagulopathy and anemia [1]. Additionally, cardiovascular comorbidities may also demand a higher than normal hematocrit. Clearly, there is a need to have an understanding of the patient's health status, the characteristics of the tumor, and the extent of the proposed operation. Of course, a discussion preoperatively with the surgeon to review the operative strategy and review the imaging is always good form.

References

1. Gruenbaum SE, Ruskin K. Red blood cell transfusion in neurosurgical patients. Curr Opin Anesthesiol. 2014;27(4):470–3.
2. Linsler S, Ketter R, Eichler H, Schwerdtfeger K, Stuedel WI, Oertel J. Red blood cell transfusion in neurosurgery. Acta Neurochir. 2012;154(7):1303–8.
3. McEwen J, Huttunen KTH. Transfusion practice in neuroanesthesia. Curr Opin Anesthesiol. 2009;22(5):566–71.

Traumatic Brain Injury: Where Do We Stand with Ketamine and Hyperventilation?

54

Corey S. Scher

Case

A 29-year-old man on his bicycle is hit by a taxi cab despite being in a New York City designated bike lane. The rider does not have a helmet on and sustains a left tibia/fibula open fracture and a large bleeding scalp laceration. The first responders place a neck collar on, start an intravenous line, and call the trauma emergency department (ED) at Bellevue Hospital to report their assessment at the site of the accident. Above all, he is unconscious, with bilateral breath sounds, strong pulses, and no apparent abdominal or chest trauma. With a Glasgow Coma Scale score less than 8, the anesthesiologist is called to intubate the patient to both protect his airway and initiate neuroresuscitation. Total body computed tomography (CT) scan is consistent with the orthopedic trauma discovered on examination and a traumatic brain injury with a parietal subarachnoid hemorrhage and midline shift. The Glasgow Coma Scale (GCS) looks at traumatic brain injury within 48 h and describes the severity (Table 54.1).

The anesthesiologist draws up ketamine for the intubation. Right away, a disagreement breaks out between the two attending anesthesiologists who assume care of the airway and venous access.

PRO Ketamine is the perfect drug for this intubation. If this trauma patient is bleeding from a site that has not been discovered yet, we are at risk for worsening hypotension. At least with ketamine, the blood pressure will not precipitously drop from the anesthetic. Above all, ketamine lowers intracranial pressure (ICP). We thought that an increased ICP was likely in this patient from the examination and history, and we can confirm this by looking at the midline shift on the CT scan.

CON Excuse me! Ketamine increases intracranial pressure!! Additionally, I believe that in the trauma patient, catecholamines are depleted and ketamine serves as a myocardial depressant.

PRO Let me address the ketamine issue. Like you, I hear from so many residents that ketamine increases ICP. It is essential to examine the current literature: Cohen et al. [1] developed a systematic search strategy and applied it to six electronic reference databases. Studies, prospective and both randomized and nonrandomized, looked at ketamine and another intravenous anesthetic agent in patients who were intubated [1]. A qualitative method was utilized to synthesize the study designs, populations of patients, outcomes, and follow-up times, because these were dissimilar in each study [1]. Of 4896 titles that were retrieved, ten studies met the inclusion criteria, reporting data on 953 patients. Two of eight studies reported small reductions in intracranial pressure within 10 min of ketamine administration, and two studies reported an increase. None of the studies reported significant differences in cerebral perfusion pressure, neurologic outcomes, ICU length of stay, or mortality [1].

In a second yet similar study, "The ketamine effect on ICP in traumatic brain injury," Zeller et al. [2] looked at multiple databases, focusing on ketamine and intracranial pressure as well as cerebral perfusion pressure: 101 adult and 55 pediatric patients were included, with no ICP increase with ketamine administration. A significant decrease in ICP with a ketamine bolus was seen in three studies. In two studies, there was an actual increase in blood pressure and cerebral perfusion pressure. This meant that there was actually a decrease in the need for vasopressors in one study. No significant adverse events related to ketamine were noted. If you look at the study, the statistics were robust in saying that ketamine lowers ICP, but not with any clinical significance. There were two studies that showed an increase

C.S. Scher (✉)
Department of Anesthesiology, Perioperative Care and Pain Medicine, New York University School of Medicine, New York, NY 10016, USA
e-mail: coreyscher@gmail.com

C.S. Scher et al. (eds.), *You're Wrong, I'm Right*, DOI 10.1007/978-3-319-43169-7_54

Table 54.1 Calculating severity of traumatic brain injury using the Glasgow Coma Scale

Eye opening
Spontaneous = 4
To speech = 3
To painful stimulation = 2
No response = 1
Motor response
Follows commands = 6
Makes localizing movements to pain = 5
Makes withdrawal movements to pain = 4
Flexor (decorticate) posturing to pain = 3
Extensor (decerebrate) posturing to pain = 2
No response = 1
Verbal response
Oriented to person, place, and date = 5
Converses but is disoriented = 4
Says inappropriate words = 3
Says incomprehensible sounds = 2
No response = 1
The severity of TBI according to the GCS score (within 48 h) is as follows:
Severe TBI = 3–8 points
Moderate TBI = 9–12 points
Mild TBI = 13–15 points

in ICP, but again, the result was not clinically significant [2]. Are we arguing over something that is of no concern?

CON The evidence level in both studies appears to be on the low side. When I was a resident back in the 1990s, I do recall that some of the literature clearly taught that ketamine increased intracranial pressure. Let me check my iPad for a second… "Ketamine is usually not administered for the anesthetic management of patients at risk of intracranial hypertension because of the reported increases in cerebral metabolism" [3]. This came from a sentinel paper by Bazin [3]. Finally, another paper [4] stated, "The effect on intracranial pressure (ICP) of ketamine as an anesthetic induction agent following pretreatment with either midazolam (ten cases) or diazepam (five cases) was investigated in unpremeditated neurosurgical patients. In all patients in the midazolam group, ICP increased following ketamine while the cerebral perfusion pressure (CPP) fell in five cases." It seems as if these historical data have now been refuted in more recent studies.

Let us move on to hyperventilation to reduce intracranial pressure. I have been doing this for years when the intracranial pressure needed to be reduced. ICP is normally 7–15 mm Hg; at 20–25 mm Hg, the upper limit of normal, treatment to reduce ICP may be needed. In traumatic brain injury, however, this becomes problematic because hyperventilation may lead to severe vasoconstriction to the injured area of the brain thus denying critically needed oxygen and leading to poor outcomes. Regional blood flow and oxygen consumption were measured during normoventilation, mild hypocapnea, and mild hypercapnea. Regional ischemia occurred in 28.9 % during normocapnea, increased to 59.4 % during mild hypercapnea, and increased to 73 % with hyperventilation and hypocapnea. Despite this strong evidence, 90 % of clinicians still hyperventilate throughout the case, as shown in one survey study in Western Europe [5]. As with every study, though, it is important to ask if this model holds up in real clinical situations.

PRO It is difficult to argue with your comments. First of all, when treating of traumatic brain injury, when the *cerebral perfusion pressure* (CPP) falls below 70 mm Hg and/or the ICP is greater than 20 mm Hg, steps must be taken to lower ICP. Maintenance of an adequate cerebral perfusion pressure is more important than control of ICP. Before getting all fancy trying to control the ICP, first try to control the mean arterial pressure (MAP). Measures to increase MAP should be instituted prior to starting more complex methods of ICP control. Elevated carbon dioxide dilates cerebral vessels thus elevating ICP. It is now standard of care to ventilate a patient to a PaCO2 of 30 mm Hg. Hyperventilation below 30 mm Hg does not increase cerebral vessel constriction. This has been shown with transcranial Doppler measurements and jugular venous saturations. It is not recommended to hyperventilate in the first 24 h after a TBI.

The true effect of hyperventilation is actually to control pH. Although the effects of hyperventilation on ICP are almost instant, they lessen over 6–24 h because the brain adjusts by normalizing the pH by fluctuating bicarbonate levels in the extracellular fluid. If hyperventilation is suddenly discontinued and normocapnia is restored too quickly, there is a rebound increase in CBF and ICP. Aggressive ICP only causes alkalosis and cerebral vessel constriction leading to ischemia of the TBI patient.

CON What do we do when the surgeon wants us to bring the paCO2 to 25 or below?

PRO Don't do it. Explain these reasons to the surgeon, and you should be on more solid ground. If you are in a situation of desperation from a "tight" brain, you must increase your level of monitoring to include both transcranial Doppler and cerebral oximetry. There is no way that you would be able to defend yourself later if you hyperventilated to a CO2 to 25. End of discussion.

Summary

When I was a resident in the early 1980s, there were hard and set rules in neuroanesthesia. Ketamine was never used in the patient with increased intracranial pressure, and persistent hyperventilation was done throughout an entire anesthetic for a neurosurgical case with elevated ICP. Old dogma dies a slow death, and I think that this pro–con discussion puts us on more solid ground with using ketamine and mild hyperventilation.

References

1. Cohen L, Athaide V, Wickham ME, Doyle-Waters MM, Rose NG, Hohl CM. Ann Emerg Med. 2015;65(1):43–51.e2. doi:10.1016/j.annemergmed.2014.06.018 (Epub 2014 July).
2. Zeller FA. The ketamine effect on ICP in traumatic brain injury. Neurocrit Care. 2014;21(1):163–73.
3. Bazin JE. Effects of anesthetic agents on intracranial pressure. Acta Anaesthesiol Scand. 1982;26(5):458–62.
4. Belopavlovic M, Buchthal A. Modification of ketamine-induced intracranial hypertension in neurosurgical patients by pretreatment with midazolam. Paediatr Anaesth. 2014;24(7):703–10. doi:10.1111/pan.12415 (Epub 2014 May).
5. Hardcastle N, Benzon HA, Vavilala MS. Update on the 2012 guidelines for the management of pediatric traumatic brain injury—information for the anesthesiologist. New York: Wiley; 2014.

Is General Anesthesia or Conscious Sedation More Appropriate for Patients Undergoing Endovascular Clot Retrieval for Acute Ischemic Stroke?

55

Elina Abramchayeva and Jinu Kim

Case

A 68-year-old man with history significant for hypertension, hyperlipidemia, and chronic lower back pain presents to the emergency department (ED) with hemiplegia of his left leg. An emergent head computed tomography (CT) scan reveals an anterior cerebral artery occlusion. The patient is brought to the interventional radiology suite for a cerebral angiogram and intra-arterial recanalization. The patient is alert and oriented, comfortable, with a benign airway examination. His last meal was 9 h prior to the procedure.

You decide to provide conscious sedation (CS) for the procedure with intermittent boluses of fentanyl. An hour into the procedure, the patient grows restless and tells you that his back is uncomfortable and he cannot lay still. The surgeon says the patient movement is interfering with his images and requests that you do something about it. You are uncomfortable with further sedating the patient without a definitive airway and proceed to intubate and start general anesthesia (GA). Your colleague comes to assist you and says under their breath, "I would have intubated from the beginning."

A number of studies have investigated the effect anesthetic technique (GA versus CS) has on patient outcomes for endovascular recanalization therapy.

Question

Should general anesthesia or sedation be used for endovascular clot retrieval for patients who have had an embolic stroke?

E. Abramchayeva (✉) · J. Kim
Department of Anesthesiology, Mount Sinai West St. Luke's Hospital, 1000 Tenth Avenue, 5th Floor, New York, NY 10019, USA
e-mail: eabramchayeva@gmail.com

J. Kim
e-mail: jikim@chpnet.org; jikdoc@gmail.com

PRO GA Although the patient is NPO, the patient is still at increased risk of aspiration, both from the stroke and secondary to the sedation he is receiving, especially in the context of supine positioning. Vomiting and aspiration of gastric contents during the procedure would necessitate emergent intubation for airway protection. Emergent intubation is not without risk, and can result in hypoxia, trauma to the cerebral circulation secondary to catheters in the intracranial circulation, further aspiration and even death, providing a valid argument for why these patients should be intubated from the beginning of the case in a controlled setting.

PRO CS Yes, emergent intubation has risks, but numerous studies have suggested that the rate of emergent intubations during conscious sedation is very low, and that those who undergo endovascular recanalization under conscious sedation have higher rates of a successful procedure and no increase in intraprocedural complications [1]. This should curb any perceived disadvantages of conscious sedation.

In addition, conscious sedation permits for continuous intraprocedural monitoring and assessment of new or worsening neurologic deficits. This continuous monitoring allows the procedure to proceed to a clinical endpoint rather than a radiologic endpoint and also provides a quicker assessment of function post-procedure [2]. This can potentially decrease the time the patient is exposed to contrast and fluoroscopy and shorten the duration of the procedure.

PRO GA General anesthesia, on the other hand, addresses one of the main disadvantages of conscious sedation, which is patient movement during the procedure. At times, it is imperative that the patient be still in order for the proceduralist to obtain adequate images of the brain for clot retrieval. Patients undergoing the intervention under conscious sedation can become agitated either because of the stroke or due to device-induced discomfort. General anesthesia avoids this situation and provides complete immobility.

C.S. Scher et al. (eds.), *You're Wrong, I'm Right*, DOI 10.1007/978-3-319-43169-7_55

Our patient began the procedure under sedation and had difficulty lying still. If that was not immediately rectified it could have resulted in catastrophic events—such as wire perforation resulting in intracranial hemorrhage or vascular injury in the form of dissection.

PRO CS General anesthesia in itself has been associated with poorer neurologic outcomes and higher mortality when compared to conscious sedation. A meta-analysis of 1956 patients for stroke intervention comparing conscious sedation and general anesthesia showed that GA is associated with lower odds of a favorable functional outcome and successful recanalization, and higher odds of mortality and respiratory complications [1].

PRO GA Just to point out, in the same meta-analysis study, when the data are adjusted for baseline preoperative neurologic status, there is no statistically significant difference in outcomes between GA and CS. There are no prospective randomized double blind trials as of yet proving improved patient outcomes with conscious sedation. Most of the studies cited by proponents of CS are retrospective and contain selection bias since most patients with high-grade or posterior circulation strokes undergo GA.

PRO CS Patients undergoing general anesthesia are more prone to hemodynamic instability during induction and emergence, which can potentially cause brain ischemia, especially in the penumbra, the vulnerable watershed areas at the periphery of the ischemic stroke. The induction phase of general anesthesia is often complicated by hypotension, which can profoundly decrease cerebral blood flow, resulting in cerebral hypoperfusion, and further exacerbating ischemic injury in the penumbra. Furthermore, inhalational anesthetics inhibit cerebral autoregulation and can also contribute to reperfusion injury. This could explain lower neurologic testing scores in patients who received GA instead of CS. Conscious sedation, on the other hand, preserves cerebral autoregulation, maintaining cerebral perfusion.

Summary

General anesthesia and conscious sedation both have potential risks for patients undergoing intra-arterial therapy for acute ischemic stroke. The anesthetic modality used should be tailored to the patient and surgeon. Factors to consider include the extent and severity of the stroke, patient comorbidities, hemodynamics and airway status.

Many studies suggest that conscious sedation is the superior anesthetic modality when compared to general anesthesia for patients undergoing neuro-interventional procedures for acute ischemic stroke. While none of these studies are prospective randomized trials, a meta-analysis of retrospective studies shows that the use of CS results in improved outcomes and lower mortality [1]. Specifically, the meta-analysis indicates that GA is associated with lower odds of favorable functional outcome, lower odds of successful recanalization, and higher odds of mortality and respiratory complications. There was no significant difference in the rate of vascular complications, total procedure duration, time to catheter insertion in the groin, and time to recanalization between the 2 groups.

However, it is important to note that there are numerous limitations in the study design that may have confounded the results. Stroke severity, for instance, is one of the confounding variables. Patients with worse initial stroke presentations, with altered mental status or those who could not protect their airway, invariably require intra-arterial therapy under GA with endotracheal intubation. Additionally, these patients also contribute to increased rates of post-treatment morbidity and mortality. Stroke location is another important variable for determination of patient outcome that was not accounted for in the meta-analysis study. Patients with posterior circulation infarcts, bulbar involvement, or basilar artery occlusion also typically require GA and often have worse outcomes [3].

Future studies comparing the outcomes of GA versus CS for patients undergoing endovascular therapy for acute ischemic stroke should be prospective and randomized and exclude patients where CS is not possible, i.e., posterior infarcts.

The current 2014 SNACC (Society for Neuroscience in Anesthesiology and Critical Care) Consensus statement recommends hemodynamic control with SBP 140–180, DBP < 105, and NIBP every 3 min [4]. This means that there should not be any delay in obtaining arterial access for BP monitoring. Oxygenation should be maintained with $SpO_2 > 92$ %, $PaO_2 > 60$, along with maintaining normocapnia. Glucose should be checked hourly, with a goal of 70–140. Glucose > 140 should be treated with IV insulin. Patients should be maintained euvolemic, and temperature should be 35–37 °C. Anticoagulation should be available, as well as protamine in the event of intracranial hemorrhage.

General anesthesia should be reserved for patients with severe neurologic deficits, posterior circulation infarcts, hemodynamic instability, airway compromise, or inability to cooperate. Meanwhile, conscious sedation may be more appropriate for patients with anterior circulation strokes, those who are cooperative, and those for whom you can protect their airway. All patients receiving conscious sedation should be prepared to convert to general anesthesia in an expeditious manner if needed.

References

1. Brinkji W, Murad MH, Rabinstein AA, Cloft HJ, Lanzino G, Kalmes DF. Conscious sedation versus general anesthesia during endovascular acute ischemic stroke treatment: a systematic review and meta-analysis. Am J Neuroradiol. 2015;36(3):525–9.
2. Abue-Chebl A, Lin R, Hussain MS, Jovin TG, Levy EI, Liebeskind DS, et al. Conscious sedation versus general anesthesia during endovascular therapy for acute anterior circulation stroke. Stroke. 2010;41:1175–9.
3. Froehler MT, Fifi JT, Majid A, Bhatt A, Ouyang M, Mcdonagh DL. Anesthesia for endovascular treatment of acute ischemic stroke. Neurology. 2012;79(13 Suppl 1):S167–73.
4. Talke PO, Sharma D, Heyer EJ, Bergese SD, Blackham KA, Stevens RD. Society for Neuroscience in Anesthesiology and Critical Care Expert consensus statement: anesthetic management of endovascular treatment for acute ischemic stroke: endorsed by the Society of NeuroInterventional Surgery and the Neurocritical Care Society. J Neurosurg Anesthesiol. 2014;26(2):95–108.

Tranexamic Acid for Major Spine Surgery

56

Sergey Pisklakov

Case

A 55-year old man presents for elective L3-L5 lumbar laminectomy with decompression. His medical history consists of hypertension, well- controlled with amlodipine. In addition, he suffers from chronic back pain due to lumbar radiculopathy and spinal stenosis. His laboratory work, including electrolytes, complete blood count, and coagulation factors, is normal. The surgeon is asking you to give the patient tranexamic acid (TXA) to reduce intraoperative bleeding. You wonder whether the benefits of TXA outweigh its downsides.

Question

Should pro-hemostatic therapy in the form of a fibrinolytic inhibitor be administered for surgical procedures with significant anticipated blood loss?

PRO: Anti-fibrinolytic agents such as tranexamic acid (TXA) are used to improve hemostasis, which may be achieved by stimulation of fibrin formation or inhibition of fibrinolysis. Simply stated, TXA maintains clot stability. Perioperative hemorrhage is a major complication following spine surgery, resulting in increased morbidity and mortality due either to the extent of the surgical intervention or to an underlying coagulation disorder [1, 2] Pro-hemostatic topical and systemic pharmacological agents provide a potential avenue for decreasing this blood loss [3]. Systemic pharmacological agents include TXA, aprotinin, aminocaproic acid (EACA), desmopressin, and recombinant factor VIIa and can be used prophylactically or if unexpected blood loss occurs [4]. Over the last decade, studies have produced evidence supporting the use of antifibrinolytic agents in a wide variety of procedures: liver transplant, obstetrics and gynecology, trauma, orthopedics, and spine surgery.

S. Pisklakov (✉)
Department of Anesthesiology, Albert Einstein College of Medicine, Montefiore Medical Center, 111 East 210th Street, Bronx, NY 10467, USA
e-mail: spisklak@montefiore.org; spisklakov@hotmail.com

CON: Identifying patients at risk is essential for the prevention of excessive blood loss. The techniques to minimize blood transfusion include positioning to minimize epidural venous bleeding, intraoperative normovolemic hemodilution, cell salvage, systemic administration of antifibrinolytic agents, minimally invasive surgery, and staging of complex procedures. TXA studies in spine surgery are limited by low patient enrollment. Furthermore, the safety of TXA and the possibility of adverse reactions in the surgical arena need further evaluation. What is the optimal intraoperative dose of TXA? The published data indicate a wide range of dosage regimens [5]. Should TXA be used in combination with other pro-thrombotic agents during surgery? There are too many questions that have not been answered.

PRO: TXA is traditionally used to reduce surgical blood loss. It can be administered orally, intramuscularly, intravenously, or topically. TXA is similar to EACA, which is a synthetic lysine analog that competitively inhibits the conversion of plasminogen to plasmin by binding to plasminogen-specific sites and preventing fibrin degradation [6]. Rather than promoting new clot formation, TXA enhances clot stability.

CON: The perioperative dosage of TXA is not standardized. It varies for different surgeries and medical conditions. The original manufacturer of TXA, Pfizer, recommends different dosages for different surgical interventions in its product insert.

PRO: The evidence that TXA reduces blood transfusion in surgical patients has been available for years. A trial of TXA by Ker et al. showed that it reduced overall blood loss by one-third [7].

C.S. Scher et al. (eds.), *You're Wrong, I'm Right*, DOI 10.1007/978-3-319-43169-7_56

In randomized clinical studies, TXA reduced perioperative blood loss compared to placebo in a variety of surgical procedures, including intracranial surgery, trauma, cardiac surgery with or without cardiopulmonary bypass, total hip and knee replacement, oral and maxillofacial surgery, craniosynostosis surgery, gastrointestinal endoscopy procedures, ear-nose-and-throat procedures, prostatectomy, and spinal surgeries. TXA is considered to be effective in trauma care. It is incorporated into the US military practice guidelines for tactical combat casualty management [8]. The effects of TXA administration on death, vascular occlusive events, and blood transfusion in trauma patients were examined in the CRASH-2 trial, which established that TXA might be life-saving. Specifically regarding spine surgery, TXA significantly reduced the percentage of patients with idiopathic scoliosis requiring blood transfusion. It also reduced intraoperative blood loss from posterior spine fusion [9] and posterior lumbar surgery [10].

CON: The efficacy of TXA varies with the type of surgery. When directly compared with similar agents, TXA was found to be at least as effective as EACA and more effective than desmopressin in surgical procedures [11]. Postoperative complications and mortality after administration of aprotinin compared to tranexamic acid were studied in cardiac surgery. Although the study was neither randomized nor double-blinded, and there was no control group, the investigators concluded that both antifibrinolytic drugs bear risks of adverse effects. Compared to TXA, aprotinin was associated with a higher incidence of complications after primary CABG surgery and a higher 1-year mortality in high-risk patients. Tranexamic acid may also have unfavorable effects after valve surgery. Both antifibrinolytic drugs bear risks of adverse effects; the benefit of any blood-sparing effect has to be balanced against the potential risks of the drugs [12]. When compared to aprotinin, TXA and aminocaproic acid are probably similarly effective in reducing bleeding and the need for blood transfusion during spinal surgery [13].

The prophylactic efficacy of TXA in spinal surgery is neither well studied nor established. The administration of a prophylactic low dose of TXA failed to have a significant effect on transfusion requirements in patients undergoing spinal fixation [14] or during surgical treatment of metastatic spine tumors [15], but was shown to be effective in reducing perioperative blood loss in cervical laminoplasty, primarily through a reduction in *postoperative* hemorrhage [16].

PRO: The overall incidence of vascular thrombosis was low or none in prospective controlled trials, retrospective studies, and case series in children and adults, including those targeted at spine surgery [13]. Most of the clinical trials and randomized studies were done on patients undergoing joint replacements. Conducted in 2012, a meta-analysis of cardiac surgery patients did not reveal an increase in the risk of deep vein thrombosis (DVT) associated with TXA administration [7].

CON: Fibrinogen levels are known to rise steadily throughout the postoperative period when Amicar is given [17]. There is a legitimate concern that TXA may cause a higher incidence of postoperative thromboembolic events. Active thromboembolic disease is a contraindication for TXA use. Pulmonary embolism (PE) and DVT [18] have been described with TXA use.

Most randomized studies showed that compared to placebo, antifibrinolytic agents, while reducing bleeding and need for transfusion in joint replacement and spine surgery [18], do not increase the risk of myocardial infarction, stroke, deep vein thrombosis, or pulmonary embolism.

However, cases of acute renal cortical necrosis have been described after TXA. In patients with renal dysfunction, TXA is associated with postoperative seizures. Multifocal myoclonus has also been described after TXA infusion, especially in patients with renal dysfunction [18]. Ligneous conjunctivitis, toxic epidermal necrolysis, central venous stasis retinopathy, disturbances of color vision, and central retinal artery occlusion may also result from TXA use.

Summary

Spinal surgery is often associated with significant bleeding requiring multiple blood transfusions. This makes antifibrinolytic agents, including TXA, potentially important adjuncts to perioperative management. However, the present role of TXA in reducing perioperative blood loss and transfusion requirements in spine surgery is not clear. The majority of research studying the role of antifibrinolytic drugs in spine surgery has had limited patient enrollment and reports mixed results. Nevertheless, accumulating evidence suggests that TXA may reduce the need for transfusion in the setting of spinal surgery. Careful assessment of risks and benefits must be evaluated on a case-by-case basis. It is important to identify the types of surgical interventions where TXA use should be advised (such as spinal fusion, spinal stenosis correction, and trauma) or discouraged (such as tumors). The dosage of TXA is not well established and varies for different procedures and medical conditions.

The effect of TXA on the occurrence of thromboembolic events, strokes, myocardial ischemia, seizures, and mortality has not been adequately evaluated and remains ambiguous. The majority of the clinical trials analyzing thromboembolic complications of TXA in surgery are either conflicting or inadequately powered and therefore insufficient to establish definitive conclusions. The published literature supports the safe use of TXA for the prevention of blood transfusion for major joint replacement procedures. Although the benefit and safety of tranexamic acid in patients undergoing major spinal fusion have yet to be thoroughly established, TXA appears to have a potential beneficial role in their management. Currently, there is no strong evidence that TXA leads to an increased rate of thromboembolic events. Future multicenter, placebo-controlled, blinded, prospective, randomized studies are needed to clarify the exact role and safety of TXA in spine surgery.

References

1. Lee MJ, Konodi MA, Cizik AM, Bransford RJ, Bellabarba C, Chapman JR. Risk factors for medical complication after spine surgery: a multivariate analysis of 1591 patients. Spine J. 2012;12:197–206.
2. Eubanks JD. Antifibrinolytics in major orthopaedic surgery. J Am Acad Orthop Surg. 2010;18:132–8.
3. Fraser IS, Porte RJ, Kouides PA, Lukes AS. A benefit-risk review of systemic haemostatic agents: part 1: in major surgery. Drug Saf. 2008;31:217–30.
4. Ortmann E, Besser MW, Klein AA. Antifibrinolytic agents in current anaesthetic practice. Br J Anaesth. 2013;111(4):549–63.
5. McCormack PL. Tranexamic Acid. Drugs. 2012;72:585–617.
6. Porte RJ, Leebeek FW. Pharmacological strategies to decrease transfusion requirements in patients undergoing surgery. Drugs. 2002;62:2193–211.
7. Ker K, Edwards P, Perel P, Shakur H, Roberts I. Effect of tranexamic acid on surgical bleeding: systematic review and cumulative meta-analysis. BMJ. 2012;344:e3054.
8. Pusateri AE, Weiskopf RB, Bebarta V, Butler F, Cestero RF, Chaudry IH, Deal V, Dorlac WC, Gerhardt RT, Given MB, Hansen DR, Hoots WK, Klein HG, Macdonald VW, Mattox KL, Michael RA, Mogford J, Montcalm-Smith EA, Niemeyer DM, Prusaczyk WK, Rappold JF, Rassmussen T, Rentas F, Ross J, Thompson C, Tucker LD, US DoD Hemorrhage and Resuscitation Research and Development Steering Committee. Tranexamic acid and trauma: current status and knowledge gaps with recommended research priorities. Shock. 2013;39:121–6.
9. Dhawale AA, Shah SA, Sponseller PD, Bastrom T, Neiss G, Yorgova P, Newton PO, Yaszay B, Abel MF, Shufflebarger H, Gabos PG, Dabney KW, Miller F. Are antifibrinolytics helpful in decreasing blood loss and transfusions during spinal fusion surgery in children with cerebral palsy scoliosis? Spine. 2012;37:E549–55.
10. Wang Q, Liu J, Fan R, Chen Y, Yu H, Bi Y, Hua Z, Piao M, Guo M, Ren W, Xiang L. Tranexamic acid reduces postoperative blood loss of degenerative lumbar instability with stenosis in posterior approach lumbar surgery: a randomized controlled trial. Eur Spine J. 2013;22:2035–8.
11. Mahdy AM, Webster NR. Perioperative systemic haemostatic agents. Br J Anaesth. 2004;93:842–58.
12. Martin K, Wiesner G, Breuer T, Lange R, Tassani P. The risks of aprotinin and tranexamic acid in cardiac surgery: a one-year follow-up of 1188 consecutive patients. Anesth Analg. 2008;107:1783–90.
13. Kuklo TR, Owens BD, Polly DW Jr. Perioperative blood and blood product management for spinal deformity surgery. Spine J. 2003;3:388–93.
14. Farrokhi MR, Kazemi AP, Eftekharian HR, Akbari K. Efficacy of prophylactic low dose of tranexamic acid in spinal fixation surgery: a randomized clinical trial. J Neurosurg Anesthesiol. 2011;23:290–6.
15. Bednar DA, Bednar VA, Chaudhary A, Farrokhyar F. Tranexamic acid for hemostasis in the surgical treatment of metastatic tumors of the spine. Spine. 2006;31:954–7.
16. Tsutsumimoto T, Shimogata M, Ohta H, Yui M, Yoda I, Misawa H. Tranexamic acid reduces perioperative blood loss in cervical laminoplasty: a prospective randomized study. Spine. 2011;36:1913–8.
17. Thompson GH, Florentino-Pineda I, Armstrong DG, Poe-Kochert C. Fibrinogen levels following Amicar in surgery for idiopathic scoliosis. Spine. 2007;32:368–72.
18. Elwatidy S, Jamjoom Z, Elgamal E, Zakaria A, Turkistani A, El-Dawlatly A. Efficacy and safety of prophylactic large dose of tranexamic acid in spine surgery: a prospective, randomized, double-blind, placebo-controlled study. Spine. 2008;33:2577–80.

Should Major Spine Surgery Patients Be Extubated in the Operating Room?

57

A. Elisabeth Abramowicz

Case

A 72-year-old woman, who is still working and enjoys physical activity, has thoracolumbar kyphoscoliosis related to degenerative spine disease. She has a history of hypertension, well controlled with a diuretic. Her quality of life has deteriorated because of back pain and posture changes, and she desires correction. She takes acetaminophen, 325 mg/oxycodone, 10 mg, every 4–6 h for back pain. In the past, she had a 2-level anterior cervical discectomy and fusion and a hysterectomy. She is scheduled for an 8-level spinal decompression, fusion, and instrumentation with a 2-level pedicle osteotomy.

Her height is 5′4″ and weight is 180 lbs. Hemoglobin (Hgb): 12.7 g/dL. Creatinine: 1.3 mg/dL. Blood pressure (BP): 140/89. Heart rate: 76. Electrocardiogram (EKG): sinus rhythm at 65/min, left ventricular hypertrophy with non-specific ST segment and T wave changes.

The surgery lasted 7 h, with the patient positioned prone on a Jackson table. Multimodal neurophysiological monitoring was used. The head was resting on a foam pillow. The intubation was difficult with a Cormack-Lehane class III view of the larynx on direct laryngoscopy, but she was successfully intubated on the second attempt using a video laryngoscope with a 7.0-mm ID Mallinckrodt Lo-Pro endotracheal tube. Her anesthetic consisted of sufentanil, propofol, and ketamine infusions. She was given a continuous infusion of tranexamic acid throughout the surgery. The blood loss was estimated to be 3000 mL. There were periods of hypotension, which responded to phenylephrine and volume expansion. Phenylephrine was infused continuously from midway through the surgery. The patient received 500 mL of 5 % albumin, 5400 mL of crystalloids, 3 units of packed red blood cells (PRBCs), and 900 mL of cell saver blood. The urine output was 600 mL. The surgery ended at 10:15 p.m., at which time the Hgb was 9.1 g/dL and the pressors had been discontinued.

A. Elisabeth Abramowicz (✉)
Department of Anesthesiology, New York Medical College, Westchester Medical Center, 100 Woods Rd., Macy 2391, Valhalla, NY 10595, USA
e-mail: APABRAMO@montefiore.org; elisabeth.abramowicz@gmail.com

Question

Should this patient be awakened and extubated in the operating room (OR)?

PRO: Stable major spine surgery patients should be extubated in the OR.

Complex or major spine surgery is poorly defined. It implies fusion and instrumentation, usually in the prone position. A high number of levels fused and a severe deformity that requires an osteotomy correlate with the length of surgery and the blood loss [1, 2].

Degenerative spine disease, spondylosis, is common in the aging population. Major elective surgery requires thorough preoperative preparation with risk stratification. The RCRI (Revised Cardiac Risk Index) categorizes all spine surgery as intermediate risk procedures. However, in a group of patients undergoing complex spine surgery, the RCRI performed no better than chance in identifying those patients who developed perioperative cardiac complications [3]. This type of surgery has an inherent risk of complications, including death. The Scoliosis Research Society Morbidity and Mortality Database reported 2 deaths per 1000 adult patients [4]. The highest risk procedures included spine fractures and kyphosis and scoliosis correction. The main causes of death were respiratory/pulmonary, cardiac, stroke, sepsis, and intraoperative blood loss. In another study, the incidence of major complications in adult spinal deformity surgery approached 8.5 % [5].

There are 3 other types of complications that are particularly prevalent in major spine surgery in the prone position: airway edema; postoperative visual loss (POVL), specifically posterior ischemic optic neuropathy (PION) [6, 7]; and

C.S. Scher et al. (eds.), *You're Wrong, I'm Right*, DOI 10.1007/978-3-319-43169-7_57

awareness in the setting of total intravenous anesthesia (TIVA) [8], commonly used to facilitate motor-evoked potential (MEP) monitoring.

Anastasian [9] retrospectively examined the factors correlating with the decision to delay extubation after major spine surgery of 8-h duration or more in a series of 289 patients from one center. She found that 44 % of patients remained intubated, and the decision not to extubate correlated independently with older age, American Society of Anesthesiologists (ASA) status, procedure duration, total volume of crystalloids, and total blood volume administered. Delayed extubation also correlated independently with case end time—6 p.m. for immediate extubation versus 8 p.m. for delayed extubation on average with a mean difference in duration of 100 min. Patients who remained intubated had a threefold higher rate of postoperative pneumonia.

Management of pain after major spine surgery may be challenging, especially in patients who are not opioid naïve. Recently, there has been a trend to use multimodality pain management in this setting, aiming at reducing reliance on opioids with their attendant side effects and risks. When the preoperative daily oral dose of opioids exceeds 30 mg of morphine, equivalent, multimodality pain management should be implemented postoperatively, including gabapentinoids, nonsteroidal anti-inflammatory drugs (NSAIDs), acetaminophen, ketamine, and infiltration of extended-release local anesthetics [10].

In the elective setting, patients optimized for major spine surgery should be extubated after its conclusion in order to diminish the likelihood of postoperative respiratory complications, including pneumonia and sepsis. This is particularly important in patients with implants, as seeding of bacteria can have disastrous consequences. It appears from the analysis of Anastasian that delaying extubation is influenced by the time the intervention ends. Anesthesiologists may delay extubation for indications related to provider fatigue, decreased nursing and physician staffing, and lack of other resources after hours and, since handoff of care was more common (although not significantly so in the multivariate analysis) in the delayed extubation group, perhaps more caution in dealing with an unfamiliar patient [9].

Although patients usually disclose intraoperative awareness many days after surgery, the NAP5 group identified a group of patients whose recall was probably related to post-anesthesia care, especially if they remained intubated [8]. Unless fully discussed with the patient preoperatively, postoperative intubation and ventilation may be a source of major distress.

Postoperative visual loss (POVL) becomes apparent once the patient has recovered sufficiently from anesthesia to appreciate visual field defects. In the worst-case scenario, blindness is complete and bilateral. In many instances, however, visual loss is unilateral and/or partial. Posterior ischemic optic neuropathy (PION) is considered irreversible. However, if discovered early, visual loss due to cortical blindness or acute angle glaucoma, both rare but potentially reversible, may be diagnosed and treated. Clearly, there could be a benefit to the patient if awakening from anesthesia were immediate.

Multimodality pain management with the stated goal of decreasing opioid dosage makes sense only in the awake patient; after all, we are guiding narcotic administration based on the patient's subjective pain assessment. Similarly, early detection of dyspnea in pulmonary embolism, chest pain in a coronary syndrome, or neurological deterioration in an ischemic stroke is more likely to lead to a focused and successful intervention. Let us remember that these complications may occur in up to 8.5 % of major spine surgery patients [5].

A minor reason not to delay intubation is related to the Lo-Pro endotracheal tube, often used for routine surgery because of low cost. These high-pressure, low-volume cuffed tubes are not designed for prolonged intubation because the cuff pressure is high enough to damage the tracheal mucosa. Who measures tracheal cuff pressure in the OR?

Lastly, it is important to perform a neurological examination after extensive spine surgery to identify potentially correctable neural compression. Postoperative hematoma may develop, albeit very rarely, after all monitoring has been discontinued. Rapid decompression could save cord function.

CON: Major spine surgery patients should remain intubated after lengthy, bloody interventions.

Although good data are lacking, resuscitation from blood loss in the prone position, especially during lengthy surgery, leads to airway edema. It is not uncommon to observe conjunctival edema and its partial prolapse. This is indicative of dependent mucosal edema and perhaps of the risk of airway obstruction after extubation. Various techniques have been proposed to identify high-risk patients. Laryngeal ultrasound is gaining popularity, but it cannot evaluate the oropharynx and palate. The cuff-leak test, from qualitative to quantitative, where the tidal volume deficit is measured with the cuff deflated while the patient is mechanically ventilated, has been used. However, it is neither perfectly sensitive nor specific [11]. Within a few hours, with the patient supine and with head elevation, the facial edema subsides. Why not wait until then to extubate the patient?

Patients with lumbar spondylosis often present difficulties in endotracheal intubation: Spondylosis affects the cervical spine as well, and limits neck extension, especially when a previous decompression and fusion has taken place. Waiting for a few hours before extubation until any ongoing blood loss from the large postoperative wound has abated, and other potential complications have declared themselves, prevents emergent reintubation in this difficult setting. In its extubation guidelines, the Difficult Airway Society (UK) [12] recommends that "patient factors"—cardiovascular, respiratory, metabolic/temperature, and neuromuscular—be optimized before extubation. How can one be certain that the patient has been optimized mere minutes after returning to the supine position? Delaying extubation until the hemoglobin and blood gas values have been reviewed and corrected seems like a reasonable plan. Core temperature may also drop significantly in a cold OR during wound cleaning and dressing. The guideline further recommends that if reintubation may be potentially difficult or oxygenation uncertain, the patient should be considered for the high-risk extubation pathway, which includes delaying extubation until an informed judgment is made that it is safe to remove the endotracheal tube, and all the necessary adjunct devices as well as personnel are available for reintubation if necessary.

Restricting crystalloids [6] and keeping the Jackson table in reverse Trendelenburg are 2 commonly used techniques to minimize the risk of orbital venous congestion and to reduce the risk of PION [7]. This position, however, contributes to a decrease in venous return to the heart and amplifies the decrease in cardiac output, which is common in the prone position [13]. Pressors are commonly necessary during prolonged major surgical interventions. Intravascular volume repletion using BP as a guide is very imperfect. Noninvasive pulse pressure and stroke volume variation monitors are sometimes used, but they work only in mechanically ventilated patients. It is prudent to allow time to be able to fully assess the cardiovascular performance of the mechanically ventilated patient in the supine position in the hours after surgery, when continued bleeding may occur.

Summary

The common argument that neurological evaluation must be done as soon as surgery is completed, rushing the extubation process, may be related to tradition in this era of sophisticated computed tomography (CT)-based intraoperative navigation used to place pedicle screws with continuous multimodality neurophysiological monitoring.

There should be no fast rule that all major spine surgery patients should be extubated at the conclusion of the intervention. A deliberate, guideline-based approach factoring in the general respiratory and cardiovascular patient variables as well as airway-related elements is mandatory in each case. It is probably best to make the decision to extubate in the calm after the storm.

References

1. Yu X, Xiao H, Wang R, Huang Y. Prediction of massive blood loss in scoliosis surgery from preoperative variables. Spine. 2013;38:350–5.
2. Carabini LM, Zeeni C, Moreland NC, Gould RW, Avram MJ, Hemmer LB, et al. Development and validation of a generalizable model for predicting major transfusion during spine fusion surgery. J Neurosurg Anesthesiol. 2014;26:205–2015.
3. Carabini LM, Zeeni C, Moreland NC, Gould RW, Hemmer LB, Bebawy JF, et al. Predicting major cardiac events in spine fusion patients: is the revised cardiac risk index sufficient? Spine. 2014;39:1441–8.
4. Smith JD, Saulle D, Chen CJ, Lenke LG, Polly DW Jr, Kasliwal MK, et al. Rates and cause of mortality associated with spine surgery based on 108,419 procedures. Spine. 2012;37:1975–82.
5. Schwab FJ, Hawkinson N, Lafage V, Smith JS, Hart R, Mundis G, International Spine Study Group, et al. Risk factors for major peri-operative complications in adult spinal deformity surgery: a multi-center review of 953 consecutive patients. Eur Spine J. 2012;21:2603–10.
6. Postoperative Visual Loss Study Group. Risk factors associated with ischemic optic neuropathy after spinal fusion surgery. Anesthesiology. 2012;116:15–24.
7. ASA Task Force on Postoperative Visual Loss. Practice advisory for perioperative visual loss associated with spine surgery. Anesthesiology. 2012;116:274–85.
8. Pandit JJ, Andrade J, Bogod DG, Hitchman JM, Jonker WR, Lucas N, Royal College of Anaesthetists, Association of Anaesthetists of Great Britain and Ireland, et al. 5th National Audit Project (NAP5) on accidental awareness during general anesthesia: summary of main findings and risk factors. Br J Anaesth. 2014;113:549–59.
9. Anastasian ZH, Gaudet JG, Levitt LC, Mergeche JL, Heyer EJ, Berman MF. Factors that correlate with the decision to delay extubation after multilevel prone spine surgery. J Neurosurg Anesthesiol. 2014;26:167–71.
10. Devin CJ, McGirt MJ. Best evidence in multimodal pain management in spine surgery and means of assessing postoperative pain and functional outcomes. J Clin Neurosci. 2015;22:930–8.
11. Gros A, Holzapfel L, Marqué S, Perard L, Demingeon G, Piralla B, et al. Intra-individual variation of the cuff-leak test as a predictor of post-extubation stridor. Respir Care. 2012;57:2026–31.
12. The Difficult Airway Society. https://www.das.uk.com/guidelines/das-extubation-guidelines1. Accessed May 8 2015.
13. Dharmavaram S, Jellish WS, Nockels RP, Shea J, Mehmood R, Ghanayem A, et al. Effect of prone positioning systems on hemodynamic and cardiac function during lumbar spine surgery: an echocardiographic study. Spine. 2006;31:1388–93.

General Anesthesia for Intra-arterial Stroke Treatment (Endovascular Mechanical Thrombectomy): Still Needed or a Thing of the Past?

58

A. Elisabeth Abramowicz

Case

A 74-year-old female presents with right-sided hemiplegia and aphasia. She was last seen well by her family 1 h before arrival in the emergency room (ER). They report a history of hypertension, type II diabetes, and paroxysmal atrial fibrillation. She is taking lisinopril, hydrochlorothiazide, metformin, and metoprolol. She has no known allergies and last ate 3 h ago. Height: 5′2″ and weight: 220 lbs. Vital signs: blood pressure (BP) 180/105 mm Hg, heart rate (HR) 120, respiratory rate (RR) 18, and temperature 36.7 °C.

The neurointerventional team and the anesthesiology department are contacted by the stroke neurology team for endovascular thrombectomy of the left middle cerebral artery (MCA). The patient has had a computed tomography (CT)/CT angiogram (CTA) confirming occlusion of the left MCA and is receiving intravenous tissue plasminogen activator (iv T-PA). Her electrocardiogram (EKG) shows atrial fibrillation and her blood glucose is 240 mg/dL. She arrived in the emergency room 1 h ago.

Question

What are the anesthetic management options?

The on-call anesthesiologist has no experience with acute ischemic stroke (AIS) intervention. The patient is aphasic, does not follow commands, and is somewhat agitated. She tolerated the CTA with head and torso restraints. The airway examination is limited by her lack of cooperation; the patient is obese and has good dentition. She requires full-stomach precautions.

The anesthesiologist is interviewing the family members and has learned that the patient had an uneventful total hip replacement at another institution 2 years ago.

The stroke neurologists insist that the patient be brought to the neurointerventional suite immediately, as "time is brain" and a good neurological outcome depends heavily on rapid reperfusion of the occluded MCA.

The anesthesiologist informs the family that she will administer general anesthesia because of lack of patient cooperation, morbid obesity, and a risk of aspiration. The stroke neurologist, who overhears the informed consent discussion, pulls the anesthesiologist to the side and insists that general anesthesia for endovascular thrombectomy is contraindicated in AIS because the literature is clear that it is associated with adverse neurological outcomes. The interventional neurologist joins the conversation and supports the stroke neurologist. She explains that she does not need complete immobility and that "conscious sedation" will be adequate.

PRO: General anesthesia for endovascular thrombectomy is contraindicated in AIS. Sedation is always the preferred anesthetic modality.

Although first-generation mechanical clot retrieval devices have been on the market with US Food and Drug Administration (FDA) approval since 2004, proof that endovascular mechanical thrombectomy is superior to iv t-PA alone in AIS caused by occlusion of the internal carotid artery or its major branch, the MCA, has not been evident until very recently [1–5]. The tide has turned, probably because newer thrombectomy devices, so-called stent retrievers, which restore flow faster and more effectively, have been universally adopted in the endovascular treatment of major ischemic stroke, provided recanalization can be achieved within 6 h of onset. The American Heart Association/American Stroke Association (AHA/ASA) has issued a focused update to its 2013 guidelines on early management of patients with ischemic stroke, confirming this important development [6]. It has been estimated that up to 10 %, or 60,000, of patients with acute

A. Elisabeth Abramowicz (✉)
Department of Anesthesiology, New York Medical College, Westchester Medical Center, 100 Woods Rd., Macy 2391, Valhalla, NY 10595, USA
e-mail: APABRAMO@montefiore.org; elisabeth.abramowicz@gmail.com

C.S. Scher et al. (eds.), *You're Wrong, I'm Right*, DOI 10.1007/978-3-319-43169-7_58

ischemic stroke may benefit annually from this novel treatment [7]; up to 300 centers nationwide will be needed to provide this service on demand.

There are no randomized controlled trials addressing the safety of general anesthesia and/or its components in interventions for acute ischemic stroke. There is a body of weaker evidence indicating that general anesthesia, or "the intubated state" as it has been referred to in earlier publications, results in worse neurological outcomes despite similar occluded vessel recanalization levels (Thrombolysis in Cerebral Infarction, or TICI scale); the December 2014 meta-analysis of the published retrospective, single-center, mostly small series supports this association [8]. The major criticism of the available data is that it is likely that more neurologically impaired patients with higher National Institutes of Health (NIH) Stroke Scale values, at higher risk of poor outcome at the outset, required general anesthesia. The most recent study, which analyzed a cohort of consecutive AIS patients in several centers in the Netherlands, where the type of anesthesia administered depended on each center's local protocol/preference, again indicates that general anesthesia is detrimental, even after adjustment for stroke severity [9]. The putative advantages of general anesthesia, such as immobility, decrease in motion artefacts with resultant shortening of the procedure, decreased risk of vessel perforation, decreased radiation exposure to personnel, and smaller contrast dose have not been borne out in many observational studies. Indeed, most interventionalists state that since wire and micro-catheter navigation is "blind" because of vessel occlusion, immobility does not offer the same technical advantage as in aneurysm or AVM embolization.

It is no surprise then that the AHA/ASA now recommends that "it might be reasonable to favor conscious sedation over general anesthesia during endovascular therapy for AIS" (New Recommendation, number 16, Class IIb; Level of evidence C) [6]. A proposed reason for the worsened outcomes with general anesthesia is a delay in the time from stroke to groin puncture. In an observational study from a well-run stroke center in Switzerland, general anesthesia caused a 15-min delay on average [10], while a 20-min delay was seen in the Dutch study [9]. One minute of brain ischemia destroys 2 million neurons, 714 km of myelinated fibers, and 830 billion synapses [11]. Better neurological outcomes, irrespective of other variables, occur with short stroke-to-reperfusion times.

Despite these preliminary data, it is not yet known why general anesthesia worsens neurological outcome. A retrospective study by Davis et al. [12] found that a decrease in systolic blood pressure below 140 mm Hg, common in the general anesthesia group, was independently associated with poor neurological outcome. Does it follow that, provided the BP is maintained above that level, general anesthesia is safe? Is it possible that blood pressure variability alone affects the tenuous viability of the ischemic penumbra? It has also been suggested that even modest hyperventilation during general anesthesia might be the culprit. Unspecified toxic effects of (volatile) anesthetics on the ischemic brain could also be in play. This is all conjecture at this point. The additional arguments in favor of sedation are: It allows monitoring for both worsening neurological deficit and clinical improvement, which then may serve as a treatment end-point; pain perception during wire/catheter manipulation may be used as a warning sign of vessel damage before dissection/perforation occurs; and last but not least, it provides the hemodynamic stability that is so important in the acute phase of an ischemic stroke.

CON: General anesthesia must have a place in AIS thrombectomy. Sedation cannot be safely administered to every patient.

AIS patients are old; the mean age of a stroke patient is 79 years. In 65 % of cases, patients are over 65 years of age. Comorbidities are common in this group, as they constitute risk factors for stroke. These include hypertension, diabetes, atrial fibrillation or flutter, obstructive sleep apnea, smoking, and chronic kidney disease [13]. Stroke increases the risk of seizures, neurologic deterioration, and aspiration. The emergent nature of endovascular treatment precludes a thorough preanesthetic evaluation and optimization. Left MCA syndromes cause aphasia; patients do not follow commands, nor do they understand what is being done to them. They may be agitated, which may pose a danger of neck or limb injury and loss of both intravenous and arterial access lines, and may make imaging impossible.

Administering sedation to such patients in any other circumstance would be considered risky or outright unsafe. Patients who have mental status changes are at risk for airway obstruction and aspiration, even after small doses of medication. In addition, the topography of the neurointerventional suite does not allow access to the airway. Moreover, the patient is positioned flat on a horizontal radiolucent table with a head restraint. This is a very dangerous position if regurgitation or vomiting were to occur. The table is usually poorly padded, and the massive electronic and bi-plane X-ray equipment requires cooling, creating thermal discomfort. These conditions may aggravate agitation and lack of cooperation, necessitating further doses of sedatives. The deployment of the stent portion of the thrombectomy device causes pain from intracranial vessel stretch, which is further amplified by the retrieval of the clot. Several passes of the stent retriever may be necessary before reperfusion and anticipated neurological improvement occurs.

Considering the dual problems of positional discomfort and pain from intracranial and intracerebral arterial manipulation, a good analgesic regimen is probably satisfactory in cooperative patients and avoids over-sedation, airway obstruction, and hypoventilation with hypoxemia. However, the potential complications should not be considered minor in comparison to the hemodynamic variability of general anesthesia, which can be tightly controlled. Patients with AIS who need to be immobilized for safety would need deep sedation. Instead, they deserve elective airway protection and controlled ventilation; i.e., general anesthesia.

Until randomized, controlled trials elucidate the best anesthetic management for AIS, most centers will continue to rely on local protocols. There is a strong preference for either one or the other technique; availability of consistent coverage by an anesthesiologist may be one of the defining, but unpublished, criteria. In centers that prefer "conscious sedation," emergent conversion to general anesthesia is reported in 10–13 % of cases [14]. We know from the anesthesia literature that emergency conversions carry significant risks, as they are really respiratory rescues, not controlled induction of anesthesia.

Interestingly, in his meta-analysis of retrospective case series, Brinjikji [8] found that respiratory complications, as well as death and poor neurological and angiographic outcomes, were more common in the general anesthesia group. Only 6 of 9 studies analyzed had stroke severity data; in these, patients with higher severity strokes were more likely to have had general anesthesia, indicating a selection bias and a more frequent need to protect the airway. Unlike the two studies previously quoted [9, 10], he did not find a delay in treatment associated with general anesthesia.

There is little information on optimal sedation drug selection in AIS thrombectomy. John et al. [15] retrospectively compared 35 patients receiving dexmedetomidine with 37 given propofol. Despite similar outcomes, patients receiving dexmedetomidine not unexpectedly exhibited hemodynamic instability and required large doses of vasopressors. These results, if confirmed, call into question the validity of the argument that sedation is preferable because it avoids the hemodynamic variability caused by general anesthesia.

Summary

Despite the neurologists' exhortations and the soft recommendation to "favor" sedation in the 2015 AHA/ASA guidelines, there are many unanswered questions [16]. Because of a lack of quality prospective data, the choice of anesthetic technique is best left to the anesthesiologist, who must identify and communicate the contraindications to sedation to the treating team, while being aware of the technical aspects of the procedure and respecting the local preference-guided protocol.

References

1. Berkhemer OA, Fransen PS, Beumer D, van den Berg LA, Lingsma HF, Yoo AJ, MR CLEAN Investigators, et al. A randomized trial of intraarterial treatment for acute ischemic stroke. N Engl J Med. 2015;372:11–20.
2. Demchuk AM, Menon BK, Eesa M, Rempel JL, Thornton J, Roy D, ESCAPE Trial Investigators, et al. Randomized assessment of rapid endovascular treatment of ischemic stroke. N Engl J Med. 2015;372:1019–30.
3. Campbell BC, Mitchell PJ, Kleinig TJ, Dewey HM, Churilov L, Yassi N, EXTEND-IA Investigators, et al. Endovascular therapy for ischemic stroke with perfusion-imaging selection. N Engl J Med. 2015;372:1009–18.
4. Saver JL, Goyal M, Bonafe A, Diener HC, Levy EI, Pereira VM, SWIFT PRIME Investigators, et al. Stent-retriever thrombectomy after intravenous t-PA vs. t-PA alone in stroke. N Engl J Med. 2015;372:2285–95.
5. Jovin TG, Chamorro A, Cobo E, de Miquel MA, Molina CA, Rovira A, REVASCAT Trial Investigators, et al. Thrombectomy within 8 hours after symptom onset in ischemic stroke. N Engl J Med. 2015;372:2296–306.
6. Powers WJ, Derdeyn CP, Biller J, Coffey CS, Hoh BL, Jauch EC, American Heart Association Stroke Council, et al. AHA/ASA focused update of the 2013 guidelines for the early management of patients with acute ischemic stroke regarding endovascular treatment. Stroke. 2015;46(10):3020–35.
7. Furlan AJ. Endovascular therapy for stroke—it's about time. N Engl J Med. 2015;372:2347–9.
8. Brinjikji W, Murad MH, Rabinstein AA, Cloft HJ, Lanzino G, Kallmes DF. Conscious sedation versus general anesthesia during endovascular acute ischemic stroke treatment: a systematic review and meta-analysis. Am J Neuroradiol. 2015;36:525–9.
9. Van Den Berg LA, Koelman DL, Berkhemer OA, Rozeman AD, Fransen PS, Beumer D, MR CLEAN Pretrial Study Group; Participating centers, et al. Type of anesthesia and differences in clinical outcome after intra-arterial treatment for ischemic stroke. Stroke. 2015;46:1257–62.
10. Brekenfeld C, Mattle HP, Schroth G. General is better than local anesthesia during endovascular procedures. Stroke. 2010;41:2716–7.
11. Saver JL. Time is brain—quantified. Stroke. 2006;37:263–6.
12. Davis MJ, Menon BK, Baghirzada LB, Campos-Herrera CR, Goyal M, Hill MD, Calgary Stroke Program, et al. Anesthetic management and outcome in patients during endovascular therapy for acute stroke. Anesthesiology. 2012;116:396–405.
13. Go AS, Mozaffarian D, Roger VL, Benjamin EJ, Berry JD, Blaha MJ, American Heart Association Statistics Committee and Stroke Statistics Subcommittee, et al. Heart disease and stroke statistics-2014 update: a report from the American Heart Association. Circulation. 2014;129:e28–292.
14. Soize S, Kadziolka K, Estrade L, Serre I, Bakchine S, Pierot L. Mechanical thrombectomy in acute stroke: prospective pilot trial of the solitaire FR device while under conscious sedation. Am J Neuroradiol. 2013;34:360–5.
15. John S, Somal J, Thebo U, Hussain MS, Farag E, Dupler S, et al. Safety and hemodynamic profile of propofol and dexmedetomidine during intra-arterial acute stroke therapy. J Stroke Cerebrovasc Dis. 2015;24(10):2397–403.
16. Grotta JC, Hacke W. Stroke neurologist's perspective on the new endovascular trials. Stroke. 2015;46:1447–52.

Is It Better to Perform a Craniotomy for Brain Tumor Resection Awake?

59

John L. Ard Jr. and Irene Kim

Case

A 44-year-old, otherwise healthy, right-handed woman presents to the emergency room after having her first seizure in a restaurant. A computed tomography (CT) scan of her head revealed a 2-cm by 4-cm mass in her right parietal lobe.

Her neurosurgeon recommends a craniotomy for resection of her tumor and diagnosis of tumor type.

The patient, who is the mother of 2 small children, had a relative who had a brain tumor removed while "awake." The procedure went well and the relative left the hospital 2 days after surgery. Although she is fearful of an awake procedure she wants to get home as soon as possible to care for her children. She wonders if she can avoid general anesthesia and have her tumor taken out "awake" as well.

Her neurosurgeon has done a few awake cases, but only when the tumor was located in an eloquent area of the brain, which this tumor is not. The surgeon consults his anesthesia colleague.

Question

Are outcomes just as good or better after awake craniotomies?

PRO: Recently a number of prospective and retrospective studies compared craniotomy for tumor resection under general anesthesia versus an "awake" technique [1]. The awake craniotomy patients had shorter hospital stays with fewer neurologic deficits. Most of these cases involved tumors near eloquent areas (language or motor), but the benefit to patients was so great that an awake technique should be considered for all craniotomies.

CON: Most of those studies are retrospective or nonrandomized [1]. In the meta-analysis [1], the awake group was younger and had more frontal and temporal tumors compared to the general anesthesia group. It is difficult to overcome selection bias in these studies as patients with sleep apnea, morbid obesity, anxiety, speech or language problems would not be suitable candidates for an awake technique.

PRO: In 2014, a case series of very sick patients having awake craniotomies was published [2]. The patients were able to tolerate the procedure and did well afterward. Only a few neurosurgical centers perform all craniotomies "awake" [3]. Perhaps anesthesiologists don't have to be so selective about who gets an awake craniotomy.

CON: We still lack randomized trials. It's easy enough to publish a series where all patients do well, likely introducing publication bias. The failures are just not mentioned.

PRO: The awake group may do better because they avoid general anesthesia agents or at least receive these agents at lower doses [4]. For instance, both inhaled and intravenous anesthetics have profound cardiac and vasoactive effects. The awake craniotomy anesthetic, in contrast, produces less hypotension; this is undoubtedly good for maintaining cerebral perfusion. Awake craniotomy also avoids mechanical ventilation and resulting barotrauma, which releases cytokines and initiates an inflammatory cascade.

CON: There is some evidence in the literature that commonly used anesthetics such as propofol or sevoflurane have toxic effects on organs such as the lungs, heart, and brain. But it is certain that hypoxia and hypercarbia are bad for these organs as well. Episodes of desaturation occur in

J.L. Ard Jr. (✉)
Department of Anesthesiology, New York University Langone Medical Center, 550 First Avenue, New York, NY 10016, USA
e-mail: john.ard@nyumc.org

I. Kim
Department of Neurosurgery, New York University Langone Medical Center, 462 First Avenue, NB-7S4, New York, NY 10010, USA
e-mail: irenekim514@gmail.com

C.S. Scher et al. (eds.), *You're Wrong, I'm Right*, DOI 10.1007/978-3-319-43169-7_59

awake craniotomies. The unsecured airway could also increase the likelihood of aspiration pneumonitis.

PRO: General anesthetics affect immune function [4]. The inhaled agent halothane suppresses natural killer cell activity, and isoflurane adversely impacts the peripheral helper-T lymphocyte ratio after craniotomy. Commonly used opioids such as fentanyl and morphine decrease cellular and humoral immunity [5]. An awake craniotomy relies on local anesthetics for pain control, so the use of narcotics and inhaled anesthetics is reduced or eliminated.

CON: These are interesting research findings and may one day change how we practice anesthesia in patients with all types of cancer. Unfortunately, there is a lack of randomized controlled trials to confirm that any of this makes a difference in patient outcome. Additionally, the local anesthetics used for the scalp block are cardiotoxic and neurotoxic in high doses.

Concession from PRO: There will always be patients who require general anesthesia such as the very young or those who refuse to undergo an awake procedure. There is a lack of solid evidence to indicate that an awake technique is as safe as general endotracheal anesthesia for this type of case.

Concession from CON: Although the evidence for performing more craniotomies awake is mostly retrospective, the possibility of better outcomes without an increase in complications should push anesthesiologists to perform and publish the necessary clinical trials.

References

1. Brown T, Shah AH, Bregy A, Shah NH, Thambuswamy M, Barbarite E, et al. Awake craniotomy for brain tumor resection: the rule rather than the exception? J Neurosurg Anesthesiol. 2013;25:240–7.
2. Garavaglia M, Das S, Cusimano M, Crescini C, Mazer D, Hare G, Rigamonti A. Anesthetic approach to high-risk patients and prolonged awake craniotomy using dexmedetomidine and scalp block. J Neurosurg Anesthesiol. 2014;26:226–33.
3. Serletis D, Bernstein M. Prospective study of awake craniotomy used routinely and nonselectively for supratentorial tumors. J Neurosurg. 2007;107:1–6.
4. Meng L, Berger MS, Gelb AW. The potential benefits of awake craniotomy for brain tumor resection: an anesthesiologist's perspective. J Neurosurg Anesthesiol. 2015;27(4):310–7.
5. Meserve JR, Kaye AD, Prabhakar A, Urman RD. The role of analgesics in cancer propagation. Best Pract Res Clin Anaesthesiol. 2014;28:139–51.

Nitrous Oxide in Neuroanesthesia: Does It Have a Place?

60

Elizabeth A.M. Frost

Case

You had rather hoped that you would be assigned to the aneurysm clipping this morning. After all, operative aneurysms are becoming increasingly rare now that the interventionalists are getting so good at coiling. However, the case has been given to one of the older members of the department, who has more experience with craniotomies. And here you are with the short eye cases. So between cases you decide to wander into the neuro room, just to see how things are going. To your horror you realize that your colleague has dialed in nitrous oxide 60 % with the isoflurane!

Question

Will his choice of anesthesia adversely impact the patient's neurologic outcome?

PRO (You): What are you doing? Don't you know how bad nitrous oxide is for maintenance of stable intracranial dynamics?

CON (Your Colleague): I've been doing craniotomies this way since you were in kindergarten, and I have never had a problem. I'm using N_2O so she wakes up quickly and that makes my surgeon happy so he can check her out early… none of this "days on a ventilator" stuff.

PRO: Well. It's time you listened to a little science and changed. You are right that early studies suggested that N_2O was pharmacologically inert and provided good analgesia. So it became a background gas. But as long ago as 1939, Courville described adverse effects [1]. Almost 80 years ago he demonstrated decisively that asphyxic damage to the brain is a frequent consequence of N_2O [1]. And while the use of N_2O in neuroanesthesia has been debated for years, studies reviewed by Lam and Mayberg and Culley [2, 3] confirm that N_2O cannot be considered safe for all patients—especially neurosurgical patients—and that its inclusion should be a conscious act rather than a reflex.

CON: Oh, I know all that. And if you are quoting history, let me remind you of Clement's book from the same era extolling the virtues of N_2O as the sole agent [4]. My patient was stable before I started. She knew her name and almost got the date right. The patient had just a little weakness in her left arm. Sure she had a bad headache. Don't we all? Given the norm around here, I thought she was pretty good. Vital signs were no problem… I mean she is a bit old at 60 and she was anxious, so a blood pressure of 170/95 and a few ectopic beats were no big deal.

PRO: How do you know that the hypertension and dysrhythmias were not due to raised intracranial pressure? What was her Hunt and Hess classification score? You know that those numbers are used as a predictor of severity of injury and outcome, ranging from 1 = mild symptoms going up to 5 = a decerebrate, comatose patient [5]. Sounds like your patient was between a 2 and a 3, which is just on the cusp of where we could make a significant difference in outcome" [5].

CON: Hardly matters. Neuro said to give mannitol and furosemide before incision, anyway.

PRO: So it seems she does have significant neurologic symptoms. Nitrous oxide is an NMDA antagonist and as such has a real potential to exert neurotoxic effects. It is a direct cerebral vasodilator and also increases metabolism, thus increasing intracranial pressure. In fact, 66 % N_2O was shown to increase mean intracranial pressure (ICP) by

E.A.M. Frost
Icahn Medical Center at Mount Sinai, 1 Gustav L Levy Place, New York, NY, USA10029

E.A.M. Frost (✉)
2 Pondview West, Purchase, NY 10577, USA
e-mail: elzfrost@aol.com; elizabeth.frost@mountsinai.org

C.S. Scher et al. (eds.), *You're Wrong, I'm Right*, DOI 10.1007/978-3-319-43169-7_60

27 mmHg in patients with neurologic damage. Autoregulation is also impaired. And on top of that, there is quite a bit of mounting evidence that nitrous oxide in combination with isoflurane might induce apoptosis and increase beta amyloid protein levels [6], which are known to be toxic to the immature brain. And before you say anything, I know these are in vitro studies on fetal mice cell cultures and may not be relevant to human brains. Still it is evidence that N_2O can exert damaging effects at some point during development.

CON: So what? A little increase in cerebral blood flow I can manage with some hyperventilation! And I am glad you agree that mice are not humans. Those studies just don't apply. My patient is a grown woman, not a fetus or neonate!

PRO: But back to your hyperventilation. That causes cerebral ischemia by itself. Soukup and colleagues showed that decreasing $PaCO_2$ by 20 % (that is, from 40 to 32 mmHg) resulted in a decrease in cerebral blood flow (CBF) from 30 to 25 ml/100 g/min and decreased the brain tissue partial pressure of oxygen ($ptiO_2$) by 25 % [7].

CON: Back off. I am delivering 40 % oxygen, and the pulse oximeter is reading 97 %.

PRO: OK. Let's consider some of the other effects of N_2O on the nervous system. Did you find out if the surgeon is planning on monitoring any evoked potentials?

CON: That's only for back surgery.

PRO: Not at all…evoked potential monitoring is widely used to detect neural damage throughout the nervous system. Nitrous oxide can have profound effects on the electroencephalogram (EEG) and can depress all evoked potentials. And while it is most likely an anticonvulsant, withdrawal may elicit convulsive activity.

CON: You clearly don't like my choice of anesthetic here.

PRO: No, I don't given that this is someone who already has sustained a major intracranial insult. Your technique might well work for a short non-neurosurgical procedure, but it is just not the best technique here. In fact, Hancock and Nathanson after a review of the literature concluded that remifentanil should be substituted for N_2O for the "at risk" brain [8]. Also, diuretics and hyperventilation shrink the brain. When the surgeon comes to close, air will be trapped intracranially. Because the blood/gas solubility coefficient of N_2O is 30 times that of nitrogen, the number of N_2O molecules given up by the blood to the air within the cranium exceeds the number of molecules of nitrogen and oxygen absorbed by the blood. Thus, a tension pneumocephalus will develop and is only very slowly absorbed.

CON: Maybe the surgeon will leave a drain in?

PRO: Not likely. Moreover, while many of the inhalation agents, including the isoflurane you are using, have been shown to have cerebral protective effects, nitrous oxide will eliminate those beneficial actions. Another study by Pasternak et al. compared 199 patients who were given N_2O during intracranial aneurysm clipping with 242 who received other techniques [9]. Those who received N_2O were at significantly higher risk of developing delayed ischemic neurologic deficits.

References

1. Courville CB. Untoward effects of nitrous oxide. Mountain View: Pacific Press Publishing Association; 1939.
2. Lam AM, Mayberg TS. Use of nitrous oxide in neuroanesthesia: why bother? J Neurosurg Anesthesiol. 1992;4(4):285–9.
3. Culley DJ. Nitrous oxide in neuroanesthesia: tried and true or toxin? Anesthesiology. 2008;108:553–4.
4. Clement FW. Nitrous oxide–oxygen anesthesia. Philadelphia: Lea and Febiger; 1939.
5. Hunt WE, Hess RM. Surgical risk as related to time of intervention in the repair of intracranial aneurysms. J Neurosurg. 1968;28(1):14–20.
6. Zhen Y, Dong Y, Wu X, Xu Z, Lu Y, Zhang Y, et al. Nitrous oxide plus isoflurane induces apoptosis and increases beta-amyloid protein levels. Anesthesiology. 2009;111(4):741–52.
7. Soukup J, Bramsiepe I, Brucke M, Sanchin L, Menzel M. Evaluation of a bedside monitor of regional cerebral blood flow as a measure of CO_2 reactivity in neurosurgical intensive care patients. J Neurosurg Anesthesiol. 2008;20(4):249–55.
8. Hancock SM, Nathanson MH. Nitrous oxide or remifentanil for the "at risk" brain anaesthesia. Anaesthesia. 2004;59:313–5.
9. Pasternak JJ, McGregor DG, Lanier WL, Schroeder DR, Rusy DA, Hindman B, IHAST Investigators, et al. Effect of nitrous oxide use of long term neurologic and neuropsychological outcome in patients who received temporary proximal artery occlusion during cerebral aneurysm clipping surgery. Anesthesiology. 2009;110(3):563–73.

Should We Treat Hypertension Immediately Before Electroconvulsive Therapy?

61

Elana B. Lubit

Case

A 70-year-old man admitted with refractory major depression is scheduled for electroconvulsive therapy (ECT). He has hypertension and coronary artery disease, s/p myocardial infarction (MI), and stent 10 years ago. His cardiologist writes that he is stable on medications (lisinopril, aspirin, and escitalopram). He is thin, with a normal airway. Blood tests are within normal limits, and electrocardiogram (ECG) shows sinus rhythm with old Q-waves in inferior leads.

You have not anesthetized anyone for ECT since your residency, so a colleague, who has been doing ECT cases for 20 years, is standing by to help. Your patient stares silently at the ceiling as you apply the monitors. His heart rate is 98, and his blood pressure is 180/110. Your colleague glances at the numbers and waits for your response.

Questions

Is it safe to proceed with ECT if the patient has elevated heart rate and blood pressure? Should you try to control the numbers before treatment? If so, with what?

You step away from the bedside for a word with your colleague.

> Can we continue?" you ask. "Uncontrolled hypertension is a risk factor for cardiac complications, right?

Your colleague shrugs. "Probably not, in an otherwise stable patient," she replies. "Besides, if we canceled ECT for every acutely hypertensive patient, we'd miss many chances to save lives. Let's do this."

PRO: "The fact that a patient is acutely hypertensive before induction doesn't mean he's going to have a problem. A meta-analysis of perioperative studies showed an increase in transient effects—lability, dysrhythmias, and ischemia—when patients started out with systolic blood pressure above 180 or diastolic above 110. But the analysis showed no change in outcome based on initial blood pressure. Moreover, there was no evidence that postponing surgery for blood pressure control led to any difference in outcome" [1].

CON: "So? What makes you think that a meta-analysis of surgical patients is relevant to ECT? People's vital signs go crazy with ECT. Bradycardia, tachycardia, hypertension—even in patients who start out normal! Surely ECT is a special high-risk situation."

PRO: "Not really. We get too anxious about these numbers. The duration of ECT-related lability is rarely more than 10 min, usually fewer, and it seems pretty benign. A review of 17,400 ECTs at the Mayo Clinic found only 1 (non-fatal) cardiac arrest; the other complications were transient arrhythmias or transient respiratory events. All the transient complications together affected fewer than 1 % of patients [2]. Also, a recent Danish review found no deaths related to ECT in almost 100,000 treatments [3]. So ECT is extremely safe. It's really a low-risk procedure."

CON: "Even so. You're talking about all ECT patients. Don't you think the ECT patients with uncontrolled hypertension represent a high-risk subgroup? Our patient has coronary disease too!"

PRO: "Well, some smallish studies in the 1990s (fewer than 100 patients) compared high-cardiac-risk ECT patients to other ECT patients, and the groups differed only in transient complications, such as chest pain or dysrhythmias without

E.B. Lubit
Department of Anesthesiology, New York University School of Medicine/Bellevue Hospital Center, 550 First Avenue, Room TH 530, New York, NY 10016, USA

E.B. Lubit (✉)
134 West 93rd Street, Apt. 2E, New York, NY 10025, USA
e-mail: Lubit@nyumc.org

C.S. Scher et al. (eds.), *You're Wrong, I'm Right*, DOI 10.1007/978-3-319-43169-7_61

sequelae. I admit there haven't been large studies of specific high-risk subgroups. But so many depressed patients have major comorbidities, I suspect most ECT patients belong to one medical risk group or another! So those low complication rates probably do apply here."

CON: "OK, so let's say we can proceed safely. It still seems like we ought to do something for his blood pressure before we get started."

At this point, the attending psychiatrist asks whether you are planning to treat the patient or merely have a seminar. You request a few more minutes. The psychiatrist leaves to make phone calls.

The patient does not move at all. "He's always like that," says the psychiatric nurse. "That's why we're here."

You turn back to your colleague.

"So, let's treat his blood pressure," you suggest. "After all, we know that treating hypertension reduces a patient's overall risk of stroke and cardiac death [4], even if we can't prove it reduces peri-ECT risk. How about a beta-blocker?"

PRO: "No," your colleague replies, "I think we're better off leaving him alone. Remember, this is his first ECT treatment, so the psychiatrist has to titrate the stimulus to find the seizure threshold. If there's no seizure, the unopposed vagal effect of the stimulus can cause severe bradycardia. Do we really want to give a beta-blocker right before that happens? I once gave a patient a metoprolol premed, and after 1 stimulus without a seizure he went completely asystolic. Never again!"

CON: "So how about a peripheral vasodilator?"

PRO: "What, and send his heart rate over the top before we've even started ECT?"

CON: "A calcium-channel blocker then."

PRO: "Diltiazem shortens seizure duration."

CON: You sigh, and check another blood pressure: 185/105. Heart rate still in the 90s.

"How about this, then," you propose, "Let's treat his blood pressure and give him another day to stabilize. We can start ECT in 2 days." You are not surprised when your colleague shakes her head.

PRO: "I say we do it now. Remember, we can treat the pressure as soon as the seizure begins. I don't think he's at risk for any serious complication if we proceed now, and this depression is keeping him in a state of devastating pain. We are looking at a person in agony, like someone screaming with pain on a battlefield. Do we say, 'you'll need to scream another couple of days?' However long he's been depressed, however long he's been catatonic—he's in our hands now and he's in terrible pain. I say, this is not elective."

CON: "We're medical doctors, not psychiatrists. If he suffers another 2 days of depression, that's a psychiatric problem. If he has a cardiac complication, we will have harmed him."

PRO: "But delaying ECT may reduce his chances of cure" [2].

CON: "How about you put your name on this case, since you're so confident about this?"

PRO: Your colleague smiles sympathetically. "I understand. Nobody wants to harm a patient, and this is your first ECT as an attending. But we're helping save a life here. Let's go."

She signs the chart and turns to the patient. The psychiatrist has returned and places the ECT electrodes while you place an IV.

Treatment begins. Etomidate… succinylcholine… The blood pressure comes down a bit while you mask-ventilate the patient. Right unilateral stimulus… no seizure. The heart rate and blood pressure drop to 50 and 110/60. You watch the screen. The psychiatrist increases the current for the second stimulus… this time the patient seizes. Suddenly, his heart rate is 130, blood pressure is 200/120, and you see ST depressions. Your colleague gives esmolol; the vital signs and ECG normalizes in 5–10 min. Now the patient is breathing; soon he opens his eyes. You scan his face, but he is still impassive.

"No miracles on the first day," remarks the nurse. "But he's on his way now. Thank you for your help."

Summary

Moderate preinduction hypertension is nearly always benign in ECT patients; we may not be justified in delaying the case. Moreover, given the unpredictability of vital signs after induction—especially in ECT with titration, when a seizure may not occur—we may do best not treating preinduction blood pressure, but rather waiting until after the seizure begins.

We are naturally loath to bring a patient with high blood pressure into an elective procedure. Perhaps, then, we should consider these cases semi-elective, if not emergent. If we consider the agony of depression, and the risk of failure associated with delaying treatment, we may be more willing to proceed.

Finally, the ubiquitous caveat of our profession: We must always consider the individual case when we determine our plan. Some cases will still warrant waiting for medical stabilization, and we will have to judge which ones they are.

References

1. Howell SJ, Sear JW, Foëx P. Hypertension, hypertensive heart disease and perioperative cardiac risk. Br J Anaesth. 2004;92:570–83.
2. Nuttall GA, Bowersox M, Douglass SB, McDonald J, Rasmussen LJ, Decker PA, et al. Morbidity and mortality in the use of electroconvulsive therapy. J ECT. 2004;20:237–41.
3. Østergaard SD, Bolwig TG, Petrides G. No causal association between electroconvulsive therapy and death. J ECT. 2014;30:263–4.
4. American College of Cardiology/American Heart Association Task Force on Practice Guidelines. ACC/AHA 2007 guidelines on perioperative cardiovascular evaluation and care for noncardiac surgery. Circulation. 2007;2007(116):e418–500.

Part VII
Transplant

Viscoelastic Testing in Liver Transplantation

62

Cynthia Wang

Case

A 57-year-old female with alcoholic cirrhosis presents for an orthotopic liver transplantation. Her pre-transplant hospital course has been prolonged and complicated. She has been intubated for respiratory failure and has had sepsis that is currently resolving but remains on a low-dose norepinephrine infusion. She is in renal failure secondary to a combination of hepatorenal syndrome and acute tubular necrosis and is on continuous renal replacement therapy. She has a history of a repaired ruptured duodenal ulcer, and her portal vein is thrombosed. Her calculated model for end-stage liver disease (MELD) score is 45. Following a very difficult and bloody hepatectomy, the graft is finally reperfused. The surgeon mentions that he does not see clot forming in the surgical field and asks what you "can give to make the bleeding better." You have already administered almost 100 units of blood and fresh frozen plasma (FFP), 2 packs of platelets, and 2 packs of cryoprecipitate.

Question

Do the prothrombin time (PT), partial thromboplastin time (PTT), and international normalized ratio (INR) accurately reflect the patient's true coagulation status? What about fibrinogen levels?

PRO: PT, PTT, and INR testings are widely available, relatively quick, and inexpensive ways of assessing the intrinsic and extrinsic pathways. PT and particularly INR have historically been accurate indicators of the severity of liver disease. PTT, on the other hand, may detect congenital factor deficiencies, particularly since it is usually normal or near normal in liver disease. Fibrinogen levels over 100 mg/dL are generally a reliable indicator that the patient has adequate fibrinogen to initiate coagulation [1]. Low levels, on the other hand, may be a clue that hyperfibrinolysis is present.

It has been suggested that clot formation times on thromboelastometry tracings are the reflective of, or may be a substitute for, PT and PTT values [2]. However, other studies have tried to correlate the results of viscoelastic testing with conventional coagulation tests such as PT, PTT, and INR and failed to demonstrate a positive correlation [3]. Overall, various types of thromboelastography have been shown to correlate poorly with PT and PTT levels [4]. Given these limitations, thromboelastometry should be utilized as a test to supplement conventional laboratory testing rather than as a replacement for the traditional values.

CON: Conventional coagulation tests performed in plasma samples have been shown to have little correlation with bleeding or the need for transfusion in liver transplantation [5]. Patients with end-stage liver disease exhibit not only a deficiency of procoagulants and antifibrinolytic factors, but also a decrease in anticoagulants and profibrinolytics. Thus, in addition to being at risk for bleeding, patients carry the additional risk of thromboembolic complications. During orthotopic liver transplantation, evaluation of the patient's coagulation status is complicated by blood loss, the possibility of massive transfusion, and the stress of surgery. This, in conjunction with the dynamic nature of coagulopathy during the liver transplantation, makes the utility of conventional coagulation tests limited at best.

The international normalized ratio (INR) was developed in the 1980s in order to standardize therapeutic anticoagulation with vitamin K antagonists. The INR is calibrated on healthy volunteers, not on the patients with end-stage liver disease. Furthermore, there can be significant inter-laboratory variability depending on which thromboplastin reagent is used

C. Wang (✉)
Department of Anesthesiology and Pain Management, University of Texas Southwestern Medical Center, 5323 Harry Hines Blvd, Dallas, TX 75390, USA
e-mail: Cynthiawang2@utsouthwestern.edu; cynwang14@hotmail.com

C.S. Scher et al. (eds.), *You're Wrong, I'm Right*, DOI 10.1007/978-3-319-43169-7_62

for testing. Thus, INR testing in cirrhotic patients may lead to imprecise and unreliable results. Neither INR nor PT values have been shown to predict bleeding in the patients with liver disease. In fact, the American Association for the Study of Liver Diseases practice guidelines for the performance of liver biopsies states that there is no PT or INR level that clearly predicts bleeding before or after biopsy [6]. Similarly, PTT levels usually do not reflect the degree of liver dysfunction and therefore have limited utility. Low fibrinogen levels are often seen in stable, nonbleeding cirrhotic patients. Thus, they may not predict the propensity to bleed nor are they predictive of disseminated intravascular coagulation in cirrhotic patients. Fibrinogen is also an acute phase reactant, so levels may vary widely during liver transplantation, rendering isolated results unreliable.

Question

The bleeding continues, and surgeon is asking if you can consider giving a dose of tranexamic acid. Is thromboelastometry a superior test of coagulation than conventional laboratory tests?

PRO: Thromboelastometry provides a comprehensive analysis of coagulation defects in patients with liver disease. It is performed in whole blood whereas conventional coagulation tests are performed in plasma samples. Theoretically, because testing is done in the whole blood, all the components of coagulation are analyzed. Conventional laboratory coagulation assays use turbidimetry—or the "cloudiness" of the sample—to detect clot characteristics. Viscoelastic testing, however, is capable of detecting mechanical properties of the clot, such as clot firmness, which is dependent on fibrinogen and platelet levels and functions. Furthermore, it demonstrates clot evolution; over time, a thromboelastometry tracing can show dissolution of the clot. If it occurs earlier rather than later, hyperfibrinolysis may be a source of abnormal bleeding. Clot evolution is displayed in real time, and enough information may be obtained from the tracing within as little as 10 min in order to make significant management decisions. Conventional coagulation testing, on the other hand, may require 30–60 min, depending on the laboratory, before results can be obtained. Thus, by the time results are available, the coagulation status may have changed dramatically, particularly in the dynamic setting of liver transplantation. I predict that future well-done studies will show that thromboelastometry-guided transfusion practices will reduce the overall use of blood products in liver transplantation.

CON: Despite the advantages of viscoelastic studies, there are disadvantages and potential limitations to thromboelastometry. For one, viscoelastic tests measure the coagulation status in a cuvette in a static environment that is dramatically different from whole blood flowing through an endothelialized blood vessel. Furthermore, viscoelastic testing systems demand operator expertise. Tests run by untrained personnel without an established quality assurance protocol are bound to be inaccurate and imprecise. There are many technical variations in running the test, each of which may show a different result. Thromboelastometry machines also require daily calibration (sometimes multiple). Failure to maintain and calibrate the device may result in inaccuracies. In addition to requiring trained personnel to perform the examination, interpretation of tracings also demands experience and expertise.

Although thromboelastometry shows clot formation and dissolution in real time, the entire test may not yield results any more quickly than standard coagulation tests. A test takes 30–60 min to complete, a time frame in which most laboratories are able to process conventional coagulation tests.

Summary

Although the use of viscoelastic testing does not completely eliminate the utility of conventional coagulation testing, it has been shown to streamline transfusion practices during liver transplantation, which will ideally decrease overall transfusion requirements. As we transition into an age of transfusion medicine in which the use of FFP is replaced by factor concentrates, viscoelastic testing may begin to play a greater role. That said, conventional coagulation testing remains valuable, particularly in settings in which thromboelastometry is inaccessible. Obtaining reliable and precise thromboelastograms requires a considerable amount of technical and interpretative expertise that may be unavailable at some centers. The two testing modalities each offer insight into the different aspects of a very complex coagulation process in the patient with end-stage liver disease.

References

1. Northup PG, Caldwell SH. Coagulation in liver disease: a guide for the clinician. Clin Gastroenterol Hepatol. 2013;11:1064–74.
2. Bolliger D, Seeberger MD, Tanaka KA. Principles and practice of thromboelstography in clinical coagulation management and transfusion practice. Transfus Med Rev. 2012;26:1–13.

3. Ganter MT, Hofer CK. Coagulation monitoring: current techniques and clinical use of viscoelastic point-of-care coagulation devices. Anesth Analg. 2008;106:1366–75.
4. Roullet S, Pillot J, Freyburger G, Biais M, Quinart A, Rault A, Revel P, Sztark F. Rotation thromboelastrometry detects thrombocytopenia and hypfibrinogenaemia during orthotopic liver transplantation. Br J Anaesth. 2010;104:422–8.
5. Herbstreit F, Winter EM, Peters J, Hartmann M. Monitoring of haemostasis in liver transplantation: comparison of laboratory based and point of care tests. Anaesthesia. 2010;65:44–9.
6. Rockey DC, Caldwell SH, Goodman ZD, Nelson RC, Smith AD. American Association for the Study of Liver Disease. AASLD position paper: liver biopsy. 2009.

Antifibrinolytics in Liver Transplantation 63

Cynthia Wang

Case

A 27-year-old male with a history of liver transplantation as a child for biliary atresia presents for retransplantation secondary to graft failure due to chronic rejection. Upon presentation to the operating room, his Model for End-Stage Liver Disease (MELD) score is 36. He is oliguric and has just begun single-pass dialysis. He is not intubated and not on any vasopressor infusions. His platelet count is 45,000, his international normalized ratio (INR) is 2.1, and his fibrinogen levels are 95 mg/dL. Since this is a redo liver transplantation, you place 2 large bore central venous catheters in anticipation of massive bleeding and transfusion requirements. The surgeon asks you if it would be appropriate to administer tranexamic acid prophylactically in order to minimize bleeding risk.

PRO: It is a well-known fact that hyperfibrinolysis can contribute significantly to bleeding and increased transfusion requirements during liver transplantation. Increased plasminogen activator activity accompanied by decreased activity of various inhibitors of fibrinolysis result in excessive breakdown of fibrin. Clinically, this manifests as diffuse raw surface, non-surgical bleeding. Due to these processes, antifibrinolytics have long played a significant role in liver transplantation in attempts to decrease the risk of bleeding and need for massive transfusion. Some, however, have argued that there has been a paucity of clear evidence for the efficacy of antifibrinolytics in liver transplantation [1]. Others have pointed out that the use of these agents may increase the risk of perioperative thromboembolic complications in the liver transplant population [1]. However, a meta-analysis performed by Molenaar et al. of 23 studies involving a total of 1,407 patients who received either aprotinin or tranexamic acid for liver transplantation suggested that both agents reduced transfusion requirements compared to control groups [2]. At the same time, the analysis did not show any increase in incidence of hepatic artery thrombosis, venous thromboembolism, or perioperative mortality. Multiple prospective, randomized, controlled trials have shown a decrease in blood transfusion requirement in patients receiving antifibrinolytics when compared to placebo [2]. Thus, administering an antifibrinolytic when massive bleeding is anticipated may be clinically appropriate.

CON: Despite the compelling conclusions reached from the large meta-analysis mentioned above [2], it is important to note that it was based on a number of underpowered studies, which may exaggerate the difference in results between study groups. Thus, the fact that the group did not find differences between the groups does not indicate that there is no increase in the risk of thrombotic events associated with the use of antifibrinolytic agents. Furthermore, although aminocaproic acid is frequently used, there have been few studies that show definitive benefit for patients who receive this agent during transplantation.

Liver transplantation patients bleed for a variety of reasons, and hyperfibrinolysis is only one of them. They suffer from thrombocytopenia/thrombocytopathia, dilutional coagulopathy, hypothermia-related coagulopathy, and surgical bleeding. Prophylactic administration of antifibrinolytic agents may be misdirected in clinical situations in which hyperfibrinolysis is not the primary reason for uncontrollable raw surface bleeding; in fact, it may prove deleterious to the patient, potentially resulting in thromboembolic complications [3]. There have been many case reports of thromboembolism in patients undergoing liver transplantation who received antifibrinolytic agents. In fact, it has been postulated that these complications are probably under-reported or underestimated; a number of subclinical cases of thromboembolic events likely occur perioperatively without being recognized or reported.

C. Wang (✉)
Department of Anesthesiology and Pain Management, University of Texas Southwestern Medical Center, 5323 Harry Hines Blvd, Dallas, TX 75390, USA
e-mail: Cynthiawang2@utsouthwestern.edu; cynwang14@hotmail.com

C.S. Scher et al. (eds.), *You're Wrong, I'm Right*, DOI 10.1007/978-3-319-43169-7_63

Renal complications have been associated with aminocaproic acid, possibly due to acute tubular necrosis, renal infarction, myopathy- or pigment-induced renal insufficiency, glomerular capillary thrombosis, or obstruction of the upper urinary tract [3]. Patients who receive aminocaproic acid may suffer from severe proteinuria and/or myoglobinuria from myonecrosis, for which the only definitive treatment is hemodialysis. Renal complications have also been reported with aprotinin, [3] which may have a direct toxic effect on the proximal tubular cells. Furthermore, patients who have received aprotinin in the past may have a propensity for hypersensitivity reactions.

Question

You tell the surgeon that perhaps it is better to delay administration of an antifibrinolytic until after the hepatectomy—during the anhepatic or postreperfusion phase. You also recommend that a thromboelastogram be obtained prior to administration of the agent. When you call the pharmacy for tranexamic acid, you are told that the pharmacy is out of tranexamic acid and only has epsilon-aminocaproic acid (EACA) in stock. Are the 2 agents equivalent?

PRO: Antifibrinolytic agents fall into 2 categories: lysine analogues and serine protease inhibitors. Lysine analogues competitively inhibit the binding of plasminogen to lysine residues on the surface of fibrin, thereby preventing the conversion of plasminogen to plasmin. Serine protease inhibitors suppress fibrinolysis by inhibiting tissue plasminogen activator production. Both tranexamic acid and EACA are lysine analogues. EACA was the first antifibrinolytic used in liver transplantation. In the 1980s, Kang et al. reported 20 patients who developed severe fibrinolysis (out of a group of 97 undergoing liver transplantation) who were all treated with EACA [4]. All patients demonstrated improvement in hyperfibrinolysis as demonstrated by thromboelastography [4]. Likewise, the use of tranexamic acid was also first reported in the liver transplantation population in the 1980s, although it was not studied until later. In 1996, Boylan et al. reported a double-blinded, placebo-controlled study of a series of 45 cases that showed decreased intraoperative blood loss and reduced platelet, cryoprecipitate, and plasma transfusion requirements in patients who received tranexamic acid compared to the placebo group [5]. This is one of many studies that have shown a beneficial effect of tranexamic acid on blood loss and transfusion requirements during liver transplantation.

CON: Although both EACA and tranexamic have similar mechanisms of action, there are significant differences between the 2 agents that must be taken into consideration. Tranexamic acid is 6–10 times more potent than EACA [3]. Although both drugs are excreted in the urine, EACA has been shown to be associated with significant renal morbidity. Trials involving tranexamic acid and EACA in liver transplantation are difficult to compare since dosing regimens vary widely from group to group. Over the last decade, many placebo-controlled trials involving tranexamic acid and aprotinin have been published. However, EACA has been studied only in one randomized, controlled trial, which incidentally concluded that EACA offered no benefit compared to placebo [6]. It is difficult to equate the 2 agents as there have been no head-to-head trials comparing the efficacy and safety profiles of tranexamic acid and EACA.

Summary

The use of antifibrinolytics in liver transplantation remains a hotly debated topic. Although some have demonstrated a clear reduction in transfusion requirements for patients who have received antifibrinolytics, case reports of sometimes fatal thromboembolic complications make the routine administration of these agents questionable. As more studies related to the use of antifibrinolytics in the transplant population emerge, it is prudent to use them judiciously and with guidance from coagulation and viscoelastic testing.

References

1. Xia VW, Steadman RH. Antifibrinolytics in orthotopic liver transplantation: current status and controversies. Liver Transpl. 2005;11:10–8.
2. Molenaar IQ, Warnaar N, Groen H, TenVergert EM, Slooff MJH, Porte RJ. Efficacy and safety of antifibrinolytic drugs in liver transplantation: a systematic review and meta-analysis. Am J Transplant. 2007;7:185–94.
3. Porte RJ. Antifibrinolytics in liver transplantation: they are effective, but what about the risk-benefit ratio? Liver Transpl. 2004;10:285–8.
4. Kang Y, Lewis JH, Navalgund A, Russell MW, Bontempo FA, Niren LS, et al. Epsilon-aminocaproic acid for treatment of fibrinolysis during liver transplantation. Anesthesiology. 1987;66(6):766–73.
5. Boylan JF, Klinck JR, Sandler AN, Arellano R, Greig PD, Nierenberg H, et al. Tranexamic acid reduces blood loss, transfusion requirements, and coagulation factor use in primary orthotopic liver transplantation. Anesthesiology. 1996;85(5):1043–8; discussion 30A–31A.
6. Dalmau A, Sabate A, Acosta F, Garcia-Huete L, Koo M, Sansano T, et al. Tranexamic acid reduces red cell transfusion better than aminocaproic acid or placebo in liver transplantation. Anesth Analg. 2000;91:29–34.

Would You Recommend Accepting a "Donation After Cardiac Death" Liver?

64

Corey S. Scher

Case

At 3 in the morning, the telephone rings 5 times before it is picked up by the anesthesiologist.

> Robert, this is your friend Elizabeth. Sorry to wake you but as you know, my aunt needs a liver transplant, and we are trying to decide if she should accept a liver from a donation after cardiac death (DCD) patient. The surgeons are giving us all this information, but I want to know from the anesthesiologist's perspective as well before we make a decision as a family.

Question

Would you recommend that your colleague's family member who needs a transplant accept a "donation after cardiac death" liver?

PRO: As you know, the 3 types of livers available are: (1) living donor, (2) donation after cardiac death (DCD), and (3) donation after brain death (DBD). Since your aunt has designated you in writing as her health care proxy, I will discuss her medical details with you. When your aunt potentially had a liver donor last week from a DBD donor, as you know, that liver was suboptimal. Your aunt has a Model for End-Stage Liver Disease (MELD) score around 50. Her chance of passing away without a transplant within 3 months is greater than 80 %. She has hepatorenal syndrome and is due for hemodialysis today. The cause of her end-stage liver disease is hepatitis C. Her transhepatic internal jugular portal caval shunt (TIPS) is not functioning, and disease has left her with ascites, bilateral pleural effusions, and a pulmonary artery (PA) pressure of 40/22. Hemodialysis during the case is arranged so that the anesthesiologist will not be burdened with hyperkalemia that is nearly impossible to treat. Most of the electrolytes will be normal throughout the case thanks to dialysis. As you know, that liver came from a patient who is in North Carolina. The Organ Procurement and Transplantation Network (OPTN) and the United Network Organ Sharing (UNOS) group are regulatory agencies that have divided the country into 11 regions [1]. We are region 9 (New York), and North Carolina is in region 11. This means that all transplant centers in region 11 had turned this liver down. Why?

Simply, it could be a suboptimal liver after biopsy or the donor may have an unusual blood type that no one in the region had. In essence, there are many reasons that a liver may get turned down by an entire region and accepted by a center from a different region. In most cases, if the region has centers that have a small patient load, they need excellent outcomes and will not take organs that may be suboptimal leading to a questionable result. Many small volume centers cannot risk a suboptimal outcome that may occur for a liver that is donated after cardiac death. Simply stated, not every transplant center has the resources and experience to procure and deliver a liver with minimal ischemic times.

As the UNOS agent told us, the DBD donor last week had a subarachnoid bleed and had a respiratory arrest while at home. Doing the math, it took 10 min for first responders to get into that patient's home, 3 min to assess the situation, and 8 min to get the patient intubated and on 100 % oxygen. Totaling these numbers, the warm ischemic time was therefore 21 min. After 2 weeks, the patient had no neurologic recovery and a computed tomography (CT) scan of the head revealed a huge bleed in the temporal lobe and a subarachnoid bolt measured an intracranial pressure of 25 (normal in the supine patient is 7–15). A craniectomy was performed to relieve pressure and there was no clinical improvement in neurologic status. Two independent clinicians agreed that this was consistent with brain death. Once this decision is made, the liver can be procured with no

C.S. Scher (✉)
Department of Anesthesiology, Perioperative Care and Pain Medicine, New York University School of Medicine, New York, NY 10016, USA
e-mail: coreyscher@gmail.com

C.S. Scher et al. (eds.), *You're Wrong, I'm Right*, DOI 10.1007/978-3-319-43169-7_64

further ischemic time. I think that the liver took a big hit from the original incident of hypoxia in the home and the CT scan revealed a fatty liver. Since statistics count, the centers in region 9 did not want to take the risk. Some centers take the liver to examine, get pathology involved, and then make a decision. It can be a tough call, because some of the borderline livers do fine.

Based on you wanting the best for your aunt, though, "some do fine" is not exactly a ringing endorsement! I think that the right DCD liver is now acceptable as there is a nationwide shortage of organs and with a MELD score of 50, her time is clearly running out and if you wait, she may become just too sick to endure the trials and tribulations of the surgery and the normal stormy postoperative course.

CON: On the other hand, DCD cases are fraught with ethical issues. The procurement process itself means that 4/5 times I get called in for a DCD case, it is cancelled.

I will explain the process to you and you can decide the medical and ethical issues for DCD donation. When it is clear that a patient who is not brain dead, who is usually intubated, and possibly on vasoactive agents (e.g., epinephrine, norepinephrine, vasopressin) will not recover, the family works with the medical team on making a decision to withdraw care. The term "to withdraw care" in a patient who is technically alive puts clinicians and family together on an ethically charged slippery slope. The proper terminology is to "provide comfort care." Anything that makes the patient comfortable such as extubation is considered. It is essential that the surgeons doing the procurement do not introduce themselves as involved with transplant until there is complete agreement with the managing physicians and family to transition over to comfort care. The extubation is done in the operating room, and in some protocols, the use of vasoactive agents is discontinued. Narcotics and benzodiazepines are administered if the patient appears uncomfortable or struggling. Depending upon state or center regulatory rules, heparin may be given to prevent clots forming in organs designated for procurement. It is always hoped that the patient's heart stops shortly after extubation to cut down on the dreaded "warm ischemia" time.

From an organ procurement perspective, the ideal would be to cut down the "warm ischemia" time to zero by immediately flushing the patient with University of Wisconsin solution as soon as he is extubated, replacing the blood with preservative. This action, however, is considered to be a homicide.

The liver is somewhat resilient; therefore, more ischemic time is allowed than would be for, say, the small bowel for a small bowel transplant. The waiting time for the heart to stop is not unlimited. If the heart does not stop after 45 min, the patient is returned to the intensive care unit, and no organ procurement will be performed. Comfort care is continued in the unit.

The organ procurement team is very careful to avoid even the remote chance that this could be a breach of regulatory protocols. As soon has the heart stops, there is a 5 min "no touch" period as autoresuscitation can occur. The warm ischemia time consists of this 5 min plus the time from extubation to asystole (during which the patient who was extubated is alive but may have low oxygen saturation). After the 5 min "no touch" period, a large bore arterial catheter is placed and organs are flushed with University of Wisconsin solution, which both arrests metabolism and preserves the organ to some degree. Cold ischemia time is the time from the University of Wisconsin solution flush until the liver arrives at the destination hospital where it is prepared on ice before it is ready to be sewn in. Under the present rules, there is controversy. The bile duct is very sensitive to any form of ischemia. While it may look pristine when it is being sewn in, months down the line you may find a stricture severe enough that a new liver may be needed.

This is so much more challenging than a simple brain dead donor. Upon unclamping all of the vascular anastomoses, the DCD liver will have a reperfusion injury even if it is a fairly normal liver. I look at the surgical field. A lack of firmness in the liver is a good sign. Firmness in the liver implies that blood flow is meeting resistance. I keep my central venous pressure (CVP) low to allow blood to flow easily through the new liver. I try to minimize vasopressors and use calcium to increase cardiac contractility rather than epinephrine or norepinephrine. Vasopressors will increase resistance to flow. Usually reperfusion hypotension requires at most a few hits of a vasopressor and rarely an infusion.

You can imagine what we must see on reperfusion to a DCD liver that has had an ischemic injury. The liver invariably becomes firmer than baseline and often looks mottled for the first half hour. Much time is spent using a Doppler to assess perfusion of the hepatic artery and portal vein. Because the liver is suboptimal, coagulation is suboptimal. The appearance of bile is very reassuring after reperfusion. We cross our fingers hoping that bile will start to be excreted in a patient with a DCD liver. While I am not sure whether there are data on blood products, in the DCD liver with an ischemic injury we seem to use the same amount of blood products after reperfusion as we do during the anahepatic phase. While everyone is worried about overcorrection and hypercoagulation with the use of fresh frozen plasma (FFP), cryoprecipitate, and prothombin complex concentrates, this seems to be less of a problem in DCD cases. In summary, we sweat these cases out.

CON: The facts are that overall survival rates from DCD donors (71 % at 1 year and 60 % at 3 years) were significantly inferior to those from DBD donors (80 % at 1 year and 70 % at 3 years) [2]. The 2 biggest factors that are responsible for this difference are thermal injury and ischemia.

PRO: While these numbers are almost alarming, the future appears to include more DCD donors as there is so much more availability than DBD donors. Your aunt could die waiting.

CON: Perhaps the possibility of a living related donor could be explored further. I had a case the other day of an 8-kg baby with biliary atresia. The baby was unfortunate because his parents were talked into refusing the Kasai procedure to give him a better chance of receiving a transplant (increasing his MELD score moves him up on the transplant list). It is my understanding that the child is now comatose, and with no correctly sized deceased donors available, his mother has agreed to donate a portion of her liver. Luckily, she is the correct blood type, and sizing measurements are favorable. DBD cases are rare in the pediatric population. Kids just do not face catastrophic injuries or illnesses often enough to make a pool of donors. Receiving a matched living donation from a family member or friend poses a threat to both the donor and recipient. The donor takes the risk that she will not have enough liver left to survive. The recipient takes the risk that despite best preoperative efforts to estimate sizing, the donated lobe will end up being an incorrect size when actual placement is attempted. Anesthesia in these cases is complicated by difficulties in gaining adequate intravenous access and the ever-difficult pediatric arterial line.

Summary

The liver transplant or solid organ transplant program is a huge endeavor that involves countless professionals including hepatologists, transplant surgeons, anesthesiologists, pathologists, coordinators, psychiatrists, cardiologists, social workers, physical therapists, and pulmonologists. With a shortage of organs, there is a strong push to have the strict regulations that go with DCD cases reviewed by both people in the medical field and those outside the field. Some future steps that would allow for advancement would include allowing arterial flush lines in place, mandatory procurement from surgeons who are at the same professional level as those transplanting organs, discovery of essential therapies to lessen reperfusion syndrome, and liberalizing some of the IRB regulations to permit increased clinical research.

References

1. Mateo R, Cho Y, Singh G, Stapfer M, Donovan J, Kahn J, et al. Risk factors for graft survival after liver transplantation from donation after cardiac death donors: an analysis of OPTN/UNOS data. Am J Transplant. 2006;6(4):791–6.
2. Manzarbeitia CY, Ortiz JA, Jeon H, Rothstein KD, Martinez O, Araya VR, et al. Long-term outcome of controlled, non-heart-beating donor liver transplantation. Transplantation. 2004;78(2):211–5.

65 Should Only Patients Who Are Medically Optimized Receive a Liver Transplant?

Corey S. Scher

Case

A 42-year-old with alcohol-induced end-stage liver disease has been listed by United Network Organ Sharing (UNOS) for a liver transplant. His end-stage liver disease resulting in severe cirrhosis is a threat to his life while he is on the waiting list. In short, he is likely to die waiting. His Model for End-Stage Liver Disease (MELD) score is 35.

A consult note to his private medical doctor by the multiple members of a liver transplant section included the following: "The end-stage of liver damage is cirrhosis. Cirrhosis frequently shows up insidiously with minor laboratory abnormalities, such as slight thrombocytopenia or mild increases in aspartate aminotransferase. Imaging and percutaneous liver biopsy confirm the diagnosis. Ideal management involves treatment for alcoholism; management of ascites, variceal bleeding, and encephalopathy; regular screening for hepatocellular carcinoma; treatment of infections; immunization; and attention to nutrition and general health. Effective treatment is focused on the cause, which may stop disease progression, stabilize function of the liver, and abolish or postpone the need for liver transplant."

Of note, the consult specifically states that "sobriety, while important, is not a must."

Question

Is it right for this patient to receive a liver transplant if he has not achieved sobriety?

CON: No. It seems to make sense that a patient who carries a diagnosis of substance abuse, particularly an alcoholic, must have embraced sobriety by having gone through a well-respected program and must be sober for 6 months. Zero alcohol ingestion, along with perfect compliance with antirejection medications, is needed to give the liver the best long-term success. I know it is ethically charged, but the information we have seems to indicate that the most successful treatment for alcoholism is sobriety.

PRO: Any addiction treatment is marked by short moments of success and long moments of relapse. If he embraces treatment, the success rate is excellent and if he does not, the success rate is low. The treatment of the chronic disease of addiction does not end with a liver transplant but is a separate medical problem that requires years of treatment. If the patient buys into addiction treatment, it is ongoing for the rest of his life. Why draw a line in the sand for sobriety when it can be dealt with after transplant or while he is waiting on the liver transplant list? Six months of sobriety means only 6 months of sobriety. In reality, the transplant and sobriety are really two separate issues that should not be lumped into one. True, his lack of sobriety may be looked at by regulatory agencies and make him move down the liver transplant waiting list, but it shouldn't mean that he can't be listed at all.

CON: Donated livers vary greatly in quality. There are several ways of categorizing donors. The cadaveric donor is simply brain dead, but liver perfusion is not compromised. The second type is donation after cardiac death, which is ethically charged as this involves patients who are not brain dead but will die and are not conscious. They are taken to the operating room and are extubated. Time from extubation is recorded and when and if there is asystole, the liver is procured after an additional 5 min "no touch" period. In these cases, the liver to be donated may have been ischemic for more time than it can tolerate. Many centers do not do this type of procurement as the outcome of the transplant may be compromised. I believe he would be offered a "donation after cardiac death" liver before a "donation after brain death" liver. The third type of donation is a part of a liver from a healthy person to the recipient. While the recipient's

C.S. Scher (✉)
Department of Anesthesiology, Perioperative Care and Pain Medicine, New York University School of Medicine, New York, NY 10016, USA
e-mail: coreyscher@gmail.com

C.S. Scher et al. (eds.), *You're Wrong, I'm Right*, DOI 10.1007/978-3-319-43169-7_65

MELD score determines, for the most part, where they are on the list, the alcoholic should not receive the perfect donor.

PRO: With proper care, this patient may have many good years ahead of him [1].

Improvement strategies include the following:

1. Create a network of family and friends who will help and encourage the patient to attend appointments and comply with treatment.
2. Evaluate cardiac function and the presence of pericardial and pleural fluid. In a patient with liver disease, the heart will not tolerate stress as well. Perform an echocardiogram and stress test.
3. Treat portal hypertension. If untreated, this condition leads to esophageal varices, ascites, and intestinal bleeding. Consider accomplishing this with a TIPS procedure (transjugular intrahepatic portosystemic shunt). This is a synthetic conduit within the liver connecting the inflow portal vein and the outflow hepatic vein.
4. Electrolytes—mental fuzziness can be caused by hyponatremia, and this can be treated with vasopressin antagonists.
5. Band esophageal varices.
6. Pulmonary hypertension can keep someone off of the transplant list. Stated simply, in a patient with a pulmonary artery pressure greater than 60, the liver will swell with reperfusion during the transplant, severely compromising transplant success. Sildenafil can be started, sometimes decreasing pulmonary hypertension enough to qualify the patient for the transplant list.
7. Evaluate for intrapulmonary shunt. This involves the deoxygenated blood from the right heart bypassing gas exchange before returning to the left heart.
8. Hepatorenal syndrome—This involves kidney dysfunction in patients with liver failure, and patients may eventually receive a combined kidney–liver transplant. It is characterized by severe vasoconstriction in the kidneys, as well as splanchnic vasodilatation. Treatment is terlipressin, a vasopressin analogue, which constricts the splanchnic bed to squeeze the blood into the renal vascular bed. It works in a small subset of patients, but most patients eventually return to their baseline hepatorenal state and require dialysis. The exact cause in patients with severe liver disease is unknown. Even if a combined liver–kidney transplant is needed, having some kidney function is beneficial and also helps to decrease the inevitable hyperkalemia that occurs during transplant from packed red blood cell transfusion.
9. Encephalopathy—This is due to hyperammonemia, although the exact mechanism is unclear. Antibiotics serve to cut down on bowel flora and thus blood ammonia levels. Lactulose also helps to decrease bowel flora by increasing motility. Encephalopathy ranges from mild cognitive changes to frank coma. Surgeons and hepatologists would be reluctant to transplant a patient in a coma.
10. Anemia—from bleeding varices, low platelet counts from portal hypertension, and generalized marrow suppression. Chronic anemia should be treated with either stimulants of the bone marrow or blood transfusion so that patients enter the operating room with maximal oxygen delivery to tissues [1].

CON: I do not think that optimization is always the right thing. I once took care of a baby who had biliary atresia. The therapeutic option was a Kasai procedure, which is when bowel is sewn to the porta hepatis. This allows bile to drain, jaundice to disappear, and nutritional status to be optimized. If the child gains enough weight, the child can receive a transplant from a donation by one of the parents. Recurrent cholangitis, unfortunately, can occur as an ongoing process in these patients.

I do remember a family who refused the Kasai with the mindset being as the child gets sicker, he or she would move up quickly on the transplant list. The fact is that there is a tremendous shortage of child donors and the parents may not have the anatomy and circulation status to permit donation of their own livers. In this case, the child grew sicker and did move up the list. By the time he was first on the list, he was close to death as neither parent could donate. When the child was brought to the operating room for a transplant, he had a cardiac arrest on induction. CPR was successful and the child's transplant proceeded without incident. The parents took a huge risk and succeeded by getting a transplant significantly earlier than if he had the Kasai. They were victorious by the skin of their teeth.

In adults, there have also been documented cases of patients who deliberately withdrew optimization in favor of moving up the list. With an enormous shortage of donor organs, it makes sense to get somewhat sicker to have access to a liver quicker. The list is a slippery slope and sometimes a fictitious MELD score is reported, especially when surgeons are incentivized to perform surgery. While the United Network Organ Sharing guidelines are strict, they are not always followed.

PRO: I believe that optimization should occur. In 2011, the US Food and Drug Administration (FDA) approved for the first time direct-acting antivirals (DAAs) for the treatment of hepatitis C. DAAs, including protease inhibitors, block enzymes that the hepatitis C virus uses to multiply [2]. More options have been approved since then. The genotype of the virus will determine for which combination of drugs the patient is eligible. By the time the patient has cirrhosis, the patient may have no detectable virus but the complications of cirrhosis remain. The new liver may thrive, but the effects of the end-stage cirrhotic state will remain and transplant will be needed; these medications are very expensive and not readily available to the underserved population.

Summary

Refusing optimization treatment for end-stage liver disease may make a patient move up on the liver transplant list; however, he or she could easily die from concurrent complications such as bleeding. Optimization allows, in the long run, a healthier patient for this high-risk case. Refusing treatment in order to move up the list is dangerous if not irresponsible as a patient increases his or her chances of becoming de-listed from becoming too ill to endure the transplant. I do not think a patient or parent of a child should even be offered the option of not being optimized.

References

1. Schiano TD, Bourgoise T, Rhodes R. High risk liver transplant candidates: an ethical proposal on where to draw the line. Liver Transplant. 2015;21(5):607–11.
2. Webster DP, Klenerman P, Dusheiko GM. Hepatitis C. Lancet. 2015;385(9973):1124–35.

Is the Model for End-Stage Liver Disease (MELD) Score the Best Way to Evaluate Liver Transplant Patients Preoperatively?

66

Benjamin Heller and Jeron Zerillo

Case

A 52-year-old male with a past medical history of hepatitis C cirrhosis, hypertension, hyperlipidemia, and a body mass index of 34 presents for deceased donor liver transplantation. He has been on the liver transplant list for 6 months. His international normalized ratio (INR) is 2.1, creatinine is 1.6, and total bilirubin is 8.4, and he has never undergone renal replacement therapy. As a result, his preoperative Model for End-Stage Liver Disease (MELD) score is 27. In the holding area, he responds appropriately to most questions, although his wife reports that he has seemed more confused in the past 2 days. On physical exam, you note that the patient is diffusely jaundiced, has spider angiomas, and has marked ascites.

Your resident, who has done a thorough history and physical, asks you whether this patient is sick enough to appropriately utilize such a precious resource.

Question

Is the MELD score the best way to evaluate liver transplant patients preoperatively?

PRO: This patient can best be evaluated for a liver transplant by utilizing the MELD score, which was originally created to predict survival in patients with portal hypertension undergoing transjugular intrahepatic portosystemic shunt [1]. However, it has since been adopted by the United Network of Organ Sharing (UNOS) to prioritize patients for liver transplantation. The MELD system utilizes objective measures, thereby decreasing the likelihood of skewing organ allocation inappropriately by the use of subjective criteria. With historic allocation systems that utilized subjective measures, practitioners could claim that patients were encephalopathic when they were not. MELD scoring, on the other hand, emphasizes 3 of the most important criteria in disease severity for cirrhotics and provides an objective value that can be compared against other patients with end-stage liver disease. It is calculated using the following formula:

$$\begin{aligned}\text{MELD} = 9.57 \times \text{Log}_e(\text{creatinine}) + 3.78 \\ \times \text{Log}_e(\text{total bilirubin}) + 11.2 \\ \times \text{Log}_e(\text{INR}) + 6.43.\end{aligned}$$

The following apply to MELD scoring:

- UNOS has set the lower limit of creatinine, INR, and bilirubin at 1, so there are no negative values.
- UNOS has capped the upper limit of creatinine at 4. Additionally, if a patient has received hemodialysis twice in the previous 7 days, he/she is scored with this value whatever the creatinine level.
- Scores range from 6 to 40 and are used to predict 3-month mortality, while the patient is on the wait list [2].

CON: While the MELD score has been used for allocation since 2002 [1], it is not without its limitations. Although widely used as a predictor of survival, even its creators admit that the survival of 15–20 % of patients cannot be accurately predicted by this scoring system [1]. Furthermore, while the MELD score can accurately predict mortality for patients on the liver transplant waiting list, it has not been found to accurately predict mortality after liver transplant, likely due to a variety of factors such as donor characteristics,

B. Heller
Department of Anesthesiology, Icahn School of Medicine at Mount Sinai, 1 Gustave L. Levy Place, New York, NY 10029, USA
e-mail: Benjamin.Heller@mountsinai.org

J. Zerillo (✉)
Department of Anesthesiology, Division of Liver Transplantation, Icahn School of Medicine at Mount Sinai, 1 Gustave L. Levy Place, 8th Floor, New York, NY 10029, USA
e-mail: Jeron.zerillo@mountsinai.org

C.S. Scher et al. (eds.), *You're Wrong, I'm Right*, DOI 10.1007/978-3-319-43169-7_66

experience of the surgeons and anesthesiologists [3], and unanticipated postoperative complications [1].

PRO: Prior to the MELD score, the Child-Turcotte-Pugh (CTP) score was used to assess patients undergoing liver transplantation. This scoring system has 5 categories: total bilirubin, serum albumin, prothrombin time (PT) (or INR), ascites, and hepatic encephalopathy (Table 66.1) [4]. Each category is assigned a value from 1 to 3, with 3 being the most severe for a maximum score of 15 [4]. Many clinicians consider the subjective categories of ascites and hepatic encephalopathy, combined with an absence of evaluation of renal function, to be the major drawbacks of this scoring system.

Most studies have indicated that the MELD score has yielded results superior to the Child-Turcotte-Pugh score in predicting patients' risk of mortality [1]. Furthermore, renal function is an established marker of prognosis in patients with cirrhosis [5], and the CTP score lacks these data. The new MELD system has eliminated waiting time as a criterion for transplant [5]. This allows sicker patients, once listed, to be considered earlier for transplantation, which helps to maximize justice, one of the main values of modern-day medical ethics.

CON: The MELD score cannot predict post-liver transplant survival [5]. If the purpose of liver transplantation is long-term survival, then the scoring system should ideally reflect postoperative survival as well. This would help to ensure the best possible use of a scarce resource. Part of maximizing justice is making sure that organs do not go to waste; therefore, postoperative survival should be considered. In the future, donor characteristics may be weighed more heavily, as the relationship between donor and recipient is of paramount importance. Additionally, since sarcopenia has recently been demonstrated to be an independent risk factor for wait-list mortality, its incorporation into organ allocation systems may improve organ matching [6].

PRO: With any system, unanticipated events peri- and postoperatively can affect the success of liver transplantation even in the best of candidates. There is no way to predict the future and to expect any preoperative scoring system to do so is unrealistic. What the MELD system does is quantify how sick patients are preoperatively. While the CTP system does the same thing, it is less objective and more user dependent. The MELD score creates a uniform, objective scoring system that can equally risk-stratify a patient in a small, local hospital in rural Wisconsin as well as in a large tertiary care center in New York City. When the MELD system was adopted for organ allocation, the average MELD at time of transplantation increased from 18.5 to 24.1, with the first decrease in wait-list mortality/patient removal for extreme illness since the inception of the list [2].

CON: Exceptions to the MELD system are becoming increasingly common. Patients with hepatocellular carcinoma (HCC) do not inherently have high MELD scores, but given certain criteria can benefit greatly from liver transplantation [2]. These patients may be granted "exception" points to their MELD score (such that their minimal starting MELD is 22, and then 3 points may be added every 3 months to account for potential tumor progression), increasing their likelihood of receiving a transplant. These HCC exceptions do not maximize the benefit of transplants, as life-years gained after transplant in these patients is less, since they likely would have survived longer than their non-exception equally MELD scored counterparts [2].

PRO: This is an issue that, at present, is widely debated. The addition of exception points for HCC patients is currently under review and may change in the near future, with proposals that include capping this patient population at 34 points [7], a level that would preclude them from taking part in the Share 35 liver region sharing program.

CON: Furthermore, patients that are candidates for re-transplantation are given a MELD score, which can be misleading. Studies have shown that patients undergoing

Table 66.1 The Child-Turcotte-Pugh (CTP) score to assess patients undergoing liver transplantation

	Total Bilirubin (mg/dl)	Serum Albumin (g/dl)	INR	Ascites	Hepatic encephalopathy
1 point	<2	>3.5	<1.7	None	None
2 points	2–3	2.8–3.5	1.7–2.3	Mild	Grade I–II
3 points	>3	<2.8	>2.3	Moderate to Severe	Grade III–IV

INR international normalized ratio

re-transplantation have a worse prognosis than those undergoing primary procedures [5]. Even for patients with the same MELD score, studies have shown survival was significantly lower for those undergoing re-transplantation than for primary transplant patients [8].

Summary

MELD-based scoring is the best available system because it has improved organ allocation since its implementation [9]. The patient in this vignette demonstrates the stigmata of end-stage liver disease such as ascites and hepatic encephalopathy, which is not unusual for those who present for liver transplantation. The answer to the resident about whether the patient is sick enough to appropriately utilize such a precious resource is that according to the objective qualifications outlined in the MELD score, he is.

While the MELD system is our best means of allocating liver grafts, it should remain constantly under review to maximize justice and optimize patient outcomes as our understanding of perioperative risk factors improves. Regardless of the scoring system used, we must continue to improve our ability to match organs to those patients who will benefit most, which may result in transplantation of increasingly sicker patients. As a result, communication with the surgeon and the transplant team is essential, and extreme intraoperative vigilance is a necessity. Ultimately, the anesthesiologist can play a critical role in the success of these surgeries, regardless of the scoring system utilized [3].

References

1. Kamath PS, Kim WR. The model for end-stage liver disease (MELD). Hepatology. 2007;45(3):797–808.
2. Wagener G, editor. Liver anesthesiology and critical care medicine. New York, NY: Springer; 2013. p. 48–81.
3. Hofer I, Spivak J, Yaport M, Zerillo J, Reich DL, Wax D, DeMaria S Jr. Association between anesthesiologist experience and mortality after orthotopic liver transplantation. Liver Transpl. 2015;21:89–95.
4. Pugh RNH, Murray-Lyon IM, Dawson JL, Pietroni MC, Williams R. Transection of the oesophagus for bleeding oesophageal varices. Br J Surg. 1973;60(8):646–9.
5. Cholongitas E, Marelli L, Shusang V, Senzolo M, Rolles K, Patch D, Burroughs AK. A systematic review of the performance of the model for end-stage liver disease (MELD) in the setting of liver transplantation. Liver Transpl. 2006;12:1049–61.
6. Tandon P, Ney M, Irwin I, Ma MM, Gramlich L, Bain VG, et al. Severe muscle depletion in patients on the liver transplant wait list: its prevalence and independent prognostic value. Liver Transpl. 2012;18:1209–16.
7. Organ Procurement and Transplant Network. At-a-Glance: Proposal to Cap the HCC Exception Score at 34.: US Department of Health & Human Services. http://optn.transplant.hrsa.gov/PublicComment/pubcommentPropSub_330.pdf. Published March 14, 2014. Accessed 3 Nov 2015.
8. Watt K, Lyden E, McCashland T. Poor survival after liver retranplantation: is hepatitis C to blame? Liver Transpl. 2003;9:1019–24.
9. Coombes J, Trotter JF. Development of the allocation system for deceased donor liver transplantation. Clin Med Res. 2005;3:87–92.

A Small Bowel Transplant for a Patient with Scleroderma: Once Again on the Slippery Slope Both Clinically and Ethically

67

Corey S. Scher

Case

A 55-year-old gentleman with a 30-year history of diffuse scleroderma presents for a small bowel transplant. His rapidly progressive autoimmune disease includes his entire gastrointestinal tract, liver, lungs, skin, and joints. He is brought to the holding area, and the chart includes the following preoperative assessment by organ system:

1. Raynaud's phenomenon: This is the presenting symptom in 70 % of scleroderma patients and occurs in 95 % at some time during their illness: pitting ulcers on the fingertips including skin and mucosal telangiectasia.
2. Cardiovascular: dysrhythmias and syncope due to conduction abnormalities, hypertension, and congestive heart failure (CHF).
3. Digestive: gastro-esophageal reflux disease, bloating, indigestion, loss of appetite, diarrhea alternating with constipation, sicca syndrome, and its complications, loosening of teeth and hoarseness due to acid reflux.
4. Pulmonary: progressively worsening shortness of breath, chest pain caused by pulmonary hypertension, and dry persistent cough due to interstitial lung disease.
5. Musculoskeletal: joint and muscle aches, loss of range of motion, carpal tunnel syndrome, and muscle weakness.
6. Genitourinary: scleroderma renal crises and kidney failure.
7. Other: facial pain due to trigeminal neuralgia, hand paresthesias, headache, stroke, fatigue, calcinosis, and weight loss.

His evaluation includes:

- Abdominal computed tomography (CT) scan
- Barium enema
- Blood tests for liver function, electrolytes, kidney function, and antibodies to certain viruses
- Colonoscopy
- Electrocardiogram (ECG) and echocardiogram
- Endoscopy
- Motility studies
- Ultrasound of the circulatory system
- Upper gastrointestinal and small bowel X-ray series

Additional test results include:

1. Pulmonary function tests indicated less than 50 % of predicted in all values.
2. Chest X-ray revealed significant cardiomegaly and decreased pulmonary markings.
3. Increased values on liver function tests, reflecting invasion of the liver by scleroderma along with total parenteral nutrition induced cirrhosis.
4. Upper endoscopy revealed a "hard, tube-like structure with no sphincters."
5. Double balloon enteroscopy revealed a rock-solid small bowel with a paucity of normal villi.
6. Anemia.
7. Glomerular flow rate 20 % of predicted.

On examination, he was unable to breathe through his nose and showed an extremely limited mouth opening of 1–2 finger breadths. His skin was hard as stone, and he held a tissue over his mouth as bile continuously poured out. His only intravenous access was a peripherally inserted central catheter (PICC) line near his right axilla that was dedicated to total parenteral nutrition (TPN) and did not run spontaneously. ENT and the cardiopulmonary pump team were notified about the potential for a lost airway.

PRO: The patient is here and we must move forward. It is what it is, a situation where it is almost impossible to avoid

C.S. Scher (✉)
Department of Anesthesiology, Perioperative Care and Pain Medicine, New York University School of Medicine, New York, NY 10016, USA
e-mail: coreyscher@gmail.com

C.S. Scher et al. (eds.), *You're Wrong, I'm Right*, DOI 10.1007/978-3-319-43169-7_67

complications related to anesthesia and obviously to the transplant surgery.

CON: This procedure should not be done. His pulmonary function and renal status make his 6-month survival quite limited. Is there a backup recipient in the hospital so that his organ does not go to waste? We are not helping this patient. We are only going to speed up his dying process and make him even more miserable, if that is possible.

PRO: The surgeons are ready to move forward with this case and, unlike the extensive list of patients waiting for a liver transplant, there are not many patients who are eligible for this small bowel.

CON: I cannot imagine intubating him without serious aspiration.

PRO: It is unlikely that we will be able to topicalize him for an awake intubation. Nebulized lidocaine or spraying-as-you-go are 2 approaches that will not work. I would like to give him small incremental doses of ketamine and see how far that takes us. We will start out by giving 0.2 mg of glycopyrrolate to dry him out.

CON: Dry him out? He has a river of bile that continuously flows from his bowel to his mouth. That is why glycopyrrolate and spray-as-you-go will not work. Blocking the recurrent laryngeal and the internal branch of the superior laryngeal nerves and the back of the throat cannot be attempted as we cannot feel his cricoid cartilage or hyoid bone. And his small mouth opening prohibits gargling with viscous lidocaine. ENT thinks that an awake tracheostomy is needed with cardiac surgery backup because of the possible need for a sternotomy. How did we get into this?

PRO: I am going to do the ketamine thing and hope for the best. It is a no-win situation. I was in many no-win situations in Iraq and many did work out.

CON: Will you allow the resident to do the fiberoptic or will you just take it yourself and get it over with one way or another?

PRO: The resident gets first crack as he is excellent with the scope. We will pre-oxygenate for 5 min through his mouth as his nose is blocked. Then I will count to 10. If the resident is not close, we will pre-oxygenate again. We will give ketamine in 20 mg increments and start when 80 mg are in.

CON: How can you let a resident do this? If there was ever one for an attending this is it.

PRO: I am sorry, but I have to start this case and I am going to do it the way I want. Let's bring him to the operating room (OR) and start by putting monitors on. We are going straight to the right internal jugular with the ultrasound. If visualization is good, we will double-stick the neck and place 1 wire for a triple lumen and 1 for a 9.0 French introducer. As with many patients with autoimmune diseases, he may be hypercoaguable and we may not see any viable vessels.

CON: You are better off sticking him with the long large-bore needle as the angiocath in the kit may not be strong enough for his widespread sclerosis. The downside is that the neck may be like a rock, and if you insert a wire in the neck, then you have to confirm the wire is properly placed, which requires you to insert the angiocath over the wire, pull the wire out, and then hook up IV tubing for manometry to see the venous tracing before placing the actual venous catheter. You will also need to place an arterial line. The more steps you take the more chances for infection or worse, a mistake.

PRO: The double stick was easy but dilating required so much more force than I would normally apply that it made me feel nervous. We will use the triple lumen for drugs and the introducer for volume. Actually, before we deal with the airway, let's stick the left neck for another introducer.

CON: You have a bad case of being overconfident if not crazy!

PRO: Here is the plan. Let's give him 2 mg of midazolam to offset possible hallucinations from the ketamine. I will titrate the ketamine to be able to pry the mouth open to fit an Ovassapian airway. If he does not tolerate the airway, I will titrate 20 mg at a time until he does. I will use the airway to place an orogastric tube so I can get whatever I can out of his gastrointestinal tract. I do not look at this as a full stomach but rather an entire GI tract that has no sphincters or barriers [1].

CON: There is over a liter of bilious fluid coming out. You better leave that tube in on suction during the intubation. I am starting to shake watching your resident pick up the fiberoptic scope.

PRO: After 20 more milligrams of ketamine, I am pleasantly shocked as it took the resident 30 s to intubate. I need to take the scope for myself and examine as much of the lung for bile as possible.

CON: It will be hard to tell if the bile that you see is the result of aspiration that just happened during the intubation or nothing more than his ongoing daily aspiration of bile. Does it even matter if he is oxygenating well?

PRO: The paper on "The Strategy of Mechanical Ventilation in ARDS: 2012 Update" (from ARDSNET.org) strongly implies that early employment of low-volume ventilation in patients at risk protects a significant number of them from contracting acute respiratory distress syndrome (ARDS). There was close to a 10 % reduction in ARDS-related mortality. This patient is at high risk for ARDS and my sense is that both acute and chronic bilious aspiration is what is going on. We will bring the tidal volumes down to 6–8 ml/kg ideal body weight.

CON: This patient will become wildly atelectatic at 6 ml/kg ventilation, with an increase of pulmonary vascular resistance and inevitable hypoxia. He will need many recruitment breaths to make a dent in the respiratory acidosis that will evolve. I would not pick this patient for your "clinical trial." I would volume-control ventilate the patient with a pressure limit of 25. That dose could be similar to the 6–8 cc ARDSNET recommendation [2]. The key to survival if the surgical technique is well done will be related to complications of immunosuppression. Iatrogenic atelectasis with potent immunosuppressants is a setup for life-threatening pneumonia. These patients do poorly without an immune system, and your ARDSNET ventilation is not seeing the big picture here.

PRO: There are several big ticket items that must addressed, namely blood product administration, monitoring for clot stability, and avoidance of reperfusion injury to preserve the new graft. The components of reperfusion injury and attempts to control it in liver transplantation are clearer than in the small bowel. We do take the big leap and view the pathophysiology similarly.

In essence, reperfusion of the graft leads to a massive inflammatory response and disturbance of the microcirculation in the new small bowel. The cause is multifactorial, but both warm and cold ischemic times are certainly factors. If the reperfusion injury is massive, the newly created vascular grafts could clot, compromising viability. In liver transplantation, unclamping of new vascular grafts often leads to severe hypotension, requiring a short course of vasopressors. Inflammatory mediators are vasodilators, and the loss of nitric oxide is the main player in unstable vital signs. A similar but less profound hemodynamic response occurs with reperfusion of a small bowel graft. Gut flow is severely compromised by vasopressors, and they are given as a last resort.

CON: In summary, we are going to spend hours and dollars on a man who might make it through the surgery but will present on postop day one with 1 or all of 3 possible clinical scenarios that act like the same thing: (1) acute rejection, (2) inflammatory or iatrogenic bowel perforation, and (3) clots in the microcirculation or the major vascular anastomoses. It is likely that you will be giving anesthesia again within hours of the end of the initial case.

PRO: Once we go back to the OR, we may not find any of the aforementioned possibilities and we are then stuck with hemodynamic instability and a rising lactate. The old saying is that the longer you are on the ventilator the longer you will remain on the ventilator. The anesthesiologists and surgeons often have only 1 shot at this and you are right that take backs to the OR increase the chance of his demise.

Fast Forward to Postop Day #3

CON: The patient has now gone back to the OR 3 times for anastomotic leaks, vascular compromise, and an exploration solely based on rising lactate. He is now on a norepinephrine infusion. His arterial blood gases (ABGs) and chest X-ray (CXR) are consistent with ARDS. He has already received 40 units of packed red blood cells (PRBCs) and 55 units of fresh frozen plasma (FFP) with multiple rounds of platelets. He is dying [3].

PRO: The survival rate in high-volume small bowel transplant centers is almost 80 % at the end of the first year with morbidity and mortality most often related to severe immunosuppression; we just have to have him turn around.

CON: Look at the big picture here. He cannot survive. We should provide comfort care or, in more frank although improper terminology "withdraw care."

Summary

This is an ethically charged case as the patient's lung function is poor, his kidney and liver are compromised, and his "new" small bowel will lack normal motility. He might have been a better candidate months ago when his systemic sclerosis was not that bad. The anesthesiologist should have made a more forceful appeal for the involvement of an ethics consult as he knew from the beginning he was providing care that would hasten the patient's death.

References

1. Llanos JC, Ruiz P, Takahashi H, Delacruz V, Bakonyi Neto A. Outcome of pigs with short gut syndrome submitted to orthotopic intestinal transplantation. Acta Cir Bras. 2015;30:143–50.
2. Davies SW, Leonard KL, Falls RK Jr, Mageau RP, Efird JT, Hollowell JP, et al. Lung protective ventilation (ARDSNet) versus airway pressure release ventilation: ventilatory management in a combined model of acute lung and brain injury. J Trauma Acute Care Surg. 2015;78(2):240–51.
3. van Dijk G, Hilhorst M, Rings E. Liver, pancreas and small bowel transplantation: current ethical issues. Best Pract Res Clin Gastroenterol. 2014;28(2):281–92.

Part VIII
Critical Care

Should Steroids Be Used in Septic Shock?

68

Samion Shabashev

Case

You are rounding on an elderly woman in the intensive care unit (ICU) when John, one of your residents, presents a case.

"This is a 76-year-old female with a past medical history of type 2 diabetes who presented to the emergency department with a 3-day history of fever, chills, dysuria, flank pain, and altered mental status," John says. "Upon admission her vitals were: temperature 39.5 °C, heart rate 126, blood pressure 70/42, and respiration of 20 breaths per minute, and oxygen saturation of 99 % on 4 L nasal cannula. On physical exam she is an ill-appearing elderly women with an altered mental status, who appears dehydrated and is warm to the touch. Lab work is significant for white blood count of 17,000 mg/dL with predominant polymorphonuclear neutrophils shift, hemoglobin and hematocrit are 15 g/dL and 44 %, and chemistry panel with elevated BUN/Creatinine levels of 50 and 2.2 mg/dL, respectively. The urinalysis is consistent with a urinary tract infection. The patient was given 2 L of lactated Ringer's in the emergency room with minimal improvement in blood pressure. She was subsequently started on broad-spectrum antibiotics, a norepinephrine infusion, and admitted to the intensive care unit."

John then continues his assessment and plan for the patient. "Since the patient presented with signs and symptoms that fulfill the systemic inflammatory response syndrome (SIRS) criteria and the patient is hemodynamically unstable requiring vasopressor support for acute circulatory collapse secondary to the infection, I believe this patient is in septic shock."

John says, "My management for this patient is to continue with broad-spectrum antibiotics and then narrow down the antibiotics once culture sensitivities come back. I will continue with crystalloid fluid resuscitation as needed, and continue with a norepinephrine drip for blood pressure support until we can start weaning it down."

Question

At this point, Peter, another resident, intervenes to ask a question. "Since sepsis is driven by a systemic inflammatory response in which production of inflammatory cytokines plays a large role, wouldn't it make sense to give this patient a steroid to help reduce her inflammatory response?"

CON: John replies, with only the slightest hint of eye roll, "Steroids are anti-inflammatory drugs that modulate gene expression for suppressing the immune system response. This effect might decrease the effectiveness of immune system's response against microbial infections. Corticosteroids can also mask some symptoms of infection and can potentially lead to superimposed infections in this patient."

PRO: Peter replies patiently, "Yes, John, but recently there has been data that demonstrated that low-dose hydrocortisone treatment in patients with septic shock have improved hemodynamic parameters, inhibited systemic inflammation, and prevented overwhelming compensatory anti-inflammatory response, and maintained Th1-related immune responsiveness" [1].

CON: "On the contrary!" exclaims John, "the CORTICUS trial (a multicenter, prospective randomized, double-blind, placebo-controlled trial) showed that there was no significant difference in 28-day mortality between those treated with placebo (36 %) and those who received hydrocortisone (39.2 %) (with $P = 0.069$). There was also no significant difference in either hospital or ICU mortality in this study (31.5 % placebo vs 34.3 % hydrocortisone, $P = 0.51$). The hydrocortisone group also had more episodes of superinfection, including new sepsis and septic shock" [2].

S. Shabashev (✉)
Department of Anesthesia, New York University Langone Medical Center, 333 East 38th Street, New York, NY 10016, USA
e-mail: Samion.Shabashev@nyumc.org

C.S. Scher et al. (eds.), *You're Wrong, I'm Right*, DOI 10.1007/978-3-319-43169-7_68

PRO: Peter continues to keep his cool as he proceeds with his point of view. "Despite this information, there have still been various studies that have shown a decrease in the time necessary to reverse septic shock with the use of low-dose steroids. In fact, in that same CORTICUS study, they demonstrated significantly shorter times to reversal of shock in the group treated with hydrocortisone as compared to the placebo group (3.3 vs 5.8 days with $P < 0.001$)" [2].

CON: "I don't know about you, Peter," says John, "but I just don't feel comfortable giving my patient medication that has so much controversy as to its efficacy. From what I've read there is still controversy on how effective steroids are in septic shock. In addition, from all the main studies that I've read, the treatment with steroids did not modify the duration of shock and the mortality of septic shock enough to convince me to start using them in this patient" [3].

PRO: Peter once again replies patiently, "I agree, John, there is no evidence to use steroids in EVERY patient with SIRS criteria or sepsis. However, there is a plethora of research that supports the hypothesis that it would be appropriate to reserve low-dose steroid therapy for patients with septic shock whose blood pressure is poorly responsive to aggressive fluid and vasopressor therapy alone, as in this patient."

CON: "Can you give me an example?" asks John.

PRO: After a moment of thought, Peter then proceeds with an answer. "Well, according to one paper I read, the use of low-dose corticosteroids in septic patients restores cardiovascular homeostasis, terminates systemic and tissue inflammation, restores organ function, and prevents death [4]. According to the author, corticosteroids should be initiated only in patients with sepsis who require 0.5 μ(mu) g/kg/min or more of norepinephrine and should be continued for 5–7 days except in patients with poor hemodynamic response after 2 days" [4].

Summary

The Final Verdict

The use of corticosteroids in septic patients has been a controversial subject for many years. Originally, a short course of high-dose corticosteroids (>300 mg hydrocortisone daily) was tried. However, subsequent studies showed no benefit from this regimen and actually demonstrated an increased mortality due to increased superinfection-related deaths. This in turn led to a Grade-A recommendation by the Surviving Sepsis Campaign (SSC) guidelines *against* the use of high-dose corticosteroids [5]. Thereafter, some experts began to use the adrenocorticotropic hormone (ACTH) stimulation test to identify subpopulations of "responders" and then discontinue steroid therapy in these patients. However, this approach has also been shown to be ineffective due to the inability to accurately distinctly indentify between responders and nonresponders. Thus, the most recent SSC guidelines discourage using the ACTH stimulation test to identify the subset of adults with septic shock who should receive hydrocortisone (Grade-2B recommendation) [6]. This brings us to the most contemporary role of steroids in septic patients. More recently, studies that used lower doses of hydrocortisone for longer durations have shown promising results in certain subsets of septic patients [2]. In patients with septic shock that are unresponsive to IV fluid resuscitation and vasopressors, the addition of low-dose corticosteroids (hydrocortisone 200 mg/daily, for 7 days) has been shown to be safe, is associated with lower mortality, and leads to improved rates of shock reversal, ultimately to a decreased ICU length of stay.

References

1. Keh D, Boehnke T, Weber-Cartens S, Schulz C, Ahlers O, Bercker S, et al. Immunologic and hemodynamic effects of "low-dose" hydrocortisone in septic shock. Am J Respir Crit Care Med. 2003;167(4):512–20.
2. Sprung CL, Annane D, Keh D, Moreno R, Singer M, Freivogel K, CORTICUS Study Group, et al. Hydrocortisone therapy in patients with septic shock. N Engl J Med. 2008;358(2):111–24.
3. Raurich JM, Llompart-Pou JA, Ibáñez J, Frontera G, Pérez O, García L, et al. Low-dose steroid therapy does not affect hemodynamic response in septic shock patients. J Crit Care. 2007; 22(4):324–9.
4. Annane D. Corticosteroids for severe sepsis: an evidence-based guide for physicians. Ann Intensive Care. 2011;1(1):7.
5. Dellinger RP, Carlet JM, Masur H, Gerlach H, Calandra T, Cohen J, Surviving Sepsis Campaign Management Guidelines Committee, et al. Surviving sepsis campaign guidelines for management of severe sepsis and septic shock. Crit Care Med. 2004;32(3):858–73.
6. Dellinger RP, Levy MM, Rhodes A, Annane D, Gerlach H, Opal SM, Surviving Sepsis Campaign Guidelines Committee including the Pediatric Subgroup, et al. Surviving sepsis campaign: international guidelines for management of severe sepsis and septic shock: 2012. Crit Care Med. 2013;41(2):580–637.

69 Should Extracorporeal Membrane Oxygenation Be Used for the Early Treatment of Acute Respiratory Distress Syndrome?

Melissa M. Anastacio and Scott A. Falk

Case

A 48-year-old African American man with a medical history notable for asthma, chronic obstructive pulmonary disease (COPD), and active tobacco use presented to his primary care physician (PCP) with a 5-day history of progressive shortness of breath, productive cough, generalized malaise, and body aches. He traveled to Florida 1 week prior to presentation and was exposed to "moldy" water due to flooding of his basement the preceding week. He denied any recent sick contacts. At his PCP's office, his room air oxygen saturation was 78 %.

A chest radiograph (Fig. 69.1a) taken in the emergency department demonstrated a right middle lobe opacity concerning for community-acquired pneumonia. He was admitted, placed on supplemental oxygen, and treated with levofloxacin.

Over a 5-day period, hypoxemia worsened with escalation of noninvasive (CPAP with FiO_2 100 %, inhaled epoprostanol) to invasive ventilation (bilevel, 100 % FiO_2, tidal volume of 450, high/low PEEP of 30/0, and pressure support of 13 with a PaO_2:FiO_2 ratio of 78). Chest radiographs (Fig. 69.1b, c) showed progressive development of diffuse ground glass opacities confirmed by a chest computed tomography (CT) scan (Fig. 69.2), all concerning for acute respiratory distress syndrome (ARDS). An extensive infectious and rheumatologic workup failed to identify a causative agent. Antimicrobial coverage was broadened to vancomycin and piperacillin/tazobactam.

Question

As the patient continued to worsen, the clinicians asked themselves: Should extracorporeal membrane oxygenation (ECMO) be used for the early treatment of ARDS?

PRO: Acute respiratory distress syndrome (ARDS) is associated with significant morbidity and mortality. Extracorporeal membrane oxygenation (ECMO) is a therapeutic option in the management of severe ARDS. The concept of "lung rest" underlies the potential benefit of ECMO in the management of severe ARDS.

CON: Yes, but inconsistencies in the literature have made the definitive role of ECMO in ARDS management difficult to establish.

ARDS is classically defined as the acute onset of hypoxemia and bilateral pulmonary infiltrates consistent with pulmonary edema in the absence of left heart failure [1]. In an attempt to address validity issues with the original definition, the ARDS Task Force refined the definition and further classified ARDS according to the degree of hypoxemia: mild ($200 < PaO_2:FIO_2 \leq 300$), moderate ($100 < PaO_2:FIO_2$ 200), and severe ($PaO_2:FIO_2 < 100$) [2]. Associated mortality rates were 27, 35, and 45 %, respectively [2]. The most common etiology of acute respiratory failure was infectious with bacterial pneumonia, the most frequently encountered pathology followed by viral pneumonia, while less common causes were sepsis, trauma, and pulmonary emboli [3–6].

ARDS is associated with significant mortality rates and the majority die because of refractory hypoxemia [2, 7, 8]. For survivors, the morbidity remains significant with diminished quality of life that can persist for years [8, 9].

M.M. Anastacio
Department of Surgery, Medstar Washington Hospital Center, 110 Irving Street, NW, Room 4B 42, Washington, DC 20010, USA
e-mail: Melissa.M.Anastacio@medstar.net; manastacio@hotmail.com

S.A. Falk (✉)
Department of Anesthesiology and Critical Care, Hospital of the University of Pennsylvania, 3400 Spruce Street, Dulles 680 F, Philadelphia, PA 19104, USA
e-mail: falks@uphs.upenn.edu; Scott.Falk@uphs.upenn.edu

C.S. Scher et al. (eds.), *You're Wrong, I'm Right*, DOI 10.1007/978-3-319-43169-7_69

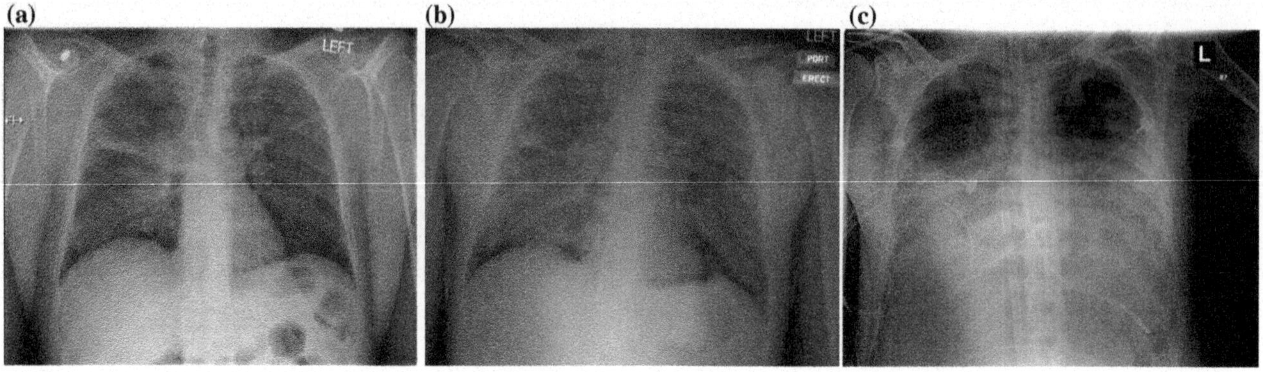

Fig. 69.1 Serial chest radiographs from **a** the day of presentation to the emergency department, **b** prior to and **c** after ECMO initiation demonstrate progressive worsening bilateral pulmonary infiltrates

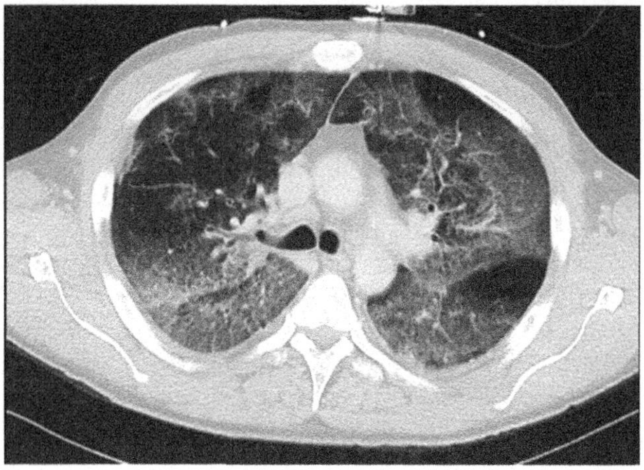

Fig. 69.2 Computed tomography scan of the chest demonstrates bilateral ground glass opacities, interseptal thickening, and bilateral atelectasis

The average annual medical cost for survivors is 2–4 times greater than for healthy individuals [10].

PRO: Key concepts to the management of ARDS involve treatment of the underlying cause and supportive care, but the hallmark is utilization of lung-protective strategies including low tidal volume, low pressure, permissive hypercapnia, and minimal oxygen, all to limit ventilator-associated lung injury and oxygen toxicity [3]. The ARDSNet trial demonstrated significant reduction in mortality from 39 to 31 % with the use of low tidal volumes and permissive hypercapnia; however, outcomes remained poor [3]. If conventional ventilation failed, more advanced ventilator modes such as a high frequency oscillator or airway pressure release ventilation or adjuncts such as steroids or nitric oxide could be utilized—although there has been no data to prove their efficacy in ARDS. It was at this extreme end of the spectrum that ECMO emerged as a potentially lifesaving alternative for the management of severe ARDS.

ECMO is an extracorporeal circuit that provides cardiac and/or pulmonary support. It has been utilized in both pediatric and adult populations, for emergent cardiac support, and severe respiratory failure [11]. A venous outflow cannula placed in the internal jugular vein or femoral vein removes blood, which is passed through a membrane oxygenator where gas exchange occurs. It is then recirculated back into the body through an inflow cannula in the femoral vein (VV ECMO) or through a central artery (femoral artery or axillary artery) (venoarterial/VA ECMO). For severe ARDS, both VV and VA ECMO have been utilized, though VV ECMO is more commonly used. As a result of advances in ECMO technology and its greater availability, ECMO cannulation can be perceived as straightforward. However, it is associated with potentially serious complications (vascular injury, stroke, bleeding, infection, and extremity ischemia) and requires a skilled multidisciplinary team of specialized physicians, perfusionists, nurses, and ancillary staff [12]. Additionally, it requires a tremendous amount of resources and finances from ECMO institutions.

With severe ARDS, ECMO has the advantage of facilitating lung-protective strategies, correcting hypoxemia and hypercarbia while providing target organ recovery and maintaining adequate whole-body organ perfusion.

CON: Fine, but did you examine the actual data? The data on the benefits of ECMO have been less than conclusive and fraught with many issues. Developed in the early 1970s, the first randomized controlled trial utilizing VA ECMO in ARDS patients demonstrated poor outcomes (close to 90 % mortality in both the control and ECMO groups) [13]. As a result, the concept of ECMO in ARDS fell out of favor.

PRO: It is important to note, however, that this study was performed prior to the improved understanding of ARDS, development of lung-protective strategies, and advancements in ECMO technology. Since then, several institutional experiences with ECMO have been published. They provide a generally favorable view of ECMO's benefit in ARDS patients.

CON: Yes, but this study is limited—it is retrospective and observational and has inconsistent methodologies.

PRO: Let's look at more recent literature. The largest single-institution experience comes from the University of Michigan. Based on data from 255 patients with severe ARDS placed on ECMO over a 14-year period, the overall survival to hospital discharge was 52 %, a rate similar to contemporary programs [12, 14]. This data reflected experience before and after the launch of lung-protective ventilation strategies. The CESAR trial is the only other randomized control trial that evaluated primary outcomes (death or severe disability) at 6 months from hospital discharge for ARDS patients who were randomized to either conventional medical management or transfer to an ECMO center for consideration of ECMO [15]. Survival rates without disability at 6 months post-discharge were statistically higher for ARDS patients who received ECMO consideration (63 vs 47 % for the conventional group). Additionally, a gain of 0.03 in quality-associated life years was gained at 6 months. Further stimulating growing interest in ECMO's role with ARDS came with the outbreak of H1N1 influenza that demonstrated survival rates in the 70 percentile range in patients rescued with ECMO [16, 17]. Both the CESAR trial and experience with H1N1 influenza outbreak also highlighted the importance of referral to ECMO-specialized centers.

CON: Fine, but What is the best way to even implement an ECMO program? ECMO's use in the management of ARDS has been plagued by the absence of consensus guidelines for indications, contraindications, and even management. Although the Extracorporeal Life Support Organization (ELSO) published general guidelines for indications and contraindications for ECMO support, the ELSO stresses that they do not reflect standard-of-care practices nor do they reflect consensus guidelines [18]. Published criteria in the literature reflect variations across institutions, across nations, and over time.

Further complicating the discussion is the absence of agreement on the role of specific patient factors such as age, body mass index, preexisting chronic medical conditions (including malignancy, COPD, renal or liver disease, malnutrition, or immune compromised state), and the presence and severity of acute extrapulmonary dysfunction in the decision algorithm for ECMO consideration. All of these factors inherently increase one's risk for complications including death. Frequently cited independent predictors of mortality pre-ECMO are as follows: age, sex, the presence of chronic diseases such as diabetes, COPD, and acute extrapulmonary organ dysfunction (namely renal and hepatic), severity of illness based on scoring systems (APACHE, SOFA, PRESERVE, MODS), degree of acidosis (pH <7.10), PaO_2:FiO_2 ratio, and number of ventilator days [4–6, 12, 19].

PRO: Yes, but ECMO itself could potentially assist patients in avoiding the worsening of these comorbidities. ARDS-related complications include worsening hypoxemia and hypercarbia, progression to non-recoverable lung function and extrapulmonary organ dysfunction (hemodynamic instability, renal or liver dysfunction). The number of ventilator days prior to ECMO initiation has consistently been cited as an independent predictor of mortality (typically greater than 7–10 days) [4–6, 9, 12]. ECMO may be able to ameliorate the development of acute extrapulmonary organ dysfunction and can shorten overall ventilator days, but would have no influence on other fixed patient variables.

CON: However, other issues remain unanswered. Namely, what constitutes "early" initiation? Is it based on the number of days on the ventilator? Is it based on when ARDS is diagnosed, which is problematic because it can be misdiagnosed or diagnosed late? Additionally, When should that phone call be made to an ECMO-based institution for assistance or transfer? Who should perform ECMO cannulation? Oftentimes, patients are placed on ECMO at the referring hospital and then transferred for further management. Should only the ECMO center actually place patients on ECMO so that transferred patients can be properly evaluated? Despite well-established literature, there are inconsistencies in the real-life practice of ARDS management. There are also differences in the experience of diverse hospital systems in the management of critically ill patients and in the understanding and utilization of ECMO. Inconsistencies and lack of standardized practices may contribute to mortality seen in severe ARDS and in ECMO patients.

Consensus More important than addressing earlier ECMO utilization, we should all consider the even greater benefit of early referral or transfer to an ECMO center. The benefit would not only be from the ECMO expertise and infrastructure but the overall higher level of knowledge provided by physicians in such referral centers in the management of complex patients such as the ARDS population. Their expertise may even obviate the need for ECMO if proper management strategies are employed, avoiding certain device-associated complications that only increase patient morbidity and mortality. Additionally, ECMO centers should take a more active role in educating surrounding referral hospitals.

Follow-up

On hospital day 7, the patient was transferred to a tertiary referral center and placed on veno-venous ECMO (VV ECMO) via the right internal jugular vein and the right femoral vein. Transesophageal echocardiogram demonstrated an ejection fraction of 65 % with normal biventricular function. Mechanical ventilator settings were minimized. Additional interventions included escalation of antimicrobials, the addition of an antifungal agent and steroids, and utilization of a combination of neuromuscular blockade, sedative, and analgesic infusions of varying duration. He was decannulated from ECMO on the 22nd day, undergoing a percutaneous tracheostomy in the interim. He did not suffer any extrapulmonary organ damage or ECMO-related complications. He was ultimately liberalized from the ventilator and discharged from the hospital for extensive physical rehabilitation.

Summary

ECMO is a valuable, potentially lifesaving alternative to conventional management of severe ARDS. However, its efficacious use is fraught with many unanswered questions, inconsistent data, and potentially morbid complications. Although early institution of ECMO in ARDS patients may be lifesaving, the data are inconclusive.

References

1. Bernard GT, Artigas A, Brigham KL, Carlet J, Falke K, Hudson L, et al. Report of the American-European Consensus conference on acute respiratory distress syndrome: definition, mechanisms, relevant outcomes, and clinical trial coordination. Consensus Committee. J Crit Care. 1994;9:72–81.
2. Definition Task Force ARDS, Ranieri VM, Rubenfeld GD, Thompson BT, Ferguson ND, Caldwell E, Fan E, et al. Acute respiratory distress syndrome: the Berlin definition. JAMA. 2012;307(23):2526–33.
3. [no authors listed] Ventilation with lower tidal volumes as compared with traditional tidal volumes for acute lung injury and the acute respiratory distress syndrome. The Acute Respiratory Distress Syndrome Network. N Engl J Med. 2000;342:1301–1308.
4. Pappalardo F, Pieri M, Greco T, Patroniti N, Pesenti A, Arcadipane A, et al. Italian ECMOnet. Predicting mortality risk in patients undergoing venovenous ECMO for ARDS due to influenza A (H1N1) pneumonia: the ECMOnet score. Intensive Care Med. 2013;39:275–81.
5. Schmidt M, Zogheib E, Rozé H, Repesse X, Lebreton G, Luyt CE, et al. The PRESERVE mortality risk score and analysis of long-term outcomes after extracorporeal membrane oxygenation for severe acute respiratory distress syndrome. Intensive Care Med. 2013;39:1704–13.
6. Rock A, Hraiech S, Masson E, Grisoli D, Forel JM, Boucekine M, et al. Outcomes of acute respiratory distress syndrome patients treated with extracorporeal membrane oxygenation and brought to a referral center. Intensive Care Med. 2014;40:74–83.
7. Rubenfeld GD, Caldwell E, Peabody E, Weaver J, Martin DP, Neff M, et al. Incidence and outcomes of acute lung injury. N Engl J Med. 2005;353(16):1685–93.
8. Stapleton RD, Wang BM, Hudson LD, Rubenfeld GD, Caldwell ES, Steinberg KP. Causes and timing of death in patients with ARDS. Chest. 2005;128:525–32.
9. Heddridge MS, Tansey CM, Matté A, Tomlinson G, Diaz-Granados N, Cooper A, et al. Canadian Critical Care Trials Group. Functional disability 5 years after acute respiratory distress syndrome. N Engl J Med. 2011;364:1293–304.
10. Rubenfeld GD, Herridge MS. Epidemiology and outcomes of acute lung injury. Chest. 2007;131:554–62.
11. Extracorporeal Life Support Organization. ELSO registry report. International summary. https://www.elso.org/Registry/Statistics/InternationalSummary.aspx. Ann Arbor, MI. July 2015. Accessed 16 Aug 2015.
12. Hemmila MR, Rowe SA, Boules TN, Miskulin J, McGillicuddy JW, Schuerer DJ, et al. Extracorporeal life support for severe acute respiratory distress syndrome in adults. Ann Surg. 2004;240:595–605.
13. Zapol WM, Snider MT, Hill JD, Fallat RJ, Bartlett RH, Edmunds LH, et al. Extracorporeal membrane oxygenation in severe acute respiratory failure. A randomized prospective study. JAMA. 1979;242:2193–6.
14. Brogan TV, Thiagarajan RR, Rycus PT, Bartlett RH, Bratton SL. Extracorporeal membrane oxygenation in adults with severe respiratory failure: a multi-center database. Intensive Care Med. 2009;35(12):2105–14.
15. Peek GJ, Mugford M, Tiruvoipati R, Wilson A, Allen E, Thalanany MM, et al. CESAR trial collaboration. Efficacy and economic assessment of conventional ventilator support versus extracorporeal membrane oxygenation for severe adult respiratory failure (CESAR): a multicenter randomized controlled trial. Lancet. 2009;374:1351–63.
16. ANZIC Influenza Investigators, Webb SA, Pettilä V, Seppelt I, Bellomo R, Bailey M, et al. Critical care services and H1N1 influenza in Australia and New Zealand. N Engl J Med. 2009;2009 (361):1925–34.
17. Patrorriti N, Zangrillo A, Pappalardo F, Peris A, Cianchi G, Braschi A, et al. The Italian ECMO network experience during the 2009 influenza A (H1N1) pandemic: preparation for severe respiratory emergency outbreaks. Intensive Care Med. 2011;37:1447–57.
18. Extracorporeal Life Support Organization (ELSO) guidelines for adult respiratory failure version 1.3. December 2013. https://www.elso.org/Portals/0/IGD/Archive/FileManager/989d4d4d14cusersshyerdocumentselsoguidelinesforadultrespiratoryfailure1.3.pdf Accessed 16 Aug 2015.
19. Chiu LC, Tasi FC, Hu HC, Chang CH, Hung CY, Lee CS, et al. Survival predictors in acute respiratory distress syndrome with extracorporeal membrane oxygenation. Ann Thorac Surg. 2015;99:243–50.

What Is the Most Effective Initial Resuscitation for the Septic Shock Patient?

70

Howard Nearman

Case

A 67-year-old 88 kg man with a past medical history of coronary artery disease and heart failure with a reduced ejection fraction (rEFHF) underwent a Whipple procedure 2 weeks ago for a duodenal adenocarcinoma. His postoperative course was uneventful, and he was discharged home a week later. He now presents to the emergency department with complaints of fever, malaise, and abdominal pain. His vital signs include a temperature of 101.2 °F, pulse of 112, and a blood pressure of 82/46. In keeping with the most recent Surviving Sepsis Campaign International Guidelines for Management of Severe Sepsis and Septic Shock [1], cultures are obtained and the patient is started on empiric broad-spectrum antibiotics. Fluids are started, and he is quickly admitted to the intensive care unit (ICU) for stabilization before further diagnostic and/or source control procedures are performed.

Question

What is the most effective initial resuscitation for the septic shock patient?

PRO (ICU Attending): We have started treatment in short order and need to follow the guidelines by providing early goal-directed therapy (EGDT) [2]. Let us place an arterial line, a central venous catheter and measure a blood lactate level. Since the patient is hypotensive, we can give 30 mL/kg of a crystalloid solution and push the central venous pressure (CVP) above 8 mmHg. Our goals are to achieve a mean arterial pressure (MAP) of at least 65 mmHg and get the central venous oxygen saturation ($ScvO_2$) above 70 %. We can continue to give fluids as long as there is hemodynamic improvement, such as increase in blood pressure or decrease in tachycardia. If our fluid resuscitation does not get the MAP above 65 mmHg, we may have to consider adding a norepinephrine drip.

CON (ICU Fellow): With all due respect, I have concerns aggressively pushing fluids in a patient with rEFHF and I think we need to take a look at some of the newer data. There are 2 large studies recently published that do not totally support EGDT as defined in the Surviving Sepsis Campaign. The ARISE trial found that EGDT in septic shock patients did not reduce all-cause mortality at 90 days and that the EGDT group actually received a larger volume of resuscitative fluid and were more likely to receive vasopressors than the usual-care group [3]. Similarly, the ProCESS trial also found that protocol-based resuscitation of septic shock patients did not improve outcomes at 90 days. In addition, they noted no difference in the need for organ support [4]. Furthermore, both studies demonstrated that measuring central venous pressure (CVP) and central venous oxygen saturation, although safe, is not necessary for successful resuscitation.

PRO (ICU Attending): OK. Good to know. We can still press on with our fluid resuscitation while assessing response to volume. Let us hang normal saline and follow MAP, CVP, and heart rate.

CON (ICU Fellow): I am not a big fan of normal saline in the critically ill. Infusing large quantities of normal saline with a chloride concentration of 154 meq/L will result in hyperchloremic acidosis, which cannot be good for the unstable septic patient. In fact, a recent study in septic patients found those who received balanced fluids had lower

H. Nearman (✉)
Department of Anesthesiology and Critical Care,
Hospital of the University of Pennsylvania, 3400 Spruce Street,
Philadelphia, PA 19104, USA
e-mail: Howard.nearman@uphs.upenn.edu;
Howard.Nearman@uhhospitals.org

H. Nearman
Department of Anesthesiology and Perioperative Medicine,
University Hospitals Case Medical Center, 11100 Euclid Avenue,
Cleveland, OH 44106, USA

C.S. Scher et al. (eds.), *You're Wrong, I'm Right*, DOI 10.1007/978-3-319-43169-7_70

in-hospital mortality; in fact, the larger the proportion of balanced fluids compared with normal saline, the lower the mortality [5].

PRO (ICU Attending): Ringer's Lactate it is then. We can run in 30 mL/kg and then assess MAP. We should also re-measure blood lactate if the initial level was >4 mmol/L.

CON (ICU Fellow): Do you think it is a good idea to administer more than 2.5 L of fluid in a patient with a history of systolic heart failure? Can't we better tailor our resuscitation goals?

PRO (ICU Attending): Well, we need to normalize perfusion. I suppose we can closely assess response to fluid as we resuscitate to see if we have reached our goal of a CVP of 8 mm Hg.

CON (ICU Fellow): I am not sure that with respect to fluids in sepsis, more is necessarily better—especially in this patient with a history of congestive heart failure. And I really do not think that CVP is the best indicator of volume responsiveness.

Regarding total fluids administered, in a retrospective review of 350 septic patients treated in accordance with the Surviving Sepsis Campaign guidelines, a more positive fluid balance at 24 h significantly increased the risk of in-hospital mortality [6]. In sepsis, hypoperfusion results in capillary endothelial leak, and administered fluid will accumulate in the interstitial space. This will interfere with diffusion of nutrients from the intravascular space, leading to organ dysfunction. But if we really need to give fluid, let us do it quickly. There is data demonstrating that the higher the proportion of total fluid that is received within the first 3 h of onset of sepsis was associated with decreased hospital mortality [7].

PRO (ICU Attending): All right. I can buy that. Let us push fluid quickly, but we need to figure out when enough is enough—when our patient will no longer be preload responsive. You are not a big fan of using CVP as a guide to fluid resuscitation I take it?

CON (ICU Fellow): We can agree that the only reason to give fluid is to increase stroke volume. CVP has been widely accepted as a valid indicator of intravascular volume, being mentioned prominently in the Surviving Sepsis Guidelines. However, CVP is a static indicator, and a systemic review has concluded that CVP is not a reliable gauge of volume status in the critically ill, nor can it be used reliably to predict responsiveness to fluid therapy [8]. The efficacy of fluid challenges in producing a beneficial hemodynamic response is better assessed using minimally invasive cardiac output monitors that track changes in stroke volume dynamically and in real time [9].

If we do not achieve our hemodynamic goals with judicious fluid resuscitation, then we will need to start vasopressors and/or inotropes.

PRO (ICU Attending): It is always a tough call on how to balance achieving goal MAP between administration of fluids and the use of vasopressors. I know that fluid resuscitation is clearly the initial treatment, but I am not comfortable sitting on a MAP <65 mmHg for very long waiting for fluids to take effect.

CON (ICU Fellow): And I agree with that. In general, it seems that starting vasopressors early rather than later leads to better outcomes. Recent data from a retrospective cohort study showed that for every 1-h delay in starting norepinephrine during the first 6 h of onset of sepsis, there was a 5.3 % increase in mortality. Patients who had norepinephrine started within the first 2 h had significantly lower lactate levels, required less total norepinephrine in the first 24 h, and had lower 28-day mortality rates [10]. It is also possible that earlier vasopressor use allowed for lower fluid volumes needed to reach hemodynamic goals. Specifically, with respect to this patient with rEFHF, we may see improved outcomes by providing pure inotropic support early and optimizing cardiac output with dobutamine for instance, rather than from a pure vasoconstrictor like vasopressin, which may serve only to increase afterload and stress his failing heart without improving overall perfusion. Current guidelines are unable to consider exceptions for all potential circumstances and only provide a "one size fits all" approach.

PRO (ICU Attending): All right. I assume you will want to use norepinephrine as the initial agent as it is the vasopressor recommended by the Surviving Sepsis Guidelines.

CON (ICU Fellow): Not necessarily. I mean, I know what the guidelines say, but I am not convinced. There was an article out many years ago that found that endogenous vasopressin plasma levels in hypotensive septic shock patients receiving catecholamines were inappropriately low [11]. More recently, a retrospective cohort study evaluated septic shock patients who received monotherapy with either norepinephrine or vasopressin as initial vasoactive therapy. The results demonstrated that vasopressin was noninferior to norepinephrine for the achievement of MAP goal [12]. A definitive randomized controlled trial of vasopressin versus norepinephrine as initial therapy is currently underway and hopefully will provide a definitive answer [13].

PRO (ICU Attending): Well, I am glad that we had this discussion. It certainly seems that the optimal initial resuscitation of septic shock patients—with the exception of antibiotics and source control, of course—may not necessarily be exactly as defined in the 2012 Surviving Sepsis Guidelines. Apparently, there is a lot of new data that need to be analyzed with respect to fluids, monitoring and hemodynamic therapy.

CON (ICU Fellow): As a matter of fact, that is exactly what is happening now. Dr. Dellinger, the lead author on the 2012 Guidelines, has recently published an update looking at some of these controversies [14]. We have made a lot of headway into improving the outcome for our patients in septic shock, but more work lays ahead. Prospective randomized controlled trials are difficult due to the range of disease presentations, origins of the septic process, and definition of measured outcomes.

References

1. Dellinger RP, Levy MM, Rhodes A, Annane D, Gerlach H, Opal SM, Surviving Sepsis Campaign Guidelines Committee including the Pediatric Subgroup, et al. Surviving Sepsis Campaign: international guidelines for management of severe sepsis and septic shock. Crit Care Med. 2013;41(2):580–637.
2. Rivers E, Nguyen B, Havstad S, Ressler J, Mussin A, Knoblich B, Early Goal-Directed Therapy Collaborative Group, et al. Early goal-directed therapy in the treatment of severe sepsis and septic shock. N Engl J Med. 2001;345(19):1368–77.
3. Peake SL, Delaney A, Bailey M, Bellomo R, Cameron PA, Cooper DJ, ARISE Investigators, ANZICS Clinical Trials Group, et al. Goal-directed resuscitation for patients with early septic shock. N Engl J Med. 2014;371(16):1496–506.
4. Yealy DM, Kellum JA, Huang DT, Barnato AE, Weissfeld LA, Pike F, ProCESS Investigators, et al. A randomized trial of protocol-based care for early septic shock. N Engl J Med. 2014;370 (18):1683–93.
5. Raghunathan K, Shaw A, Nathanson B, Stürmer T, Brookhart A, Stefan MS, et al. Association between the choice of IV crystalloid and in-hospital mortality among critically ill adults with sepsis. Crit Care Med. 2014;42(7):1585–91.
6. Sadaka F, Juarez M, Naydenov S, O'Brien J. Fluid resuscitation in septic shock: the effect of increasing fluid balance on mortality. J Intensive Care Med. 2014;29(4):213–7.
7. Lee SJ, Ramar K, Park JG, Gajic O, Li G, Kashyap R. Increased fluid administration in the first three hours of sepsis resuscitation is associated with reduced mortality: a retrospective cohort study. Chest. 2014;146(4):908–15.
8. Marik PE, Monnet X, Teboul J. Hemodynamic parameters to guide fluid therapy. Ann Intensive Care. 2011;1(1):2–9.
9. Marik PE, Lemson J. Fluid responsiveness: an evolution of our understanding. Br J Anaesth. 2014;112(4):617–20.
10. Bai X, Yu W, Ji W, Lin Z, Tan S, Duan K, et al. Early versus delayed administration of norepinephrine in patients with septic shock. Crit Care. 2014;18(5):532.
11. Landry DW, Levin HR, Gallant EM, Ashton RC, Seo S, D'Alessandro D, et al. Vasopressin deficiency contributes to the vasodilation of septic shock. Circulation. 1997;95(5):1122–5.
12. Daley MJ, Lat I, Mieure KD, Jennings HR, Hall JB, Kress JP. A comparison of initial monotherapy with norepinephrine versus vasopressin for resuscitation in septic shock. Ann Pharmacother. 2013;47(3):301–10.
13. Gordon AC, Mason AJ, Perkins GD, Ashby D, Brett SJ. Protocol for a randomized controlled trial of VAsopressin versus Noradrenaline as Initial therapy in Septic sHock (VANISH). BMJ Open. 2014;4(7):e005866.
14. Dellinger RP. The Surviving Sepsis Campaign: Where have we been and where are we going? Cleve Clin J Med. 2015;82(4):237–44.

71 Should Patients with Acute Respiratory Distress Syndrome Be Placed in the Prone Position to Improve Ventilation?

Arati Patil

Case

We always had a variety of critically ill patients in the surgical intensive care unit: trauma, postoperative, cardiac, vascular, and postoperative respiratory failure patients. Although most of the patients were memorable, one in particular has stood out to me throughout the years.

James was young, only aged 22 years. His mother had passed away in the year prior to his admission, and he started drinking heavily after that life-altering event—up to 1 L of vodka a day. Prior to his alcohol abuse, he had been completely healthy. He presented to the hospital with severe mid-epigastric pain and was quickly diagnosed with pancreatitis. James was admitted to the surgical intensive care unit due to the severity of his pancreatitis and risk for alcohol withdrawal. He decompensated very quickly and needed to be intubated the evening of his admission and soon thereafter developed systemic inflammatory response syndrome (SIRS).

During the course of his admission, he developed acute respiratory distress syndrome, or ARDS. At first, his ARDS was manageable. We followed the ARDS Network protocol, and he was "stable." However, as his pancreatitis worsened, his ARDS followed suit and he required increasing ventilator support. During rounds, we discussed management options of his pancreatitis and ARDS as it was quickly becoming apparent that his condition was deteriorating.

Placing James in the prone position for his ARDS was brought up and it initiated some intense debate during rounds. It was not merely a ventilator change or medication order we were talking about. In the end, we decided to perform a literature search in order to bring some evidence-based medicine to the table and help us make an informed decision.

A. Patil (✉)
Department of Anesthesiology, Perioperative Care and Pain Medicine, New York University Langone Medical Center, 550 First Avenue, TH 530, New York, NY 10016, USA
e-mail: arati.m.patil@gmail.com

Question

Should patients with ARDS be placed in the prone position?

PRO: During rounds, I stated, "I read that prone positioning improves arterial oxygenation, positive end-expiratory pressure (PEEP) induced alveolar recruitment, and drainage of secretions. The improvement in arterial oxygenation stems from an improvement in ventilation/perfusion mismatch as there is better ventilation in the perfused lung areas. Prone positioning can also prevent ventilator-induced lung injury by decreasing overdistention and increasing alveolar recruitment. This homogenizes the strain induced by mechanical ventilation and decreases the overall stress on the lungs. Wouldn't it then be indicated in patients with ARDS?" [1].

CON: One of the team members responded, "The improvement in arterial oxygenation and decrease in ventilator-induced lung injury is valid, but does it actually make a difference in the patient's outcome and is it worth the risks?"

> "Prone positioning is not indicated for ALL patients with ARDS because there are absolute contraindications. These include burns and open wounds on the face, pelvic fractures, spinal instability, and increased intracranial pressure. There are complications from prone positioning as well. We need to consider the risk of facial edema, pressure sores, desaturation during the turning process, loss of the airway, and damage to important lines. I certainly want to avoid reintubating a patient or replacing lines". [2]

PRO: I responded, "I understand your concern, but there are hazards to all types of treatment modalities. Facial edema resolves when the patient no longer requires prone positioning, and pressure necrosis can be prevented by protective covering and careful positioning. The desaturation during the positioning process is typically transient and does not

C.S. Scher et al. (eds.), *You're Wrong, I'm Right*, DOI 10.1007/978-3-319-43169-7_71

require intervention. There is a risk of loss of the airway and lines, but with careful positioning this can be prevented.

> As for outcomes, in 2013 the *New England Journal of Medicine* published the large (466 patients) prospective randomized-controlled PROSEVA trial, which showed that for patients with severe ARDS, prone positioning significantly decreased 28-day (16 % in the prone group vs 32.8 % in the supine group) and 90-day mortality. The benefits certainly outweigh the risks!" [3]

CON: My team member responded, "Sure that was an interesting study, but we need to keep in mind that the trial only studied patients with severe ARDS, defined as a partial pressure of arterial oxygen (PaO_2) to fraction of inspired oxygen (FiO_2) ratio of less than 150 mmHg, a FiO_2 of at least 0.6, PEEP of at least 5 cm H_2O, and a tidal volume close to 6 ml per kg of predicted body weight. If James doesn't meet that criteria, he might not benefit from prone positioning. Also, the PROSEVA trial patients were intubated and mechanically ventilated for ARDS for less than 36 h prior to being enrolled in the study."

PRO: "OK. We can check to see if our patient meets that criteria. Regardless, we should consider prone positioning for our severe ARDS patients in this ICU. The study also showed there was a significant increase in rate of successful extubations in the prone group!"

CON: "The ICUs where the study was performed used prone positioning in daily practice for 5 years. We have not performed prone positioning in our ICU before. Our staff would have to be trained. We may have a higher risk of complications from prone positioning due to our lack of experience."

Concession from PRO: "I agree that we should not implement prone positioning without training. Let's get started with planning sessions for our staff in the classroom and with the human patient simulator."

Summary

Although in my patient's case, we did not use prone positioning as an ARDS treatment, it is an important topic to consider. It is evident that prone positioning in patients with severe ARDS can decrease mortality, and each ARDS patient needs to be looked at independently to consider whether prone positioning will be beneficial. It is important that intensive care units become familiar with prone positioning and require classroom and hands-on education on this topic in order to offer it in a safe and effective manner.

References

1. Guerin C, Baboi L, Richard JC. Mechanisms of the effects of prone positioning in acute respiratory distress syndrome. Intensive Care Med. 2014;40(11):1634–42.
2. Benson AB, Albert RK. Prone positioning for acute respiratory distress syndrome. Clin Chest Med. 2014;35(4):743–52.
3. Guérin C, Reignier J, Richard JC, Beuret P, Gacouin A, Boulain T, et al. PROSEVA Study Group. Prone positioning in severe acute respiratory distress syndrome. N Engl J Med. 2013;368(23):2159–68.

What Is the Best Strategy for Ventilation in Acute Respiratory Distress Syndrome?

72

Lee Stein

Case

A 52-year-old man who was a pedestrian struck by a car is a patient in your intensive care unit (ICU). No history is known, and no one has been able to reach his family. The impact was mainly on his left chest and abdomen, and the patient required intubation upon arrival to the emergency department. A computed tomography (CT) scan upon admission showed a pulmonary contusion, along with 2 rib fractures. The patient's condition has been worsening, and a chest X-ray (CXR) shows complete whiteout of both lungs. A partial pressure of oxygen/inspired fraction of oxygen (PaO_2/FiO_2) ratio of 90 is calculated, and the diagnosis of severe acute respiratory distress syndrome (ARDS) is made.

Questions

How should we ventilate patients with acute respiratory distress syndrome? Should we use a high positive end-expiratory pressure (PEEP) or low PEEP strategy? Should we use spontaneous or passive mechanical ventilation?

PRO: I think we can both agree to start with a lung protective strategy, as it's been widely accepted that this reduces mortality in patients with ARDS [1]. What that means is that we will ventilate the patient using a low-tidal volume strategy and try to limit our plateau pressures to as low as possible, not exceeding 30 cm H_2O. I believe we should also use a high PEEP and keep the patient sedated and muscle relaxed to use passive mechanical ventilation.

L. Stein
Department of Anesthesiology, New York University/Bellevue, 550 First Avenue, New York, NY 10016, USA

L. Stein (✉)
5 Peter Cooper Road, Apt 3E, New York, NY 10010, USA
e-mail: Lee.stein@nyumc.org

CON: Yes, I do agree that we should limit our tidal volumes to 6 mL/kg of ideal body weight and increase respiratory rate to maintain an adequate minute ventilation, as well as limit plateau pressures. However, I disagree with the use of high PEEP and passive mechanical ventilation. I believe low PEEP would be safer for the patient. Also, the patient will be better off spontaneously breathing, in order to maintain muscle tone and avoid deconditioning!

PRO: Well, I'll explain why I think high PEEP is a better strategy first. In ARDS, you lose a significant amount of lung volume because of fluid, consolidation, and atelectasis. We need to try to maximize the viable lung available for gas exchange by using higher pressures to keep alveoli open. This also helps prevent constant opening and collapsing of alveoli, which causes further damage [2]. A high PEEP strategy will improve the chances of survival for our patient.

CON: I don't think that it will. The evidence does not show any difference in mortality between a high PEEP strategy and a low PEEP strategy. A high PEEP strategy may help keep more alveoli open in certain areas of the lung, but will also cause over-distention in other areas leading to barotrauma. Very high intra-thoracic pressure may also negatively affect hemodynamics by impairing venous return to the heart [2]. Multiple randomized controlled trials seem to indicate that there is no difference in mortality between the 2 strategies. The largest of them, the Lung Open Ventilation Study, had 983 patients and showed that there was no difference in all-cause hospital mortality in patients with ARDS who were ventilated with high PEEP or low PEEP [3].

PRO: There is a meta-analysis that combined the data from 3 randomized controlled trials (RCTs), including the Lung Open Ventilation Study, which looked at high PEEP versus low PEEP in patients with lung injury who were ventilated with lung protective strategies. All of this data analyzed together showed that for patients with ARDS, there was an improvement in mortality with a high PEEP strategy [4].

C.S. Scher et al. (eds.), *You're Wrong, I'm Right*, DOI 10.1007/978-3-319-43169-7_72

Patients with ARDS had better oxygenation and were more likely to achieve unassisted breathing earlier. The paper also showed this was not associated with an increase in adverse effects, such as causing pneumothorax or requiring vasopressors [4].

CON: It's interesting to see that although individual studies showed no difference, for patients with ARDS (i.e., more severe lung damage), there was a decrease in mortality in the high PEEP group. However, there still is too much conflicting evidence on the subject. Part of the problem may be that each individual's injury and lung pathology may have a different threshold for finding the right balance of PEEP, where oxygenation is improved, but over-distention does not cause harm [2]. Perhaps all of our studies looking at entire populations of patients show no difference in mortality because they combine data points from a heterogeneous group. There are many ideas for individualized strategies for determining the ideal amount of PEEP. I recently read a pilot study where PEEP was set based on the static compliance of a patient's lung [5]. The authors showed that there was decreased organ dysfunction versus the group with FiO_2-guided PEEP settings. There was also a non-statistically significant trend toward decreased mortality in the group with PEEP set based on lung static compliance [5]. With further research, maybe we will find a method of individualization that will significantly decrease mortality.

PRO: OK, I will agree that an individualized strategy would likely result in the best outcomes. It's not yet possible to say what might be the best method though. Research is ongoing as to which measure should determine optimal PEEP: static compliance as you mentioned, pressure-volume curves, esophageal pressure as a surrogate for pleural pressure, or even directly measuring lung volume with nitrogen washout [2]. Studies haven't established what may work and what may not.

CON: You also mentioned that we should keep the patient sedated and muscle relaxed with passive mechanical ventilation. My concern is that without use of the diaphragm, you may get atrophy and weakness [2]. This would make it harder to wean the patient from the ventilator and could result in a longer hospital course. There is also evidence that spontaneous breathing with ventilator support can reduce lung inflammation and improve oxygen delivery [2]. I've even heard concerns that the use of non-depolarizing muscle relaxants can cause long-term problems with weakness.

PRO: This is completely wrong! It is better to keep the patient muscle relaxed and on passive mechanical ventilation. First, there is evidence that in severe ARDS, maintaining spontaneous ventilation may actually cause increased damage to the lung, although the evidence is from animal models [6]. Even so, the cause of the worsening lung injury was likely from an increase in transpulmonary pressure induced by the forceful spontaneous breathing effort [6]. Secondly, based on the evidence, you are wrong to say that use of muscle relaxants might cause long-term weakness in survivors of ARDS. In a prospective study looking at lung injury survivors, Fan et al. [7] showed that while there was significant morbidity from long-term ICU-related weakness, muscle relaxant use was not an associated factor. In a meta-analysis looking at neuromuscular blocking agents in ARDS, this was again shown to be the case. In that study, short infusions of cisatracurium were not associated with an increase in ICU-acquired weakness [8]. In each of the studies included in the meta-analysis, the infusion of cisatracurium was for 48 h. Even more importantly, however, that same meta-analysis showed that the use of cisatracurium in patients with ARDS was associated with a decrease in mortality and barotrauma [8]! So, I would argue that we should muscle relax our patient with a cisatracurium infusion and he will be less likely to have lung injury and more likely to survive.

CON: I will concede that the evidence shows that in severe ARDS, it is beneficial to use a neuromuscular blocking agent and this certainly applies to our patient. One caveat is that these are associations—a randomized controlled trial or large population database study is still needed for definitive proof. The evidence is less clear for mild-to-moderate ARDS and maintaining ventilator-assisted spontaneous ventilation in those cases could be more beneficial [2]. So what consensus have we arrived at?

PRO: Based on our discussion, I think that we can finally agree on how to best ventilate the patient. We will, of course, use a low-tidal volume strategy and limit our tidal volumes to 6 mL/kg of ideal body weight. We will use an individualized protocol for determining the proper PEEP for our patient, which will help us take into account the severity of his injury, and will try to find the right balance between keeping alveoli open and promoting gas exchange without causing over-distention and barotrauma. Although there is little evidence on the best individualization strategy, we can use a strategy based on static compliance because it showed a statistically significant reduction in organ dysfunction. Finally, the patient will be kept on passive mechanical ventilation with a cisatracurium infusion, which has been shown to decrease mortality and barotrauma in severe ARDS, and has not been associated with an increased risk for ICU-related weakness.

References

1. Petrucci N, De Feo C. Lung protective ventilation strategy for the acute respiratory distress syndrome. Cochrane Database Syst Rev. 2013;2:CD003844.
2. Rittayamai N, Brochard L. Recent advances in mechanical ventilation in patients with acute respiratory distress syndrome. Eur Respir Rev. 2015;24:132–40.
3. Meade MO, Cook DJ, Guyatt GH, Slutsky AS, Arabi YM, Cooper DJ, et al. Ventilation strategy using low tidal volumes, recruitment maneuvers, and high positive end-expiratory pressure for acute lung injury and acute respiratory distress syndrome: a randomized controlled trial. JAMA. 2008;299(6):637–45.
4. Briel M, Meade M, Mercat A, Brower R, Talmor D, Walter S, et al. Higher vs lower positive end-expiratory pressure in patients with acute lung injury and acute respiratory distress syndrome: systematic review and meta-analysis. JAMA. 2010;303(9):865–73.
5. Pintado MC, dePablo R, Trascasa M, Milicua JM, Rogero S, Daguerre M, et al. Individualized PEEP setting in subjects with ARDS: a randomized controlled pilot study. Respir Care. 2013;58(9):1416–23.
6. Yoshida T, Uchiyama A, Matsuura N, Mashimo T, Fujino Y. Spontaneous breathing during lung-protective ventilation in an experimental acute lung injury model: high transpulmonary pressure associated with strong spontaneous breathing effort may worsen lung injury. Crit Care Med. 2012;40(5):1578–85.
7. Fan E, Dowdy DW, Colantuoni E, Mendez-Tellez PA, Sevransky JE, Shanholtz C. Physical complications in acute lung injury survivors: a 2-year longitudinal prospective study. Crit Care Med. 2014;42(4):849–59.
8. Alhazzani W, Alshahrani M, Jaeschke R, Forel JM, Papazian L, Sevranksy J, Meade MO. Neuromuscular blocking agents in acute respiratory distress syndrome: a systematic review and meta-analysis of randomized controlled trials. Crit Care. 2013;17:R43.

Is a Single Dose of Etomidate for Rapid Sequence Intubation (RSI) Safe in the Critically Ill Patient?

73

Matt Bilbily

Case

A 64-year-old man admitted for exacerbation of chronic obstructive pulmonary disease (COPD) is now septic and failing noninvasive mask ventilation and requires intubation. He has a full-stomach.

The attending anesthesiologist asks the resident, "What method would you like to use to intubate this patient?"

"I think I will perform direct laryngoscopy after rapid sequence induction (RSI) and go with the most commonly used induction agent for RSI, 0.3 mg/kg intravenous (IV) etomidate," the resident answers. "I think this is a good choice because after my single induction dose of etomidate there will be minimal changes in heart rate and stroke volume. Additionally, etomidate is unlikely to cause a harmful drop in blood pressure.""You make a good argument for etomidate. However, are you at all concerned about its effect on adrenal suppression in an intensive care unit patient?" asks the attending.

The resident now recalls from his readings that etomidate is known to suppress the normal cortisol production of the adrenal glands through inhibition of 11-beta-hydroxylase enzyme. However, he admits that he is not sure whether a single dose of etomidate is enough to result in clinically significant adrenal suppression.

Question

Is a single dose of etomidate for RSI safe in the critically ill patient?

CON: "A single dose of etomidate for RSI has been shown to suppress the adrenal production of cortisol," the attending says. "A prospective study of 40 non-septic critically ill patients receiving etomidate for RSI showed that within 12 h of receiving etomidate 80 % of patients met the diagnostic criteria for adrenal suppression. However, by 48 h, this number decreased to 9 %" [1].

PRO: "Has etomidate-induced adrenal suppression in critically ill patients been shown to lead to worse patient outcomes?" asks the resident.

Concession from CON: "Single-dose etomidate for RSI in critically ill patients has not been shown to increase mortality compared to other induction agents," the attending admits. "In the Cochrane collaboration, Bruder and colleagues did a meta-analysis of 7 randomized control trials looking at critically ill patients requiring RSI, with a census of 772 patients [2]. They found no significant difference in mortality when comparing the 390 patients receiving etomidate to the 382 patients receiving other induction agents, with an odds ratio of 1.17 at 95 % CI.

"However, be mindful that no RCT to date has been adequately powered to detect mortality difference so you must still be cautious."

"This report also looked at secondary outcomes including: sequential organ failure (SOFA) score, ICU length of stay (LOS), hospital LOS, duration of mechanical ventilation, and duration of vasopressor support among others. After reviewing the included studies, the authors concluded no significant difference in any of these secondary outcomes with the exception of the SOFA score. As you know, the SOFA score ranges from 0 (good organ function) to 24 (worse organ function). In one of the included RCTs, which compared etomidate versus ketamine for RSI of critically ill patients, the mean difference in score was found to be 0.7 (95 % CI). In the original paper, this result was not deemed statistically significant, however, in this meta-analysis they found statistical significance but concluded that the difference was not clinically meaningful" [2].

PRO: "Would it be a good idea to supplement corticosteroids after etomidate administration to 'counteract' the adrenal suppression?" asks the resident.

CON: "It seems like a logical course of action, however, a randomized control trial done in critically ill non-septic shock patients showed no benefit to this therapy," says the

M. Bilbily (✉)
Department of Anesthesiology, Kingston General Hospital, 76 Stuart Street, Kingston, ON K7L 2V7, Canada
e-mail: bilbilym@kgh.kari.net

C.S. Scher et al. (eds.), *You're Wrong, I'm Right*, DOI 10.1007/978-3-319-43169-7_73

attending. "In this study they administered an infusion of hydrocortisone or placebo after a single induction dose of etomidate. They found no difference in the SOFA score, ICU length stay, number of ventilator days, or 28 day mortality. On the other hand they did show a decreased requirement for norepinephrine in patients receiving hydrocortisone" [3].

PRO: The resident concludes that based on the evidence to date, the use of etomidate in critically ill patients does suppress the adrenal production of cortisol but does not seem to increase mortality, organ system dysfunction, or health-care resource utilization. He realizes that this question is being investigated on an ongoing basis but feels comfortable with using etomidate as the induction agent for this critically ill patient.

Summary

Pro Concession

The attending suggests that perhaps the best solution to the controversy is to avoid RSI and etomidate altogether. Reviewing the patient's chart, it becomes clear that the patient's deterioration has been gradual over hours, and that the need for intubation is urgent, not emergent. With the patient still able to maintain tolerable saturations on supplemental oxygen, and not yet on vasopressors for sepsis, they formulate an alternative plan together to intubate using awake direct laryngoscopy after thorough airway topicalization with nebulized lidocaine and minimal sedation.

References

1. Vinclair M, Broux C, Faure P, Brun J, Genty C, Jacquot C, et al. Duration of adrenal inhibition following a single dose of etomidate in critically ill patients. Intensive Care Med. 2008;34:714–9.
2. Bruder EA, Ball IM, Ridi S, Pickett W, Hohl C. Single induction dose of etomidate versus other induction agents for endotracheal intubation in critically ill patients. Cochrane Database Syst Rev. 2015;1:CD010225.
3. Payen JF, Dupuis C, Trouve-Buisson T, Vinclair M, Broux C, Bouzat P, et al. Corticosteroid after etomidate in critically ill patients: a randomized controlled trial. Crit Care Med. 2012;40:29–35.

Should Intensive Care Unit Patients Be Deeply Sedated? 74

Caitlin J. Guo

Case

A 75-year-old man is admitted to the surgical intensive care unit (ICU) after an emergent laparotomy for perforated bowel. His medical history includes hypertension, diabetes, coronary artery disease, and previous alcohol abuse. On arrival to the ICU, he is acidotic and in septic shock, requiring norepinephrine and vasopressin infusions. Progressively over the next few hours in the ICU, vasopressor support has decreased and lactic acidosis is improving, but he now has acute respiratory distress syndrome (ARDS) and is being mechanically ventilated with lung protective ventilation. It is expected that his length of mechanical ventilation will exceed 48 h.

Question

Should this ICU patient be deeply sedated?

PRO: Yes, pain is the most common issue patients recall after discharge from the ICU, and it is commonly associated with the endotracheal tube and mechanical ventilation. For this reason, traditionally, deep sedation has been used in the ICU.

CON: No, recently, there has been an increasing body of evidence that a daily wake-up and lightening of sedation are associated with better clinical outcomes.

PRO: Why would we want our patients to be more aware of their situation and surroundings?

CON: Most ICU stays have multiple phases. The early phase is generally brief but active, involving many interventions and procedures, followed by a longer convalescence. Should we tailor our sedation accordingly?

PRO: Possibly, but this is difficult to do. Historically, ICU sedation practices stemmed from intraoperative anesthetic care at a time when ventilators could only deliver mandatory breaths. Deep sedation was thus required to maintain synchrony between the patient and the ventilator. The use of neuromuscular blockade was common. And when agitation was observed, sedatives were used to induce deep sedation to prevent self-harm when the patient would accidentally remove vascular lines and the endotracheal tube.

To further complicate matters, assessing pain in the ICU is challenging. Self-reported pain scales for awake patients cannot be validated in the ICU. Objective measures such as heart rate and blood pressure can be difficult to interpret and are frequently confounded by the underlying medical condition. There are many reasons why patients may experience pain: blood draws, mechanical ventilation, placement of vascular lines, Foley catheters, and skeletal and muscular pain from immobility and pressure ulcers. Short-term sequelae of untreated pain may include an increase in the stress response, inflammation, and impairment of the immune system, predisposing patients to infection and poor wound healing. Long-term consequences include chronic pain, anxiety, and post-traumatic stress disorder. For these reasons, many providers favor the strategy of deep sedation.

The Society of Critical Care Medicine practice guidelines on sedation from 1995 to 2002 favored this approach, with liberal benzodiazepine infusions. Because many patients have significant cognitive and physical impairment after ICU discharge, the addition of post-traumatic stress would be cruel and should be avoided if possible.

CON: With the advent of the modern ventilator modes, mechanical ventilation is no longer a reason for deep sedation.

C.J. Guo (✉)
Department of Anesthesiology, Perioperative Care and Pain Medicine, New York University Langone Medical Center, 550 First Avenue, New York, NY 10016, USA
e-mail: Caitlin.Guo@nyumc.org

C.S. Scher et al. (eds.), *You're Wrong, I'm Right*, DOI 10.1007/978-3-319-43169-7_74

PRO: It is important to note that patients may have a medical indication for continuous deep sedation, which may include intracranial hypertension, severe respiratory failure, profound hemodynamic instability, status epilepticus, deliberate hypothermia, concurrent use of neuromuscular blockade, and critical lines and drains that require protection.

In our patient who underwent a laparotomy and was in septic shock requiring aggressive hemodynamic support, the argument could be made that he should be deeply sedated because of his severe hemodynamic instability. Any coughing on the endotracheal tube can cause a vagal response and compromise his cardiac function. In addition, a patient who has recently received large-volume resuscitation for septic shock following bowel surgery is at risk of abdominal compartment syndrome. Light sedation can increase the likelihood of ventilator dyssynchrony and increased intrathoracic pressure and can mimic abdominal compartment syndrome. A hemodynamically unstable patient who is in shock and requiring active resuscitation and interventions should be deeply sedated.

CON: Traditional ICU sedation is comprised of short-acting benzodiazepines and opiates, but the context-sensitive half-life of these drugs is greatly increased with a continuous infusion. During the time when these medications are wearing off, patients are at the highest risk for developing delirium, a form of acute cerebral dysfunction. The incidence is reported to be as high as 70 % in ventilated patients. The clinical hallmarks of delirium include decreased attention span, inability to comprehend surroundings, and waxing and waning alertness. The 2 major subtypes are hypo- and hyperactive delirium, and some patients may have both. Regardless of type, delirium is associated with increased short- and long-term morbidity and mortality. Many ICU survivors are found to have permanent loss of memory and reasoning power. Recent long-term studies have shown that a fair number of patients meet the criteria for delirium long after they are discharged from the ICU. Lighter sedation is better. In the last 15 years, evidence from randomized trials demonstrated that a daily wake-up paired with trials of spontaneous breathing have been associated with better clinical outcomes, less delirium, and fewer ventilator and ICU days than deep sedation. The results were first demonstrated in a landmark study: "Daily Interruption of Sedative Infusions in Critically Ill Patients Undergoing Mechanical Ventilation" [1]. They showed that daily interruption of sedation significantly reduced mechanical ventilation and ICU days and was associated with less neuroimaging. Subsequent large randomized studies have confirmed similar findings: the "Awakening and Breathing Controlled Trial" [2] and the "A Protocol of No Sedation for Critically Ill Patients Receiving Mechanical Ventilation: a Randomized Trial" [3]. All groups were treated for pain. In contrast to deep sedation, light sedation was not associated with additional short-term adverse effects or long-term psychiatric outcomes.

While most of the original trials studied daily wake-up, recent trials focused on targeted light sedation: "Daily Sedation Interruption in Mechanically Ventilated Critically Ill Patients Cared for with a Sedation Protocol" [4]. The Canadian Critical Care Trials Group showed that there was no additional benefit when daily wake-up was added to a protocol that minimized the level of sedation. Coupled with the newer generation of ventilators that are capable of delivering synchronized breaths, the development of shorter acting sedatives and early mobility programs has dramatically changed the practice of ICU sedation. Routine use of heavy sedation in ventilated patients is no longer favored. The goal is to have calm, lucid patients who are able to cooperate with their care.

Propofol and dexmedetomidine have gained popularity over benzodiazepines after a number of randomized trials demonstrated a shorter duration of mechanical ventilation and ICU length of stay, according to a 2015 Cochrane Review [5]. There seems to be some reduction in the risk of delirium, but the heterogeneity among the studies was high. The most common side effect associated with dexmedetomidine is bradycardia. There is no evidence that dexmedetomidine impacts mortality. In anesthesia literature, dexmedetomidine has been increasingly used for procedural sedation in lieu of propofol because of a better hemodynamic profile and less respiratory depression.

The most recent sedation practice guideline [6] by the Society of Critical Care Medicine calls for the aggressive monitoring and treatment of pain, agitation, and delirium, rather than masking the symptoms with sedatives. Some of the major recommendations are as follows:

1. Treat pain first.
2. Routine use of ICU sedation scores such as SAS (Sedation-Agitation scale) and RAAS (Richmond Sedation-Agitation scale) when administering sedatives.
3. Minimize benzodiazepines as the primary choice of sedative because of the increased association with delirium.
4. Monitor delirium with ICU-CAM (Confusion Assessment Method for the ICU).
5. Prevent ICU delirium with nonpharmacological measures.

In the past decade, as the overall trend moved away from heavy sedation, many have started evaluating nonpharmacological methods of reducing delirium. These methods include frequent reorientation, noise reduction, visual and hearing aids, and sleep promotion. Early ICU mobility programs are also safe and feasible. They consist of activities from passive range of motion to ambulating with a ventilator. Studies that couple lightened sedation with early mobility have demonstrated better functional outcome at discharge. Integrated programs such as the ABCDEF bundle by the ICU Delirium and Cognitive Impairment Study Group [7] are leading efforts to reduce delirium through these multidisciplinary approaches.

Back to our patient who underwent a laparotomy for perforated bowel: Following a few hours of additional resuscitation after arrival to the ICU, his hemodynamic status improved on decreased inotropic support. We anticipate our patient will need prolonged mechanical ventilation because of his acute lung injury. Our approach to sedation should incorporate a multimodal approach to minimize his ventilator time and ICU stay. Targeted light sedation with early mobility will benefit this patient greatly. In addition, optimal pain control is crucial as inadequate pain relief may delay weaning him from the ventilator. A regional anesthetic such as an epidural can be utilized to reduce the quantity of systemic opiates he receives. Side effects from large doses of opiates include sedation and delay of return of bowel function. Nonpharmacological measures such as promoting a day/night circadian cycle, along with frequent reorientation, may help prevent delirium. Finally, early mobility can prevent skeletal muscular weakness.

Summary

Growing evidence suggests that management of sedation and delirium has important effects on clinical outcome. Guidelines have evolved from deep sedation to daily wake-up and trials of spontaneous breathing to a more comprehensive approach to managing pain, agitation, and delirium. It seems that best practices are achieved with protocols that assess depth of sedation and pain, targeting appropriate sedatives and opiates. When administered, sedation should be kept to the minimum necessary to ensure patient safety and comfort. When possible, nonpharmacological methods should be utilized to minimize delirium.

The pendulum for sedation practice has been shifting over the past decade. Different stages of ICU care may require different levels of sedation. During the early active phase when there are multiple interventions and active resuscitation, deep sedation is a reasonable approach. During the convalescent phase when the patient remains critically ill but stable, light sedation paired with early mobility should be emphasized.

References

1. Kress JP, Pohlman AS, O'Connor MF, Hall JB. Daily interruption of sedative infusions in critically ill patients undergoing mechanical ventilation. N Engl J Med. 2000;342:1471–7.
2. Girard TD, Kress JP, Fuchs BD, Thomason JW, Schweickert WD, Pun BT, et al. Efficacy and safety of a paired sedation and ventilator weaning protocol for mechanically ventilated patients in intensive care (Awakening and Breathing Controlled trial): a randomized controlled trial. Lancet. 2008;371(9607):126–34.
3. Strome T, Martinussen T, Toft P. A protocol of no sedation for critically ill patients receiving mechanical ventilation: a randomized trial. Lancet. 2010;375(9713):475–80.
4. Mehta S, Burry L, Cook D, Fergusson D, Steinberg M, Granton J, et al. Daily sedation interruption in mechanically ventilated critically ill patients cared for with a sedation protocol, a randomized controlled trial. JAMA. 2012;308(19):1985–92.
5. Chen K, Lu Z, Xin YC, Cai Y, Chen Y, Pan SM. Alpha 2 agonist for long-term sedation during mechanical ventilation in critically ill patients. Cochrane Database Syst Rev. 2015;1:CD010269.
6. Barr J, Fraser GL, Puntillo K, Ely EW, Gelinas C, Dasta JF, et al. Clinical practice guideline for the management of pain, agitation, and delirium in adult patients in the intensive care unit. Crit Care Med. 2013;41:263–306.
7. ICU Delirium and Cognitive Impairment Study Group. "ABCDEF Bundle." www.icudelirium.org. Accessed 3 Nov 2015.

Is There Any Advantage to Albumin Over Crystalloid for Volume Resuscitation?

75

Michael J. Naso

Case

A 55-year-old male presents to the trauma bay after being involved in a motor vehicle accident while intoxicated. He is well known to the emergency department for multiple alcohol-related admissions, and has a past medical history of smoking, hypertension, mild renal insufficiency, and abnormal liver function tests and coagulation studies. He has sustained multiple fractures, is intubated for airway protection, and has a Glascow Coma Score of 8 on arrival. A chest tube is placed in the trauma bay for suspicion of pneumothorax, and a massive transfusion protocol is initiated. He is stable enough to be brought for a pan-computed tomography (CT) scan, which reveals a traumatic brain injury (TBI). At this point he deteriorates hemodynamically and the neurosurgical and trauma teams rush the patient to the operating room for emergent craniotomy and exploratory laparotomy.

Now in the operating room with invasive lines and monitors, the patient is requiring vasopressors/inotropes to maintain adequate mean arterial pressures (MAP) after resuscitation has begun with liters of crystalloid and blood products. Should you as the anesthesiologist administer albumin to replete the intravascular volume, improve the stroke volume index, and reduce cerebral edema?

Question

Is there any reason to administer albumin in addition to standard resuscitation with crystalloids, blood products, vasopressors, and inotropes?

PRO: A drug usage evaluation (DUE) revealed in 2009 that only 53 % of albumin use met the current criteria and 70 % of the albumin was used by 3 services (medicine, transplant, and cardiothoracic surgery) [1]. Guidelines for the Use of Albumin were developed by the University Hospital Consortium, published in the *Archives of Internal Medicine* and most recently revised in 2010 [1]. They address 12 indications for albumin use and often did not follow the US Food and Drug Administration (FDA)-approved recommendations as first-line therapy. Non-protein colloids such as hetastarch and dextrans were offered as first-line, less costly alternatives. This treatment paradigm has shifted in recent years as these colloids have become notoriously implicated with renal failure, hypersensitivity, and increased risk of bleeding. The DUE clearly shows that clinicians were not considering the use of albumin as a viable alternative even for FDA-approved indications [1].

It is my opinion that with the competition from other colloids, the use of albumin is not being considered in the acutely ill patients who need emergent cardiovascular resuscitation.

The FDA indications for albumin include hemorrhagic and maldistributive shock, hepatic resection, burns, cerebral ischemia or hemorrhage, cardiac bypass surgery, nutritional intervention, acute nephropathy/nephrotic syndrome, hyperbilirubinemia of the newborn, ascities/cirrhosis/spontaneous bacterial peritonitis/hepatorenal syndrome, organ transplant, plasmapheresis, and acute respiratory distress syndrome (ARDS).

CON: Multiple clinical trials have failed to consistently demonstrate any difference between colloid and crystalloid in the treatment of septic shock [2–4]. A Cochrane review of 24 studies suggested albumin administration resulted in a 6 % increased risk of death [5], but a larger Cochrane review in 2013 analyzed 78 randomized controlled trials looking at colloids versus crystalloids for fluid resuscitation in trauma, burns, and post-surgical patients and found no evidence that colloid administration improved mortality and that starches might actually increase the relative risk (RR) of death: RR of albumin 1 (95 % CI .92–1.09), hetastarch RR 1.1 (CI 1.02–1.1) [6]. Based on these results, the authors

M.J. Naso (✉)
Philadelphia, PA, USA
e-mail: MichaelJ.Naso@gmail.com

C.S. Scher et al. (eds.), *You're Wrong, I'm Right*, DOI 10.1007/978-3-319-43169-7_75

recommended that the use of colloids rather than crystalloids was hard to justify because of their substantially higher cost [6].

Despite albumin administration to neurosurgical ICU patients being listed as an indication, there is preliminary evidence (SAFE study) that its use is considered inappropriate. The SAFE study (saline versus albumin fluid evaluation) suggested that patients resuscitated with albumin had a higher mortality rate than those resuscitated with saline [4].

PRO: The mortality results of the SAFE trial may not be at all relevant because 28-day all-cause mortality is not an appropriate end point to assess outcomes for patients with brain injuries. A more meaningful end point for research in patients with TBI is mortality and functional neurological status at least 6 months after injury [7]. Furthermore, patients with TBI represented only 7 % of the study population [4]. The SAFE study [4] also excluded patients admitted to the intensive care unit (ICU) after cardiac surgery, liver transplantation, and burns, all of which are FDA-approved indications for treatment with albumin.

CON: The SAFE trial was a multicenter, randomized, double-blinded trial to compare saline and albumin on heterogeneous ICU patient populations and found absolutely no differences between death, single or multiple organ failure, days spent in the ICU or hospital, or days of mechanical ventilation or renal replacement therapy [4].In patients with severe traumatic brain injury (GCS score, 3 to 8), 61 of 146 patients in the albumin group (41.8%) had died at 24 months as compared with 32 of 144 in the saline group (22.2%) (relative risk, 1.88; 95% CI, 1.31 to 2.70; $P<0.001$). The authors proposed that contrary to the expectation of reduced cerebral edema from increased plasma oncotic pressure, albumin leak across the damaged blood brain barrier caused paradoxical cerebral edema. This theory was further supported by patients with intracranial pressure (ICP) monitors; the albumin group's ICPs were higher, but this needs further study [8]. Mannitol and hypertonic saline are commonly used in these patients.

PRO: True, but the CRISTAL trial, published that same year, showed no mortality differences at 28 days but a RR of death of .92 ($p = .03$) in the colloid group at 90 days, meaning that there were significantly more patients who survived 90 days in the colloid group [2]. Also in the CRISTAL trial, there were more days alive without mechanical ventilation by 7 days and 28 days ($p = .01$) and more days alive without vasopressor therapy by 7 days ($p = .04$) and by 28 days ($p = .03$) [2].

Concession from CON: The CRISTAL study population differs from other trials because it only enrolled patients with hypotension and lactic acidosis [2]. The difference in baseline hemodynamic status of patients before randomization may account for the difference in colloid resuscitation mortality from previous studies. This population may reflect the patient population that we as anesthesiologists are likely to encounter in emergent cases.

PRO: Even in the SAFE trial, whose results strongly condemned the use of albumin, patients in the colloid group received significantly less fluid volume to achieve the same hemodynamic targets than patients in the crystalloid group, while maintaining better MAP and central venous pressure (CVP) [4].

In the CRISTAL study, fluid resuscitation based on colloids administration showed a similar mortality and morbidity to a strategy based only on crystalloids and patients did not experience more complications such as kidney failure or, severe shock with multi-organ failure [2].

Concession from PRO: Hetastarch and dextrans, which are commonly administered colloids and have known negative renal impacts, showed no differences in the CRISTAL trial [2]. The lack of adverse outcomes known to be associated with hetastarch, especially in patients in shock and at high risk of acute renal injury, can be explained by exclusion of patients with chronic renal failure from the trial; hetastarch volume administration was limited to the manufacturer's guidelines, and further, colloids may prevent renal injury by improving cardiac output.

Summary

In conclusion, albumin is a safe alternative to fluid resuscitation with crystalloid only. It has no difference in mortality and can help achieve satisfactory cardiovascular end points such as mean arterial pressures with less volume, which is important in patients who may become volume overloaded. As for the patient in the scenario presented, the results of the SAFE trial subgroup analysis suggest a randomized controlled trial in patients with traumatic brain injuries will help elucidate whether a crystalloid versus crystalloid plus colloid fluid resuscitation strategy affects mortality.

References

1. Vermeulen LC, Ratko TA, Erstad BL, Brecher ME, Matuszewski KA. A paradigm for consensus. The University Hospital Consortium guidelines for the use of albumin, nonprotein colloid, and crystalloid solutions. Arch Intern Med. 1995;155:373–9 (revised 2010).

2. Annane D, Siami S, Jaber S, Martin C, Elatrous S, Declère AD, CRISTAL Investigators, et al. Effects of fluid resuscitation with colloids versus crystalloids on mortality in critically ill patients presenting with hypovolemic shock: The CRISTAL randomized trial. JAMA. 2013;310:1809–17.
3. Orbegozo Cortes D, Santacruz C, Donadello K, Nobile L, Taccone FS. Colloids for fluid resuscitation: what is their role in patients with shock? Minerva Anestesiol. 2014;80:963–9.
4. Finfer S, Bellomo R, Boyce N, French J, Myburgh J, Norton R, SAFE Study Investigators. A comparison of albumin and saline for fluid resuscitation in the intensive care unit. N Engl J Med. 2004;350:2247–56.
5. [no authors listed] Cochrane Injuries Group Albumin Reviewers. Human albumin administration in critically ill patients: a systematic review of randomized controlled trials. BMJ 1998;317:235–40.
6. Perel P, Roberts I, Ker K. Colloids versus crystalloids for fluid resuscitation in critically ill patients. Cochrane Database Syst Rev. 2013;2:CD000567.
7. Narayan RK, Michel ME, Ansell B, Baethmann A, Biegon A, Bracken MB, et al. Clinical trials in head injury. J Neurotrauma. 2002;19:503–57.
8. Gantner D, Moore EM, Cooper DJ. Intravenous fluids in traumatic brain injury: what's the solution? Curr Opin Crit Care. 2014;20:385–9.

There Is Nothing Dexmedetomidine Does that Cannot Be Done Old School

76

Hersh Patel

Case

Pediatric anesthesiology was mesmerizing. Watching the anesthesiologist use tools scaled down to facilitate management of airways the size of my pupil enticed me. More importantly, as a medical student, I was an observer and I was keen on understanding the intricacies of the magic performed behind that blue curtain. And so it was another day on my rotation as the anesthesiology team wheeled down a patient from the pediatric intensive care unit (PICU). The child was aged 3 years who was unfortunately inflicted with a relatively rare disorder known as nemaline myopathy. She lay flaccid and weak with nasal bi-level positive airway pressure (BiPAP) assisting her every breath. As I stared into the portable monitor where the pulse oximeter measured a frustrating 89 %, the attending looked at me and asked, "What are we worried about in this patient?"

As everything I learned in medical school escaped me at that very moment, my reflex fail-safe response kicked in with "airway, breathing, and circulation."

I immediately heard a pretentious chuckle behind me followed by the statement, "We're obviously worried about malignant hyperthermia."

In my short-lived years in the medical field, I've learned that modesty goes a long way at the bottom of the totem pole. The attending abruptly pulled back on the reins of the stretcher and glared back at the resident who had made the decree about malignant hyperthermia.

> There is no increased risk over the general population [1]. Our medical student is absolutely correct, airway management will be challenging when performing a bronchoscopy on a BiPAP-dependent patient like ours," the attending said.

H. Patel
Department of Anesthesiology,
New York University Langone Medical Center,
550 First Avenue, New York, NY 10016, USA

H. Patel (✉)
11 Kelly Way, Monmouth Junction, NJ 08852, USA
e-mail: hersh.patel2@nyumc.org

> "Nemaline myopathy is an autosomal recessive disease classified into 6 types based on time of onset and severity of symptoms. The most severe types have low life expectancies secondary to respiratory failure [2], but no association to malignant hyperthermia.

The challenge in this patient was maintaining sufficient ventilation while providing appropriate sedation and analgesia during a bronchoscopy. The attending had discussed managing the airway via a mask with swivel adapter connected to the anesthesia circuit to provide positive pressure ventilation throughout the case. The more challenging question became, "What anesthetics do you plan on using to provide amnesia, analgesia, and sedation while maintaining spontaneous ventilation?"

The resident promptly responded with "dexmedetomidine," which incited a clash between the old and new age of anesthetics.

Question

The attending asked, "What does dexmedetomidine do that can't be done with older drugs?"

We began by discussing the basic pharmacology of the medication. Dexmedetomidine is a highly selective alpha-2 agonist thought to have all of the properties required for sedation, analgesia, anxiolysis, sympatholysis, and opioid sparing. These effects are mediated by subset receptors: Alpha-2a promotes sedation, hypnosis, analgesia, neuroprotection, and inhibition of insulin secretion; alpha-2b centrally suppresses shivering, provides analgesia at the spinal cord, and induces vasoconstriction in the periphery; and alpha-2c modulates sensory processing, locomotor activity, and epinephrine outflow from the medulla. All 3 subtypes generally affect inhibition of norepinephrine release [3].

PRO (Resident): Dexmedetomidine allows the patient to maintain spontaneous ventilation during anesthesia.

C.S. Scher et al. (eds.), *You're Wrong, I'm Right*, DOI 10.1007/978-3-319-43169-7_76

Propofol, barbiturates, and benzodiazepines cause respiratory depression, while dexmedetomidine can even be used through tracheal extubation and beyond [4]. A key benefit of dexmedetomidine infusions is its limited effect on respiration with a wide margin of safety at higher doses [5]. It also allows for preservation of hypercapnic arousal, while decreasing apneic threshold [3].

CON (Attending): I have been using ketamine for years with the same effect. In fact, it has less cardio-depressive effects and improves bronchiole relaxation in patients prone to bronchospasm [6]. More importantly, the doses of ketamine approved by the US Food and Drug Administration (FDA) have more reliable sedative effects than dexmedetomidine.

One of the major controversies surrounding dexmedetomidine is its dosing. Many clinicians find variable response to the medication with sedation. Jones et al demonstrated that patients who received doses greater than those approved by the FDA (max 0.7 μg/kg/min) had a lower percentage of Richmond Agitation-Sedation Scale (RAAS) scores at goal and a higher percentage in the unsedated category than those receiving less than 0.7 μg/kg/min. Interestingly, the side effect profile remained constant even with these higher doses [7]. A phase 2 trial on medical ICU patients by Venn et al showed that 58 % of patients on rates as high as 2.5 μg/kg/min still required rescue doses of propofol [8].

PRO: Ketamine sounds like a good option, but if we need to intubate this patient, dexmedetomidine will attenuate the hemodynamic stress response. Another benefit of dexmedetomidine is its sympatholytic properties [9] and is commonly used as an adjunct in patients with disorders that are exacerbated by stress responses, such as urea cycle disorders. It has also been shown to reduce oxygen consumption [10], which along with the sympatholytic effects may improve cardiac outcomes [11].

CON: For years, sympatholytics such as beta-blockers have worked just fine. With chronic disease, the patient may be completely reliant on adrenergic tone for stability. How will she overcome the bradycardic and hypotensive effects of this drug? Adverse effects for dexmedetomidine include hypotension (30 %), hypertension (12 %), nausea (11 %), bradycardia (9 %), and dry mouth (3 %) [12]. Dexmedetomidine exhibits a biphasic, dose-dependent change in blood pressure in the setting of decreasing norepinephrine concentrations while progressively decreasing heart rate and cardiac output [13]. At low doses, mean arterial pressure decreases without any changes to central venous pressure or pulmonary and systemic vascular resistance. At higher doses, all of these parameters increase.

PRO: Aside from the hemodynamics, I've been told that children wake up better with dexmedetomidine and require less opioids overall. In a study performed by Shukry et al, 50 children were randomized to receive either placebo or dexmedetomidine 0.2 mcg/kg/h [14]. The study revealed a significantly lower incidence of delirium in children receiving this low-dose infusion during emergence, but no effect on pain score, time to extubation, or discharge from recovery time [14].

The opioid-sparing effects of dexmedetomidine are more controversial. The analgesic properties are thought to be spinally and supraspinally mediated through activation of alpha-2a receptors, inhibition of nociceptive signals, and release of local endorphins. Venn et al showed that dexmedetomidine in the postoperative period reduced analgesic requirements by 50 % in cardiac patients [5].

CON: Propofol, fentanyl, and midazolam can achieve similar clinical effects at lower costs [15]. Even though dexmedetomidine provides many benefits to the patient, the overall cost compared to benefits received may be unnecessarily higher. The long-term effects or benefits have not been well established and would need to be evaluated for a more comprehensive understanding of the opioid-sparing effects.

Summary

While dexmedetomidine is far from the perfect anesthetic, it provides a strong set of anesthetic qualities, including analgesia, sedation, hypnosis, anxiolysis, sympatholysis, and opioid sparing. It serves as a powerful adjunct among the anesthesia arsenal, but also requires vigilance, as with any potent chemical, especially with its tendency toward inducing bradycardia and hypotension. This short-acting, quick onset drug creates an effective respiratory milieu for spontaneous ventilation and may be advantageous for this patient, but not necessary. Each anesthetic comes with its own set of advantages and disadvantages. Optimization requires a balanced anesthetic approach, and each user will justify their own personalized technique. Until multiple studies show clear evidence of a single drug being the perfect anesthetic, controversy over the choice of anesthetic will persist.

References

1. Davis PJ, Brandom BW. The association of malignant hyperthermia and unusual disease: when you're hot you're hot or maybe not. Anesth Analg. 2009;109(4):1001–3.
2. Genetics Home Reference. Nemaline myopathy. http://ghr.nlm.nih.gov/condition/nemaline-myopathy. Accessed 4 Sept 2015.
3. Afonso J, Reis F. Dexmedetomidine: current role in anesthesia and intensive care. Rev Bras Anestesiol. 2012;62(1):118–33.

4. Panzer O, Moitra V, Sladen RN. Pharmacology of sedative–analgesic agents: dexmedetomidine, remifentanil, ketamine, volatile anesthetics, and the role of peripheral mu antagonists. Crit Care Clin. 2009;25(3):451–69 vii.
5. Venn RM, Bradshaw CJ, Spencer R, Brealey D, Caudwell E, et al. Preliminary UK experience of dexmedetomidine, a novel agent for postoperative sedation in the intensive care unit. Anaesthesia. 1999;54(12):1136–42.
6. Miller AC, Jamin CT, Elamin EM. Continuous intravenous infusion of ketamine for maintenance sedation. Minerva Anestesiol. 2011;77(8):812–20.
7. Venn M, Newman J, Grounds M. A phase II study to evaluate the efficacy of dexmedetomidine for sedation in the medical intensive care unit. Intensive Care Med. 2003;29(2):201–7.
8. Jones GM, Murphy CV, Gerlach AT, Goodman EM, Pell LJ. High-dose dexmedetomidine for sedation in the intensive care unit: an evaluation of clinical efficacy and safety. Ann Pharmacother. 2011;45(6):740–7.
9. Keniya VM, Ladi S, Naphade R. Dexmedetomidine attenuates sympathoadrenal response to tracheal intubation and reduces perioperative anaesthetic requirement. Indian J Anaesth. 2011;55(4):352–7.
10. Taittonen MT, Kirvelä OA, Aantaa R, Kanto JH. Effect of clonidine and dexmedetomidine premedication on perioperative oxygen consumption and haemodynamic state. Br J Anaesth. 1997;78(4):400–6.
11. Yu SB. Dexmedetomidine sedation in ICU. Korean J Anesthesiol. 2012;62(5):405–11.
12. Gerlach AT, Dasta JF. Dexmedetomidine: an updated review. Ann Pharmacother. 2007;41(2):245–52.
13. Ebert TJ, Hall JE, Barney JA, Uhrich TD, Colinco MD. The effects of increasing plasma concentrations of dexmedetomidine in humans. Anesthesiology. 2000;93(2):382–94.
14. Shukry M, Clyde MC, Kalarickal PL, Ramadhyani U. Does dexmedetomidine prevent emergence delirium in children after sevoflurane-based general anesthesia? Paediatr Anaesth. 2005;15(12):1098–104.
15. Naaz S, Ozair E. Dexmedetomidine in current anaesthesia practice—a review. J Clin Diagn Res. 2014;8(10):1–4.

Does Treating Systemic Inflammatory Response Syndrome Lead to Better Outcomes in Surgical Patients?

77

Nader Soliman

Case

A 40-year-old obese woman presents for a laparoscopic cholecystectomy for acute cholecystitis and cholelithiasis. The gallbladder was found to be inflamed, and the case was converted to open. The most common systemic complications of open cholecystectomy are pulmonary in nature; however, surgical procedure-related complications are also possible such as surgical site or intra-abdominal infections, a bile leak, or bleeding, all of which may produce an inflammatory response.

The inflammatory response is initiated by cytokines, which are polypeptide signaling molecules that adhere to specific receptors with an autocrine, paracrine, and/or endocrine mechanism in response to an instigating stimulus. This process is kept in check with anti-inflammatory cytokines. At times, the pro-inflammatory cytokines overwhelm the anti-inflammatory cytokines, which may lead to a systemic inflammatory response rather than a localized one. The major influential pro-inflammatory cytokines are as follows: interleukin-1 (IL-1), tumor necrosis factor-alpha (TNF-α[alpha]), interleukin-6 (IL-6), interleukin-8 (IL-8), and macrophage inflammatory protein-1α(alpha) (MIP-1alpha). The major anti-inflammatory cytokines are interleukin-10 (IL-10) and interleukin-13 (IL-13).

Systemic inflammatory response syndrome (SIRS) is defined as a systemic response to a nonspecific infectious or noninfectious insult. Examples are burns, pancreatitis, an autoimmune disorder, ischemia, or trauma. The presence of two or more of the following clinical criteria helps establish the diagnosis of SIRS: (1) body temperature >38°C (100.4°F) or <36°C (96.8°F), (2) heart rate >90 beats per minute, (3) respiratory rate more than 20 breaths per minute or hyperventilation with an arterial carbon dioxide tension (PaCO2) ≤32 mm Hg, and (4) abnormal white blood cell count (>12,000/mcL or <4000/mcL or >10 % immature [band] forms) [1–3]. This unchecked destructive response may lead to organ dysfunction and failure.

N. Soliman
Department of Anesthesiology, New York University, New York, NY 10016, USA

N. Soliman (✉)
3844 Wasatch Ave Apt 4, Los Angeles, CA 90066, USA
e-mail: solinader85@yahoo.com

Questions

Does treating SIRS lead to better outcomes in surgical patients? If so, which treatment options are most promising?

PRO: I believe that recognition and early treatment of SIRS are important to influence its natural course and decrease morbidity and mortality. Did you know that the Italian SEPSIS study showed an inverse correlation between the identification of SIRS and the development of sepsis [1]? This is why there are several different treatment strategies for SIRS including physiological, pharmacological, and/or cytokine adsorption therapy [1]. These strategies target supposed triggers, early mediators, and physiological responses to inflammation.

CON: You might be right, but what are these strategies and how do they work exactly in the treatment for SIRS and multi-organ dysfunction syndrome?

PRO: Great question Early goal-directed therapy works by optimizing cardiac pre-load, after-load, and contractility. This optimizes oxygen delivery to the heart and systemic tissues, therefore, reducing morbidity and mortality in patients with SIRS, shock, and severe sepsis [1, 2].

CON: That could possibly work, but keen recognition for signs of SIRS and quick action are of upmost importance for this strategy to be successful.

PRO: That is true! As you may know, TNF-α(alpha) is one of the major cytokines in the development and propagation

C.S. Scher et al. (eds.), *You're Wrong, I'm Right*, DOI 10.1007/978-3-319-43169-7_77

of SIRS. Its plasma levels have been found to rise rapidly when measured following any insult. Pharmacological therapies targeting pro-inflammatory cytokines have been developed in hope of treating SIRS and sepsis. In the MONARCS trial from North America, a study of 2634 septic patients using afelimomab (anti-TNF-α[alpha] Fab2 monoclonal antibody fragment) showed a significant reduction in mortality of 3.6 % [1]. It also displayed a significant reduction in levels of TNF-α(alpha) and IL-6, and rapid improvement in organ failure scores compared with placebo [1–3].

CON: I've read that trial, and these results are directed toward septic patients, not patients with only SIRS [3]. I don't think that single monoclonal therapy will be enough given the multifaceted nature of the dyscytokinaemia in SIRS.

PRO: Well, maybe you heard of antioxidant micronutrient supplementation such as selenium and glutamine in improving outcomes in patients with SIRS and sepsis. Selenium given intravenously at high doses when compared to placebo significantly improved Acute Physiology and Chronic Health Evaluation (APACHE) scores and reduced the incidence of renal failure requiring hemodialysis. Gut permeability to endotoxin may be decreased by oral glutamine, which in turn may reduce cytokine levels, as well as reduce temperature, heart rate, and leukocyte count [1]. This could be used as an adjunct to other therapies.

CON: I understand that Berger et al. claim Level A evidence for using these supplements, but the inquiry is open to the way the cytokines are actually being influenced [1]. Also, the data for oral glutamine have been inconclusive.

PRO: If a multimodal approach to SIRS therapy will be used, then the anchor to this method should be hemoadsorption technology. It has been proven that with the use of CytoSorb® (CytoSorbents Corp., Monmouth Junction, NJ), the patient's hemodynamic profile improves faster, while the need for catecholamine support decreases. This technology uses highly biocompatible and hemocompatible porous high-tech polymer beads that work during blood purification therapies by trapping and permanently eliminating molecules sized in the range of 5–60 kDa from the blood. Most cytokines fall within that range [4]. In a case study, CytoSorb was used as an adjuvant therapy in combination with continuous veno-venous hemofiltration on a patient with postoperative septic shock after undergoing a cephalic pancreatectomy. It was observed that there was a decrease in the levels of TNF-α(alpha), IL-1β(beta), and interferon-gamma (IFN-γ[gamma]) while there was an increase in IL-10 levels. This correlated with a decrease in vasopressor requirements and provided a more stable hemodynamic profile and cardiac output while normalizing the systemic vascular resistance index [4].

CON: I actually read that case report and would like to add that while the patient seemed to improve he ended up dying 24 h after the second CytoSorb was discontinued. You have mentioned several options to treat SIRS, but they have one thing in common, they lack extensive affirmative evidence for treating SIRS specifically! It just seems too early to get excited about these strategies.

Summary

The central mechanism in initiating SIRS is complex but is likely to be the secretion of cytokines anomalously. Cytokines are peptides and glycoproteins of low molecular weight, which function as intercellular mediators regulating inflammation, wound healing, local and systemic immune responses, and hematopoiesis. The resulting inflammatory response includes release of potentially harmful phospholipids, attraction of neutrophils, and activation of the complement, kinin, and coagulation cascades. Current treatments for SIRS have not shown much promise, but with a multimodal therapeutic approach and further research focused on hemoadsorption technology strategies, SIRS looks to be tamable in the near future.

References

1. Jaffer U, Wade RG, Gourlay T. Cytokines in the systemic inflammatory response syndrome: a review. HSR Proc Intensive Care Cardiovasc Anesth. 2010;2(3):161–75.
2. Born F, Pichlmaier M, Peterss S, Khaladj N, Hagl C. Systemic inflammatory response syndrome in heart surgery: new possibilities for treatment through the use of a cytokine adsorber during ECC? Kardiotechnik. 2014.
3. Toft P, Tonnesen E. The systemic inflammatory response to anesthesia and surgery. Curr Anesth Crit Care 2008;349–53.
4. Tomescu D, Dima SO, Tănăsescu S, Tănase CP, Năstase A, Popescu M. Effects of a novel cytokine haemoadsorbtion system on inflammatory response in septic shock after cephalic pancreatectomy —a case report. Rom J Anaesth Int Care. 2014;21(2):134–8.

Should Mechanically Ventilated Intensive Care Unit Patients Receive Physical Therapy?

78

Jonathan V. Feldstein

Case

An obese 45-year-old man is brought to our level-one trauma center after being struck by a car while on his motorcycle. He was in the right lane on the highway when a sleep-deprived delivery driver swerved to make the exit and clipped the victim's back tire. The focused assessment with sonography in trauma (FAST) scan in the trauma slot reveals significant abdominal bleeding. An exploratory laparotomy finds a ruptured spleen requiring splenectomy for source control. Due to bowel swelling and the patient's body habitus, the abdomen cannot be closed. A vacuum dressing is placed over the incision, and the patient is brought to the surgical intensive care unit (ICU).

The next day, a physiatrist responds to the automatically ordered rehabilitation medicine consult. He loosely outlines a rehabilitation plan for this patient, "Passive range-of-motion exercises of upper and lower extremities while patient is sedated. Progress to assisted active range of motion when patient becomes interactive. Rehab medicine to follow."

Later that afternoon when the physical therapist is making rounds in the ICU, she skips the patient's room. "He is not on my list of patients for today. The order must have gone in too late. I will see him tomorrow." When she looks into his room the following day, the nurse tells her, "He went to the operating room for an abdominal washout." Finally, on hospital day 3, the physical therapist is able to work with the patient. The patient is still requiring heavy sedation, so she attempts to do passive range-of-motion (ROM) exercises. Unfortunately, the patient's legs are too heavy for her to lift so she is only able to work on his upper extremities. Two days later, the patient is still intubated but more interactive. The physical therapist works on assisted active exercises, but again struggles to move his legs. Her note from the day reads, "Patient is not a strong candidate for physical therapy at this time. Please reconsult rehab medicine when condition improves."

J.V. Feldstein (✉)
Department of Anesthesiology, New York University Langone Medical Center, 550 First Avenue, Suite 530, New York, NY 10016, USA
e-mail: jonathan.feldstein@nyumc.org

Question

Should mechanically ventilated ICU patients receive physical therapy?

CON: The physical therapist is questioned about signing off on the patient. She states that there are many patients who need physical therapy in the hospital and her time may be better spent with those who can actively participate. She sees very little improvement in strength and functionality in her mechanically ventilated patients compared with non-critical patients in the hospital.

PRO: After a literature review, you present a few interesting papers to the physical therapist. You find multiple studies showing positive outcomes from early institution of physical therapy in mechanically ventilated and other critically ill patients. While some of the benefits may not be seen immediately, they are significant over the course of an admission. A multi-center randomized control trial by Schweickert et al. randomized 104 mechanically ventilated patients to early exercise and mobilization during daily interruption of sedation or to only daily interruption of sedation [1]. The unresponsive patients underwent passive range-of-motion and progressed to active assisted/independent exercises when they became more alert. When the patient was able, therapy sessions escalated to bed-mobility, transferring, sitting, and even as far as pre-gait/walking exercises in some patients. More patients in the intervention group returned to independent functional status at hospital discharge compared to the control group. They also found that the patients receiving early therapy had a shorter duration of delirium and more ventilator-free days than control patients had. Prolonged immobility can lead to ICU-acquired weakness, which further

C.S. Scher et al. (eds.), *You're Wrong, I'm Right*, DOI 10.1007/978-3-319-43169-7_78

hinders a return to baseline functionality. Patel et al. found that when early mobilization was used alongside intensive insulin therapy, early mobilization decreased the incidence of ICU-associated weakness while significantly decreasing insulin requirements [2].

CON: The physical therapist cannot argue with these findings and thanks you for the papers. She reminds you, though, that it is not as easy as sending a physical therapist to the ICU and starting an early mobilization program. Critically ill patients, especially those who are mechanically ventilated, pose unique safety concerns. Patients are often tethered by multiple access lines, monitors, and ventilation circuits. The disconnection of any of this equipment by a person not trained to replace it could lead to adverse events such as the interruption of vasoactive medication in a hemodynamically unstable patient. Physical therapists have little to no airway management training, making extubation a potentially more devastating event.

PRO: These concerns are valid without a doubt, but in your literature search, you also came across impressive safety data. After training physical therapists in a progressive mobilization program specifically for critical care patients, Sricharoenchai et al. reported only 34 potential safety events over the course of 5267, or 0.6 %, of all physical therapy sessions [3]. The most common events were arrhythmia (10 occurrences) and mean arterial pressures higher than 140 mm Hg (8 occurrences) or less than 55 mm Hg (5 occurrences). There were no reported extubations, removals of central venous lines, or cardiopulmonary arrests. In fact, of all these potential safety events, only 4 mandated additional treatment or cost.

CON: The physical therapist again welcomes the paper you present and reads it carefully. As she scrutinizes the methods of the paper, she notices that the ICU studied had the equivalent of 2.25 full-time equivalents of physical therapy support for 16 patients. The patients were also able to get therapy 6 days a week. This amount of staffing immediately strikes her as impressive and likely expensive. Considering the additional training and staffing needed for the study, she questions whether it would be more cost-effective to wait until the patients improve to a level of acuity that the therapists are currently equipped to handle.

PRO: You acknowledge that instituting a protocol similar to the one in the study would undoubtedly require more resources than currently being utilized. Fortunately, as daily rehabilitation is standard of care across most of Europe, several groups have shared their experiences. McWilliams et al. published a quality improvement project in which they instituted an ICU rehabilitation team [4]. Their unit designated a critical care physiotherapy specialist to lead a team that was trained in a progressive early mobilization program similar to the program described earlier. The introduction of this team was associated with a reduction in ICU length of stay by 2 days and total hospital length of stay by 5 days. McWilliams's team noted that the reduction in critical care length of stay would translate into significant financial benefits. For their 292 patient cohorts, they calculated a saving of 584 critical care bed days, which increased availability of beds for new admissions. Seemingly, the establishment of such a critical care rehabilitation team would eventually be more economical than less aggressive rehabilitation programs.

Summary

There is convincing evidence for the establishment of a critical care-specific rehabilitation team. These teams can have an impressive impact on mechanically ventilated patients, including earlier return to independent functional status, shorter duration of delirium, more ventilator-free days, decreased ICU-associated weakness, decreased ICU length of stay, and decreased hospital length of stay. While the implementation of these teams would be initially resource-intensive, the programs would likely be cost-effective in the long run.

References

1. Schweickert WD, Pohlman MC, Pohlman AS, Nigos C, Pawlik AJ, Esbrook CL, et al. Early physical and occupational therapy in mechanically ventilated, critically ill patients: a randomised controlled trial. Lancet. 2009;373(9678):1874–82.
2. Patel BK, Pohlman AS, Hall JB, Kress JP. Impact of early mobilization on glycemic control and ICU-acquired weakness in critically ill patients who are mechanically ventilated. Chest. 2014;146(3):583–9.
3. Sricharoenchai T, Parker AM, Zanni JM, Nelliot A, Dinglas VD, Needham DM. Safety of physical therapy interventions in critically ill patients: a single-center prospective evaluation of 1110 intensive care unit admissions. J Crit Care. 2014;29(3):395–400.
4. McWilliams D, Weblin J, Atkins G, Bion J, Williams J, Elliott C, et al. Enhancing rehabilitation of mechanically ventilated patients in the intensive care unit: a quality improvement project. J Crit Care. 2015;30(1):13–8.

Part IX
Ambulatory

Should Persistent Postoperative Nausea and Vomiting Delay Discharge of an Ambulatory Surgery Patient from the Post-anesthesia Care Unit?

79

David Shapiro and Andrew Goldberg

Case

A 43-year-old woman with a past medical history of menorrhagia and uterine fibroids just underwent a laparoscopic myomectomy this morning under general anesthesia. Her anesthesia care included desflurane, nitrous oxide, and intermittent boluses of fentanyl and rocuronium. She received dexamethasone before surgical incision and ondansetron 20 min prior to emergence. She woke up comfortable and without complaints. Thirty minutes into her recovery in the post-anesthesia care unit (PACU), she began to experience nausea and had 2 episodes of non-bloody, non-bilious emesis. More ondansetron was given and the patient reported slight improvement of her symptoms, but the nausea returned shortly thereafter.

Roughly 60 % of all surgeries performed in the United States occur in the ambulatory setting. Postoperative nausea and vomiting (PONV) is one of the most common complications associated with outpatient surgical procedures and is also a major factor limiting early postoperative discharge. In addition, PONV is uncomfortable for affected patients, sometimes more so than pain [1].

Studies have shown that approximately 30–60 % of patients who do not receive anti-emetic prophylaxis will experience postoperative nausea, vomiting, or both. In high-risk patients, PONV rates can be as high as 80 % [2–4]. Although the complications of PONV are rarely fatal, it can frustrate providers, decrease patient satisfaction, delay discharge, lead to unanticipated hospital admissions, increase resource utilization, and cost the healthcare system hundreds of millions of dollars annually [2].

D. Shapiro (✉) · A. Goldberg
Department of Anesthesiology, Icahn School of Medicine at Mount Sinai, 1 Gustave L. Levy Place, Box 1010 New York, NY 10029, USA
e-mail: David.Shapiro@mountsinai.org

A. Goldberg
e-mail: andrew.goldberg@mountsinai.org

Question

Can we send a stable patient with adequate pain control home from the PACU if she continues to experience nausea and vomiting several hours after her procedure?

PRO: The patient needs to be discharged! Her symptoms will resolve without further intervention. She has just about every risk factor for PONV: She just had a laparoscopic gynecological surgery; she is a relatively young woman, a non-smoker; and she received a volatile anesthetic for general anesthesia maintenance, neostigmine, as well as 200 mcg of fentanyl and 0.5 mg of hydromorphone over the past 3 h in the PACU. Is it really surprising that she is having a prolonged PACU course?

The patient has already received 2 different anti-emetics as well an additional liter of fluid in the PACU. We can only do so much for patients who are at the highest risk of PONV. While the volatile anesthetic she was given is a known risk factor for PONV, it is only thought to cause *early* PONV in the first 2 h postoperatively [5]. Therefore, by the time she gets home, her symptoms will likely improve. She just needs time.

CON: It would be unwise to send her home now. Do you really want a nauseous patient ambulating? Early ambulation, especially in patients with PONV is thought to exacerbate and prolong symptoms. We can certainly do more to try and alleviate her symptoms. Have you taken a look at the latest guidelines for PONV?

PRO: I am just following the Modified Post Anesthesia Discharge Scoring System (PADSS), which has been studied and validated. PADSS criteria include the following: (1) vital signs, (2) activity, (3) pain, (4) surgical bleeding, and (5) nausea and vomiting. Patients receive 0–2 points based on clinical status and those with PADSS scores $\geq$9 are fit for discharge [6]. Our patient scores 9 out of 10 possible points (given her moderate nausea and vomiting and

C.S. Scher et al. (eds.), *You're Wrong, I'm Right*, DOI 10.1007/978-3-319-43169-7_79

successful, although transient, relief of symptoms early in her PACU course) and therefore is fit for discharge.

CON: Yes, if you follow those guidelines, she is a candidate for discharge, but sometimes you have to do your own thinking and consider the patient's clinical context. All of medicine does not fit into an algorithm. I do not think you are doing right by the patient by sending her home at this point. We still have more to offer her to try and alleviate her symptoms. What if we send her home with the oral anti-emetics and her symptoms worsen again?

Let's examine the latest guidelines on managing PONV. First, we should reduce the amount of postoperative opioids this patient receives for her pain as these can directly increase PONV. Cancel her orders for all that fentanyl and hydromorphone. We can offer ketorolac and acetaminophen since those are opioid-sparing pain medications. Second, an anti-emetic should be given that is from a different pharmacologic class than the initial drug. Options include promethazine 6.25–12.5 mg IV, or less commonly, droperidol 0.625 mg IV. An awareness should be maintained of common side effects—both can potentiate respiratory depression, promethazine can cause hallucinations, and droperidol can lead to dysphoria. Of note, haloperidol 0.5–2 mg IM or IV can be regarded as an alternative to droperidol, but it should be noted that its use as an anti-emetic or its IV administration is considered off-label use by the US Food and Drug Administration (FDA). Finally, propofol, 20 mg IV, can be utilized as a rescue therapy [7].

PRO: We need space in the PACU for the patients currently in surgery. It costs our center thousands of dollars to pay overtime to our staff, keep our operating rooms idle, and delay surgeries because we cannot move patients from operating rooms to the PACU. In 1994, Carroll et al. looked at the costs incurred by outpatient surgical centers in managing more than 200 patients experiencing PONV by examining medication, supply, and personnel costs [8]. They found that these symptoms delayed discharge by an average of 24 min and cost the center $415 per patient in lost revenue [8]. Adjusting for the US medical inflation rate over the past 20 years, that amounts to more than $700 per patient. Over the course of an entire year in a high volume center, this can amount to hundreds of thousands, or even millions of dollars lost per year! If we keep this patient and others like her in the PACU, we will put our own center out of business.

CON: If the patient feels too uncomfortable from the nausea and vomiting to go home, we cannot discharge her. Just one poor patient experience is enough to harm our ambulatory care center's business. According to a study of 100 patients in the preoperative clinic, patients ranked vomiting and nausea the first and fourth of the 10 most undesirable postoperative outcomes, respectively [1]. In 2001, Gan et al. reported that patients were willing to shell out up to $100 of their own money to avoid feeling nauseous in the postoperative period [9]. If our patient feels this way, we cannot just send her home; we must alleviate her symptoms.

Healthcare delivery is becoming more focused on patient satisfaction, and we need to keep in mind that patients are essentially customers of our anesthesia services. Therefore, we must change our practice in order to deliver the care that patients value most. If our patient considers nausea more unpleasant than pain, we must tailor our PACU care to reflect these concerns and wishes.

Summary

Ultimately, it is at the discretion of the healthcare provider to determine when a patient is safe for discharge after ambulatory surgery. PONV risk assessment should be performed during the preoperative history and physical, and each patient should be risk stratified so that anesthetic and postoperative management plans can be created accordingly. There are numerous strategies anesthesia providers can use to prevent PONV, and several anti-emetic medications may be given to patients who experience PONV despite prophylaxis. Movement of patients through the perioperative setting is crucial to the functioning and success of an ambulatory surgery practice but patient safety and satisfaction are paramount.

References

1. Macario A, Weinger M, Carney S, Kim A. Which clinical anesthesia outcomes are important to avoid? The perspective of patients. Anesth Analg. 1999;89(3):652–8.
2. Apfel CC, Korttila K, Abdalla M, Kerger H, Turan A, Vedder I, et al. A factorial trial of six interventions for the prevention of postoperative nausea and vomiting. N Engl J Med. 2004;350 (24):2441–51.
3. Gan TJ. Postoperative nausea and vomiting–can it be eliminated? JAMA. 2002;287(10):1233–6.
4. Gan TJ, Meyer T, Apfel CC, Chung F, Davis PJ, Eubanks S, et al. Consensus guidelines for managing postoperative nausea and vomiting. Anesth Analg. 2003;97(1):62–71, table of contents.
5. Apfel CC, Kranke P, Katz MH, Goepfert C, Papenfuss T, Rauch S, et al. Volatile anaesthetics may be the main cause of early but not

delayed postoperative vomiting: a randomized controlled trial of factorial design. Br J Anaesth. 2002;88(5):659–68.
6. Marshall SI, Chung F. Discharge criteria and complications after ambulatory surgery. Anesth Analg. 1999;88(3):508–17.
7. Gan TJ, Diemunsch P, Habib AS, Kovac A, Kranke P, Meyer TA, et al. Consensus guidelines for the management of postoperative nausea and vomiting. Anesth Analg. 2014;118(1):85–113.
8. Carroll NV, Miederhoff PA, Cox FM, Hirsch JD. Costs incurred by outpatient surgical centers in managing postoperative nausea and vomiting. J Clin Anesth. 1994;6(5):364–9.
9. Gan T, Sloan F, de L Dear G, El-Moalem HE, Lubarsky DA. How much are patients willing to pay to avoid postoperative nausea and vomiting? Anesth Analg. 2001;92(2):393–400.

Should We Postpone Surgery in Patients with Uncontrolled Preoperative Hypertension?

80

Kristina Natan and Arthur Atchabahian

Case

A 67-year-old male patient with a history of hypertension (HTN) presents for total hip arthroplasty. In the holding area, his blood pressure (BP) is 220/120 on repeated measurements. You recommend that the surgery be postponed to achieve better control of the BP. The cardiologist called to consult suggests just giving some labetalol to decrease the BP, then proceeding.

Question

Should surgery be postponed for patients with uncontrolled preoperative hypertension?

PRO: You quote 2 landmark articles by Prys-Roberts et al. [1, 2] that demonstrated that patients with poorly treated hypertension are at increased risk of myocardial ischemia and hemodynamic instability.

When the cardiologist tells you that medicine has evolved since the 1970s, you also quote a 2010 paper by Wax et al. [3] that demonstrated an increase in the incidence (2.8 vs. 1.3 %) of any adverse outcome (elevated troponin and in-hospital death) in patients who underwent surgery with a systolic blood pressure (SBP) >200 mm Hg.

CON: "That may be true," replies the cardiologist, "but in that paper, the 42 patients whose surgery was canceled and who returned for surgery had an even higher rate of adverse cardiac outcomes (4.8 %) than those for whom surgery was allowed to proceed" [3].

K. Natan (✉)
Northern Valley Anesthesiology, 1500 William Floyd Parkway, Suite 302, Shirley, NY 11967, USA
e-mail: Kristinanatan@hotmail.com

A. Atchabahian
Department of Anesthesiology, New York University School of Medicine, 301 East 17th St Rm C2-222, New York, NY 10003, USA
e-mail: arthur.atchabahian@gmail.com; Atchabahian@nyumc.org

PRO: "Well," you answer, "the number of patients whose surgery was postponed is too small to make the difference statistically significant" [3].

CON: The cardiologist says, "While it is obviously true that patients with hypertension have worse outcomes, and the higher their BP, the worse the outcome, as was shown by Stamler et al. using population data [4], postponing surgery did not seem to vastly reduce the incidence of complications."

When you mention that the diastolic blood pressure (DBP) is also elevated, he sits down at the computer and retrieves a randomized controlled trial performed by Weksler et al. [5]. The authors included 989 patients with known and treated hypertension with diastolic blood pressure ranging between 110 and 130 mm Hg preoperatively, but excluded patients with target-organ damage. Patients were randomly assigned to control or study groups. Patients in the control group were admitted to the hospital for blood pressure control, and the surgery was performed once DBP was <110 mm Hg for 3 consecutive days. The study group was treated with 10 mg intranasal nifedipine for blood pressure control prior to proceeding to surgery. There were no major cardiovascular or neurological postoperative complications in either group. The hospitalization time was shorter in the study group than in the control group. Based on the results, the authors' recommendation was to proceed with surgery in patients with Stage 3 hypertension as long as there is no evidence of end-organ damage (ischemic heart disease, heart failure, cerebrovascular disease, or renal impairment) [5].

PRO: You retort, "Patients in that study do not seem very representative of reality, since there was not a single serious complication in almost 1000 patients."

You remind the cardiologist that the 2002 American College of Cardiology and American Heart Association guidelines recommended postponing elective surgery in severely hypertensive patients who have SBP > 180 mmHg or DBP > 110 mmHg [6].

C.S. Scher et al. (eds.), *You're Wrong, I'm Right*, DOI 10.1007/978-3-319-43169-7_80

CON: "That was true," he replies, "but following a meta-analysis performed by Howell et al. [7] that did not find worse outcomes in hypertensive as compared to normotensive patients, this recommendation is no longer part of more recent guidelines [8]. Howell et al. pointed out that patients would not die perioperatively from elevated BP itself, but were more likely to die from hypertension-induced comorbidities and inadequate management. Therefore, patients with target-organ damage induced by hypertension deserve more attention and perhaps should even have surgery delayed. They propose not to delay surgery, however due to a single systolic hypertension reading, since patients with severe hypertension may need 3 or more months to see significant change in cardiovascular risk factors with treatment."

Summary

Due to a lack of data and somewhat contradictory results of the existing studies, it is difficult to draw a definite conclusion about this controversial issue. There is a general consensus to proceed with the surgery in patients with mild-to-moderate hypertension without any end-organ damage. However, for severely hypertensive patients, physicians should evaluate the urgency and risks of cardiovascular complications on an individual basis. Any recommendations to proceed or postpone elective surgery should take into account the risks and benefits of each choice. Patients with end-organ damage (ischemic heart disease, heart failure, cerebrovascular disease, or renal impairment) deserve more attention and scrutiny, and delaying surgery in those patients can probably be justified.

References

1. Prys-Roberts C, Meloche R, Foëx P. Studies of anaesthesia in relation to hypertension. I. Cardiovascular responses of treated and untreated patients. Br J Anaesth. 1971;43(2):122–37.
2. Prys-Roberts C, Greene LT, Meloche R, Foëx P. Studies of anaesthesia in relation to hypertension. II. Haemodynamic consequences of induction and endotracheal intubation. Br J Anaesth. 1971;43(6):531–47.
3. Wax DB, Porter SB, Lin HM, Hossain S, Reich DL. Association of preanesthesia hypertension with adverse outcomes. J Cardiothorac Vasc Anesth. 2010;24(6):927–30.
4. Stamler J, Stamler R, Neaton JD. Blood pressure, systolic and diastolic, and cardiovascular risks. US population data. Arch Intern Med. 1993;153:598–615.
5. Weksler N, Klein M, Szendro G, Rozentsveig V, Schily M, Brill S, et al. The dilemma of immediate preoperative hypertension: To treat and operate, or to postpone surgery? J Clin Anesth. 2003;15:179–83.
6. Eagle KA, Berger PB, Calkins H, Chaitman BR, Ewy GA, Fleischmann KE, et al. American College of Cardiology; American Heart Association. ACC/AHA guideline update for perioperative cardiovascular evaluation for noncardiac surgery–executive summary: a report of the American College of Cardiology/American Heart Association Task Force on Practice Guidelines (Committee to Update the 1996 Guidelines on Perioperative Cardiovascular Evaluation for Noncardiac Surgery). J Am Coll Cardiol. 2002;39(3):542–53.
7. Howell SJ, Sear YM, Foex P. Hypertension, hypertensive heart disease, and perioperative cardiac risk. Br J Anaesth. 2004;92:570–83.
8. Fleisher LA, Fleischmann KE, Auerbach AD, Barnason SA, Beckman JA, Bozkurt B, et al. American College of Cardiology; American Heart Association. 2014 ACC/AHA guideline on perioperative cardiovascular evaluation and management of patients undergoing noncardiac surgery: a report of the American College of Cardiology/American Heart Association Task Force on practice guidelines. J Am Coll Cardiol. 2014;64(22):e77–137.

Should the Morbidly Obese Patient Be Allowed to Leave the Day of Surgery?

81

Christopher J. Curatolo and Andrew Goldberg

Case

A patient with a body mass index (BMI) of 42 just underwent an uneventful hernia repair under sedation. She is a 34-year-old woman with a history of hypertension, non-insulin-dependent diabetes, hyperlipidemia, and anxiety. The post-anesthesia care unit (PACU) attending was discussing with his resident his plan to discharge the patient later that day when another attending, who overheard this, commented that it was not appropriate to discharge such a patient. Who is correct?

Question

Should the patient be allowed to leave the day of surgery?

PRO The PACU attending pointed out that it was indeed appropriate to discharge this patient from the PACU since she had an uneventful procedure under sedation and met all of the standard discharge criteria.

CON The other attending replied that some morbidly obese patients are at increased risk of perioperative complications and should stay for a few hours in a monitored setting or even spend the entire night.

PRO The PACU attending responded that a recent study showed no difference in unplanned hospital admissions between morbidly obese and non-obese patients [1]. Additionally, as long as comorbidities are minimal or optimized before surgery, there is no reason to keep patients overnight [2].

CON But several studies have shown that obesity is a risk factor for postoperative complications, unplanned admissions, and cancellations in outpatient surgery [2, 3].

PRO Those studies aren't conclusive and haven't been reproduced [4]. Additionally, it is a huge resource burden (both in hospital space and in healthcare expenditure) to keep patients overnight simply because of their BMI.

CON That may be, but what about this patient's comorbidities? Surely you have to take that into account.

PRO All of her comorbidities were optimized so she should be allowed to go home.

CON Does the patient have obstructive sleep apnea (OSA) or is she suspected of having it?

PRO She doesn't have a history of OSA, but I am not sure if there's a possibility of it.

CON Let's do a quick assessment. The currently favored method of screening for suspected OSA is to use the STOP-Bang questionnaire [5]. It is highly sensitive, and its specificity increases considerably as the number of positive findings increases. So the more questions the patient answers positively, the more likely the patient has OSA and the greater the severity of OSA if confirmed. To summarize, the questionnaire asks the following:

- S = Snoring. Do you snore loudly (louder than talking or loud enough to be heard through closed doors)?
- T = Tiredness. Do you often feel tired, fatigued, or sleepy during daytime?
- O = Observed apnea. Has anyone observed you stop breathing during your sleep?

C.J. Curatolo (✉) · A. Goldberg
Department of Anesthesiology, Icahn School of Medicine at Mount Sinai, One Gustave Levy Place, Box 1010, New York, NY 10029, USA
e-mail: Christopher.curatolo@mountsinai.org

A. Goldberg
e-mail: andrew.goldberg@mountsinai.org

C.S. Scher et al. (eds.), *You're Wrong, I'm Right*, DOI 10.1007/978-3-319-43169-7_81

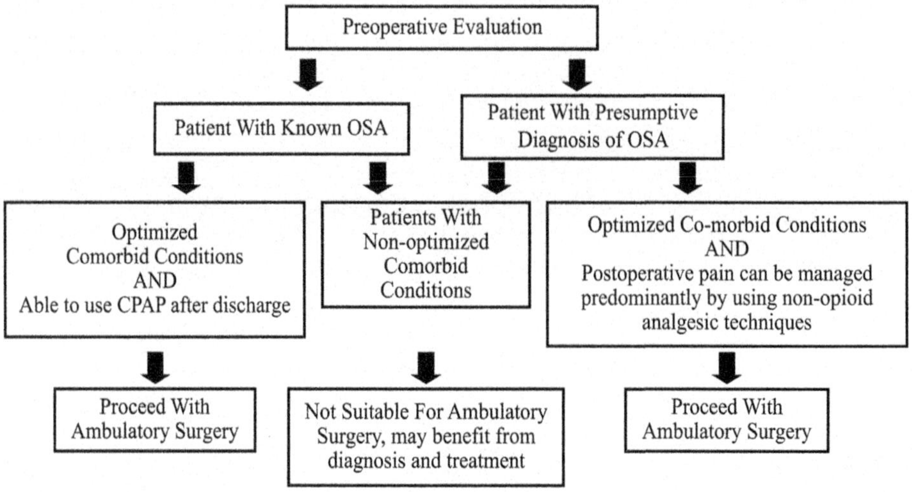

Fig. 81.1 Ambulatory surgery algorithm for patients with obstructive sleep apnea (OSA). *CPAP:* continuous positive airway pressure. Reprinted with permission from Joshi et al. [6]

- P = Pressure. Do you have or are you being treated for high blood pressure?
- B = BMI > 35 kg/m^2
- A = Age > 50 years
- N = Neck circumference > 40 cm
- G = Male gender

Three or more positive answers indicate a high risk for OSA, and 5–8 positive replies indicate a high probability of moderate-to-severe OSA.

PRO This patient scores a 6. How does this change things?

CON This patient, with a score of 6, has a high probability of moderate-to-severe OSA. This helps us because several societies have published guidelines on the approach to these patients. For example, the Society for Ambulatory Anesthesia (SAMBA) published a consensus statement in 2012 on the preoperative selection of adult patients with OSA scheduled for ambulatory surgery [6]. Additionally, the American Society of Anesthesiologists (ASA) Task Force on Perioperative Management of patients with obstructive sleep apnea published practice guidelines on the perioperative management of patients with OSA [7].

PRO So how do they recommend we handle patients like these?

CON Both societies take similar, but slightly different, approaches. SAMBA's consensus statement has us start by classifying patients into those with known OSA versus a presumed diagnosis of OSA. Next must be a discussion of whether their comorbid conditions are optimized. This is because we know that non-optimized comorbidities such as congestive heart failure and unstable angina are independent risk factors for poor outcomes. So not all patients, and especially not all morbidly obese patients, will be suitable candidates for ambulatory surgery. Next, optimized patients with OSA who are able to use a continuous positive airway pressure (CPAP) device after discharge may proceed with ambulatory surgery since we know that this greatly reduces their risk of complications. These patients should be instructed to bring their CPAP machine to the hospital and should be started on therapy immediately following surgery.

Next, let's consider patients with a presumed diagnosis of OSA, such as our patient, who screened positive with the STOP-Bang questionnaire. If the patient's comorbidities are optimized for surgery, then it must be determined whether postoperative pain can be managed predominantly using non-opioid analgesic techniques. Patients suspected of having OSA, even though not explicitly diagnosed, have an increased sensitivity to opioids. Furthermore, these patients are also more likely to hypoventilate, become apneic, and experience hypoxemia postoperatively. Together, this combination can be fatal. Therefore, if a postoperative analgesic plan can avoid opioids, then these patients may undergo ambulatory surgery. Here's a summary diagram of what we just discussed (Fig. 81.1) [6].

PRO How do the ASA practice guidelines differ?

CON According to the ASA, their guidelines include a larger sample of anesthesiologists and a broader review of scientific data than others. They say the literature itself is insufficient to state definitively whether inpatient or outpatient surgery is safer for patients with OSA. Similar to other guidelines, they list multiple factors to consider, such as OSA status, coexisting diseases, nature of surgery, type of anesthesia, need for postoperative opioids, patient age, adequacy of post-discharge observation, and the capabilities of the outpatient facility. They agree that studies report lower rates of postoperative complications when CPAP is used.

PRO What about the types of anesthesia the patients should receive?

CON Regional and other potentially opioid-sparing techniques should be considered when applicable. Patients receiving sedation should have their ventilation monitored by continuous capnography. If general anesthesia is required, a secure airway with an endotracheal tube may be preferable due to the increased risk of airway obstruction. Patients undergoing endotracheal intubation should have full neuromuscular blockade reversal, if applicable, and be extubated when awake and in a non-supine position (such as lateral or Fowler's). Risk factors for postoperative respiratory depression must be considered, including the severity of OSA, use of sedatives, administration of opioids, site and invasiveness of the procedure, and finally the potential for apnea during sleep on the third or fourth day as sleep patterns are reestablished. Comparative observational studies indicate a decrease in apneic periods when patients with OSA slept in positions other than supine.

PRO But wait, we've been talking this whole time about OSA and other comorbidities. What about her morbid obesity itself?

CON Good question. Obesity, although clearly associated with an increased number of comorbidities, does not in and of itself direct you to a particular management technique. The bigger concern is the complications of obesity itself, the most important of which is OSA.

PRO So can I discharge my patient yet?

CON Our patient underwent a relatively noninvasive procedure with minimal sedation, was medically optimized prior to surgery, and does not require postoperative opioids. Since she is at minimal risk for respiratory depression, she may be discharged home once she meets all of the standard criteria for discharge. Given her risk for OSA, however, she should be encouraged to follow-up with her primary care physician for a formal sleep study to ascertain whether she does in fact have OSA and the potential need for CPAP.

Summary

Morbid obesity is associated with multiple comorbidities that may prevent a patient from undergoing ambulatory surgery. While it is imperative that comorbidities be properly optimized prior to approving an ambulatory procedure, the most serious determination is whether the patient has suspected or known OSA. If the patient is suspected of having OSA, it is recommended that the patient not undergo ambulatory surgery unless respiratory depression-causing agents can be avoided, especially postoperatively. In the patient with known OSA, it is recommended that CPAP be used in the postoperative period and that full precautions be taken to reduce the number of apneic periods (e.g., sleeping in the non-supine position). While the literature is not conclusive, specialty and subspecialty organizations have made recommendations to help tailor care.

References

1. Hofer RE, Kai T, Decker PA, Warner DO. Obesity as a risk factor for unanticipated admissions after ambulatory surgery. Mayo Clin Proc. 2008;83(8):908–16.
2. Joshi GP, Ahmad S, Riad W, Eckert S, Chung F. Selection of obese patients undergoing ambulatory surgery: a systematic review of the literature. Anesth Analg. 2013;117(5):1082–91.
3. Arance Garcia M, Docobo Durantez F, Conde Guzman C, Perez Torres MC, Martin-Gil Parra R, Fernandez Jimenez PE. Is obesity a risk factor for complications, hospital admissions, and surgical cancellations in ambulatory surgery? Rev Esp Anestesiol Reanim. 2015;62(3):125–32.
4. Rosero EB, Joshi GP. Nationwide use and outcomes of ambulatory surgery in morbidly obese patients in the United States. J Clin Anesth. 2014;26(3):191–8.
5. Chung F, Yegneswaran B, Liao P, Chung SA, Vairavanathan S, Islam S, et al. Stop questionnaire: a tool to screen patients for obstructive sleep apnea. Anesthesiology. 2008;108(5):812–21.
6. Joshi GP, Ankichetty SP, Gan TJ, Chung F. Society for ambulatory anesthesia consensus statement on preoperative selection of adult patients with obstructive sleep apnea scheduled for ambulatory surgery. Anesth Analg. 2012;115(5):1060–8.
7. American Society of Anesthesiologists Task Force on Perioperative. Management of patients with obstructive sleep a. Practice guidelines for the perioperative management of patients with obstructive sleep apnea: an updated report by the american society of anesthesiologists task force on perioperative management of patients with obstructive sleep apnea. Anesthesiology. 2014;120(2):268–86.

Should Complementary and Alternative Medicine (CAM) Be Used for the Treatment of Postoperative Pain Following Ambulatory Surgery?

82

Dennis Grech, David Kam, and Preet Patel

Case

Following arthroscopic shoulder surgery at a multi-specialty ambulatory surgery center (ASC), a patient with a history of obstructive sleep apnea (OSA) complained to the anesthesiologist that he was feeling mild postoperative pain. Postoperative pain is a common complaint following shoulder procedures as the joint is heavily innervated and highly vascularized. The patient requested pain relief; he also expressed a desire to continue his recovery at home as originally planned. As the anesthesiologist and the patient began discussing the available pain treatment options, the patient revealed that he had terrible experiences in the past with opioid medications. Common side effects of these medications include severe nausea, vomiting, constipation, pruritus, dependence, and apnea. The anesthesiologist decided that a non-pharmacological treatment modality may be best suited for the treatment of postoperative pain in this patient.

The anesthesiologist and patient discussed a number of complementary and alternative medicine (CAM) treatment options including aromatherapy, homeopathy, massage therapy, and acupuncture before deciding on an exact treatment plan. The patient had reservations about the effectiveness of some of these therapies. He asked the doctor, "Are you sure that these will work?"

D. Grech (✉)
Department of Anasthesiology, Rutgers New Jersey Medical School, 185 South Orange Ave MSB E-5386, Newark, NJ 07103, USA
e-mail: glechde@njms.rutgers.edu

D. Kam
Department of Anasthesiology, Perioperative Medicine, and Pain Management, University of Miami, Miami, Fl, USA

P. Patel
Department of Anesthesiology and Pain Management, Rutgers Robert Wood Johnson Medical School, 125 Paterson Street, CAB 3100, New Brunswick, NJ 08901, USA
e-mail: preetpatelmd@gmail.com

Question

What are the benefits and limitations of complementary and alternative medicine (CAM)—specifically aromatherapy, homeopathy, massage therapy, and acupuncture—for the treatment of postoperative pain in the ambulatory setting?

Acupuncture

The anesthesiologist discussed each treatment modality in detail with the patient, beginning with acupuncture for postoperative pain relief. Acupuncture, a component of traditional Chinese medicine, is a popular and widely used treatment for pain and other conditions that has been employed in China for more than 3 millennia. There have been an increasing number of clinical trials evaluating the efficacy of acupuncture and related techniques as an adjuvant method for postoperative pain.

PRO: In 2008, researchers published a systematic review that quantitatively evaluated the available evidence for the efficacy of acupuncture and related techniques in postoperative pain management [1]. In this meta-analysis, they found that acupuncture and related techniques are effective adjuncts for postoperative pain management as demonstrated by a significant reduction of postoperative pain scores and opioid consumption. The opioid-sparing effect was most marked at 72 h postoperation where a 29 % reduction of morphine consumption was demonstrated. The opioid-sparing effect at 8 and 24 h was 21 % and 23 %, respectively [1]. It has been suggested that anesthesia may inhibit the effects of acupuncture and that the analgesic effect of acupuncture is progressively more evident in the postoperative period. While the reduction in pain scores achieved with acupuncture was statistically significant at 8 and 72 h, the reduction in pain intensity was moderate and it could be argued that it may not be clinically relevant. The same

C.S. Scher et al. (eds.), *You're Wrong, I'm Right*, DOI 10.1007/978-3-319-43169-7_82

applies to the small absolute reductions in opioid consumption.

However, the relative reduction in opioid consumption ranged from 21 to 29 %, which is generally considered clinically significant [1]. Furthermore, this meta-analysis showed a significant reduction in the incidence of opioid-related adverse effects, including nausea, pruritus, dizziness, sedation, and urinary retention in the acupuncture treatment group. This suggests that the opioid-sparing effects are clinically significant. The reduction in nausea, however, could also be attributed to the acupuncture itself with stimulation of some acupuncture points having anti-emetic effects. The side effects attributable to acupuncture were minimal and resolved spontaneously. This is an important consideration, since the use of some adjunct analgesics might be limited by the concern for adverse effects such as bleeding and renal dysfunction with the use of non-steroidal anti-inflammatory drugs (NSAIDs). Other studies have supported the effectiveness of acupuncture for other types of pain such as chronic knee pain.

CON: Although most studies show acupuncture to be an effective treatment modality for postoperative pain management, the exact mechanism of acupuncture analgesia remains unclear. Some proposed mechanisms include activation of the endogenous pain inhibitory system, release of endogenous opioids including β(beta)-endorphins, enkephalins, and dynorphins, and release of non-opioid substances such as serotonin, norepinephrine, and gamma-aminobutyric acid (GABA). There are also several limitations with the currently published data on acupuncture for postoperative pain management. First, there is wide variability in the acupuncture regimens, types of surgery, time of application, and duration of stimulation. Next, there is inconsistent reporting of outcome measures. There is large variation in outcome measures, and those outcomes that might be regarded as clinically significant (e.g., duration of recovery room stay and opioid-related adverse events) were inconsistently reported. Side effects related to acupuncture are also a concern and they include minor bleeding at the acupuncture site, headache, local pain, dizziness, and instantaneous bradycardia.

Homeopathy

Next, the anesthesiologist discussed the history and benefits of homeopathy for postoperative pain with the patient. Homeopathy was developed by a German physician, Samuel Christian Hahnemann (1755–1843), who described his theory of "like cures like" as the "Principle of Similars." He recorded the symptoms caused to healthy individuals by certain substances, and treated patients exhibiting those same symptoms with the matched substances. These symptoms are treated independently of their clinical diagnosis; 2 patients with the same disease may receive different treatments based on their specific symptomology.

CON: A meta-analysis of 4 randomized controlled trials (RCTs) that used St. John's wort in homeopathic form for pain after dental surgery found a benefit in pain control over placebo that was not statistically significant [2]. These studies were all well designed and blinded, but did not all control for confounders or adequately detail the homeopathic treatment regimen used. Lokken et al. performed a randomized double-blind study with crossover of patients who had bilateral molar impaction [3]. This allowed 2 identical surgeries to be performed, with postoperative analgesia provided by either homeopathy or placebo for the first surgery, and the other type for the second. The researchers found that pain after surgery was the same whether treated by homeopathy or by placebo. However, the authors noted that pain scores were low throughout the group for both surgeries and suggested that this was due to the strong belief of the study participants in the efficacy of homeopathy.

In treatment of postoperative pain in orthopedic surgeries, the use of less dilute Traumeel S was not found to be superior to placebo in patients with hallux valgus surgery [4]. The authors noted a statistically significant decrease in the daily maximum pain score on the day of operation among patients receiving the homeopathic remedy, but this effect did not extend beyond the first postoperative day. A single-center randomized study of knee ligament reconstructions found no difference in postoperative morphine consumption between those given homeopathic treatment compared to those given placebo [5]. Another randomized double-blind trial of add-on homeopathic *Arnica montana* in patients undergoing knee surgery found no statistically significant difference in pain levels compared to placebo [6]. Again, total amount of analgesics used was identical between both groups. These add-on studies may more closely represent conditions in reality, as patients commonly see both conventional physicians in addition to taking homeopathic remedies. In the case of homeopathy, this study design may be more pragmatic than the standard superiority trials commonly used to evaluate new treatment regimens.

PRO: Previous work has demonstrated that therapeutic benefits seen with homeopathy are actually from homeopathic consultations and not the remedies themselves. Homeopathic consultations involve detailed history-taking and collaboration with the patient for a personalized treatment plan. This ritual may have symbolic meaning for the patient; communication skills, empathy, hopefulness, and patient enablement all may play important roles in the pain management seen with homeopathy. Anxiety, commonly associated with pain, has been found to be relieved with the rapport that is built with homeopathic practitioners. Physicians with open minds may therefore derive benefit for their patients through complementary homeopathic consultations.

CON: Many previous studies have found equivocal evidence supporting homeopathy and further research with well-designed studies is necessary for adequate evaluation of this popular alternative therapy [7]. Often, the exact mechanisms of action are unknown resulting in skepticism and poor acceptance of the treatment modalities among physicians. Additionally, homeopathic preparations are not distributed in standardized formulations. This raises major concerns as patients may be exposed to unknown side effects and adverse drug interactions.

Massage Therapy

Next, the anesthesiologist reviewed the benefits of massage therapy with the patient. Massage is a therapeutic modality that involves manual manipulation of the soft tissues of the body. References to the use of massage as a healing art date back to at least the 8th century BCE. Massage has since been used throughout the world for the treatment of a wide range of ailments.

PRO: The benefits of massage therapy include that in general, massage is non-invasive and safe when practiced by an experienced therapist. Studies have been conducted testing the effectiveness of massage therapy in reducing postoperative pain. Taylor et al. found no statistically significant difference in postoperative pain level between complementary massage therapy, complementary vibration therapy, and usual care alone among patients who had undergone laparotomies [8]. In contrast, another randomized controlled trial found significant decreases in pain level among postoperative patients receiving adjuvant massage therapy, as well as a more rapid decrease in pain intensity [9]. Smaller studies among cardiothoracic and abdominal surgery patients have also shown reduced pain in postoperative patients who received massage therapy as compared to controls. An assessment of postoperative massage in cancer patients was conducted by Mehling et al., who found that massage used in conjunction with acupuncture was associated with 38 % of patients reporting a decrease in pain score of at least 2 points, compared with 18 % of control patients [10]. Average pain scores improved by 1.6 points in the first 3 postoperative days, compared to 0.6 points in the control group. These differences were statistically significant. Adjunctive massage therapy without acupuncture was associated with a greater improvement in pain than receiving usual care alone, but this effect was only seen the first postoperative day and the authors did not report a quantification of this decrease.

CON: Though there is emerging evidence that adjunctive massage therapy may improve surgical patients' pain scores, particularly in the early postoperative period, this is still an area of active study with no clear consensus. Among massage researchers, a controversial issue is the use of touch controls. Many trials have used a control group that does not receive any physical contact; critics of this method assert that it is important to clarify whether a massage given by an untrained individual is as efficacious as that given by a massage therapist. Furthermore, this method fails to control for the non-specific impact of touch. The recently completed Reducing End-of-Life Symptoms with Touch (REST) study, a large National Institutes of Health (NIH) phase III trial, evaluated the impact of the systematic touching of patients by hospice volunteers untrained in massage therapy [11]. These results showed statistically significant immediate and sustained improvements in pain among patients treated with simple touch alone, comparable to those treated with massage therapy. Finally, massage therapy should be limited to patients who are without coagulation disorders, low platelets, bone lesions, open wounds, or dermatitis due to the risk of adverse effects. As demand for this popular adjunctive therapy continues to grow in the USA, further large-scale research of these intriguing results is required, especially in their application to the postoperative patient population.

Aromatherapy

Finally, the patient and anesthesiologist discussed the benefits and limitations of aromatherapy. Aromatherapy utilizes essential oils distilled from plant sources for inhalation as a treatment modality; it has been practiced throughout history for a wide variety of ailments. Recent interest has fueled study into its possible uses due to the intimate links between the olfactory and the limbic systems.

PRO: There is evidence that aromatherapy decreases the intensity of postoperative pain. In 2006, Kim et al. found that aromatherapy with lavender oil after breast biopsy was not associated with a significant difference in narcotic requirements, discharge times, or pain scores [12]. However, patients treated with aromatherapy reported more satisfaction with their postoperative pain control than the control group; this difference was statistically significant.

In 2007, Kim et al. again examined the effect of aromatherapy on postoperative pain control, this time in morbidly obese patients undergoing lap-band surgery [13]. They found that lavender inhalation was associated with a statistically significant decrease in use of postoperative analgesics in general, as well as morphine in particular, when compared to the control group. These authors expressed concern that these findings could not be applied to other operations [13].

However, in 2011 aromatherapy was found to statistically significantly improve pain scores of post-Cesarean patients at a half-hour, 8 h, and 16 h from the time of intervention when compared to the control group who received an artificial neutral aromatic compound that resembled lavender essence [14]. A similar study the following year found that post-Cesarean section patients who received aromatherapy had less pain in the first 4, 8, and 12 h after first intervention, as well as decreased heart rate, decreased analgesic requirements, and increased satisfaction with pain control [15]. In the pediatric population, aromatherapy with lavender essential oils was associated with decreased oral analgesic use after tonsillectomy, but not with decreased pain intensity [16]. Use of *Rosa damascena Mill.* in postoperative pediatric patients was associated with significantly decreased pain scores as compared to patients receiving almond oil placebo [17].

CON: The anesthesiologist admitted to the patient that although numerous studies indicate a quantifiable decrease in analgesic use in postoperative patients with aromatherapy, it has not been proven to be a sufficient postoperative pain treatment option by itself; rather, aromatherapy should be used as an adjuvant with traditionally prescribed pain medications. The current data suggest that further inquiries into aromatherapy's analgesic effects are warranted in the future. Finally, side effects have also been reported with the use of certain agents; lavender oil can cause hypersomnia and using licorice for a significant time can cause hypertension.

Summary

Despite limitations, complementary and alternative medicine (CAM) can be used for the treatment of postoperative pain following ambulatory surgery. Aromatherapy has been shown to decrease the intensity of postoperative pain (decreased pain scores) following a number of surgical procedures. Homeopathic consultations have been shown to decrease patient anxiety and improve patient satisfaction. Massage therapy is a non-invasive technique that has been shown to lower pain scores as well as decrease pain intensity more rapidly when used as an adjuvant therapy. Finally, acupuncture has been shown to unequivocally reduce postoperative pain scores and reduce opioid consumption as well as opioid-related adverse events, and is associated with reduced nausea and vomiting in the postoperative state.

References

1. Sun Y, Gan TJ, Dubose JW, Habib AS. Acupuncture and related techniques for postoperative pain: a systematic review of randomized controlled trials. Br J Anaesth. 2008;101(2):151–60.
2. Raak C, Büssing A, Gassmann G, Boehm K, Ostermann T. A systematic review and meta-analysis on the use of Hypericum perforatum (St. John's Wort) for pain conditions in dental practice. Homeopathy. 2012;101(4):204–10.
3. Lokken P, Straumsheim PA, Tveiten D, Skjelbred P, Borchgrevink CF. Effect of homoeopathy on pain and other events after acute trauma: placebo controlled trial with bilateral oral surgery. BMJ. 1995;310(6992):1439–42.
4. Singer SR, Amit-Kohn M, Weiss S, Rosenblum J, Maoz G, Samuels N, et al. Traumeel S® for pain relief following hallux valgus surgery: a randomized controlled trial. BMC Clin Pharmacol. 2010;10:9.
5. Paris A, Gonnet N, Chaussard C, Belon P, Rocourt F, Saragaglia D, et al. Effect of homeopathy on analgesic intake following knee ligament reconstruction: a phase III monocentre randomized placebo controlled study. Br J Clin Pharmacol. 2008;65(2):180–7.
6. Barlow T, Downham C, Barlow D. The effect of complementary therapies on post-operative pain control in ambulatory knee surgery: a systematic review. Complement Ther Med. 2013;21(5):529–34.
7. Roberts M, Brodribb W, Mitchell G. Reducing the pain: a systematic review of postdischarge analgesia following elective orthopedic surgery. Pain Med. 2012;13(5):711–27.
8. Taylor AG, Galper DI, Taylor P, Rice LW, Andersen W, Irvin W, et al. Effects of adjunctive Swedish massage and vibration therapy on short-term postoperative outcomes: a randomized, controlled trial. J Altern Complement Med. 2003;9(1):77–89.
9. Mitchinson AR, Kim HM, Rosenberg JM, Geisser M, Kirsh M, Cikrit D, et al. Acute postoperative pain management using massage as an adjuvant therapy: a randomized trial. Arch Surg. 2007;142(12):1158–67.
10. Mehling WE, Jacobs B, Acree M, Wilson L, Bostrom A, West J, et al. Symptom management with massage and acupuncture in postoperative cancer patients: a randomized controlled trial. J Pain Symptom Manage. 2007;33(3):258–66.
11. Kutner JS, Smith MC, Corbin L, Hemphill L, Benton K, Mellis BK, et al. Massage therapy versus simple touch to improve pain and mood in patients with advanced cancer: a randomized trial. Ann Intern Med. 2008;149(6):369–79.
12. Kim JT, Wajda M, Cuff G, Serota D, Schlame M, Axelrod DM, et al. Evaluation of aromatherapy in treating postoperative pain: pilot study. Pain Pract. 2006;6(4):273–7.
13. Kim JT, Ren CJ, Fielding GA, Pitti A, Kasumi T, Wajda M, et al. Treatment with lavender aromatherapy in the post-anesthesia care unit reduces opioid requirements of morbidly obese patients undergoing laparoscopic adjustable gastric banding. Obes Surg. 2007;17(7):920–5.
14. Hadi N, Hanid AA. Lavender essence for post-cesarean pain. Pak J Biol Sci. 2011;14(11):664–7.
15. Olapour A, Behaeen K, Akhondzadeh R, Soltani F, Al Sadat Razavi F, et al. The effect of inhalation of aromatherapy blend containing lavender essential oil on cesarean postoperative pain. Anesth Pain Med. 2013;3(1):203–7.
16. Soltani R, Soheilipour S, Hajhashemi V, Asghari G, Bagheri M, Molavi M. Evaluation of the effect of aromatherapy with lavender essential oil on post-tonsillectomy pain in pediatric patients: a randomized controlled trial. Int J Pediatr Otorhinolaryngol. 2013;77(9):1579–81.
17. Marofi M, Sirousfard M, Moeini M, Ghanadi A. Evaluation of the effect of aromatherapy with Rosa damascena Mill. on postoperative pain intensity in hospitalized children in selected hospitals affiliated to Isfahan University of Medical Sciences in 2013: a randomized clinical trial. Iran J Nurs Midwifery Res. 2015;20(2):247–54.

Pros and Cons of a Freestanding Ambulatory Surgery Center (ASC) Versus a Hospital-Based Operating Room

83

Dennis Grech, Preet Patel, and David Kam

Case

A 25-year-old healthy male patient with no significant past medical history visits his doctor after a right knee injury 1 week ago. The patient says to the doctor, "I was playing basketball with my buddies last week when I heard a pop and felt a lot of pain in my knee." After a visit to the local emergency room following the incident, the patient was told that he had a torn meniscus in his right knee and would need corrective surgery. The patient is visiting his doctor today in order to determine the next step. He asks the doctor, "Where's the best place to go to get my knee fixed?".

Question

What are the benefits and limitations of having surgical procedures performed in a freestanding ambulatory surgery center (ASC) as opposed to a hospital-based operating room (OR)?

As the patient and his doctor discuss their options, the doctor says, "You can get the procedure done at a freestanding ambulatory surgery center just down the road. I think it is the best choice for you."

PRO: The doctor's recommendation to have the procedure performed at a freestanding ASC is a sensible decision for a multitude of reasons. First, according to a study published in 2010, which examined Medicare data on common ambulatory procedures in Florida, ASCs are more efficient than hospital-based operating rooms [1]. A second study from 2012 compared ambulatory surgical visits of Medicare beneficiaries between hospital-based ORs and freestanding ASCs [2]. The main outcomes of interest, including time in surgery, time in operating room, time in postoperative care, and total perioperative time, were significantly shorter in freestanding ASCs than in hospital-based ORs. However, the authors admit that it is unclear how much of the difference was the result of efficiency versus patient selection.

A major study published in 2015 by Kadhim et al. which compared surgical time and operating room efficiency for primary anterior cruciate ligament reconstruction (ACLR) between inpatient and ambulatory facilities within the same institution, found that despite the fact that the same surgeon performed the same surgery at facilities owned by the same institution and primarily working in a single OR, there were differences in OR procedure time and work efficiency [3]. ACLR procedures at the ASC were of shorter duration than those at the inpatient OR ($p < 0.0001$). The median turnover time was also significantly longer at the inpatient facility compared with the ambulatory facility. In fact, if 2 procedures were performed consecutively, the surgical day lasted for 6 h at the ASC compared with 9 h at the hospital.

In addition to being more efficient, ASCs are also associated with a lower cost per case [1]. Koenig et al. studied the impact of the growth of ASCs on total Medicare procedure volume and ASC market share from 2000 to 2009 for 4 common outpatient procedures: cataract surgery, upper gastrointestinal procedures, colonoscopy, and arthroscopy [4]. ASC growth was not significantly associated with Medicare volume, except for colonoscopy. An additional ASC operating room per 100,000 population results in a 1.8 % increase in colonoscopies performed in all outpatient settings. The study demonstrates that continued growth of ASCs could reduce Medicare spending, because ASCs are

D. Grech (✉)
Department of Anesthesiology, Rutgers New Jersey Medical School, 185 South Orange Ave, MSB E-5386, Newark, NJ 07103, USA
e-mail: grechde@njms.rutgers.edu

P. Patel
Department of Anesthesiology and Pain Management, Rutgers Robert Wood Johnson Medical School, 125 Paterson Street, CAB 3100, New Brunswick, NJ 08901, USA
e-mail: preetpatelmd@gmail.com

D. Kam
Department of Anesthesiology, Perioperative Medicine, and Pain Management, University of Miami, Miami, FL, USA

C.S. Scher et al. (eds.), *You're Wrong, I'm Right*, DOI 10.1007/978-3-319-43169-7_83

paid a fraction of the amount paid to hospital outpatient departments for the same services.

Finally, ASCs are not only more efficient and potentially cheaper, but studies have also shown that they achieve a high level of patient satisfaction [5]. Gardner et al. examined differences in patient anxiety and patient satisfaction among patients who experienced surgery at a hospital-based OR versus a freestanding ASC. Forty-seven participants completed the State Trait Anxiety Inventory and Press Ganey Ambulatory Surgery Survey. Patients at both types of facilities experienced moderate levels of preoperative anxiety and were highly satisfied with care received. No significant differences were found in preoperative anxiety, overall satisfaction with care, or overall satisfaction with nursing care. The site where the surgery was performed may not be a determining factor in patient anxiety or satisfaction levels.

CON: While ASCs have many advantages, these facilities also have some drawbacks. According to Hollenbeck et al. ASCs may spur higher overall procedure utilization and thus lead to greater overall health care costs [1]. These investigators used the State Ambulatory Surgery Database of the State of Florida to identify Medicare-aged patients undergoing 4 common ambulatory procedures in 2006, including knee arthroscopy, cystoscopy, cataract removal, and colonoscopy. Ultimately, they found that "the presence of an ASC is associated with higher utilization of common outpatient procedures in the elderly. Whether ASCs are meeting unmet clinical demand or spurring overutilization is not yet clear" [1].

With the continued growth of ASCs, the need for accreditation has become paramount, as accreditation allows for the assessment of clinical practice, improves accountability and better ensures quality of care [6]. In some states, ASC accreditation by a recognized organization is mandated, but in others, it is voluntary. Accreditation provides external validation of safe practices, benchmarking performance against other accredited facilities, and demonstrates to patients and payers the facility's commitment to continuous quality improvement.

Freestanding ASCs also have obvious limitations when compared to hospital-based ORs and inpatient facilities. Freestanding ASCs are generally limited to low- to moderate-risk surgeries as well as low- to moderate-risk patients. High-risk surgeries involve the major organs, brain, sinuses, hip, knee, limb amputations, and the head and neck. Most of these procedures must be performed at inpatient facilities as close monitoring and pain control are needed postoperatively. High-risk patients often have significant uncontrolled comorbidities. Classic examples include patients with renal failure, congestive heart failure (CHF), chronic bronchitis and emphysema (COPD), liver disease, uncontrolled diabetes mellitus (DM), hypertension (HTN), cancer, and morbid obesity. Patients with any of these comorbidities must meet with an anesthesiologist in the preoperative testing clinic, as they are more likely to have a complicated and prolonged recovery, which may require highly trained medical care from multiple specialists. A recent study at the University of Michigan identified specific risk factors that increase the risk of poor outcomes postoperatively: history of cancer, paraplegia, old age (>81), renal failure/dialysis, current steroid use, COPD, and history of stroke [7]. This study suggests that these patients may be more safely cared for if their surgery is performed as an inpatient.

The American Society of Anesthesiologists has identified many characteristics to help predict a difficult airway, including small mouth opening, prominent front teeth, history of neck surgery and/or radiation, limited range of neck motion, inability to see the uvula and tonsils when opening the mouth, and a small chin. Patients with Modified Mallampati classification III–IV are at greater risk for intra- and postoperative complications, which inpatient facilities would be more prepared to manage effectively.

Finally, many ASCs are privately owned and the oversight of a large institution is absent. In these circumstances, it becomes easier to sacrifice patient safety in order to maximize profits. For example, patients may be encouraged by the staff at freestanding ASCs to leave the PACU early. If discharged too soon, patients may experience discomfort during a prolonged drive home, nausea in transit and while at home, trouble changing blood-soaked dressings, difficulty walking to and using the bathroom, as well as more serious medical complications such as bleeding and infection. By recovering from surgery at an inpatient facility, patients can avoid comfort issues as well as have readily available access to medical specialists, imaging modalities, and enhanced postoperative pain management. Additionally, the resources may not exist to treat any serious complications that may occur, and an ambulance ride is required to take the patient to a facility with a higher level of care.

Summary

Advances in the safety of surgical technology and anesthesia medications have allowed ambulatory surgery to become the fastest growing type of surgery in the USA. Patients now have the ability to choose between freestanding ASCs and traditional hospital-based operating rooms for a wide variety of ambulatory surgical procedures. Freestanding ASCs offer many advantages over hospital-based ORs including increased efficiency, lower costs, and similar patient anxiety and satisfaction scores. However, concerns that they may be spurring overutilization, lack the same rigorous accreditation process of hospitals, and are generally unable to handle high-risk patients and perform high-risk procedures limit their appeal.

References

1. Hollenbeck BK, Hollingsworth JM, Dunn RL, Zaojun Y, Birkmeyer JD. Ambulatory surgery center market share and rates of outpatient surgery in the elderly. Surg Innov. 2010;17(4):340–5.
2. Hair B, Hussey P, Wynn B. A comparison of ambulatory perioperative times in hospitals and freestanding centers. Am J Surg. 2012;204(1):23–7.
3. Kadhim M, Gans I, Baldwin K, Flynn J, Ganley T. Do surgical times and efficiency differ between inpatient and ambulatory surgery centers that are both hospital owned? J Pediatr Orthop. 2015.
4. Koenig L, Gu Q. Growth of ambulatory surgical centers, surgery volume, and savings to medicare. Am J Gastroenterol. 2013;108(1):10–5.
5. Gardner TF, Nnadozie MU Sr, Davis BA, Kirk S. Patient anxiety and patient satisfaction in hospital-based and freestanding ambulatory surgery centers. J Nurs Care Qual. 2005;20(3):238–43.
6. Urman RD, Philip BK. Accreditation of ambulatory facilities. Anesthesiol Clin. 2014;32(2):551–7.
7. Mathis MR, Naughton NN, Shanks AM, Freundlich RE, Pannucci CJ, Chu Y, et al. Patient selection for day case-eligible surgery: identifying those at high risk for major complications. Anesthesiology. 2013;119(6):1310–21.

Part X
Acute Pain

Can a Regional Anesthetic Affect the Development of Phantom Limb Pain?

84

Christopher DeNatale

Case

A 62-year-old man presents for urgent amputation of his right lower extremity distal to the knee for progressive gangrene and necrosis. The patient had several previous procedures related to complications of peripheral vascular disease including lower extremity angiograms, femoral stents, and a bi-aorto femoral bypass. The patient has significant preoperative ischemic pain, with a large neuropathic component, and he asks you if there is anything you can do to decrease his likelihood of developing chronic pain after the amputation. After an amputation, there is the possibility that the patient will develop stump pain, phantom limb pain, and even phantom limb sensations. These symptoms can develop soon after the surgery.

Questions

Does a regional anesthetic for limb amputation surgery prevent or alter the development of phantom limb pain (PLP)? Can anything else be done to prevent PLP?

PRO: Although the evidence is controversial, I would perform a regional anesthetic because there is minimal risk, and the potential benefit is enormous.

CON: I don't know of any conclusive study that points to benefits specifically from a single regional anesthetic. Nikolajsen et al. did not demonstrate a difference in chronic phantom or stump pain by using an epidural perioperatively for pain control. They used a comprehensive technique, placing the epidural almost a day prior to the surgery, and left the catheter in place to manage acute pain for several days. The pain was well controlled preoperatively with the epidural, but no long-term benefits were seen in preventing phantom limb or stump pain [1]. Although they were successful in treating acute pain, the absence of long-term benefits and the risk of complications would not lead me to place an epidural routinely for limb amputations. These patients are often also anticoagulated, increasing the risk of epidural hematoma, sometimes to unacceptable levels. The only reason I would do an epidural or regional block would be for acute pain control.

We can improve phantom limb pain simply by achieving adequate perioperative pain control, either with or without an epidural. In their study, Karanikolas and colleagues examined the use of regional versus intravenous patient-controlled analgesia (IV PCA) in the preoperative, intraoperative, and postoperative periods. They found there was no benefit from placing an epidural during any of the 3 stages. A decreased incidence of phantom limb pain, persisting 6 months after the amputation, was found in all groups as long as there was adequate perioperative pain control. No matter what the perioperative plan (epidural or IV PCA), adequate perioperative pain management was the only measure demonstrated to decrease the incidence, intensity, and frequency of phantom limb pain [2]. So the benefit appears to be independent of the epidural.

PRO: If a peripheral nerve catheter can control postoperative pain for a longer duration and to a greater extent than intravenous narcotics, chronic pain could potentially be mitigated via this mechanism. A small study looked at placing a perioperative lower extremity perineural catheter, which was kept in place for a median duration of 30 days. The patients in the intervention study group reported decreased severe phantom limb pain and sensation, even 12 months after the infusion of local anesthetics was discontinued [3].

CON: How practical is that study? Is it safe to leave a peripheral nerve catheter in for a month? Prevention of any

C. DeNatale (✉)
Department of Anesthesiology, Perioperative Care and Pain Medicine, New York University Langone Medical Center, 550 First Avenue, New York, NY 10016, USA
e-mail: Christopher.denatale@nyumc.org

C.S. Scher et al. (eds.), *You're Wrong, I'm Right*, DOI 10.1007/978-3-319-43169-7_84

potential deleterious effect is the first objective of any treatment. There are many problems related to leaving in a perineural catheter for 30 days postoperatively, as shown by the author's reports such as inadvertent removal and infection. Nevertheless if these findings are true, there will be a need for developing methods of safely leaving a perineural catheter in place that long.

PRO: Phantom limb pain is difficult to treat with the current modalities. Any means to prevent the development of PLP would prove extremely helpful to patients undergoing amputation of an extremity. I will speak to the patient, but I feel that a peripheral nerve catheter, even if kept only for a short duration has potential benefits with limited side effects.

In cases of existing PLP, a perineural infusion for only 6 days has also shown possible benefit. Patients reported some improvement in their phantom limb pain even extending out to 1 year after this shorter local anesthetic infusion [4]. I would not make a postoperative peripheral nerve catheter the standard of care on the basis of only a few patients, but this study points to an area that may provide benefit and clearly needs to be explored more thoroughly. Again, I will discuss the anesthetic options with the patient but I would like to plan on a regional anesthetic for optimal pain control and hopefully as a preventive measure to mitigate the likelihood of developing PLP.

Summary

There is no clear consensus about the most beneficial way to approach patients undergoing amputation who are at risk for phantom limb pain. Although there is an interest in exploring postoperative regional anesthesia, there are no clear recommendations at this time. Currently the best management is to treat acute pain appropriately, by IV PCA, epidural, or peripheral regional anesthesia, which may have a beneficial effect on preventing chronic phantom limb pain.

References

1. Nikolajsen L, Ilkjaer S, Christensen J, Kroner K, Jensen T. Randomized trial epidural bupivacaine and morphine in prevention of stump and phantom pain in lower-limb amputation. Lancet. 1997;350:1353–7.
2. Karanikolas M, Aretha D, Tsolakis I, Monantera G, Kiekkas P, Papadoulas S, et al. Optimized perioperative analgesia reduces chronic phantom limb pain intensity, prevalence, and frequency. Anesthesiology. 2011;114(5):1144–54.
3. Borghi B, D'Addabbo M, White P, Gallerani P, Toccaceli L, Raffaeli W, et al. The use of prolonged peripheral neural blockade after lower extremity amputation: the effects on symptoms associated with phantom limb syndrome. Anesth Analg. 2010;111(5):1308–15.
4. Ilfeld B, Moeller-Bertram T, Hanling S, Tokarz K, Mariano E, Loland V, et al. Treating intractable phantom limb pain with ambulatory continuous nerve blocks: a pilot study. Pain Medicine. 2013;14:935–42.

85 Charcot–Marie–Tooth Disease and Regional Anesthesia: Is Perioperative Neuraxial Analgesia Really Contraindicated?

Magdalena Anitescu

Case

A 65-year-old male is scheduled for a 3-h open cholecystectomy and hemicolectomy. His electronic medical records are sparse. After meeting the patient in the preoperative holding area and discussing his case with the surgical service, you learn that the patient has had multiple abdominal surgeries for small bowel obstruction of unknown origin. Three years ago, Charcot–Marie–Tooth (CMT) disease was diagnosed. He has early leg fatigue and difficulty walking and usually requires a wheelchair. The cardiologists who evaluated him preoperatively did not recommend cardiac testing in preparation for surgery because his cardiac risk is low. A review of the computed tomography (CT) scan shows many abdominal adhesions encasing the transverse colon, cecum, and gallbladder, and extensive fibrous tissue that may indicate subacute small bowel obstruction. During an open lysis of adhesions performed two-and-a-half years ago, the patient was given an epidural, which offered excellent pain relief.

Question

Given the patient's excellent experience with epidural analgesia and in view of the expected length of surgery, would you consider placing a neuraxial catheter for this patient with a congenital neuromuscular disorder?

PRO: The patient had excellent results with a previous epidural. He is scheduled for an incision from the xiphoid process to 5 cm under the umbilicus. At risk for severe postoperative pain, he is the perfect candidate for an epidural catheter for perioperative pain control, especially after undergoing open hemicolectomy and cholecystectomy [1].

CON: Good points, but the patient has a neuromuscular disorder. CMT is a progressive congenital disease associated with distal–proximal progression of muscle weakness. In severe cases, weakness of the axial muscles contributes to scoliosis and pulmonary restriction [2]. This patient has not been evaluated recently by a neurologist. Thus, we do not know how advanced his disease is. If the patient experiences severe muscle weakness after an epidural is placed, how will we determine whether the weakness is associated with CMT or with a complication of the neuraxial procedure?

PRO: Excellent points, but CMT is a genetically heterogeneous disorder that can be diagnosed based on its common phenotypical picture: progressive peroneal muscle weakness and atrophy. The symptoms of CMT vary from very mild to severe. The critical form of this condition, CMT Type I, has an onset during adolescence. It is associated with serious musculoskeletal and respiratory comorbidities. CMT Type I neuropathy occurs before the skeletal growth spurt. As a consequence, the axial skeleton is weakened with subsequent scoliosis and restrictive lung disease. The milder form of this genetic disorder, CMT Type II, occurs around the fifth to seventh decade of life. Clinical manifestations show a slower onset and are slowly progressive, with mild weakness [3].

CON: Patients who undergo extensive surgery are at high risk of experiencing severe postoperative pain. A comprehensive perioperative regimen for pain control should be planned, involving multimodal analgesic therapy; epidural analgesia may be only 1 of the many tools necessary to treat postoperative pain in this patient. One may argue that in the presence of a neuromuscular disorder, an epidural may be contraindicated. Modalities involving intraoperative ketamine and lidocaine infusions may prove beneficial. Ketamine, at a rate of 0.5 mg/kg/h, may decrease the need for opioids and result in better pain scores [4].

M. Anitescu
Department of Anesthesia and Critical Care, University of Chicago Medicine, 4851 S. Maryland Ave, MC 4028, Chicago, IL 60637, USA

M. Anitescu (✉)
5513 S. Kimbark Ave, Chicago, IL 60637, USA
e-mail: Manitescu@dacc.uchicago.edu

C.S. Scher et al. (eds.), *You're Wrong, I'm Right*, DOI 10.1007/978-3-319-43169-7_85

PRO: In older adults with marginal cognitive dysfunction, ketamine infusions at high rates may predispose to significant perioperative delirium. A neuraxial technique may still be superior, especially if the continuous infusion contains only an opioid and not a local anesthetic. A detailed preoperative evaluation and documentation of baseline neurological function is required in this patient to sort out potential postoperative adverse events.

CON: Patients with a neurological disorder may be exposed to the "double-crush" phenomenon when a neuraxial procedure is performed. With preexisting neural compromise, patients may be more susceptible to injury than their normal counterparts when exposed to a secondary neurological insult at another site. It is possible that in those select patients, the spinal cord may be significantly injured during traumatic needle or catheter placement, especially when sensation is limited by the underlying neuropathy[5]. The patient may be unable to report paresthesias after needle or catheter placement.

PRO: Although in some select cases neuraxial analgesia may be contraindicated, the overwhelming evidence supports the many benefits of epidural perioperative analgesia in major surgery [6].

Summary

Neuraxial epidural infusions with local anesthetics and/or opioids are excellent analgesic techniques for a variety of surgical procedures. In patients with baseline neuromuscular disorders, careful neurological examination and an understanding of etiology prognosis and stage of disease are essential in weighing the risks and benefits of a neuraxial technique.

In mild, stable neuromuscular disorders such as CMT Type II, epidural analgesia may be beneficial preoperatively, especially if only opioid solutions are used. The addition of a local anesthetic (LA) to the epidural solution should be carefully considered. A LA has effects on the fibers already injured by the underlying disease. Custom-made solutions with a low concentration of LA may be better tolerated by patients with neuromuscular diseases, because they may have less impact on the sensory, autonomic, and motor fibers blocked during neuraxial anesthesia.

In severe neuromuscular disorders such as CMT Type I, the analgesic plan may involve alternative multimodal techniques such as intraoperative infusion of lidocaine and ketamine, temporary use of perioperative long-acting medications such as methadone, or preemptive administration of membrane stabilizers such as gabapentin or pregabalin. The anesthesiologist must weigh the risks and benefits of a neuraxial procedure for patients suffering from various neuromuscular disorders whether congenital or acquired.

References

1. White PF, Kehlet H. Improving postoperative pain management: what are the unresolved issues? Anesthesiology. 2010;112:220–5.
2. Bösenberg A, Larkin K. Anaesthesia and Charcot-Marie-Tooth disease. South Afr J Anaesth Analg. 2006;12(4):131–3.
3. Pareyson D, Marchesi C. Diagnosis, natural history and management of Charcot-Marie-Tooth disease. Lancet Neurol. 2009;8:654–67.
4. Bell RF, Dahl JB, Moore RA, Kalso E. Perioperative ketamine for acute post-operative pain: a quantitative and qualitative systematic review. Acta Anesthesiol Scand. 2005;49:1405–28.
5. Klingler W, Lehmann-Horn F, Jurkat-Rott K. Complications of anesthesia in neuromuscular disorders. Neuromuscul Disord. 2005;15:195–206.
6. Pöpping DM, Elia N, Van Aken HK, Marret E, Schug SA, Kranke P, et al. Impact of epidural analgesia on mortality and morbidity after surgery: systematic review and meta-analysis of randomized controlled trials. Ann Surg. 2014;259:1056–67.

Positional Headache Without a Previous Lumbar Puncture: Would a Blood Patch Be Useful?

86

Magdalena Anitescu

Case

You are paged by a neurology colleague who asks you to perform an epidural blood patch (EBP) for a 30-year-old female with severe, debilitating positional headache. You agree to evaluate the patient but do not commit to an intervention yet. The patient has been suffering from acute onset of severe positional headaches for 1 month. She was initially treated by her primary care physician with ibuprofen and hydrocodone but these medications offered little relief. Her pain is throbbing, severe, and primarily temporal, less so in the frontal and occipital areas. The pain is much worse when she sits and stands and decreases slightly when lying flat. No other symptoms are found. She states that she can no longer care for her 4 children because of debilitating pain.

Question

In view of a positional headache without a history of dural puncture and possible idiopathic intracranial hypotension (IIH), would an epidural blood patch (EBP) confirm the diagnosis and provide effective pain relief?

PRO: The neurologist who accompanies her insists you perform the EBP emergently since he is convinced that the patient has IIH [1]. The clinical presentation of this patient is consistent with IIH, a condition that manifests with new onset of severe positional headache without a history of dural puncture, that occurs within 15 min of sitting or standing. He insists that, in his experience, no medications can help this kind of pain and the most effective treatment is a lumbar epidural blood patch.

M. Anitescu
Department of Anesthesia and Critical Care, University of Chicago Medicine, 4851 S. Maryland Ave, MC 4028, Chicago, IL 60637, USA

M. Anitescu (✉)
5513 S. Kimbark Ave, Chicago, IL 60637, USA
e-mail: Manitescu@dacc.uchicago.edu

CON: In spite of the possibility of IIH, the location of the headache is somewhat unusual. The patient complains of headache primarily in the temporal area and not in the classically described fronto-occipital distribution. While IIH is still the likely diagnosis, other conditions may be associated with these symptoms, like postural orthostatic tachycardia (POTS). Diabetes insipidus and cervicogenic pain can also mimic the positional headache of IIH [2]. Those conditions would not respond well to the epidural blood patch (EBP) and as such other investigations are needed for proper diagnosis in our case.

PRO: Headache is a common symptom that brings patients to a general practitioner's office; however, positional headaches are generally rare. The idiopathic intracranial hypotension (IIH) syndrome has specific diagnostic criteria:

1. Orthostatic headache
2. At least 1 of the following:
   (a) Low opening cerebrospinal fluid (CSF) pressure (<60 mm H2O)
   (b) Sustained improvement after epidural blood patch (EBP)
   (c) Demonstrated active leak of cerebrospinal fluid
   (d) Signs of intracranial hypotension on cranial magnetic resonance imaging (MRI)
3. No history of dural puncture
4. No other disease

The EBP is essential for both diagnosing and treating IIH [3].

CON: Without imaging studies, the risk of an EBP outweighs its benefits if there is an incorrect diagnosis. When EBP was used to treat positional headache in IIH, there were several reports of rebound intracranial hypertension immediately after the blood was injected into the epidural space. Intracranial hypo- and hypertension are both usually associated with severe headaches, whose character

C.S. Scher et al. (eds.), *You're Wrong, I'm Right*, DOI 10.1007/978-3-319-43169-7_86

may sometimes be confusing. Shifting from low to high intracranial pressure may be associated with change in location of the headache. IIH is usually associated with occipital pain; intracranial hypertension is localized more in the frontal areas and retro-orbital region. New onset nausea, vomiting, and blurred vision after a blood patch may help diagnose this complication [4]. Imaging tests are needed to confirm the diagnosis.

PRO: Several diagnostic imaging studies have been used since the description of the syndrome. In a patient with severe positional headache but no history of dural puncture of any kind, suspicion of IIT should be confirmed with invasive and non-invasive imaging. Since invasive diagnostic studies primarily involve a dural puncture, imaging tests should be the first choice. An MRI may show the signs of low pressure in IIH, often known as SEEPS [5]:

1. Subdural fluid collection
2. Enhancement of the pachymeninges
3. Engorgement of the venous structures
4. Pituitary hyperemia
5. Sagging of the brain

An MRI can be a diagnostic tool in IIH, but it is unclear whether it confirms the diagnosis. Many tests utilized in diagnosing the IIH have various sensitivities and specificities. No one best test is available.

CON: With recent technological advances, imaging tests have gained momentum in diagnosing IIH. When MRI is coupled with intracranial venography, the diagnostic value of the test is enhanced [6]. A radionuclide cisternogram is currently 1 method of confirming the diagnosis of IIH. In conjunction with spine MRI for the presence of collected fluid, it allows correct visualization of the CSF leak and is therefore essential in directing the correct placement of the EBP [5].

PRO: So, if we identify the level of a CSF leak we can actually placc thc EBP. The supposed mechanism of action is gelatinous tamponade of the dural leak, followed by fibrin deposits and fibroblastic activity. Another postulated mechanism of action may be restriction of CSF flow within the spinal epidural space, which interferes with CSF absorption. I would vote for performing an EBP as quickly as possible.

CON: All treatment modalities in IIH start with a conservative regimen. As with a post dural puncture headache, the headache in IIH may resolve with rest, caffeinated beverages, increased fluid intake, and abdominal binders. Those methods are intended to increase CSF pressure at the site of the leakage and thus relieve the headaches to some extent. Other treatments include administration of intravenous caffeine or theophylline for their effects on adenosine receptors. The resulting vasoconstriction decreases intracranial blood flow and venous engorgement.

Only about 60 % of patients have both initial and long-term relief after a first EPB. A second EBP can be applied as early as the fifth day following the first injection in patients with severe symptoms [2]. To optimize the effect, the EBP must be placed as close as possible to the leak [7]. Infusion of saline or artificial CSF may offer limited benefit. Surgical intervention is a last resort, reserved for refractory cases with massive dural defect.

Summary

IIH is a syndrome of positional headache in the absence of a dural puncture. In many cases, it is difficult to diagnose and can be confused with other conditions causing headache. Diagnosis requires invasive and noninvasive imaging tests such as brain MRI with venogram, radionuclide cisternogram, and lumbar puncture with opening CSF pressure. EBP is the mainstay of treatment but is often less effective than it is for postdural puncture headache. Many times 2 or even 3 EBPs are needed for effective resolution of symptoms. Surgical treatments are reserved for refractory cases.

References

1. Schievink WI. Spontaneous spinal cerebrospinal fluid leaks and intracranial hypotension. JAMA. 2006;295(19):2286–96.
2. Schievink WI, Deline CR. Headache secondary to intracranial hypotension. Cure Pain Headache Rep. 2014;18:245–52.
3. Schievink WI, Dodick DW, Mokri B, Silberstein S, Bousser MG, Goadsby PJ. Diagnostic criteria for headache due to spontaneous intracranial hypotension: a perspective. Headache. 2011;51: 1442–4.
4. Kranz PG, Amrhein TJ, Gray L. Rebound intracranial hypertension: a complication of epidural blood patching for intracranial hypotension. Am J Neuroradiol. 2014;35:1237–40.
5. Wiesemann E, Berding G, Goetz F, Windhagen A. Spontaneous intracranial hypotension: correlation of imaging findings with clinical features. Eur Neurol. 2006;56:204–10.
6. Maralani PJ, Hassanlou M, Torres C, Chakraborty S, Kingstone M, Patel V, et al. Accuracy of brain imaging in the diagnosis of idiopathic intracranial hypotension. Clin Radiol. 2012;67:656–63.
7. Benzon HT, Nemickas R, Molloy RE, Ahmad S, Melen O, Cohen B. Lumbar and thoracic epidural blood injections to treat spontaneous intracranial hypotension. Anesthesiology. 1996;85:920–2.

Single-Dose Epidural Morphine or Patient-Controlled Epidural Analgesia (PCEA) for Post-Cesarean Pain Control?

87

Lucia Daiana Voiculescu, Olga Eydlin, and Joseph Thomas Largi

Case

A 32-year-old G3P1 female with a body mass index (BMI) of 40 presents for elective, repeat cesarean delivery. The patient denies other comorbidities, but her husband states that she snores loudly at night and notes pauses in her nighttime breathing. The patient reports that after her previous cesarean delivery, the epidural catheter impeded her ability to interact with the baby. Her right leg was numb and weak, and she could not get up to go to the bathroom. The skin around the catheter insertion remained red, swollen, and painful for a few days. Overall, it was "very uncomfortable." As a consequence, she asks you if it would be possible to have the catheter removed immediately after surgery.

Prior to the procedure, an L3/4 epidural catheter is inserted, and a surgical block is achieved using 20 mL of 2 % lidocaine with 1:200,000 epinephrine. The cesarean delivery proceeds without complications. However, the patient's oxygen level is in the low 90 s during the case, requiring supplemental oxygen via nasal cannula and placement of the patient in reverse Trendelenburg position. At the end of the surgery, the anesthesia team discusses the postoperative plan for the epidural catheter and pain management.

L.D. Voiculescu (✉) · O. Eydlin · J.T. Largi
Department of Anesthesiology, Perioperative Care and Pain Medicine, New York University School of Medicine, 550 First Avenue, New York, NY 10016, USA
e-mail: lucia.voiculescu@nyumc.org

O. Eydlin
e-mail: Olga.Eydlin@nyumc.org

J.T. Largi
e-mail: Joseph.Largi@nyumc.org

Question

Single-dose epidural morphine or patient-controlled epidural analgesia (PCEA) for post-cesarean pain control?

PRO: In recent years, the number of cesarean births in the USA has significantly increased in 2011 accounting for 33 % of total deliveries [1, 2]. The postoperative pain associated with this intervention is usually moderate to severe and gradually subsides after 40–48 h.

Neuraxial administration of morphine before removing the epidural catheter at the end of the surgery is a technique used frequently for post-cesarean analgesia. A single dose of epidural morphine produces adequate analgesia for up to 24 h without significant sedation, hemodynamic effects, or impairment of neuromuscular function [3–9].

A prospective, randomized, double-blind study by Kumarasamy et al. evaluating 60 ASA 1 and 2 patients who underwent cesarean deliveries compared the effectiveness and duration of analgesia with epidural morphine, 4 mg versus 5 mg, for postoperative pain relief. Five milligrams of morphine provided longer analgesia and was more effective in providing postoperative pain control [4]. This study notes that there was no excessive sedation or respiratory depression with either dose in these patients.

CON: Based on BMI, this patient meets the criteria for clinically severe obesity. Her history of snoring, nighttime witnessed apneic events, and dozing off frequently during the daytime is suspicious for obstructive sleep apnea (OSA), even though she has never been formally tested [10]. Administering epidural morphine, an opioid associated with delayed respiratory depression, to a patient already at risk for obstruction (due to her body habitus and symptoms of OSA), increases the risk of postoperative complications.

A recent meta-analysis by El-Solh et al. [11] showed that patients with OSA have "an almost 2.5-fold increased risk of developing postoperative respiratory failure." In a closed claims analysis, Lee et al. [12] found that "the vast majority" of opioid-induced respiratory depression events occurred

C.S. Scher et al. (eds.), *You're Wrong, I'm Right*, DOI 10.1007/978-3-319-43169-7_87

within 24 h of surgery, and a significant number involved epidural opioid administration. Obesity and OSA both increase the risk of respiratory depression when neuraxial opioids are used [12, 13]. In addition, along with the normal physiologic changes of pregnancy, obesity can result in rapid desaturation and difficult ventilation if respiratory depression occurs. After epidural morphine administration, all patients should be monitored for a minimum of 24 h [13].

PRO: PCEA patients should also be monitored for as long as the catheter is in place. Patients should be evaluated periodically for the efficacy of analgesia as well as potential complications (hematoma, epidural abscess, skin infection, catheter migration, etc.). Although the PCEA may result in better pain control beyond the first 24 postoperative hours, the equipment used and the specialized personnel involved in the process make this analgesic modality more expensive [14].

In the past, this patient experienced some catheter-related problems: unilateral, deep anesthesia (probably due to catheter migration), and superficial cellulitis at the insertion site. Removing the catheter at the end of the procedure will decrease the potential for such unpleasant results.

After the surgical block resolves, the patient will be able to stand and walk without weakness, numbness or proprioceptive deficit. Early ambulation leads to greater patient satisfaction. Further, it also could prevent deep venous thrombosis (DVT) [15]. After cesarean delivery, this obese patient has an increased risk of early venous thromboembolism [16, 17]. Removing the catheter at the end of the procedure means that a greater range of antithrombotic agents can be prescribed within hours of the surgery.

Superficial cellulitis or deep infection can be avoided by early removal of the catheter [18, 19]. If PCEA is chosen, the risk of infection needs to be minimized by maintaining a closed system, with a limited number of catheter manipulations and inspecting the insertion site every 8 h [20].

CON: While epidural morphine can provide good postoperative analgesia, many side effects are possible including nausea, vomiting, pruritus, sedation, urinary retention, and respiratory depression [3, 6, 8, 14]. These are concerns that must be considered and discussed with the patient prior to administering any medication. The risks of respiratory depression and nausea, vomiting, or pruritus are dose related, being higher with doses exceeding 4 mg of morphine [4, 6]. The study by Kumarasamy et al. demonstrated that the incidence of postoperative nausea and vomiting (PONV) as well as pruritus was significantly higher in patients who received higher doses of morphine (5 mg) than lower doses (4 mg). Specifically, 72 and 82 % of patients who received 5 mg of epidural morphine experienced PONV and pruritus, respectively. In contrast, 16 and 29 % of patients who received 4 mg of epidural morphine had PONV and pruritus, respectively [4]. This study evaluated relatively healthy patients with a mean weight of approximately 68 kg and mean height of approximately 156–158 cm. Further studies evaluating the use of epidural morphine in obese patients for post-cesarean analgesia are warranted.

PRO: The patient had a poor experience during her previous epidural, and care should be taken to avoid further problems. However, many of the side effects of epidural morphine are treatable should they arise. Pruritus is secondary to the μ (mu)-agonist property of morphine and should be treated with low-dose intravenous naloxone. Diphenhydramine will only produce sedation; it does not help to alleviate pruritus as it is not related to histamine release. Nausea can be treated with several medications and techniques including ensuring adequate hydration and administering appropriate antinausea medications, such as ondansetron.

CON: Epidural analgesia (opioids, local anesthetics, or a combination of both) is a very effective and safe way to control postoperative pain from cesarean delivery. After the neuraxial catheter is removed, the analgesic options become limited, although the patient would be able to receive acetaminophen and ketorolac if there are no contraindications. Intravenous or oral opioids could produce satisfactory analgesia; however, systemic opioids may make the mother sleepy and dizzy and may sedate the baby via her breast milk. Epidural PCA provides better postoperative pain control than parenteral or neuraxial opioids [14]. Retaining the catheter and infusing low-dose fentanyl and bupivacaine should not prevent the patient from ambulating while achieving good analgesia.

The obstetrics and anesthesia teams as well as nursing staff discussed the potential benefits and risks of the available postoperative analgesia regimens with the patient. They counseled the patient about the potential risk of respiratory depression from epidural morphine and possible challenges in satisfactorily controlling her pain, particularly toward the end of the first postoperative day [14]. The patient decided to keep the epidural catheter, and the team set up an epidural PCA with low-dose fentanyl and bupivacaine.

Summary

As the incidence of obesity in the general population is increasing, including in women of childbearing age, it is very important to choose a postoperative pain management regimen that optimizes analgesia while minimizing side effects in the obese parturient population. It is essential to achieve good pain control after cesarean delivery in order to improve maternal–infant bonding. Adequate analgesia permits early ambulation and discharge, which may lead to greater patient satisfaction. Each patient should be evaluated on a case-by-case basis by the interdisciplinary team of anesthesia, obstetrics, and/or pain management.

Epidural PCA with local anesthetics and opioids is effective and tolerated well by most patients. Initial placement and maintenance of PCEA requires specialized equipment as well as personnel trained in catheter management, making this modality more expensive.

Single-shot epidural morphine provides adequate postoperative pain control, especially in the first 20–24 h. Its use is limited by the high frequency of side effects, such as nausea, vomiting, pruritus, sedation, urinary retention, and respiratory depression.

Multimodal opioid-sparing regimens, such as acetaminophen and/or ketorolac, in conjunction with epidural analgesia (PCA or single-dose morphine at the end of the surgery) should be employed whenever possible. Further large, double-blind studies are necessary to evaluate the safety and efficacy of epidural morphine in diverse categories of postpartum patients.

References

1. Hamilton BE, Martin JA, Ventura SJ. Births: preliminary data for 2012. Natl Vital Stat Rep. 2013;62(3):1–20.
2. Witt WP, Wisk LE, Cheng ER, Mandell K, Chatterjee D, Wakeel F, et al. Determinants of cesarean delivery in the US: a lifecourse approach. Matern Child Health J. 2015;19(1):84–93.
3. Kotelko DM, Dailey PA, Shnider SM, Rosen MA, Hughes SC, Brizgys RV. Epidural morphine analgesia after cesarean delivery. Obstet Gynecol. 1984;63(3):409–13.
4. Kumarasamy S, Choy YC. Epidural morphine for postoperative analgesia after caesarean section. Acute Pain. 2008;10(3–4):117–21.
5. Youssef N, Orlov D, Alie T, Chong M, Cheng J, Thabane L, Paul J. What epidural opioid results in the best analgesia outcomes and fewest side effects after surgery?: a meta-analysis of randomized controlled trials. Anesth Analg. 2014;119(4):965–7.
6. Bonnet MP, Mignon A, Mazoit JX, Ozier Y, Marret E. Analgesic efficacy and adverse effects of epidural morphine compared to parenteral opioids after elective caesarean section: a systematic review. Eur J Pain. 2010;14(9):894.e1–9.
7. Gambling D, Hughes T, Martin G, Horton W, Manvelian G. A comparison of Depodur, a novel, single-dose extended-release epidural morphine, with standard epidural morphine for pain relief after lower abdominal surgery. Anesth Analg. 2005;100(4):1065–74.
8. Martin R, Lamarche Y, Tétrault JP. Epidural and intrathecal narcotics. Can Anaesth Soc J. 1983;30(6):662–73.
9. Rosen MA, Hughes SC, Shnider SM, Abboud TK, Norton M, Dailey PA, Curtis JD. Epidural morphine for the relief of postoperative pain after cesarean delivery. Anesth Analg. 1983;62(7):666–72.
10. Finkel KJ, Searleman AC, Tymkew H, Tanaka CY, Saager L, Safer-Zadeh E, et al. Prevalence of undiagnosed obstructive sleep apnea among adult surgical patients in an academic medical center. Sleep Med. 2009;10:753–8.
11. Hai F, Porhomayon J, Vermont L, Frydrych L, Jaoude P, El-Solh AA. Postoperative complications in patients with obstructive sleep apnea: a meta-analysis. J Clin Anesth. 2014;26(8):591–600.
12. Lee LA, Caplan RA, Stephens LS, Posner KL, Terman GW, Voepel-Lewis T, Domino KB. Postoperative opioid-induced respiratory depression: a closed claims analysis. Anesthesiology. 2015;122(3):659–65.
13. American Society of Anesthesiologists Task Force on Neuraxial Opioids, Horlocker TT, Burton AW, Connis RT, Hughes SC, Nickinovich DG, Palmer CM, et al. Practice guidelines for the prevention, detection, and management of respiratory depression associated with neuraxial opioid administration. Anesthesiology. 2009;110(2):218–30.
14. Vercauteren M, Vereecken K, La MM, Coppejans H, Adriaensen H. Cost-effectiveness of analgesia after Caesarean section. A comparison of intrathecal morphine and epidural PCA. Acta Anaesthesiol Scand. 2002;46(1):85–9.
15. Francis C. Prophylaxis for thromboembolism in hospitalized medical patients. N Engl J Med. 2007;356:1438–44.
16. Tepper NK, Boulet SL, Whiteman MK, Monsour M, Marchbanks PA, Hooper WC, et al. Postpartum venous thromboembolism: incidence and risk factors. Obstet Gynecol. 2014;123(5):987–96.
17. Gadsen J, Hart S, Santos AC. Post-cesarean delivery analgesia. Anesth Analg. 2005;101(5 Suppl):S62–9.
18. Yuan H, Zuo Z, Yu K, Lin W, Lee H, Chan K. Bacterial colonization of epidural catheters used for short-term postoperative analgesia. Anesthesiology. 2008;108:130–7.
19. Dawson S. Epidural catheter infections. J Hosp Infect. 2001;47(1):3–8.
20. Brooks K, Pasero C, Hubbard L, Coghlan RH. The risk of infection associated with epidural analgesia. Infect Control Hosp Epidemiol. 1995;16(12):725–8.

Is Opioid Avoidance Warranted for a Patient with Obstructive Sleep Apnea in the Postoperative Period?

88

Lucia Daiana Voiculescu and Olga Eydlin

Case

A 55-year-old man with a body mass index (BMI) of 46, obstructive sleep apnea (OSA) non-compliant with home continuous positive airway pressure (CPAP), hypertension, type 2 diabetes, and gastroesophageal reflux presents for laparoscopic cholecystectomy.

On examination, the patient has redundant neck tissue, a full beard, a large tongue, and a Mallampati class 3 airway. Anticipating a possible difficult airway, the anesthesia team brings a video laryngoscope into the room. After induction, the patient is difficult to ventilate, requiring an oral airway, jaw thrust, and 2-person ventilation. Direct laryngoscopy is challenging. Intubation is achieved using the video laryngoscope.

Thirty minutes into the case, the surgical team decides to convert the procedure to open cholecystectomy because of difficult visualization. The rest of the operation goes smoothly. As the surgeons are getting ready to close the abdomen, they ask the anesthesiologist to give the patient a "good amount" of fentanyl so that he will be comfortable in the postanesthesia care unit (PACU). The anesthesiologist is concerned about systemic opioid analgesia for this morbidly obese patient with OSA and a difficult airway. He suggests a ketamine infusion instead to minimize postoperative opioid requirements.

Question

Is opioid avoidance warranted for the OSA patient in the postop period?

L.D. Voiculescu (✉) · O. Eydlin
Department of Anesthesiology, Perioperative Care and Pain Medicine, New York University School of Medicine, 550 First Avenue, New York, NY 10016, USA
e-mail: lucia.voiculescu@nyumc.org

O. Eydlin
e-mail: Olga.Eydlin@nyumc.org

OSA is a common sleep-associated breathing disorder that is caused by repetitive partial or complete obstruction of the upper airway, resulting in episodes of apnea, hypercarbia, and oxygen desaturation during sleep. It is associated with excessive daytime sleepiness, fatigue, and impaired concentration. Obesity is the most important risk factor for OSA [1, 2]. Patients with OSA also have an increased hazard of developing perioperative cardiopulmonary complications [2, 3]. Bariatric surgery and difficult intubation are known to further increase the risk of postoperative events [2].

PRO: "The anesthetic and analgesic plan should be focused on avoiding agents and techniques with known potential for worsening hypoventilation and hypoxemia," says the anesthesiologist. "Morbidly obese patients with sleep apnea are at increased risk of developing apneic episodes and hypercarbia when opioids are used for pain relief. In the immediate postoperative period, systemic opioids should be carefully titrated. Pulse oximetry should be closely monitored, and supplemental oxygen considered" [2, 3].

> Furthermore, should these patients become apneic in the PACU, airway management may be problematic. Our patient was already difficult to ventilate and intubate in the operating room despite having the appropriate team and necessary equipment.

Hence, the anesthesiologist suggests that a strategy to minimize opioids, such as a ketamine infusion, should be considered [2–6].

CON: The surgeon interjects, "In all my years of practice, I have never used a ketamine infusion to treat postoperative pain. I plan to place the patient on a fentanyl patient-controlled analgesia (PCA), as I typically do for my laparotomy patients. Also, my nurses and residents are not familiar with ketamine dosing and side effects, therefore, the risk of errors would be high."

He refers to a prospective analysis by Leape et al. that found that lack of knowledge of a drug to be the most common proximal cause of medication error in the hospital setting. Incorrect dosage, frequency, and route of administration

C.S. Scher et al. (eds.), *You're Wrong, I'm Right*, DOI 10.1007/978-3-319-43169-7_88

were among the frequent mistakes identified in that analysis [7]. It is known that opioid and non-opioid analgesics are among the "high-alert" or "high-risk" drugs often involved in medication-related adverse events. Off-label use (such as the administration of ketamine for postoperative analgesia) also increases the possibility of a negative outcome [8].

The surgeon emphasizes, "I have been able to achieve good pain control with fentanyl. Fentanyl's pharmacodynamics are well known and suitable for this specific post-surgical pain. The analgesic effects are rapid. On a fentanyl PCA, the patient can be transferred to a regular room where SpO_2 monitoring and supplemental oxygen can be provided. In contrast, a ketamine infusion would require the patient to be admitted to the intensive care unit, with additional cost and possible personal financial burden."

PRO: The anesthesiologist points out that every patient does not fit into a "cookie-cutter" postoperative order list. "Ketamine may be a suitable alternative or additive to opioids in providing postoperative analgesia in selected patients (elderly, opioid sensitive or resistant, those with OSA or known difficult airway, etc.).

"Ketamine is an analgesic and dissociative anesthetic that acts on various receptors, including the *N*-methyl-D-aspartate (NMDA) receptor, opioid, and some monoaminergic receptors. [9] Through non-competitive NMDA receptor antagonism, ketamine may decrease windup (progressive increase in pain signals caused by repeated nociceptive stimuli) and central sensitization (heightened sensitivity to pain), as well as opioid-induced hyperalgesia. It is recognized to have an opioid-sparing effect. Perioperative intravenous ketamine decreases pain intensity and opioid consumption for up to 24–48 h postoperatively [5, 6, 10, 11].

A meta-analysis by Bell et al. concluded that "ketamine in subanesthetic doses is effective in reducing morphine requirements in the first 24 h after surgery." The review determined that patients receiving a combination of ketamine and morphine experience a significant reduction in postoperative nausea and vomiting, possibly due to a morphine-sparing effect [6]. Small doses of ketamine produce analgesia while preserving respiratory drive. Additionally, in low doses, it produces bronchodilatation and mild respiratory stimulation. Ketamine is also advantageous in that it protects upper airway patency in patients with OSA [5].

CON: The surgeon raises the concern that patients on ketamine may have unpleasant psychotomimetic side effects such as hallucinations, "out of body" experiences, disturbing dreams, and irrational behavior.

"While premedication with benzodiazepines can provide some protection against hallucinations, this may not always be complete [10]. Midazolam and other benzodiazepines may also cause respiratory depression, especially if administered in association with opioids," he argues.

PRO: The anesthesiologist counters, "While it is certainly possible to have unpleasant dreams and hallucinations from ketamine, these side effects are more common after large doses of ketamine rather than from low-dose infusions. The side effects associated with subanesthetic doses of ketamine are mild or absent [6, 11] and frequently are further reduced by premedication with a low dose of midazolam [11]. Additionally, while postoperative pain control with fentanyl is well established, its analgesic effects are often limited by adverse effects such as drowsiness, respiratory depression, nausea, vomiting, and constipation. Opioid-induced airway obstruction is of special concern in morbidly obese patients with OSA [5]. A multimodal opioid-sparing approach can help minimize some of these unwanted effects."

CON: "While it is possible that ketamine may decrease postoperative pain scores and opioid requirements," the surgeon says, "I'm concerned that there is no reversal agent for ketamine. My team is familiar with diagnosing and treating opioid-induced respiratory depression and sedation. Naloxone is available on the floor and can be immediately administered to reverse the unwanted effects. Should the patient receive too much ketamine in the absence of a reversal agent, supportive care and time would be the only treatment solution."

Going further, both teams agreed that an in-depth discussion between the surgical and anesthesia teams is necessary for optimal patient care and that every patient should be evaluated on a case-by-case basis. After much debate, they decided to treat this patient with acetaminophen, ketorolac, and a fentanyl PCA. The team chose not to start ketamine immediately in an attempt to avoid a costly ICU admission, but they left the option of a ketamine infusion open if the patient's pain was not adequately controlled with the above regimen.

Summary

The continuous advances made in perioperative medicine in tandem with the evolution of surgical techniques have led to increasingly complex patients undergoing surgery. This diverse patient population poses a clinically challenging environment for postoperative pain management. Elderly or frail patients, patients sensitive or resistant to opioids, and patients with OSA or a difficult airway represent only a few categories in which the opioid-sparing effect of ketamine may be considered. Each patient should be managed on a case-specific basis. Multimodal analgesia with ketamine, non-steroidal anti-inflammatory drugs (NSAIDs), acetaminophen, or other adjuvant agents should be considered whenever possible to reduce the amount of systemic opioids. Careful discussion and effective communication among perioperative teams is necessary to achieve the safest level of care.

References

1. Masood A, Phillips B. Sleep apnea. Curr Opin Pulm Med. 2000;6:479–84.
2. Porhomayon J, Nader ND, Leissner KB, El-Solh AA. Respiratory perioperative management of patients with obstructive sleep apnea. J Intensive Care Med. 2014;29(3):145–53.
3. Rösslein M. Perioperative management of adult patients with obstructive sleep apnea. Anasthesiol Intensivmed Notfallmed Schmerzther. 2015;50:174–82.
4. Thangathurai D, Roffey P. Postoperative pain relief with ketamine in patients with central sleep apnea. J Clin Sleep Med. 2009;5:480.
5. Alvarez A, Singh PM, Sinha AC. Postoperative analgesia in morbid obesity. Obes Surg. 2014;24:652–9.
6. Bell RF, Dahl JB, Moore RA, Kalso E. Perioperative ketamine for acute postoperative pain. Cochrane Database Syst Rev. 2006 Jan 25;(1):CD004603.
7. Leape LL, Bates DW, Cullen DJ, Cooper J, Demonaco HJ, Gallivan T, et al. Systems analysis of adverse drug events. ADE Prevention Study Group. JAMA. 1995;274(1):35–43.
8. Benjamin DM. Reducing medication errors and increasing patient safety: case studies in clinical pharmacology. J Clin Pharmacol. 2003;43:768–83.
9. Kapur S, Seeman P. NMDA receptor antagonists ketamine and PCP have direct effects on the dopamine D(2) and serotonin 5-HT (2)receptors-implications for models of schizophrenia. Mol Psychiatry. 2002;7(8):837–44.
10. Elia N, Tramèr MR. Ketamine and postoperative pain—a quantitative systematic review of randomised trials. Pain. 2005;113(1–2):61–70.
11. Garg N, Panda NB, Gandhi KA, Bhagat H, Batra YK, Grover VK, et al. Comparison of small dose ketamine and dexmedetomidine infusion for postoperative analgesia in spine surgery—a prospective randomized double-blind placebo controlled study. J Neurosurg Anesthesiol. 2016;28(1):27–31.

Part XI
Regional

Is Spinal or Epidural Anesthesia Contraindicated in a Patient with Multiple Sclerosis?

89

Uchenna O. Umeh

Case

An obese 31-year-old female with relapsing-remitting multiple sclerosis (MS) since the age of 23 has multiple inactive brain lesions on magnetic resonance imaging (MRI). She has no current neurologic impairment or disability. She is pregnant with twins and now presents to the labor and delivery floor with contractions.

Her obstetrician has discussed the labor plan with you; the likelihood of a cesarean delivery in her case is very high. Her airway exam revealed a Mallampati class IV airway with a thick neck. You spoke to the patient about a labor plan that includes an epidural anesthetic during her attempt at vaginal delivery. If there would be a need for an emergent cesarean delivery, a spinal anesthetic was also discussed with the patient.

She is agreeable to both options and says, "My sister is a nurse. She tells me that general anesthesia in pregnant patients is very risky and could lead to death. My sister also says that if I have general anesthesia, my babies will be exposed to all the medications that you give me. I really don't want that, Doctor."

Multiple sclerosis is an autoimmune disorder affecting the central nervous system. First described in 1868 by Jean-Martin Charcot, MS develops from the formation of lesions in the brain or the spinal cord along with inflammation and destruction of the neuronal myelin sheath. These plaques typically affect the white matter of the optic nerve, brain stem, basal ganglia, and spinal cord. The peripheral nervous system is rarely involved. The disease usually begins between 20 and 50 years of age and is twice as common in women as in men. Pregnancy is associated with improvement of symptoms although relapse can occur in the first 3 months following surgery [1]. Although pregnancy does not seem to worsen or speed the course of MS, delivery may be more challenging in these patients for several reasons. Muscle weakness and nerve damage from MS may affect the parturient's ability to push when needed. This makes cesarean delivery, or forceps or vacuum-assisted delivery, more likely.

Your colleague, an experienced anesthesiologist, is also covering the labor and delivery floor that afternoon. He heard about your patient with MS, and he noticed you planned to place a combined spinal/epidural for labor. He approaches you and says, "Are you really going to do a spinal or an epidural in this patient? She has multiple sclerosis, why would you risk it? You are just waiting for a lawsuit!"

Question

Is spinal or epidural anesthesia safe in a patient with multiple sclerosis?

PRO: "Epidural and/or spinal anesthesia are preferable in a pregnant patient who may present with a possible difficult airway," you say. After regional anesthesia, the incidence of worsening neuropathy in patients with a preexisting neuropathy is 0.4 % [2]. The majority of cases is likely due to the fact that injured nerves are more vulnerable to compressive trauma [2]. Repeated attempts at intubation, especially in the obstetric population, may increase the risk of hypoxia, laryngeal edema, airway trauma, and bleeding, as well as pulmonary aspiration. A recent retrospective review of cesarean delivery with general anesthesia was compared with an age-matched group of female patients undergoing non-obstetrical abdominal or gynecologic surgery. With rapid-sequence induction, the rate of poor laryngoscopic view in parturient women undergoing cesarean delivery was 14/851 compared to the 4/814 in the non-pregnant

U.O. Umeh
Department of Anesthesiology, Perioperative Care and Pain Medicine, New York University Langone Medical Center/Hospital for Joint Disease, 301 East 17th Street, New York, NY 10016, USA

U.O. Umeh (✉)
103-06 220th Street, Queens Village, NY 11429, USA
e-mail: Uchenna.Umeh@nyumc.org

C.S. Scher et al. (eds.), *You're Wrong, I'm Right*, DOI 10.1007/978-3-319-43169-7_89

group. Failed intubation occurred in 3 patients undergoing C-section and in only 1 non-obstetric patient [3]. The potentially increased risk of maternal morbidity or mortality during intubation of the pregnant patient is a great reason to avoid general anesthesia.

CON: Your colleague responds, "I strongly disagree! After the publication of the American Society of Anesthesiologists' (ASA) practice guidelines for the management of the difficult airway and the improvement in airway management equipment, it is safer to intubate potentially difficult patients. Airtraq, Glidescope, or awake fiberoptic intubation techniques are safer methods of securing the patient's airway. Rescue devices such as the laryngeal mask airway and the combitube are also helpful in an emergency situation when necessary. Remember, patients with preexisting neurological conditions such as multiple sclerosis may be at increased risk of regional anesthesia-related nerve injury on the basis of the 'double crush' theory, which hypothesizes that nerves that are already compromised are more vulnerable to injury at another site. Specifically in MS, the demyelinated neurons appear susceptible to local anesthetic toxicity, which can increase the conduction blockade. The administration of local anesthetics systemically or during neuraxial anesthesia can unmask silent demyelinated plaques, resulting in exacerbation of the patient's symptoms."

PRO: "But these symptoms are usually transient and reversible and do not imply deterioration of the underlying condition. A study of the influence of pregnancy and delivery on the clinical course of MS found that epidural anesthesia was not predictive of relapse [1]. Despite the increased risk of exacerbation in the first 3 months postpartum, of the 227 women enrolled, 72 % did not experience a relapse during this period. Overall, the relapse rate post-delivery was similar to the pre-pregnancy year. The 3 factors associated with likelihood of postpartum relapse were an increased relapse rate in the pre-pregnancy year, an increased recurrence rate during pregnancy, and a higher Kurtzke Disability Status Scale (DSS) [1]. Essentially, the study showed that women with more severe MS and frequent recurrences in the past were likely to have more relapses during- and post-pregnancy regardless of epidural placement. In my opinion, the risk of attempting intubation in this potentially difficult patient outweighs the risk of placing an epidural or spinal anesthetic in an obese patient with a MP IV airway. Although developing temporary neurologic deficits is not favorable, it is not as catastrophic as losing the airway in a pregnant patient."

CON: "Again, a spinal or epidural in this patient population is not as innocuous as you make it seem. Patients with preoperative neurologic injury undergo further nerve damage more readily from needle and catheter placement, local anesthetic systemic toxicity, and vasopressor-induced ischemia if epinephrine is used in the local anesthetic solution. In an obese patient, the spinal or epidural presumably will be more technically difficult, likely requiring multiple attempts. This increases the chance of needle trauma to the nerve roots as they exit from the spinal cord and travel through the epidural space."

PRO: "Another reason to avoid general anesthesia is to minimize fetal drug exposure and the potential risk of hypoxia and fetal distress if one is unable to secure the patient's airway. Under general anesthesia, the fetus is exposed to intravenous anesthetics. Most induction agents, with the exception of etomidate and ketamine, can cause hypotension after bolus administration, increasing the risk of uteroplacental insufficiency. Administration of opioids increases the likelihood of respiratory depression and possible low Apgar scores post-delivery. With regional anesthesia, the overall risks to the mother and fetus are lower. Although a spinal or epidural technique is usually associated with hypotension, early hydration and treating low blood pressure with ephedrine and/or phenylephrine as needed may ameliorate this."

Summary

Ultimately, the decision to place a spinal or epidural in patients with multiple sclerosis should be made on a case-by-case basis. There are limited studies on spinal and epidural anesthesia in this patient population, and further research is needed to help establish clear guidelines. If a spinal or epidural is planned, the patient's preoperative neurologic examination must be documented and the patient must be made aware of the risk of possible relapse and/or exacerbation of MS symptoms. Concerns for MS exacerbation after spinal or epidural anesthesia should be addressed by involving the patient in the decision-making process about the choice of anesthetic.

References

1. Vukusic S, Hutchinson M, Hours M. Pregnancy and multiple sclerosis (The PRIMS study): clinical predictors of postpartum relapse. Brain. 2004;127(6):1353–60.
2. O'Neal MA, Chang L. Postpartum spinal cord, roots, plexus and peripheral nerve injuries involving the lower extremities: a practical approach. Anesth Analg. 2015;120(1):141–8.
3. Heinrich S, Irouschek A, Prottengeier J. Adverse airway events in parturient compared to non-parturient patients. Is there a difference? Results from a quality management project. J Obstet Gynaecol Res. 2015;41(7):1032–9.

90 The Scanner, the Twitcher, or Both: How Best to Perform Peripheral Nerve Blocks?

Junping Chen

Case

I have a high comfort level with performing peripheral nerve blocks using an ultrasound-guided technique. Recently, I took care of a morbidly obese patient for an arthroscopic-assisted revision of a rotator cuff repair. While discussing the anesthetic plan, I started to prepare the ultrasound equipment.

This quiet patient suddenly blurted, "For the nerve block, I prefer a 'twitch' rather than a 'scan' technique. Are you a scanner or a twitcher?" Before I even began to process his question, he continued, "Seven years ago, when I came for the same shoulder surgery, the anesthesiologist scanned my neck with a machine and poked me with a so-called echogenic needle numerous times for more than half an hour. It was painful. My neck and bed were soaked with bloody jelly, yet he still could not find the right place. Eventually, a second physician came with a small box and with a single needle pass, he made my shoulder jerk. After that, my shoulder and arm were numb for rest of the day."

While I was trying to explain to the patient the benefits and advantages of using an ultrasound, my supervising anesthesiologist quickly set up the nerve stimulator and performed the block. Apparently, my supervising anesthesiologist had been in this situation many times before, especially during the beginning of the ultrasound-guided nerve block era. The nerve stimulator has a 30-year history of proficient use, but lately has fallen out of favor.

Question

Are ultrasound-guided peripheral nerve blocks more efficient and successful than those placed utilizing nerve stimulators?

J. Chen (✉)
Department of Anesthesiology, Mount Sinai St. Luke's and Mount Sinai West Hospital, 1000 10th Avenue, New York, NY 10019, USA
e-mail: jchen@chpnet.org

PRO: With ultrasound guidance, the precise location of a nerve is identified, rather than using anatomical landmarks to indirectly infer the point of needle insertion. The use of ultrasound results in the use of smaller volumes of local anesthetics, faster regional anesthetic onset times, and fewer block failures. Ultrasound also allows the visualization of adjacent anatomical structures, such as blood vessels and pleura, thus reducing the complication rate [1].

CON: Peripheral nerve blocks always work, as long as you deposit an appropriate dose of local anesthetic in the right place. A peripheral nerve stimulator is inexpensive and easy to transport, maintain, and store.

PRO: The case was started uneventfully, with the patient requiring only light sedation for anxiolysis in addition to the surgical anesthesia provided by the Interscalene Block. I quietly asked my supervising anesthesiologist, "Sure, there may have been difficulty scanning an obese patient seven years ago when we were just starting to use ultrasound for nerve blocks. Ultrasound technology has improved over the years and now can produce high-quality images. We have also gained experience in its use, developing specific ultrasound block techniques that result in more successful blocks, such as, the transverse abdominus plant block, the adductor canal block, and the pectoral block." [2].

CON: "I agree with you," my supervising anesthesiologist said. "Better equipment could improve success. However, we, the operators, are the ultimate key in achieving the best outcome. That is what I always emphasize: operator, operator, and operator."

PRO: Being somewhat skeptical of what my supervising anesthesiologist said, I continued, "What about safety? Isn't it obviously safer with the direct visualization of anatomical structures under real-time ultrasound imaging? As a patient, would you really want a blind inference of the nerve's

C.S. Scher et al. (eds.), *You're Wrong, I'm Right*, DOI 10.1007/978-3-319-43169-7_90

whereabouts with nerve stimulation? Many clinicians believe that ultrasound-guided nerve block can minimize nerve injury."

CON: "Evidence, evidence, and evidence." My supervising anesthesiologist increased his voice. "Where is the scientific evidence that supports your claim?" He types the keywords "ultrasound guided nerve block and associated complications" into the nearest computer search engine. Immediately, a long list appears as follows: nerve injury, spinal cord injury, intravascular and epidural space injection, pneumothorax, carotid dissection, and local anesthetic systemic toxicity, among others.

He continues, "Even prospective trials in current literature do not support the claim that the use of ultrasound guidance decreases the incidence of neural injury associated with peripheral nerve blocks. One example of many is *A Prospective, Randomized, Controlled Trial Comparing Ultrasound Versus Nerve Stimulator Guidance for Interscalene block for Ambulatory Shoulder Surgery for Postoperative Neurological Symptoms* [3]. In this carefully designed prospective study, authors did not observe significant differences between these two techniques in block failures, patient satisfaction or incidence, and severity of postoperative neurological symptoms."

PRO: "True, many reports show complications with ultrasound-guided techniques. However, the scientific value of a case report or a small observational study is limited. This is because the incidence of significant nerve injury is extremely low and the study's sample size limits the capacity to detect the difference. Furthermore, some nerve injuries presumably due to nerve block are impossible to distinguish from other causes of injury, such as positioning, the tourniquet, secondary injury from tissue swelling, or from the surgery itself. On the other hand, experience and advances with the new technology result in better images and improved needle visualization, certainly reducing the complication rate. I personally believe that the advantages of ultrasound will eventually lead to its implementation as the standard of care. For example, an analogous case, the pulse oximetry has been adopted as one of a few standard monitors in modern anesthesia care because of its obvious function despite a lack of adequate scientific evidence that it improves perioperative mortality" [4].

"Historically, there is no sufficient evidence for a nerve stimulator's superiority to the paresthesia technique, which involved finding the correct anatomic landmark and directly contact the target nerve to elicit a paresthetic response. However, this method was replaced by the nerve stimulation technique, and trainees are no longer taught this older method." [5].

CON: At this point, my supervising anesthesiologist could not restrain himself. "Why do we still encounter so many complications when we have used ultrasound so extensively in the last decade? Of my twenty years of clinical practice in this institution, I have observed three cases of postoperative nerve damage (one was a severe and permanent brachial plexus palsy) under ultrasound guidance in the last five years, while I do not recall any cases of permanent nerve injury in the past when we used nerve stimulator (personal observation in a single hospital). Although this may well relate to the increasing numbers of regional anesthetics and vigilant monitoring/reporting, one of the reasons, I believe, is that we've moved from the immobile needle technique of nerve stimulation to the mobile needle approach in ultrasound guidance." "During peripheral nerve block with nerve stimulation, one will keep the needle static for the injection of anesthetic after eliciting an acceptable motor response. During ultrasound guidance, people tend to move the needle around the target to achieve the 'ideal' block. Common wisdom says the more you manipulate and reposition the needle, the greater the chance you might puncture these vulnerable structures."

PRO: "It is Murphy's Law. If there is a wrong way to do thing, then someone will do it eventually. People believe that most of the bad outcomes are operator's deficiency rather than inherent defects of ultrasound-guidance techniques." I reply, "This is the reason that many experts advocate the importance of appropriate training and the establishment of a standard technique for block performance and monitoring devices."

CON: "Our institute is an excellent regional anesthesia center. Did you know that we have purchased ten nerve stimulators and only three ultrasound machines in the last few years? Doesn't this imply that the nerve stimulators still play a role in peripheral nerve blocks in our institute?" my supervising anesthesiologist pointed out.

PRO: "Ultrasound-guided nerve block will not preclude the use of a nerve stimulator. Instead, they should be used simultaneously. The nerve stimulator now should serve as a warning monitor of needle-nerve contact rather than act as the nerve locator itself. Nerve stimulating perhaps can provide some hints to indicate whether the needle is near the nerve even if it cannot actually identify intraneural needle placement. As you know, intraneural needle placement also may not be realized during an ultrasound-guided technique due to poor needle tracking skills and failure to observe the needle tip. The nerve stimulating can also compensate for the anatomical difficulties in scanning patients, for example, the patient we just encountered. Additionally, ultrasound artifacts are real. Anisotropy, a slight change in the angle of the ultrasound transducer or beam results in a dramatic change in the structure of the image, is one example of interpretation errors. Nerve stimulation may help to identify the nerve in this situation."

CON: "To prevent nerve damage, ultrasound images, to some extent, help visualize the nerve-needle interaction, avoid nerve punctures, and avoid intraneural injection. Nerve stimulation, even at lower currents (<0.2 mA), is less sensitive and more uncertain. The paresthesia method is the least sensitive of all [6]. It makes sense that all three used together must be equal or greater to one alone for detecting needle-nerve contact."

Summary

Our goal is to minimize the possibility for patient injury. At the present time, while there is no "perfect" monitor for avoiding nerve injury during peripheral nerve block, combining nerve stimulation and ultrasound techniques, along with having an awake patient who is able to identify a paresthesia upon needle-nerve contact, is our best method for avoiding adverse events.

References

1. Salinas FV, Hanson NA. Evidence-based medicine for ultrasound-guided regional anesthesia. Anesthesiol Clin (1932–2275). 2014;32(4):771–87.
2. Cataldo R, Carassiti M, Costa F, Martuscelli M, Benedetto M, Cancilleri F, et al. Starting with ultrasonography decreases popliteal block performance time in experienced hands: a prospective randomized study. BMC Anesthesiol. 2012;12:33.
3. Liu SS, Zayas VM, Gordon MA, Beathe JC, Maalouf DB, Paroli L, et al. A prospective, randomized, controlled trial comparing ultrasound versus nerve stimulator guidance for interscalene block for ambulatory shoulder surgery for postoperative neurological symptoms. Anesth Analg. 2009;109(1):265–71.
4. Pedersen T, Nicholson A, Hovhannisyan K, Møller AM, Smith AF, Lewis SR. Pulse oximetry for perioperative monitoring. Cochrane Database Syst Rev. 2014; 3:CD002013.
5. Liguori GA, Zayas VM, YaDeau JT, Kahn RL, Paroli L, Buschiazzo V, et al. Nerve localization techniques for interscalene brachial plexus blockade: a prospective, randomized comparison of mechanical paresthesia versus electrical stimulation. Anesth Analg. 2006;103(3):761–7.
6. Abdallah FW, Chan VW. Monitoring intraneural needle injection: work in progress. Anesth Analg. 2014;118(3):504–6.

Do We Know the Mechanism of Intravenous Lipid Emulsion (ILE) Therapy for High Blood Levels of Local Anesthetics?

91

Olga Ferreira Martins

Case

A 60-year-old man presented for arthroscopic shoulder surgery for a torn rotator cuff. His medical history was significant for coronary artery disease and hypertension. He had a myocardial infarct 8 years prior to admission followed by percutaneous transluminal coronary angioplasty. His medications included metoprolol and aspirin. His preoperative electrocardiogram (EKG) revealed a right bundle branch block and changes associated with an old anterior wall myocardial infarct. He agreed to regional anesthesia with sedation, and an interscalene block was planned.

When he arrived in the operating room (OR), we applied standard monitors and placed a 20-gauge IV in his right arm. His vital signs were the following: blood pressure, 130/82; heart rate, 72; respiratory rate, 12; and SpO_2, 100 % on room air. We administered midazolam, 2 mg IV, and placed a face mask with 2L O_2. He was properly positioned, and the area draped and prepped. The brachial plexus was identified using ultrasound, and 20 ml of local anesthetic solution (0.5 % bupivacaine) was injected over 3 min in 5-ml boluses after aspiration.

A few seconds after we completed the block, the patient developed a tonic–clonic seizure. We immediately increased the oxygen flow and administered another 5 mg midazolam IV. The seizure stopped, but about 1 min later, he was seizing again. I gave propofol, 100 mg IV. Suddenly, the EKG showed asystole, the blood pressure was undetectable, and we were unable to palpate a carotid or femoral pulse. We started CPR immediately and intubated the patient. We resuscitated the patient for 20 min, giving large doses of epinephrine and vasopressin, while simultaneously making plans to institute cardiopulmonary bypass. One of the anesthesia residents, who had recently completed simulation training in which a case of local anesthetic systemic toxicity (LAST) was presented, proposed treating him with IntraLipid (Fresenius Kabi, Uppsala, Sweden). We bolused 100 mg through the peripheral IV and continued CPR. Within 15 s, the sinus rhythm returned and the blood pressure and pulse were again detectable. We started a continuous infusion of IntraLipid at 18 ml/min and transferred him to the ICU for further monitoring. The patient was extubated and did well overnight. He was discharged home the following day.

The next day, I run into my attending. "I'm excited to write up our successful use of IntraLipid to treat LAST."

But he's doubtful. "How can we know it was the IntraLipid and not one of the numerous concurrent therapies we tried? We don't even know how IntraLipid works."

Question

Do we know the mechanism of intravenous lipid emulsion (ILE) therapy for high blood levels of local anesthetics?

PRO: Since the first report of successful use of ILE for acute bupivacaine-induced cardiac arrest was published in 2006, there have been dozens of case reports of successful treatment of LAST with IntraLipid, currently the predominant brand of lipid emulsion used. It has been successfully used to treat a wide range of patients, including a 2-day-old neonate and a 92-year-old woman. Patients like ours, with underlying heart disease such as coronary artery disease and baseline conduction defects, have been shown to be at increased risk for local anesthetic-induced cardiotoxicity [1].

CON: But the level of evidence is case reports. It's much less rigorous than evidence from prospective, randomized clinical trials. The evidence is fraught with a number of biases, including underreporting of failed outcomes.

O.F. Martins (✉)
Department of Anesthesiology, Perioperative Care and Pain Medicine, New York University Langone Medical Center, 550 First Avenue, 5th Floor, New York, NY 10016, USA
e-mail: olga.martins@nyumc.org

C.S. Scher et al. (eds.), *You're Wrong, I'm Right*, DOI 10.1007/978-3-319-43169-7_91

PRO: There are also a number of animal and in vitro studies that have been published investigating the mechanism of ILE. In fact, animal models have shown benefit in treating a variety of other drug overdoses, and ILE has been used to successfully treat toxicity from a range of lipophilic drugs with disparate pharmacologic profiles [1]. Tricyclic antidepressants and verapamil are the 2 most common drug classes that emergency medicine providers have successfully treated with ILE. These and other successes have led emergency physicians to recommend stocking ILE near all resuscitation rooms for toxicologic emergencies [2].

CON: Still, how can we explain that ILE can reverse toxicity caused by an array of drugs that lack a common mechanism?

PRO: There are a number of mechanisms proposed for the effects of lipid emulsion. Partitioning (the so-called lipid sink phenomenon) is the predominant theory. It suggests that ILE provides a lipid mass that binds the toxin and pulls the drug from the target tissue, thus reversing the toxicity. Since the brain doesn't rely on fatty acid metabolism to an appreciable degree, ILE's successful treatment of neurotoxicity in addition to cardiotoxicity provides indirect evidence for this theory [1, 2].

CON: But doesn't the list of drugs you mentioned also include water-soluble drugs, such as beta-blockers and lamotrigine? The "lipid sink" theory doesn't explain those.

PRO: The effects of ILE may not be limited to 1 mechanism alone, and studies have shown other plausible mechanisms for the effects of lipid emulsion. The large lipid load has been shown to offset the potent inhibition of fatty acid metabolism by local anesthetics and to provide a sustained fatty acid source to myocytes under toxic conditions. In addition to enhancing fatty acid metabolism, ILE has been shown to have cytoprotective effects, reducing mitochondrial permeability and apoptosis, and direct membrane effects, reducing the local anesthetic inhibition of cardiac sodium channels [1].

Concession from CON: Significant research exists to provide plausible mechanisms for ILE therapy, and ongoing work continues to explore the multifaceted ways in which ILE therapy works to reverse diverse drug toxicities. While we may not yet know fully how ILE works, the increasing number of case reports makes it clear that ILE is a useful therapy in the treatment of LAST as well as other toxic overdoses.

Summary

Although the exact mechanism of intravenous lipid therapy is yet to be fully elucidated, the 100-plus published case reports provide valuable clinical insight. Clinician education and awareness of this treatment are critically important to patient outcomes.

It is important to recognize that pharmacologic treatment of LAST is different from other cardiac arrest scenarios and to be familiar with the established treatment guidelines published by the American Society of Regional Anesthesia and Pain Medicine (ASRA). Specifically, avoid propofol for seizure suppression if the patient is showing signs of cardiovascular instability. When managing cardiac arrhythmias, avoid vasopressin, calcium channel blockers, β(beta)-blockers, or local anesthetics and reduce individual epinephrine doses to <1 mcg/kg [3].

Don't forget to post any LAST event at www.lipidrescue.org and to report the use of lipid to www.lipidresigstry.org [3]. In the absence of prospective human clinical trials, these data can help us further identify factors in treatment that improve patient survival and outcomes.

References

1. Weinberg G. Lipid emulsion infusion: resuscitation of local anesthetic and other drug overdose. Anesthesiology. 2012;117:180–7.
2. Cao D, Heard K, Foran M, Koyfman A. Intravenous lipid emulsion in the emergency department: a systematic review of the literature. J Emerg Med. 2015;48:387–97.
3. Neal JM, Mulroy MF, Weinberg GL. American Society of Regional Anesthesia and Pain Medicine checklist for managing local anesthetic systemic toxicity: 2012 version. Reg Anesth Pain Med. 2012;37:16–8.

Secrets Behind Keeping Your Block Catheter Working

92

Minda L. Patt

Case

A 20-year-old man was brought to the emergency room after being hit by an industrial garbage truck going 20–30 mph. The driver of the truck was emergently braking, but hit the patient as he was running and stumbling in unpredictable directions while attempting to cross the street. The patient admitted to having used cocaine and consuming several drinks of alcohol prior to the event.

He suffered extensive soft-tissue injury of the right distal lower extremity, including a degloving injury of the ankle with tendon, muscle, and bone exposed. Prior to the operating room (OR), the patient had loss of sensation over the right 4th and 5th toes and was unable to extend them. He went to the OR emergently for irrigation and debridement.

On the third postoperative day, the plastic surgery team performed a 9-h procedure for closure of the open wound and soft-tissue reconstruction. This included further debridement of nonviable tissue, a rectus abdominis muscle free-flap reconstruction and revascularization, and split thickness skin grafting. The patient remained in the post-anesthesia care unit (PACU) for flap checks every 30 min overnight and then hourly checks starting on postoperative day 1. Activity was restricted to bed rest, with leg elevation to avoid pressure, and a forced-air warming device on at all times. The patient suffered in bed with a hydromorphone IV patient-controlled analgesia (PCA), his pain scores hovering around 8 out of 10, and from interrupted sleep and severe constipation, while the plastic surgery team worried about the viability of the graft. I am consulted by plastic surgery for pain management, and ideally a continuous peripheral nerve block (cPNB). A colleague tersely replies to plastics that if they wanted a nerve block, they should have consulted prior to surgery because "Now the patient has a delicate graft and a known nerve injury!"

Questions

How do you place a catheter in a patient with such high acuity of care and ensure that it functions effectively? Is it worth the risk given known complications such as catheter failure and infection? Once placed, how can it be maintained to ensure prolonged efficacy of the continuous block technique?

PRO: I pull my colleague aside and tell him, "The nerve injury is well documented in the patient's medical record as having resulted from the initial injury. There's literature to support and refute the 'double crush phenomenon' (which postulates that someone with a nerve injury is at a higher risk of a second injury to the same nerve), but in his situation, I believe the block will actually promote healing. Studies show that because regional anesthesia diminishes the systemic stress response, the resultant vasodilation improves blood flow to the free flap and improves microvascular flow distribution within the flap [1]. Complications of catheters are minor, and when they occur, don't result in long term sequelae."

I show my colleague a study on the safety of peripheral nerve catheters in children. After more than 2000 catheters were placed using varying techniques, in some cases without ultrasound, there were no reports of persistent neurologic problems [2]. It also stated that catheter problems were common but minor in severity and that these findings were in line with adult studies.

"More than the nerve injury, I'm concerned about this graft viability when I position him to get to the back of his thigh for a sciatic block. I'm going to need the plastic surgery team at the bedside. They'll assist in positioning and monitoring to assure there's no pressure on the graft, and

M.L. Patt (✉)
Department of Anesthesiology, New York Presbyterian Hospital, Weill Cornell Medicine, 525 East 68th Street, Box 124 New York, NY 10065, USA
e-mail: mip9098@med.cornell.edu

C.S. Scher et al. (eds.), *You're Wrong, I'm Right*, DOI 10.1007/978-3-319-43169-7_92

that it remains adequately elevated to avoid engorgement. Also, they can check pulses pre- and post-procedure."

I contact the team and they agree that their presence during the manipulation of the extremity is safest. I start setting up for an ultrasound-guided popliteal block.

CON: "It sounds like you're adding a lot of risk to this tenuous graft. Why go through all the trouble? Especially when everyone knows continuous nerve block catheters are finicky—they leak, they disconnect, dressings come off, and they frequently fail. He's already missed out on preemptive analgesia. You're getting yourself into a mess. Like I said, the block should have been placed prior to OR."

PRO: "But he is in a lot of pain now! Any effort toward sparing opioids and employing multimodal analgesia is warranted. There's evidence that intense analgesia immediately after surgery can decrease the incidence or severity of chronic pain [3]. Because peripheral nerve blocks can potently inhibit postsurgical nociceptive input over the course of multiple postop days, they can prevent the 'wind up' or central sensitization that results in primary and secondary hyperalgesia. Without a block, this guy will have more opioid consumption, gain tolerance, possibly have longer-term outpatient use or dependence, and may even develop opioid-induced hyperalgesia. Plus, he's incredibly constipated! Yes, the sooner the better, but *now* is better than no block at all."

CON: "You just showed me that paper that said problems with catheters were common. What if he gets an infection in the injured extremity?"

PRO: "It said that the great majority of catheter problems result from accidental dislodgement or dislocation. The next most common complications are superficial infection and vascular puncture. Both of these had incidences of <1 % in this study, which validates the safety of their use [2]. Another study demonstrates that minor complications occur with a frequency similar to single injection blocks" [4].

I give my colleague one concession, "You're right about one thing, though. They are finicky. The most common adverse event is catheter malfunction, and it's usually from unintended dislodgment" [2]. I tell him that I have plenty of tricks up my sleeve to prevent this.

I start listing my usual arsenal of tactics, "I always use a sterile liquid adhesive like benzoin and Steri-Strips. 2-Octyl cyanoacrylate glue (e.g., Dermabond) is great too, but it's expensive and hard to get your hands on. The catheter can be looped and secured with these adhesives, and then covered with a sterile transparent occlusive dressing like Tegaderm. Ultrasound gel is your enemy here! I use it as sparingly as possible when I do a catheter and really thoroughly wipe it off. I also usually put a Tegaderm over each connection site—catheter to hub and hub to infusion tubing—to prevent disconnects and contamination on the wards. And I use the catheter anchoring device in the kit."

I show my colleague a review by Ilfeld and Enneking. "When they examined investigations of perineural infusion for home use, they found that using a combination of these maneuvers led to a catheter retention rate of 95–100 % for more than 60 h in ambulatory patients" [5].

My colleague is impressed, so I reveal a couple more of my tricks to him, "I never layer or sandwich the catheter between the multiple occlusive dressings because you're unable to separate them from one another, which can be a problem if you need to change the dressing."

CON: "You're having a hard time getting it to stay in the first place. Why would the catheter need to be redressed?"

PRO: "Well, for a couple of reasons." I explain that sometimes when the block is placed prior to the procedure, perhaps in a 'block area,' and the patient arrives to the OR, the dressing overlaps with the surgical field. "In that case, sometimes you have to redress it to optimize surgical exposure. So if you apply Tegaderms in series, fine; they can be peeled off the skin and even the catheter relatively easily. If you've applied Tegaderm on top of the catheter, then loop more catheter and Tegaderm on top of that, you've made the task of catheter repositioning potentially very difficult."

"If it suffices, though, I just place sterile towels or gauze over my dressing and then allow the surgical team to place their sterile drapes over the catheter. You can imagine a lot of catheters can become dislodged when the drapes come down. It only works if the catheter dressing is fully covered. If I do it this way, I make sure whoever is in the room when the drapes are removed is vigilant about retracting them carefully and that the whole surgical team, scrub tech and all, is well aware of the presence of a catheter."

"Also remember that tunneling helps steer the catheter and its dressing away from the surgical field, and it's another way to increase resistance to accidental dislodgement."

CON: "Another reason you might have to redress the catheter is because they leak all the time. When they leak on the wards, they're also predisposed to falling out. Then the nurses and surgeons just want them out anyway because they figure they aren't working."

PRO "That's true and important for two reasons. Recent studies have looked at whether a catheter-over-needle technique, rather than the Seldinger technique, can help prevent this [6]. In most continuous peripheral nerve block kits, the catheter has a smaller diameter than the needle, so it leaves space in the puncture wound for leakage and makes inadvertent dislodgment more likely. Unfortunately, this technology needs further investigation, but I'd love to use it. Another way to potentially decrease leakage is to decrease the basal rate while increasing the local anesthetic concentration. Some studies have shown that effects of some nerve blocks depend on the total local anesthetic dose rather than the concentration or volume; so higher concentrations of local anesthetic at lower infusion rates may be as effective as lower concentrations" [7].

CON: "So the leakage issue seems relatively unresolved. But that's not the only thing that goes wrong on the floor. Pumps malfunction or infusions run out causing unnecessary pauses, patients are rarely as comfortable as when the initial bolus was placed, or surgeons are dissatisfied with the amount of motor block and abruptly stop the infusion."

PRO: "Right. These problems are not infrequent. Catheters do need oversight and management, but this is nothing that can't be handled by an acute pain service (APS). An APS can set patient expectations, adjust infusions to optimal levels, and bolus on rounds. They should perform a physical exam and assure there are no signs of infection and dressings are intact. They're also an important liaison to the surgical team. They should communicate expected exam findings with a working block and determine the need for avoidance of motor block based on the surgeon's need for neuromonitoring."

CON: "But there are so many reports that cite an increase in visual analog scale (VAS) pain scores at 24 h after placement with catheters in place [8]. So why not just do a single shot and use additives for duration?"

PRO: "The density of block attained on initial placement is difficult to maintain. Rescue analgesia with clinician-activated boluses (CABs) by PACU nurses have been shown to optimize pain relief [8]. The CAB dose is often forgotten once the patient reaches the floor. To prevent this, I inform patients of the need for CABs and also tell the family and friends that plan to be with them postoperatively. I also consistently educate and encourage CABs by nurses on the hospital floors during APS rounds. They have less regular exposure to cPNBs and catheter management may be unfamiliar to them.

"Optimal infusion rates for different block types still need to be elucidated, but there will always be some inter-patient variability. Overall, there's strong evidence that a continuous peripheral nerve block improves postoperative analgesia and patient satisfaction while decreasing supplemental analgesic requirements and limiting opioid-related side effects. The improved analgesia can afford patients better sleep quality, ability to participate in rehabilitation, earlier functional recovery, and less chronic pain. In our patient's case, there's evidence to suggest it will promote healing."

Summary

Continuous peripheral nerve blockade is a safe and effective method that can result in potent analgesia for moderate-to-severe postoperative pain. It has proven benefit in optimizing postoperative analgesia, and the benefits may outlast the duration of the infusion. Perceived difficulty in placement, rate of catheter failure, and potential complications can lead to reluctance to employ this technique. Overall, it is a safe and effective approach for high-quality postoperative analgesia when prolonged blockade is desired. Optimal functioning of the catheter hinges on adept placement and methods for securing the catheter, good communication and coordination with the surgical team, patient education, and daily management of the catheter, ideally by an acute pain service.

References

1. Hahnenkamp K, Theilmeier G, Van Aken HK, Hoenemann C. The effects of local anesthetics on perioperative coagulation, inflammation, and microcirculation. Anesth Analg. 2002;94:1441–7.
2. Walker BJ, Long JB, De Oliveria GS, Szmuk P, Setiawan C, Polaner DM, et al. PRAN Investigators. Peripheral nerve catheters in children: an analysis of safety and practice patterns from the pediatric regional anesthesia network (PRAN). Br J Anaesth. 2015;115(3):457–62.
3. Andreae MH, Andreae DA. Regional anaesthesia to prevent chronic pain after surgery: a Cochrane systematic review and meta-analysis. Br J Anaesth. 2013;111:711–20.
4. Machi AT, Ilfeld B. Continuous peripheral nerve blocks in the ambulatory setting: an update of the published evidence. Curr Opin Anaesthesiol. 2015;28(6):648–55.
5. Ilfeld BM, Enneking FK. Continuous peripheral nerve blocks at home: a review. Anesth Analg. 2005;100:1822–33.
6. Tsui BC, Ip VH. Catheter-over-needle method reduces risk of perineural catheter dislocation. Br J Anaesth. 2014;112:759–60.
7. Madison SJ, Monahan AM, Agarwal RR, Furnish TJ, Mascha EJ, Xu Z, et al. A randomized, triple-masked, active-controlled investigation of the relative effects of dose, concentration, and infusion rate for continuous popliteal-sciatic nerve blocks in volunteers. Br J Anaesth. 2015;114:121–9.
8. Capdevila X, Pirat P, Bringuier S, Gaetner E, Singelyn F, Bernard N, et al. French Study Group on Continuous Peripheral Nerve Blocks. Continuous peripheral nerve blocks in hospital wards after orthopedic surgery: a multicenter prospective analysis of the quality of postoperative analgesia and complications in 1,416 patients. Anesthesiology. 2005;103:1035–45.

Is an Indwelling Neuraxial or Peripheral Nerve Catheter Safe in a Trauma Patient Who Needs Twice-Daily Low Molecular Weight Heparin?

93

Brooke Albright-Trainer and Robert Trainer

Case

A US serviceman suffered severe injuries to the lower extremities after stepping on a roadside bomb. He arrived at the hospital via critical care air transport having received a massive blood transfusion, a right traumatic above-the-knee amputation, and a left below-the-knee traumatic amputation, and other pelvic and abdominal injuries. Upon arrival, he was scheduled for irrigation and debridement (I&D) in the operating room (OR), followed by eventual extubation in the intensive care unit (ICU), but pain control was expected to limit his ability to wean from mechanical ventilation. The surgeon states that because he is a trauma patient with high risk of venous thromboembolism (VTE), he needs to be maintained on twice-daily (BID) low molecular weight heparin (LMWH), 30 mg subcutaneously (subq).

Considerations for this patient's acute pain management include the need for venous thromboprophylaxis, non-opiate-based pain control to help him wean from the ventilator and decrease the incidence of respiratory events, expected multiple OR visits for I&D of the extremities and need to limit repeated tracheal intubations, and pain control during prolonged rehabilitation.

Question

Is an indwelling neuraxial or peripheral nerve regional anesthesia catheter safe in a trauma patient who needs twice-daily low molecular weight heparin?

PRO: Trauma patients have a much higher risk (40–80 %) for developing a VTE than the general population [1]. Therefore, it is important that adequate chemoprophylaxis is given. Neuraxial and regional anesthesia (RA) provide some protection against VTE, but are not adequate prevention alone [2]. Despite some controversy, it may be necessary to maintain a neuraxial catheter in place, while the patient is on certain anticoagulation regimens. Although not known precisely, the risk of a subdural or epidural hematoma in a patient with an epidural on twice-daily LMWH maintenance dosing is small. If you avoid the epidural or peripheral nerve block catheters, you will need more opioids for sure. Trauma patients, however, are especially at a high risk of opioid-related complications, including death. A literature review by Weinger suggests that up to 1/300 postoperative patients require rescue doses of naloxone for respiratory depression, accounting for nearly 20,000 patients annually, of which 10 % suffer significant sequelae [3]. From the anesthesia closed claims project database of 9799 claims, three authors reviewed 357 acute pain claims between 1990 and 2009 and found that opioid-related respiratory depression likely contributed to severe brain damage or death in up to 77 % of patients [4]. I'd rather avoid the real risk of opioid-related respiratory depression than the theoretical risk of hematoma.

CON: I say, "first do no harm." An epidural or subdural hematoma could lead to paralysis for life. And what about the all-important Anesthesia Society for Regional Anesthesia (ASRA) guidelines? The guidelines are very clear that twice-daily dosing of LMWH is contraindicated in patients with "deep" regional anesthesia catheters in place, regardless of whether they are placed peripherally or in the neuraxial space [1]. There are no recommendations on "superficial" regional anesthesia catheters or blocks. The ASRA guidelines state it is necessary to discontinue the catheter at least 2 h prior to giving the first dose. However, if the patient only required once a day maintenance dosing of LMWH (i.e., 40 mg subq daily), then according to the guidelines, the catheter can safely be maintained. When the catheter needs

B. Albright-Trainer (✉) · R. Trainer
Department of Anesthesiology, Hunter Holmes McGuire VA Medical Center, 1201 Broad Rock Boulevard, Richmond, VA 23249, USA
e-mail: brooke.albright@gmail.com

R. Trainer
e-mail: Robert.trainer@gmail.com

C.S. Scher et al. (eds.), *You're Wrong, I'm Right*, DOI 10.1007/978-3-319-43169-7_93

to be placed or removed, the once-daily LMWH dose should be held for 10–12 h prior and not restarted until 4 h after the regional technique [1].

As my colleague mentioned, the use of regional anesthesia as a means to prevent VTE alone has not been shown convincingly in large trials. And I think we ALL can agree that pain control is of paramount importance.

PRO: OK, so what do you suggest then? Acetaminophen and non-steroidal anti-inflammatory drugs (NSAIDs)?

CON: You have a point, the optimal way in which to deliver optimal pain control is still in question. Many of the cited studies did not specifically mention the benefits of adjuncts such as ketamine, dexmedetomidine, gabapentin, COX-2 inhibitors, and intravenous local anesthetics. Recent evidence suggests that even single-dose immediate preoperative and intraoperative use of anti-epileptics (i.e., gabapentin, pregabalin) and ketamine can provide lasting benefits, such as decreased development of chronic pain syndromes, and in the case of ketamine, less opioid use at 6 weeks [5–7]. The timing of the use of these adjuvants can add provide long-lasting relief and avoidance of opioids without violating the ASRA guidelines.

PRO: Fine, but we are not just talking about regional anesthetic benefits in the immediate perioperative period. Trauma patients are at high risk of developing chronic pain syndromes (CPS). Continuous regional anesthetics have been shown in many studies to reduce the development of CPS. If placed early, and for an extended length of time (>3 days), regional anesthesia is believed to diminish release of pro-inflammatory cytokines, improve endogenous inhibitory factors, decrease peripheral excitatory factors, and reduce the lasting effect on neurocellular pathways for pain, thereby preventing a phenomenon known as central sensitization or "wind-up" [8–10]. By minimizing the perception of repeated noxious stimuli, non-painful pathways are strengthened over painful pathways and the development of CPS can be prevented utilizing multimodal therapies, including continuous regional anesthetic techniques.

CON: A patient with paraplegia from an epidural hematoma will wish that his anesthesiologist had cared more about safety than chronic pain.

PRO: I'm not the only one disagreeing with ASRA. Though the ASRA guidelines recommend against maintaining deep regional anesthesia catheters in patients receiving BID dosing of LMWH [1], the American College of Chest Physicians (ACCP) and the European Society of Anesthesiology (ESRA) both state in their guidelines that this technique can be safe and is permissible [11, 12]. They caution waiting 24 h, rather than 12 h, to place or remove catheters when the twice-daily prophylactic dose is used.

CON: Yes, although it is true that ESRA and ACCP agree that BID prophylactic LMWH is safe to use concomitantly while catheters are in place, the reason ASRA disagrees is because from 1993 to 1998 the USA saw a large increase in the incidence of spinal hematomas compared to European-reported incidences. This was thought to be related to the US Food and Drug Administration (FDA)-approved BID dosing of LMWH use in the USA. During that time period, the FDA MedWatch system reported more than 40 spinal hematomas, and this appeared related to the increased dose scheduling of 30 mg every 12 h [13]. This marked increase in the frequency of spinal hematomas in a 5-year span prompted reevaluation of the relative risks and benefits of indwelling neuraxial catheters in patients on twice-daily LMWH dosing. This is one reason the 1998 ASRA guidelines were created to discourage the use of neuraxial catheters during BID LMWH dosing. The guidelines still conclude that only once-daily LMWH dosing is safe in patients with catheters in place.

PRO: Furthermore, even if you do not want to place a neuraxial catheter, a peripheral nerve catheter should be strongly considered. There is scarce to no data that exist showing that peripheral nerve catheters (PNCs) lead to bleeding complications. Buckenmaier et al. [14] retrospectively looked at 187 combat casualties from 2003 to 2005 receiving a median enoxaparin dose and timing of 30 mg and 12 h after PNC placement, respectively, and showed no catheter-related bleeding complications. To look at the extreme scenario, the incidence of hemorrhagic complications during therapeutic anticoagulation with intravenous or subcutaneous heparin is <3 %; the risk associated with LMWH is even lower [11, 14]. In an extensive review of the literature, the overall calculated incidence of hemorrhagic complications associated with central neural blockade is approximated to be <1 in 150,000 epidural and <1 in 220,000 spinal anesthetics [15].

CON: The 1998 ASRA guidelines were created to discourage the use of catheters, both peripherally and neuraxially, during BID LMWH dosing. The guidelines still conclude that only once-daily LMWH dosing is safe in patients with catheters in place [1].

PRO: Before taking a "one-size fits all" approach to accepting these guidelines as medical dogma, let us take a closer look at those 40 cases of spinal hematomas, which spawned the concern regarding BID LMWH dosing with indwelling catheters. It seems that patient factors, concomitant antiplatelet or anticoagulant medication administration, or difficult neuraxial catheter placement contributed more to the development of bleeding complications than the BID-dosing regimen. Of the more than 40 reported cases of spinal hematoma from 1993 to 1998, over 70 % of them were in elderly (>77 years), female, low weight patients (<62 kg), with multiple comorbidities. Some of them were in patients with a history of ankylosing spondylitis or renal/hepatic dysfunction. Four patients had difficult/traumatic neuraxial placements resulting in a bloody tap, and more than 36 % were given other concomitant antiplatelet medications including warfarin, toradol, naproxen, aspirin, and others [16]. In 2 of the 40 patients, the dose of LMWH was greater than the recommended 30 mg BID dose. One complication resulted when the catheter was withdrawn at the peak of antiplatelet activity. Two separate studies evaluating risk factors for spinal epidural hematoma identified advanced age (>60 years) as an independent risk factor [17, 18]. From those reported cases of spinal epidural hematoma in the FDA MedWatch system, none were in young, otherwise healthy, trauma patients. Further studies should be done to examine the relationship between bleeding complications in trauma patients with BID thromboprophylaxis dosing in those with and without a regional anesthesia catheter in place. Perhaps it is true that the perceived increased risk of bleeding complications in the elderly population, or in those patients with decreased renal clearance, is too high to safely maintain regional anesthesia catheters with twice-daily LMWH dosing. In those patients with severe renal insufficiency, anti-Xa activity reaches a higher maximum level and the elimination half-life can increase from 4–6 to 16 h or longer [11]. However, young, otherwise healthy trauma patients have an extraordinarily increased risk of VTE and in most cases have adequate renal function. Based on this close examination of the evidence, it is my opinion that in young, healthy trauma patients with good renal function, I would maintain twice-daily LMWH dosing with a catheter in place. In this situation, I think that the risk of VTE complications is much higher than the risk of bleeding complications.

Summary

Trauma patients are at a very high risk of developing VTE, and morbidity and mortality from such events can be devastating. RA has been shown to be a safe and effective treatment modality and should be considered alongside other adjuncts as a method to decrease acute pain, potentially mitigate development of chronic pain, and limit the negative impact of opiate-based modalities. ASRA has strict guidelines regarding placement and maintenance of indwelling RA catheters [1], which should be considered in certain populations. However, more research needs to be performed in young, otherwise healthy trauma patients, to evaluate the bleeding risk versus VTE risk of maintaining indwelling RA catheters and receiving twice-daily dosing of LMWH. These studies must be performed before a final conclusion is drawn regarding safety and efficacy.

References

1. Horlocker TT, Wedel DJ, Rowlingson JC, Enneking FK, Kopp SL, Benzon HT, et al. Regional anesthesia in the patient receiving antithrombotic or thrombolytic therapy: American Society of Regional Anesthesia and Pain Medicine evidence-based guidelines (third edition). Reg Anesth Pain Med. 2010;35(1):64–101.
2. Rawal N. Epidural technique for postoperative pain: gold standard no more? Reg Anesth Pain Med. 2012;37(3):310–7.
3. Weinger MB, Lee LA. No patient shall be harmed by opioid-induced respiratory depression. APSF newsletter. Fall. 2011;26(2):21–40.
4. Lee LA, Caplan RA, Stephens LS, Posner KL, Terman GW, Voepel-Lewis T, et al. Postoperative opioid-induced respiratory depression: a closed claims analysis. Anesthesiology. 2015;122 (3):659–65.
5. Buvanendran A, Kroin JS. Multimodal analgesia for controlling acute postoperative pain. Curr Opin Anesthesiol. 2009;22(9):588–93.
6. Radhakrishnan M, Parmod KB, Arvind C. Effect of preemptive gabapentin on postoperative pain relief and morphine consumption following lumbar laminectomy and discectomy: a randomized, double-blinded, placebo-controlled study. J Neurosurg Anesthesiol. 2005;17(3):125–8.
7. Loftus RW. Intraoperative ketamine reduces perioperative opiate consumption in opiate-dependent patients with chronic back pain undergoing back surgery. Anesthesiology. 2010;113(3):639–46.
8. Nikolajsen L, Jensen TS. Phantom limb pain. Br J Anaesthesiology. 2001;87:107–16.
9. Pogatzki-Zahn EM, Zahn PK. From preemptive to preventive analgesia. Curr Opin Anesthesiol. 2006;19(5):551–5.
10. Woolf CJ. Central sensitization: implications for the diagnosis and treatment of pain. Pain. 2011;152(3 Suppl):S2–15.
11. Schulman S, Beyth RJ, Kearon C, Levine MN. Hemorrhagic complications of anticoagulant and thrombolytic treatment: American College of Chest Physicians Evidence-Based Clinical Practice Guidelines (8th Edition). Chest. 2008;133:257S–98S.
12. Wiebke G, Vandermeulen E, Van Aken H, Kozek S, Llau JV, Samama CM. Regional anaesthesia and antithrombotic agents: Recommendations of the European Society of Anaesthesiology. Eur J Anaesthesiol. 2010;27:999–1015.
13. Schroeder DR. Statistics: detecting a rare adverse drug reaction using spontaneous reports. Reg Anesth Pain Med. 1998;23(6 Suppl 2):183–9.
14. Buckenmaier CC, Shields CH, Auton AA, Evans SL, Croll SM, Bleckner LL, et al. Continuous peripheral nerve block in combat casualties receiving low-molecular weight heparin. Br J Anaesthesiol. 2006;97(6):874–7.
15. Horlocker TT, Wedel DJ. Anticoagulation and neuraxial block: historical perspective, anesthetic implications, and risk management. Reg Anesth Pain Med. 1998;23(6 Suppl 2):129–34.

16. FDA Anesthetic and Life Support Drugs Advisory Committee. February 5, 1998 meeting transcript. http://www.fda.gov/ohrms/dockets/ac/98/transcpt/3380t1.pdf Accessed 17 Nov 2015.
17. Sokolowski MJ, Garvey TA, Perl J 2nd, Sokolowski MS, Cho W, Mehbod AA, et al. Prospective study of postoperative lumbar epidural hematoma: incidence and risk factors. Spine. 2008;33(1):108–13.
18. Awad JN. Analysis of the risk factors for the development of post-operative spinal epidural haematoma. J Bone Joint Surg Br. 2005;87-B(9):1248–52.

94 Awake or Asleep: Can Regional Nerve Blocks Be Safely Performed in the Heavily Sedated or Asleep Patient?

Shawna Dorman

Case

A 59-year-old Spanish-speaking man presents for repair of a left torn rotator cuff. He has a history of coronary artery disease, hypertension, hyperlipidemia, and mild gastroesophageal reflux disease (GERD), which is diet controlled. He has a previous surgical history of 2 stents placed in the left anterior descending artery in 2009 and an appendectomy that was complicated by severe postoperative nausea and vomiting (PONV). He has no known allergies. His list of medications is as follows: Plavix (last taken 7 days ago), aspirin (taken the morning of surgery), Norvasc (taken the morning of surgery), and Lipitor.

Upon examination, blood pressure (BP) = 145/72, heart rate (HR) = 72, respiratory rate (RR) = 12, and oxygen saturation = 100 %. His height is 70 inches, and weight is 165 lbs. The physical examination is without abnormalities.

His airway examination shows a Mallampati II with a good range of motion of the neck and good mouth opening. All laboratory test results are normal, including platelets, prothrombin time/partial thromboplastin time (PT/PTT), and international normalized ratio (INR). His echocardiogram shows mild diastolic dysfunction, no valvular abnormalities, and an ejection fraction = 60 %. The patient has not had a repeat stress test since being re-vascularized; however, he exercises >4 metabolic equivalents (METS) daily and is asymptomatic.

The history and consent is taken via telephone translator. The patient describes his previous experience with general anesthesia as "miserable" due to severe postoperative nausea and vomiting and requests a different option. He also states he has a severe phobia of needles. Consent is obtained for an interscalene block and sedation. However, the patient requests to be asleep throughout.

The patient is taken to the operating room. Standard American Society of Anesthesiologists (ASA) monitors are placed. A 20-gauge intravenous line is placed with great difficulty due to the patient's fear of needles. The patient is lightly sedated with midazolam, 2 mg, and the interscalene block is started. However, the patient becomes extremely agitated and uncooperative as the needle enters the skin. It is very difficult to control the patient because of the language barrier. The needle is removed, and he is deeply sedated with a total of midazolam, 10 mg, and fentanyl, 100 μ(mu)g. The patient is spontaneously breathing and comfortable. An uneventful ultrasound-guided interscalene block is performed. The rotator cuff repair is performed in the beach chair position, and sedation is maintained with a propofol infusion. Postoperatively, the patient is extremely satisfied with his experience. He does not experience any postoperative nausea, has excellent analgesia for more than 24 h, and has no neurological abnormalities after the interscalene block resolves.

Question

Awake or asleep… Can regional nerve blocks be performed safely in the heavily sedated or asleep patient?

PRO: The placement of regional anesthetic blocks under heavy sedation or general anesthesia is standard of care in pediatric patients, as demonstrated in a large number of patients by the Pediatric Regional Anesthesia Network [1, 2] and should translate to adults as well. The current guidelines are based largely on expert opinion and case reports, rather than evidence-based medicine.

S. Dorman (✉)
Department of Anesthesia, New York University Langone Medical Center- Hospital for Joint Diseases, 301 East 17th Street, New York, NY 10003, USA
e-mail: Shawna.Dorman@nyumc.org

C.S. Scher et al. (eds.), *You're Wrong, I'm Right*, DOI 10.1007/978-3-319-43169-7_94

CON: While it is true that no prospective, randomized, controlled studies have been performed to evaluate the impact of anesthetic depth on the risk of complications from regional anesthesia, it is unlikely this study will ever be done: It would be extremely difficult to complete because complications such as nerve injury are rare events. Therefore, it behooves us to be conservative and performs regional techniques only in the awake patient.

PRO: Performing blocks in a heavily sedated patient or under general anesthesia actually makes it safer. It decreases the chance the patient will suddenly move, directing your needle into a dangerous/unwanted location.

CON: Heavy sedation removes the patient's ability to alert the anesthesiologist of early warning signs of local anesthetic systemic toxicity (LAST) and neurological injury.

PRO: Neither of these points has been proven in the literature. Seizures caused by local anesthetic toxicity can occur from direct intravascular injection or systemic absorption. While the patient may detect the typical central nervous system (CNS) symptoms that precede a seizure (circumoral numbness, dizziness, tinnitus, and visual/auditory changes) if plasma concentrations rise slowly, it is more likely that a direct intravascular injection will be the cause of the seizure. In that case, the patient will seize without premonitory symptoms. Seizures that result from systemic absorption will likely occur after all of the local anesthetic has been injected and the patient has been sedated for the surgery. Additionally, sedation with benzodiazepines can increase the seizure threshold and thus increase the safety margin of local anesthetics [3].

CON: Benumof described 4 cases of permanent loss of cervical spinal cord function after an interscalene block was performed under general anesthesia [4]. Any opportunity to avoid this terrible complication seems reasonable. Although one cannot prove this would not have occurred if the patients had been awake, an alert patient might have provided invaluable information about a pending nerve injury by telling the anesthesiologist of severe pain or paresthesia.

PRO: Misamore et al. published a prospective analysis that found interscalene blocks done under general anesthesia to have rates of success and adverse events similar to those of previous studies in which the block was performed in awake patients [5]. Also, paresthesias and pain have a very low sensitivity as indicators of nerve injury. Perlas et al. found only 30 of 104 patients reported a paresthesia as the needle contacted the nerve, as proven by ultrasound [6]. Moreover, it is likely that once a patient describes the typical excruciating pain from nerve injury by the needle, the damage has already occurred.

CON: While it is hard to prove that a patient complaint of pain or paresthesias can lead to fewer neurological complications, Auroy et al. found that these symptoms during the block indicated nerve injury in 100 % of cases [7]. The numbers in this study were small, but it at least suggests that paresthesias and/or pain during injection are at least associated with nerve injury. An anesthetized patient can never provide these potentially useful warning signs.

PRO: The majority of the studies evaluating complications with regional anesthesia were done with either paresthesia or nerve stimulator techniques. Ultrasound-guided blocks are likely safer, as there is direct visualization of the nerve, the needle, and the local anesthetic spread. Ultrasound also permits the use of decreased local anesthetic volumes.

CON: There is no evidence that ultrasound decreases complications. Most studies show similar complication rates to traditional nerve localization techniques [8–10].

PRO: It is true that the available literature describes intravascular injection to be the only complication decreased with the utilization of ultrasound. However, the majority of these studies were done when ultrasound for peripheral nerve blocks was in its infancy. In skilled hands, the ultrasound is likely to make peripheral nerve blocks safer. With the use of ultrasound, an anesthesiologist should feel comfortable about performing peripheral nerve blocks in the anesthetized patient. This will improve acceptance, allowing more patients to benefit from regional anesthesia.

CON: I agree that regional anesthesia may benefit many patients. However, our goal as physicians is to "first do no harm." Regional anesthesia practices should aim to limit potential complications. As summarized in the 2008 American Society of Regional Anesthesia (ASRA) advisory, peripheral nerve blocks should not routinely be performed on anesthetized patients [3]. However, I would agree that in certain patients with whom communication is difficult (due to language barrier, dementia, developmental delay, or abnormal movements), the benefits may outweigh the risk of injury, and a peripheral nerve block might be considered if it is carefully performed under heavy sedation or general anesthesia.

References

1. Taenzer AH, Walker BJ, Bosenberg AT, Martin L, Suresh S, Polaner DM, et al. Asleep versus awake: Does it matter? Pediatric regional block complications by patient state: a report from the pediatric regional anesthesia network. Reg Anesth Pain Med. 2014;39(4):279–83.
2. Taenzer AH, Walker BJ, Bosenberg AT, Krane EJ, Martin L, Polaner DM, et al. Interscalene brachial plexus blocks under general anesthesia in children: is this safe practice? A report from the pediatric regional anesthesia network. Reg Anesth Pain Med. 2014;39(6):502–5.
3. Bernards CM, Hadzic A, Santhanam S, Neal JM. Regional anesthesia in anesthetized or heavily sedated patients. Reg Anesth Pain Med. 2008;33(5):449–60.
4. Benumof JL. Permanent loss of cervical spinal cord function associated with interscalene block performed under general anesthesia. Anesthesiology. 2000;93(6):1541–4.
5. Misamore G, Webb B, McMurray S, Sallay P. A prospective analysis of interscalene brachial plexus blocks preformed under general anesthesia. J Shoulder Elbow Surg. 2011;20(2):308–14.
6. Perlas A, Niazi A, McCartney C, Chan V, Xu D, Abbas S. The sensitivity of motor response to nerve stimulation and paresthesia for nerve localization as evaluated by ultrasound. Reg Anesth Pain Med. 2006;31:445–50.
7. Auroy Y, Narchi P, Messiah A, Litt L, Rouvier B, Samii K. Serious complications related to regional anesthesia. Results of a prospective survey in France. Anesthesiology. 1997;87:479–86.
8. Sites BD, Taenzer AH, Herrick MD, Gilloon C, Antonakakis J, Richins J, et al. Incidence of local anesthestic systemic toxicity and postoperative neurological symptoms associated with 12.668 ultrasound-guided nerve blocks. An analysis from a prospective clinical registry. Reg Anesth Pain Med. 2012;37(5):478–82.
9. Bogdanov A, Loveland R. Is there a place for interscalene block performed after induction of general anesthesia? Eur J Anaesthesiol. 2005;22:107–10.
10. Neal J, Brull R, Chan VWS, Grant SA, Horn JL, Liu S, et al. The ASRA evidence-based medicine assessment of ultrasound-guided regional anesthesia and pain medicine: executive summary. Reg Anesth Pain Med. 2010;35(2 Suppl):S1–9.

95 Intraneural Injection: A Good Idea or not?

Jan Boublik

Case

A 65-year-old man is undergoing a total shoulder replacement. The surgeon objects to a continuous peripheral nerve block and your colleague taking care of the patient does not feel comfortable about the idea of additives to local anesthetics but does want the block to "last as long as possible." Another colleague, Dr. Pro, suggests an "intraneural" injection as it would "make the nerve block work quicker and last longer."

Question

What is an "intraneural" injection? Is it a good idea or not?

PRO: "As you know, Dr. Con, intraneural injection speeds up the onset of your block and also increases its duration. So you really get the 'best of both worlds' here. Besides, Bigeleisen et al. [1] showed that it is safe and does not lead to any neurological sequelae. And not even you with your fancy new ultrasound machine can really differentiate the boundaries of the brachial plexus reliably," Dr. Pro says with a smirk. "Further, Orebaugh et al. [2] observed that injecting into the nerve might occur more often than people realize."

CON: "You bring up several points. First, what constitutes an 'intraneural' injection? Every peripheral nerve, as you know, has 3 connective tissue sheaths that surround it: endoneurium, perineurium, and epineurium. The endoneurium surrounds the individual nerve fibers and Schwann cells. Meanwhile, the perineurium is a thin, multilayered connective tissue sheath that envelops groups of fascicles. The perineurium and the 'inner', interfascicular connective tissue are surrounded by the 'outer' or epifascicular epineurium, which delineates the nerve trunk and acts as protection against mechanical stress for the peripheral nerve. The epineurium itself is bound by another sheath of loose extraneural connective tissue, the paraneurium, which gives the nerve mobility within the surrounding tissue.

"As Franco adds [3], in the case of a plexus, the paraneurium is surrounded by fascia—for the brachial plexus, the prevertebral fascia. So as you see, you really want to inject sub-paraneural, as Choquet describes [4], to achieve circumferential or perivascular spread."

PRO: "That was certainly a fine description of the anatomy but, as you can clearly see in Biegleisen's paper, there was no incidence of paresthesias or dysesthesia during or after surgery, while dys- and paresthesias were commonly observed during injection. Furthermore, quantitative motor and sensory testing showed an absence of measurable neurologic injury (qualitative sensory and qualitative and quantitative motor testing) in any of the patients at 6-month follow-up, although transient neuropathies might have been missed between the 3-week and 6-month visits at the surgeon's office."

CON: "But the described swelling and interfascicular separation are clear signs of intraneural injection that have been time after time shown to lead to histological injury and clinical neuropathy. Selander et al. [5] showed in 1979 that direct needle trauma and the toxic or ischemic effects of local anesthetics are deleterious when they are injected intraneurally. Further, the fact that the brachial plexus contains a smaller ratio of connective tissue to neural structures makes it relatively more susceptible to neural damage. Moreover, the current level of resolution with ultrasound machines does not allow us to distinguish between intrafascicular and interfascicular injection."

J. Boublik (✉)
Department of Anesthesiology, Perioperative
and Pain Medicine, Stanford School of Medicine,
Stanford University, Stanford, CA 94305, USA
e-mail: jan.boublik@gmail.com; jboublik@stanford.edu

J. Boublik
Somers, NY, USA

C.S. Scher et al. (eds.), *You're Wrong, I'm Right*, DOI 10.1007/978-3-319-43169-7_95

PRO: "You are absolutely right that current ultrasound technology does not have the resolution to differentiate between injection into the stroma or a fascicle of the nerve. But intra-fascicular injection may be only 1 cause of nerve damage. For example, needle gauge and bevel type may also influence the incidence of nerve injury, and conduction deficits can occur after individual axon impalement even by microelectrodes. High injection pressures or volumes alone or in conjunction with intraneural injection [6] may be another cause of neural injury, so you cannot simply say that location alone is the culprit.

"Finally, the type and location of the nerve may influence the way ultrasound-guided injections proceed. A needle that pierces a nerve may be unlikely to puncture a fascicle, depending on the size of the nerve and the relationship of neural structures and connective tissue. Moreover, small nerves are freer to swell because they are not constrained by dense fascia. Finally, the cross-section of a peripheral nerve is comprised of approximately 50 % neurons and 50 % fat and connective tissue. Thus, there is a significant likelihood of puncturing a peripheral nerve without contacting a fascicle or damaging neurons."

CON: "That is all fine and well in a case of a peripheral nerve. For example, for an axillary block or a block of the sciatic nerve at the popliteal level, an injection into the common perineural sheath (an INTER-neural injection) can lead to quicker onset and higher success rates. However, blockade of the brachial plexus at the interscalene level, as in this case, is a very different animal. Nerve roots and trunks have larger fascicles with virtually no intraneural stroma and are much more heavily invested with fascia. Injection into these structures, even with small doses of local anesthetic, may produce high pressures and permanent injury. Furthermore, even a painless injection does not protect you from possible injury, so I would recommend being more cautious.

PRO: "I am very cautious but you are overcautious. Prior to the emergence of ultrasound, we used to safely place needles close to and probably into nerves with a nerve stimulator and rarely did we have parasthesias. When parasthesias did occur, most cases quickly resolved either immediately or within a day. If anything, ultrasound guidance while performing nerve blocks has revealed that 'intraneural' injections don't result in long-term injury and have potential benefits. Be progressive!"

CON: "The truth is we do not know how often intraneural injection leads to nerve injury. It is an unnecessary risk to take. Swelling of nerve elements in the interscalene groove is impossible to discern with the current technology and resolution of ultrasound machines whether you have an endoneural, epineural, or paraneural injection. And does it make any difference clinically? Spence et al. [7] showed that a less invasive peri-plexus injection results in sensory and motor blocks that are just as effective as injection within the brachial plexus sheath. Even if there were no consequences, the safe volume or concentration of local anesthetic remains unknown.

Piercing and injecting nerves is not progressive or therapeutic in any way. Why not just stop doing it instead of trying to convince ourselves that nerve injection and needle trauma are not so bad?

Summary

We need to balance the need and desire to inject close to the nerve with avoidance of purposeful intraneural/subepineural injection when too little is known about safety. Thus, routine "intraneural" injection cannot be recommended for peripheral nerve blockade when safe and efficacious techniques such as paraneural injections are available. At this point, if faced with swelling of the nerve and increase in pressure, it is prudent to withdraw and redirect the needle. Perivascular injection in the infraclavicular and axillary spaces, injections in a common nerve sheath (popliteal, sciatic), and "stay-away" procedures (interscalene) provide safe and effective alternatives.

References

1. Bigeleisen PE. Nerve puncture and apparent intraneural injection during ultrasound-guided axillary block does not invariably result in neurologic injury. Anesthesiology. 2006;105(4):779–83.
2. Orebaugh SL, McFadden K, Skorupan H, Bigeleisen PE. Subepineurial injection in ultrasound-guided interscalene needle tip placement. Reg Anesth Pain Med. 2010;35(5):450–4.
3. Franco CD. Connective tissues associated with peripheral nerves. Reg Anesth Pain Med. 2012;37(4):363–5.
4. Choquet O, Morau D, Biboulet P, Capdevila X. Where should the tip of the needle be located in ultrasound-guided peripheral nerve blocks? Curr Opin Anaesthesiol. 2012;25(5):596–602.
5. Selander D, Dhuner KG, Lundborg G. Peripheral nerve injury due to injection needles used for regional anesthesia. An experimental study of the acute effects of needle point trauma. Acta Anaesthesiol Scand. 1977;21:182–8.
6. Hadzic A, Dilberovic F, Shah S, Kulenovic A, Kapur E, Zaciragic A, et al. Combination of intraneural injections and high injection pressure leads to fascicular injury and neurological deficits in dogs. Reg Anesth Pain Med. 2004;29:417–23.
7. Spence BC, Beach ML, Gallagher JD, Sites BD. Ultrasound-guided interscalene blocks: understanding where to inject the local anaesthetic. Anaesthesia. 2011;66(6):509–14.

Is a Transversus Abdominis Plane (TAP) Block Better Than Surgical Field Infiltration?

96

Beamy Sharma, Uchenna O. Umeh, and Shruthima Thangada

Case

A 19-year-old male presents for repair of a right inguinal hernia. After discussing the primary anesthetic technique with the patient, he expresses concern about postoperative pain. The anesthesia team, which includes an anesthesia attending and a resident, informs the patient of the risks and benefits of a transversus abdominis plane (TAP) block for intraoperative and postoperative pain relief.

The TAP block was first described by A.N. Rafi in a letter to *Anaesthesia* in 2001 [1]. Using a landmark technique, he identified the lumbar triangle of petit in order to inject local anesthetic into the space between the internal oblique and transversus abdominis muscles, which blocked the lower intercostal nerves, the iliohypogastric nerve, and the ilioinguinal nerve. This covers the distribution of spinal nerves T_6 to L_1; therefore, it is often useful for lower abdominal surgery such as large intestinal resection, cesarean delivery, or inguinal hernia repair. Skin sensation and muscle and abdominal peritoneal pain are blocked. The risks include systemic toxicity from the local anesthetic and peritoneal injury. The femoral nerve may be involved by tracking of the local anesthetic deep to the fascia iliaca. Lastly, if it is performed prior to the surgery, the injection of local anesthetic may distort the abdominal anatomy. Relative contraindications include anticoagulation, a history of bleeding disorders, and the presence of an abdominal wall hernia, while absolute contraindications include patient refusal and localized infection [2].

The patient was interested in receiving the block. When the anesthesia team spoke to the surgeon regarding the anesthetic plan, he stated, "You can do the block for this first case for your own learning, but it does not add any benefit because I will infiltrate the wound with bupivacaine at the end of surgery."

Question

Is a transversus abdominis plane (TAP) block better than surgical field infiltration?

PRO: The TAP block decreases narcotic requirement postoperatively.

A recent study looked at 59 patients who underwent laparoscopic colorectal surgery [3]. Infiltration of the wound was performed by the surgeon in 29 patients with 25 mL of 0.25 % ropivacaine injected into the subcutaneous tissue and muscles at the mini-laparotomy incision and 5 cc at each port site. Another 30 patients underwent bilateral ultrasound-guided TAP blocks by the anesthesiologist; 10 mL of 0.25 % ropivacaine was injected at each side. Morphine patient-controlled analgesia (PCA) was used for postoperative pain control. For the first 24 and 48 h, morphine use was significantly less in the TAP block group than the surgical infiltration group: 16.6 versus 24.0 mg and 23.6 versus 31.8 mg, respectively.

B. Sharma (✉)
Department of Anesthesiology, Perioperative Care and Pain Medicine, New York University Langone Medical Center, 550 1st Avenue, New York, NY 10016, USA
e-mail: Beamy.Sharma@nyumc.org; beamy.sharma@gmail.com

B. Sharma
40 Waterside Plaza, 31F, New York, NY 10010, USA

U.O. Umeh
Department of Anesthesiology, Perioperative Care and Pain Medicine, New York University Langone Medical Center/Hospital for Joint Disease, 301 East 17th Street, New York, NY 10016, USA
e-mail: Uchenna.Umeh@nyumc.org

U.O. Umeh
103-06 220th Street, Queens Village, NY 11429, USA

S. Thangada
Department of Anesthesiology, New York University Langone Medical Center, 309 5th Avenue, Apt. 4C, New York, NY 10016, USA
e-mail: midazgal@gmail.com

C.S. Scher et al. (eds.), *You're Wrong, I'm Right*, DOI 10.1007/978-3-319-43169-7_96

CON: The TAP block does not decrease narcotic use when combined with multimodal pain relief.

Another study compared pain scores and morphine use in patients who underwent open radical prostatectomy and received a TAP block, surgical infiltration, or placebo [4]. However, in this study, all patients received oral gabapentin, paracetamol, and ibuprofen preoperatively, and continued to receive paracetamol and ibuprofen regularly postoperatively. Pain scores and morphine use did not differ among any of the 3 groups at 24 h. This indicates that multimodal therapy provides similar pain relief to invasive methods using blocks or wound infiltration.

CON: The decreased narcotic use is not clinically significant and does not compensate for the increased operating room time.

In the earlier study [3], it took 14.7 min on average to perform a TAP block, while only 4.0 min were needed to perform surgical infiltration. That is an extra 10 min spent in the operating room, usually with the patient still under general anesthesia. Furthermore, there were no significant differences in length of hospital stay, incidence of nausea or vomiting, or ileus.

PRO: Larger studies need to be performed to demonstrate clinical significance.

I believe decreased morphine use correlates with improved pain control, which can translate to improved patient satisfaction. The TAP block is operator-dependent; as it is used with increased frequency and becomes more routine in lower abdominal procedures, the speed of performing the block should increase and the time difference minimized. Lastly, while there was no significant decrease in incidence of nausea, vomiting or ileus, fewer patients suffered from these effects. A larger study may actually show a significant reduction, which then will clearly have a direct financial benefit from decreased length of stay in the hospital or recovery room.

In terms of the time spent in performing the block, while it is significantly longer than performing surgical field infiltration, the additional time is not really significant. The few extra minutes will not permit scheduling an additional case in the same block time. Furthermore, as anesthesiologists become more familiar with performing the block and it is incorporated as an intrinsic part of the procedure, the entire process will become more efficient.

CON: Patients are put at an unnecessarily increased risk for at most a minimal decrease in postoperative pain.

The greatest risk of surgical infiltration is systemic toxicity from the local anesthetic; however, this is more theoretical than clinical as there have been no complications cited in the literature. However, complications have been described with TAP blocks. A more common risk, accidental motor block of the femoral nerve, will actually prolong the hospital length of stay. Furthermore, block failure is also common, especially among obese patients—a growing percentage of the surgical population. Thus, these patients will have undergone a procedure that carries risk and does not provide any additional benefit. Although narcotics carry a risk of respiratory depression, there is an antidote, naloxone, that is easily available and its administration is familiar to most physicians.

PRO: A TAP block provides a relatively safe alternative for patients in whom alternative methods of pain control are contraindicated.

In the literature, few complications have actually been associated with TAP blocks. Three cases were reported of systemic toxicity and 3 had a motor femoral nerve block associated with an ilioinguinal/iliohypogastric block. Additionally, the use of ultrasound has increased the success of TAP blocks. Infiltration of the local anesthetic can be directly visualized, increasing the precision of its spread. Consequently, the incidence of associated risks is also decreased.

Furthermore, a TAP block is a safer alternative for patients at risk from alternative forms of pain control. For example, patients who are taking anticoagulants and thus cannot receive a neuraxial block, patients who have a history of narcotic abuse or increased narcotic requirements, patients with acute or chronic kidney disease, or patients at risk of hypoxia (e.g., from obstructive sleep apnea) would benefit greatly from decreased use of or avoiding narcotics altogether.

CON: Narcotics and other forms of intravenous oral analgesics can provide more prolonged relief than a single TAP block.

A TAP, if effective, provides only a few hours of postoperative pain relief and even less if it is performed preoperatively. Furthermore, the pain relief is not titratable. Narcotics and other adjuvant analgesics provide hours of relief. Shorter-acting medications, such as fentanyl, are easily titratable based on patient comfort and respiratory rate.

PRO: The use of liposomal bupivacaine can provide pain relief for up to 72 h.

Liposomal bupivacaine (Exparel®) has recently been approved for use in TAP blocks. It is administered in the same way as other local anesthetics. It has been shown to provide pain relief for up to 72 h. The expansion of its use can significantly reduce narcotic consumption and have potentially greater long-term benefits such as quicker return of bowel function and decreased length of stay.

Also, with a well-functioning acute pain team, TAP blocks can be repeated once patients are out of the operating room. The performance of the block is by no means confined to the operating room, as the only equipment needed is an ultrasound in addition to the block supplies.

Summary

The TAP block provides an alternative in analgesia for lower abdominal surgeries. This block is not the best alternative for all patient populations, such as in patients with difficult abdominal anatomy or coagulopathy. However, it has a significant role in patients in whom one would want to avoid narcotic use, including patients with heavy narcotic requirements or those prone to the respiratory depressive effects of narcotics. (i.e., elderly, obese, OSA patients).

At this time, clinical studies showing the benefits of a TAP block have mixed results, and the positive results do not extend to relevant clinical benefit. However, larger studies need to be performed to get a consensus on outcomes such as decreased length of stay in the recovery room or hospital, decreased incidence of nausea and vomiting, and quicker return of bowel function. Furthermore, as the TAP block is performed more frequently, the benefits should also become more evident. There should be decreased rates of block failure, decreased rates of complications, and improved efficiency in performing the block.

Lastly, the advent of liposomal bupivacaine in TAP blocks has a great deal of potential benefit. There are no additional risks associated with it. Its efficacy up to 72 h can strengthen the possible clinical benefits. Again, larger studies still need to be performed to objectively outline its outcomes.

References

1. Rafi AN. Abdominal field block: a new approach via the lumbar triangle. Anaesthesia 2001;56(10):1024–6.
2. Harmon D, Barrett J, Loughnane F, Finucane BT, Shorten G. Peripheral nerve blocks and peri-operative pain relief. 2nd ed. Philadelphia: Saunders Ltd.; 2011.
3. Park JS, Choi GS, Kwak KH, Jung H, Jeon Y, Park S, et al. Effect of local wound infiltration and transversus abdominis plane block on morphine use after laparoscopic colectomy: a nonrandomized, single-blind prospective study. J Surg Res. 2015;195(1):61–6.
4. Skjelsager A, Ruhnau B, Kistorp TK, Hvarness H, Mathiesen O, Dahl JB. Transversus abdominis plane block or subcutaneous wound infiltration after open radical prostatectomy: a randomized study. Acta Anaesthesiol Scand. 2013;57:502–8.

Is Point-of-Care (POC) Coagulation Testing Worthwhile Before Regional or Neuraxial Anesthesia?

97

Paul Shekane

Case

A 58-year-old man is brought into the trauma center with a crush injury of his bilateral lower extremities after a steel beam fell on him at a construction site. After responding to the page reporting the level-1 trauma, you evaluate whether the patient will need to go to the operating room (OR) emergently. Arriving at the trauma unit, you get a report from the emergency medical services (EMS) stating that this man has a history of coronary artery disease (CAD) with a drug-eluting stent (DES) placed 8 months ago and that he is on both aspirin and clopidogrel. He also has obstructive sleep apnea (OSA) and sleeps with continuous positive airway pressure (CPAP) at night. He just quit smoking last year after smoking 2 packs per day for 35 years. On the stretcher, you see a man that is at least 120 kg with a thick neck and a Mallampati IV airway.

The surgery team tells you that there is no way to salvage his right foot and that he needs an urgent below-knee right-side amputation and open reduction and internal fixation of his left first through third metatarsals.

You call the anesthesia technician to get ready for an awake fiberoptic intubation, and you call your attending to go over the anesthetic plan. You then proceed to explain to the patient what an awake fiberoptic intubation is and why it has to be done in this situation. Once the patient hears the words "awake" and "breathing tube," he becomes very anxious. He states, "I had a hernia surgery once and they just gave me a back injection to make me numb. Can't you do that again?"

Your attending arrives and you recount the patient's history. Your attending states, "A neuraxial technique would be ideal in this case, however, he has been taking aspirin and clopidogrel and there may be an increased risk of epidural hematoma."

Question

Is point-of-care coagulation testing worthwhile before regional and neuraxial anesthesia?

CON: You cite recent American Society of Regional Anesthesia (ASRA) 2010 guidelines, "Clopidogrel should be discontinued for 7 days prior to neuraxial blockade and if a neuraxial block is indicated between 5 and 7 days, normalization of platelet function should be documented [1]. Point of care (POC) coagulation testing is not standard of care yet and even if normal POC coagulation is documented, we would still be technically going against the current ASRA guidelines."

PRO: Your attending states, "Those guidelines are recommendations based on the collective experience of experts in neuraxial anesthesia and anticoagulation and are based on case reports and clinical series mostly. The decision to perform regional or neuraxial anesthesia should be made on an individual basis and after weighing the small risk of spinal hematoma (1 in 150,000 for epidural and less than 1 in 220,000 for spinal anesthetics for non anticoagulated patients) with the benefits of the regional anesthetic for that patient. I came across a case report in which a patient who, despite stopping clopidogrel 7 days prior to a combined spinal-epidural anesthetic for a knee arthroplasty, still developed an epidural hematoma [2]. We need a fast POC test that can tell us how well the patient's coagulation system works that can help us decide if it would be safe to perform a regional or neuraxial anesthetic."

CON: You ask your attending, "Why can't we just transfuse platelets and then perform neuraxial anesthesia?"

P. Shekane (✉)
Department of Anesthesiology, New York University Langone Medical Center, 550 1st Avenue, New York, NY 10016, USA
e-mail: Paul.Shekane@nyumc.org

C.S. Scher et al. (eds.), *You're Wrong, I'm Right*, DOI 10.1007/978-3-319-43169-7_97

PRO: Your attending then counters by saying, "How many units do you need to reverse dual antiplatelet therapy?"

CON: After thinking for a few seconds you can't recall any in vivo studies addressing this issue. Also patients will have a normal platelet count on laboratory analysis.

PRO: "With each unit of platelets you transfuse you expose the patient to unnecessary risks of platelet transfusion including transfusion-related acute lung injury, bacterial contamination, transfusion reaction, administrative errors, and cost."

"What if there was a way to determine if platelet transfusion was even necessary with a quick POC test to determine platelet function and guide preoperative and even intraoperative transfusion? An example of this is rapid thromboelastography (r-TEG), in which a small sample of blood is taken from the selected person and rotated gently to imitate sluggish venous flow and activate coagulation while a thin wire probe is used to measure, which the clot forms around. Another option is Sonoclot®, a device that uses a small vibrating probe in a coagulating blood sample and measures the changing opposition to movement to determine platelet function."

CON: "For most patients that need neuraxial or regional anesthesia a simple history and physical can trump the need for any coagulation tests. Are they even worth the cost and hassle?" you wonder. "The charge for rapid TEG ($317) was similar to the combined costs of getting a prothrombin time (PT), patrial thromboplastin time (PTT), international normalized ratio (INR), platelet count, and fibrinogen ($286). However, this does not take into consideration the cost of stat laboratory technicians who are needed to be able to run the POC coagulation test in the trauma slot or emergency department or the expense of every 8-h quality control that is recommended by the manufacturer [3]."

PRO: "An important advantage of whole blood clotting analysis is that standard laboratory coagulation tests (PT, PTT, INR, fibrinogen) each give you information about specific aspects of the clotting cascade while whole blood clotting analysis provides a picture of the entire clotting process and how each aspect interacts with another to form a clot. Doesn't that information seem more important?"

CON: The original TEG was initially used for coagulation monitoring during liver transplantation and has grown to provide valuable information in the trauma/critical care, cardiovascular surgery, and obstetric anesthesia settings. You remember your hematology module from second year of medical school and remember that the TEG tracing gives you information about fibrin formation (R time), acceleration of fibrin buildup and cross-linking (α[alpha] angle), platelet–fibrin interactions (maximum amplitude, MA), and fibrinolysis [3].

PRO: "It turns out the original TEG is limited in its ability to detect impairment in platelet function induced by anti-platelet agents [4]," your attending explains. "This limitation was addressed with the development of the Platelet Mapping Assay, but that takes longer and costs more."

Summary

"Since we do not have an evidence-based answer to this question, the risks and benefits of each approach have to be weighed and presented to the patient. We can increase the odds of a favorable outcome by performing a POC coagulation test."

You present both options to the patient, and he is satisfied with the risk of combined spinal-epidural (CSE) anesthesia for this surgery. You perform a rapid thromboelastography, which does not indicate a clinically significant coagulopathy. The CSE is performed without complication, and the patient tolerates the procedure without any anesthetic or surgical complications. The patient was continued on his dual antiplatelet therapy and monitored in the step-down unit until it came time to remove the epidural catheter, when another TEG was performed, which enabled safe catheter removal.

References

1. Horlocker TT, Wedel DJ, Rowlingson JC, Enneking FK, Kopp SL, Benzon HT, et al. Regional anesthesia in the patient receiving antithrombotic or thrombolytic therapy: American Society of Regional Anesthesia and Pain Medicine Evidence-Based Guidelines (Third Edition). Reg Anesth Pain Med. 2010;35(1):64–101.
2. Tam NL, Pac-Soo C, Pretorius PM. Epidural haematoma after a combined spinal–epidural anaesthetic in a patient treated with clopidogrel and dalteparin. Br J Anaesth. 2006;96(2):262–5.
3. Holcomb JB, Minei KM, Scerbo ML. Admission rapid thrombelastography can replace conventional coagulation tests in the emergency department: experience with 1974 consecutive trauma patients. Ann Surg. 2012;256(3):476–86.
4. Enriquez LJ, Shore-Lesserson L. Point-of-care coagulation testing and transfusion algorithms. Br J Anaesth. 2009;102(4):492–8.

98 Should a Peripheral Nerve Block Be Placed in an Anticoagulated Patient?

Kiwon Song and Katherine Chuy

Case

A 38-year-old female, G2P0010, 12 weeks pregnant, presents with an open right radial fracture after falling on a muddy sidewalk. She has a history of left lower extremity deep venous thrombosis (DVT) after taking oral contraceptives. Because of this, she was placed on subcutaneous enoxaparin sodium (a low molecular weight heparin), which she has injected every 12 h for the last 3 months. She took her last dose 5 h prior to her arrival at the hospital and reported her last meal as 6 h before her admission. She received morphine in the emergency room to alleviate her pain.

Due to the high risk of infection secondary to the contaminated injury, the orthopedics team determines emergent surgery is necessary. The patient is worried that general anesthesia may negatively affect her pregnancy. She suffered a spontaneous abortion 3 years ago, and it took many consultations with her infertility specialist for her to become pregnant again. She says she would do anything to avoid general anesthesia and the risk of losing her baby or exposing it to potential long-term detrimental effects.

Questions

Should a peripheral nerve block be performed in an anticoagulated patient?

CON: Many would favor a general anesthetic in patients scheduled for emergency surgery. This patient has several factors that increase her risk for pulmonary aspiration, including the fact that she is not NPO by guidelines. Pain and discomfort from trauma, pregnancy, and recent narcotic administration can further delay gastric emptying [1]. The safest option would be a general anesthetic that isolates the lungs from the stomach with an endotracheal tube and excludes the use of potentially teratogenic medications. At this point, the priority is with the adult patient and ensuring that she gets through the surgery with minimal risk. Furthermore, this patient is on an anticoagulant. Performing a regional nerve block places her at risk for bleeding if a vessel is punctured.

PRO: On the other hand, one can argue that a carefully performed regional nerve block eliminates the need to manipulate the airway or sedate the patient if she can otherwise stay awake and still for this procedure. The nerve block will render her arm insensate, providing adequate surgical anesthesia. In an awake, cooperative patient, airway reflexes remain intact. Furthermore, avoiding general anesthesia reduces potential risk to the growing fetus, especially in the first trimester [2]. *N*-Methyl-D-aspartate (NMDA)-type glutamate and γ(gamma)-aminobutyric (GABA) receptors are located throughout the central nervous system. Anesthetic agents interact with these receptors, which play an integral role in neuronal synaptogenesis, differentiation, and survival during development. Animal studies showed accelerated neuronal apoptosis in immature rodent brains exposed to anesthetic agents [2]. While these results should not be extrapolated to humans, and no drug has been directly correlated with danger to the growing human fetus, limiting fetal exposure to anesthetic medications might optimize fetal outcome.

If performed under ultrasound guidance, a nerve block can offer optimal surgical anesthesia for a cooperative patient who does not require sedation. It is particularly

K. Song (✉) · K. Chuy
Department of Anesthesiology, Perioperative Care and Pain Medicine, New York University Langone Medical Center, 550 First Avenue, New York, NY 10016, USA
e-mail: ikiwon@yahoo.com; Kiwon.Song@nyumc.org

K. Chuy
e-mail: Katherine.chuy@nyumc.org

K. Chuy
320 Center Street, Englewood Cliffs, NJ 07632, USA

C.S. Scher et al. (eds.), *You're Wrong, I'm Right*, DOI 10.1007/978-3-319-43169-7_98

helpful in cases in which multiple factors may place patients at risk for aspiration or other complications of general anesthesia. Ultrasound allows visualization of the block needle, blood vessels, target nerves, and surrounding structures. It also provides useful information regarding possible anatomical variations. The needle tip can be precisely guided close to the targeted nerve or plexus without coming into direct contact with it, thereby limiting intraneural injury. This aids in achieving the optimal position for local anesthetic deposition while minimizing the risk of accidental vascular puncture. Important steps to ensure correct and safe positioning of the needle include aspiration to confirm the absence of blood, constant observation of needle tip advancement, local anesthetic spread around the nerves, and avoidance of pressing too hard on the ultrasound, which may lead to a false absence of the veins [3].

Studies have shown ultrasound guidance correlates with fewer vascular punctures, fewer needle passes to achieve a successful block, and a reduced dose of local anesthetic without compromising the quality or duration of anesthesia [3]. Case reports also describe successful ultrasound-guided peripheral nerve blocks without hemorrhagic complications in patients receiving anticoagulants or those with coagulopathies [4].

CON: It is important to note, however, that the success of the block depends on the professional's experience and comfort level [4]. Reports of intravascular injection appear to be associated with inexperience and imperfect technique [5].

A patient who is anticoagulated has a high risk of bleeding and hematoma formation. This may lead to nerve compression and ischemia, thereby resulting in sensory or motor deficits or possible blood transfusion, which carries its own risks. There are technical issues with ultrasound, such as limited resolution, and suboptimal technique such as the needle tip not being fully visualized. This can lead to complications and is not worth the risk [3]. In a patient who has a good airway by examination, it is more comfortable to provide a protected airway rather than risk unnecessary bleeding.

Question

Does being on anticoagulants really increase the risk of hematoma formation in peripheral nerve blocks? Isn't this mainly a concern for neuraxial blocks?

CON: The patient is at risk of hemorrhagic complications if a vessel is punctured. If a block is performed in an anatomical area that is noncompressible, it can cause compression of nearby structures and other complications. A recent study reported a 3.2 % rate of vascular puncture when residents used the ultrasound in conjunction with a nerve stimulator [6].

PRO: If a peripheral nerve block is performed carefully with strict ultrasound guidance, the risk of vascular injury is low, even for an anticoagulated patient. The previously mentioned study that described blood vessel puncture involved residents, and thus, inexperience may have played a role [6]. In contrast, another study in which specialist anesthesiologists or senior residents with experience in regional anesthesia performed blocks with ultrasound guidance found that the procedures resulted in no vascular puncture [7].

Currently, there are no investigations that examine the frequency and severity of neurovascular complications in anticoagulated patients following peripheral blocks under ultrasound guidance. However, according to a few published case reports, these blocks can be safely and effectively administered without complications in these patients, with direct visualization of vascular and neural structures under ultrasound [4, 8, 9]. It is also notable that although several cases of vascular injury with or without resultant nerve dysfunction have been reported following peripheral blocks, neurologic recovery was complete within 6–12 months in all patients [10, 11]. Furthermore, the largest study performed to assess the risk of major bleeding after peripheral nerve block found that this occurred after psoas compartment or lumbar sympathetic blocks, not superficial nerve blocks [10, 11].

Question

If a supraclavicular or infraclavicular nerve block is considered to be in a noncompressible location, then an axillary block could be an option. However, this involves more needle passes. Would this increase the risk of vessel puncture?

PRO: Supraclavicular and infraclavicular blocks both have the advantage of easy accessibility to the brachial plexus. However, the subclavian vasculature is very difficult to effectively compress in the event of accidental vascular puncture. Therefore, an ideal ultrasound-guided block in an anticoagulated patient should be performed in a location where compression is possible. Furthermore, when performing a supraclavicular or infraclavicular block, the pleura is very close to the nerve, making pneumothorax another possible risk [7]. Although axillary blocks require more needle passes than a supra- or infraclavicular nerve block, the axillary vessels are easy to compress and there is no pleura to avoid, thus decreasing the risk of pneumothorax or hemothorax [8]. This rationale was reported in a case study of a patient with a left-ventricular assist device who was anticoagulated with warfarin sodium and required a wrist arthroscopy for a septic joint [8].

CON: One may argue that an anticoagulated patient can still bleed significantly even if compression of the source is possible. Close postoperative monitoring following any kinds of peripheral nerve blocks in these patients can allow early evaluation of neurologic deficits and early intervention [10, 11]. New onset or increasing pain or tenderness at the site, a drop in hemoglobin or blood pressure, or a new sensory or motor deficit may indicate underlying hematoma [9]. While computed tomography (CT) provides a definite diagnosis of bleeding, ultrasound can also aid to rule out superficial expanding hematomas [9].

Question

In the Third Consensus Conference on Regional Anesthesia and Anticoagulation, the American Society of Regional Anesthesia and Pain Medicine (ASRA) Practice Guidelines recommended that peripheral nerve blocks should follow the same guidelines as neuraxial injections. For someone on a therapeutic dose of low molecular weight heparin, this means waiting 24 h after the last dose to perform a block. Doesn't performing a peripheral nerve block in this case go against these recommendations?

CON: ASRA consensus statements are determined by a group of recognized experts in the field of regional anesthesia. Their guidelines are determined by evidence-based reviews, as well as the group's evaluation of case reports, clinical series, pharmacology, hematology, and risk factors for surgical bleeding [10, 11]. If ASRA recommends that peripheral nerve blocks should not be performed in anticoagulated patients, many practicing anesthesiologists would follow this recommendation. Again, there have been case reports of hematoma formation in patients who have been anticoagulated, leading to complications mentioned earlier [12].

PRO: Note, however, that ASRA states that the low number of case reports of hemorrhagic complications from peripheral nerve blocks is insufficient to make definitive statements. It is a Grade IC recommendation, meaning that, while there is general agreement, the recommendations stem from case reports and expert opinion because data about safety and/or risk of antithrombotic agents are sparse [12]. Some may find this advice to be very restrictive, applying only to deep plexus blocks in noncompressible regions, such as the lumbar plexus [12]. If the same guidelines are applied to all peripheral nerve blocks, the restrictions may become excessive.

Due to the current lack of good data, there is no consensus about the indications for ultrasound-guided peripheral nerve blocks in patients with coagulopathies or who are on anticoagulants [4]. In contrast to ASRA, the Austrian and Brazilian Societies currently recommend that the use of superficial peripheral nerve blocks guided by ultrasound in anticoagulated patients is relatively safe [13]. Complex cases arise, and the decision to perform a nerve block on a patient receiving antithrombotic therapy should be made individually. A number of case reports of ultrasound-guided peripheral nerve blocks in the presence of antithrombotic treatments or coagulopathies have been published and their rationale in decision making described [4, 8, 9]. In discussions with the patient and surgeon, one should weigh the low but potential risk of bleeding against the benefits of regional anesthesia, considering issues such as the experience of the professional performing the block, patient comorbidities, risks and benefits of other anesthesia options, and the urgency of surgery [4, 10, 11].

Summary

The development of ultrasound has greatly impacted the field of regional anesthesia. The ability to directly confirm anatomical structures and needle placement aids in the safety of peripheral nerve blocks, improving success and reducing complications [3]. Ultimately, good image acquisition relies on the capabilities of the monitor, operator skill, interpretation of images, and performance of the block with good needle visibility and hand/eye coordination [3]. In complex cases in which regional anesthesia can offer a significant benefit, it still has to be carefully planned. Risks and benefits of anesthetic options should be analyzed and discussed with the patient and the surgeon. Currently, there are no published prospective randomized controlled trials studying peripheral nerve blocks on patients on antithrombotic therapy that aid in setting definitive guidelines. Because the rate of hemorrhagic complications remains extremely low, large sample sizes would be required to determine the safety of performing blocks in these patients. In the future, development of more echogenic needles and of ultrasound monitors with better resolution or 3-dimensional imaging may further help in precise application of regional nerve blocks. Until further studies can determine definitive guidelines, certain ultrasound-guided superficial peripheral nerve blocks may be considered in patients on antithrombotic therapy and should be performed by an experienced specialist.

References

1. Cohen N. Aspiration: is there an optimal management strategy? In: Fleisher LA, editor. Evidence-based practice of anesthesiology. 2nd ed. Philadelphia: Saunders-Elsevier; 2009. p. 329.
2. Reitman E, Flood P. Anaesthetic considerations for non-obstetric surgery during pregnancy. Br J Anaesthesiol. 2011;107(Suppl 1): i72–8.
3. Warman P, Nicholls B. Ultrasound-guided nerve blocks: efficacy and safety. Best Pract Res Clin Anaesthesiol. 2009;23(3):313–26.
4. Ferraro LHC, Tardelli MA, Yamashita AM, Cardone JDB, Kishi JM. Ultrasound-guided femoral and sciatic nerve blocks in an anticoagulated patient. Case reports. Rev Bras Anestesiol. 2010;60(4):422–8.
5. Chin KJ, Chan V. Ultrasound-guided peripheral nerve blockade. Curr Opin Anaesthesiol. 2008;21(5):624–31.
6. Orebaugh SL, Williams BA, Kentor ML. Ultrasound guidance with nerve stimulation reduces the time necessary for resident peripheral nerve blockade. Reg Anesth Pain Med. 2007;32:448–54.
7. Gurkan Y, Acar S, Solak M, Toker K. Comparison of nerve stimulation vs. ultrasound-guided lateral sagittal infraclavicular block. Acta Anaesthesiol Scand. 2008;52(6):851–5.
8. Trunfio G, Yaguda B, Saunders P, Feierman D. Ultrasound-guided axillary block in an anticoagulated patient after Heartmate II implantation. Open J Anesthesiol. 2014;4:159–62.
9. Tantry PT, Kadam D, Shetty P, Bhandary S. Combined femoral and sciatic nerve blocks for lower limb anaesthesia in anticoagulated patients with severe cardiac valvular lesions. Indian J Anaesthesiol. 2010;54(3):235–8.
10. Horlocker TT. Regional anaesthesia in the patient receiving antithrombotic and antiplatelet therapy. Br J Anaesthesiol. 2011;107(Suppl 1):i96–106.
11. Horlocker TT, Wedel DJ, Rowlingson JC, Enneking RK, Kopp SL, Benzon HT, et al. Regional anesthesia in the patient receiving antithrombotic or thrombolytic therapy: American Society of Regional Anesthesia and Pain Medicine Evidence-Based Guidelines (3rd ed.). Reg Anesth Pain Med. 2010;35(1):64–101.
12. Benzon HT. Regional anesthesia in the anticoagulated patient. The New York School of Regional Anesthesia. 2013 Sept 20. http://www.nysora.com/mobile/regional-anesthesia/foundations-of-ra/3300-ra-in-anticoagulated-patient.html. Accessed 27 April 2015.
13. Fonseca NM, Alves RR, Pontes JPJ. SBA Recommendations for regional anesthesia safety in patients taking anticoagulants. Braz J Anesthesiol. 2014;64(1):1–15.

Are the Benefits of Stimulating Peripheral Nerve Block Catheters Worth the Risks?

99

Agathe Streiff and Junping Chen

Case

You and a colleague are called to the emergency room (ER) to assess a patient, who was sent by her surgeon because of a stuck nerve block catheter. The patient had a total shoulder replacement surgery five days ago and was discharged with a home infusion pump system connected to an interscalene catheter for pain control. In the ER, the patient is found to be calm but worried. Her left arm is neurologically intact. She tells you that her husband and her surgeon had attempted to pull out the catheter as instructed, but there was a lot of resistance. Her surgeon told her that the retained catheter may need to be removed by surgical exploration in order to avoid nerve injury, but that she should first be evaluated by the anesthesiology team. You examine and tug the catheter, which does not budge.

Under ultrasound, you see a hyperechoic catheter and its coiled wire tip, which is lodged in the neuromuscular structures between the scalene muscles. It is clear that the catheter is a stimulating type, and that its exposed tip has reacted with and adhered to the tissue. Your colleague asks you why the patient's anesthesia team had opted for a stimulating peripheral nerve catheter, as opposed to the more common non-stimulating catheter.

Question

Are the benefits of stimulating peripheral nerve block catheters worth the risks?

A. Streiff (✉)
Department of Anesthesiology, Mount Sinai St. Luke's and Mount Sinai West Hospital, 1000 Amsterdam Ave, New York, NY 10019, USA
e-mail: astreiff@chpnet.org

J. Chen
Department of Anesthesiology, Mount Sinai St. Luke's and Mount Sinai West Hospital, 1000 10th Avenue, New York, NY 10019, USA
e-mail: jchen@chpnet.org

PRO: You reply that stimulating catheters consist of a wire-reinforced catheter body, including a metal coil tip. The rationale for using stimulating catheters is that in order to achieve an optimal motor response, the tip of the catheter must lie very close to the nerve. Injection of local anesthetic in this location should, therefore, produce an effective nerve block. Compared to non-stimulating catheters, which are advanced blindly after locating the desired area, a stimulating catheter allows clinicians to confirm using nerve stimulation that the tip of the catheter is in close proximity to the target nerves. When we place peripheral nerve catheters, we advance the catheter blindly past the needle tip in the hopes that the catheter remains close to the nerve root after retracting the needle. It is challenging to keep the tip in the desired location during the removal of the needle. The optimal length that a catheter should be advanced past the needle remains unknown. Intuitively, however, increasing the insertion distance increases the chance of the catheter coiling, knotting, and ultimately failing. A stimulating nerve catheter, on the other hand, allows the practitioner to adjust the catheter tip using a nerve stimulator, ensuring that it stays near the nerves of interest. Furthermore, stimulating catheters can be visualized with ultrasound, providing the practitioner additional feedback on its location.

CON: Everything you mention is true, especially for practitioners who still use nerve stimulators only to place nerve catheters. However, in current regional anesthesia practice, ultrasound guidance for nerve blocks has become mainstream. You might have heard about the "hydrodissection" and "hyperechoic flash" techniques. One can detect the catheter tip in real time within a fluid collection while injecting fluid through the catheter, or watching for a hyperechoic flash when injecting air. These techniques allow practitioners to locate non-stimulating catheter tips that otherwise would be invisible, and allow adjustment of the catheter near the nerves. Non-stimulating catheters are inexpensive and cause less tissue irritation and fibrogenesis compared to the metal tip of stimulating catheters.

C.S. Scher et al. (eds.), *You're Wrong, I'm Right*, DOI 10.1007/978-3-319-43169-7_99

PRO: To most well-trained regional anesthesiologists, nerve localization is not a problem. However, threading the catheter may pose a challenge. In my experience, difficulty threading a catheter occurs 10–20 % of the time. If you have used both stimulating and non-stimulating catheters, you may have experienced that threading the stimulating catheter is easier and more successful. This is because the wire-reinforced catheter contains an internal stylet that extends to 5 cm from the end of the catheter tip and is relatively rigid compared to the non-stimulating one. Being able to locate the nerve with a needle past the catheter without struggling may correlate to more successful blocks and less possibility of nerve injury due to manipulation of the needle in close proximity to the nerves. In this regard, the stiffness afforded by the wire could be another major advantage of the stimulating catheter. This characteristic is especially useful in placing the catheter in deep structures such as the lumbar plexus and for adductor canal blocks [1].

CON: I agree. However, every positive feature can result in an opposite effect. The stiffness of stimulating catheters may help for insertion, but it also increases the potential to penetrate important and vulnerable structures such as blood vessels or nerve tissue. In addition, should the wire-reinforced catheter kink, it may result in obstruction to the flow of local anesthetic. In this regard, non-stimulating catheters are more resistant to this type of failure.

PRO: While these theoretical concerns may exist, clinical evidence argues in favor of stimulating catheters. In a randomized controlled trial of 58 patients, stimulating catheters achieved a complete lumbar plexus block with a reduced volume of local anesthetic compared to non-stimulating catheters [1]. Stimulating catheters have also demonstrated reduced time to onset of surgical block and decreased postoperative pain medication requirement in hallux surgeries [2]. It is worth the expense, in my opinion.

CON: You know, one recent prospective blinded cohort study looked at stimulating catheters that were placed after interscalene nerve blocks without confirming twitches prior to securing the catheter. When they checked twitches after securing the catheter, the authors found that there was a wide range of power at which twitches were obtained, which you are saying correlates to distance from the nerve. This did not correlate with 24 h morphine consumption, which reflects the patient's pain sensitivity [3].

PRO: I also read that study; I agree it must have captured a time before any catheter tip migration could have occurred, but the final sample size was only 34 patients, and using morphine patient-controlled analgesia (PCA) to determine the intensity of surgical pain may be flawed since heterogeneous populations may consume morphine for reasons other than surgical site pain. Additionally, the duration of the loading dose of their local anesthetic, ropivacaine, could be as long as 20 h postoperatively, so I am not sure how well 24 h morphine PCA consumption correlates with postoperative pain. There are more studies, including a semiquantitative systematic review, that demonstrate that stimulating catheters provide better postoperative analgesia than conventional catheters [4].

CON: While I agree that it was a strong study, they could not assess other clinically important parameters, such as functional recovery and patient satisfaction. In another prospective randomized trial, stimulating catheters were no different from non-stimulating catheters when used without ultrasound guidance in infraclavicular blocks [5], so how can we say these catheters are better than the already existing catheters?

PRO: The study you cited followed patients for a shorter period of time, with telephone follow-ups concluding after ten days unless a complication arose. A prospective, randomized, double-blinded trial of interscalene blocks using landmark and nerve stimulation technique did show the superiority of stimulating catheters—but not the way you would think. While there was no difference in postoperative pain, stimulating catheters enabled a faster onset of motor block, and a much improved functional outcome six weeks after shoulder surgery [6]. I think that makes them considerably more advantageous.

CON: I think the literature so far is pretty divided when it comes to the superiority of stimulating versus conventional peripheral nerve catheters, especially when looking at the different types of blocks. Alright, let us suppose there is an advantage to stimulating catheters in interscalene blocks. In this case, our patient has returned to the emergency room and will now retain a bad experience from her surgery.

One institution reported five cases of patients with ambulatory stimulating catheters, which were "stuck" and not able to be removed at home, similar to our patient. In their experience, which consisted of 2,500 prior patients who had received non-stimulating catheters, they had not experienced any of these complications. They were luckily all removed using steady, continuous traction, and sometimes dilation using the reverse Seldinger technique, but in many, the wire had sheared through the catheter. The patients did not suffer any neurologic deficits and avoided surgical extraction of the catheters, but they point out that when such a return visit to the hospital is needed, much of the benefit of facilitating these ambulatory procedures is lost [7].

Another study reports a case of perineural entrapment of an interscalene stimulating catheter, which required surgical extraction under general anesthesia once the block had worn off. They suggest that the exposed metal tip of the catheter makes it especially liable to adhere to the surrounding fibrous tissue, compared to non-stimulating catheters, and they mention animal and clinical studies that support this hypothesis [8].

Summary

You both agree that these are worrying findings, and further studies to quantify the risks should be undertaken, as well as to obtain more consensus on the superiority of stimulating catheters in various blocks. You both agree that given the current known risks and case reports with stimulating catheters, you would want to exercise caution when using them in an ambulatory setting in the future, as these patients will have less supervision than those who are admitted and watched in the hospital.

You discuss these findings with the patient, as well as your plan, which is to rule out catheter-nerve entanglement and carefully detect the point of attachment under ultrasound. She understands the situation and would like to proceed. Under ultrasound guidance, you inject five mL of saline and apply gentle but firm traction, slowly increasing the force of traction while monitoring her response. After a few minutes, the fibrous tissue attached to the catheter is disrupted and the catheter comes out smoothly with the tip intact. Your patient did not experience any pain, neurologic symptoms, or changes during this time. Her physical exam remains unchanged. She thanks you and your colleague for your efforts and is discharged from the emergency room.

References

1. Cappelleri G, Ghisi D, Ceravola E, Guzzetti L, Ambrosoli AL, Gemma M, et al. A randomized controlled comparison between stimulating and standard catheters for lumbar plexus block. Anaesthesia. 2015;70:948–55.
2. Casati A, Fanelli G, Koscielniak-Nielsen Z, Cappelleri G, Aldegheri G, Danelli G, et al. Using stimulating catheters for continuous sciatic nerve block shortens onset time of surgical block and minimizes postoperative consumption of pain medication after hallux valgus repair as compared with conventional nonstimulating catheters. Anesth Analg. 2005;101:1192–7.
3. Schoenmakers K, Heesterbeek P, Jack N, Stienstra R. No correlation between minimal electrical charge at the tip of the stimulating catheter and the efficacy of the peripheral nerve block catheter for brachial plexus block: a prospective blinded cohort study. BMC Anesthesiol. 2014;14:26.
4. Morin A, Kranke P, Wulf H, Stienstra R, Eberhart LH. The effect of stimulating versus nonstimulating catheter techniques for continuous regional anesthesia: a semiquantitative systematic review. Reg Anesth Pain Med. 2010;35:194–9.
5. Dhir S, Ganapathy S. Comparative evaluation of ultrasound-guided continuous infraclavicular brachial plexus block with stimulating catheter and traditional technique: a prospective-randomized trial. Acta Anaesthesiol Scand. 2008;52:1158–66.
6. Stevens MF, Werdehausen R, Golla E, Braun S, Hermanns H, Ilg A, et al. Does interscalene catheter placement with stimulating catheters improve postoperative pain or functional outcome after shoulder surgery? A prospective, randomized and double-blinded trial. Anesth Analg. 2007;104:442–7.
7. Clendenen SR, Robards CB, Greengrass RA, Brull SJ. Complications of peripheral nerve catheter removal at home: case series of five ambulatory interscalene blocks. Can J Anesth. 2011;58:62–7.
8. Adhikary SD, Armstrong K, Chin KJ. Perineural entrapment of an interscalene stimulating catheter. Anaesth Intensive Care. 2012;40:3.

Part XII
Chronic Pain

Epidural Steroid Injection or Physical Therapy for Lumbosacral Radiculopathy Due to Disc Herniation?

100

Ryan T. Gualtier

Case

A 58-year-old male presents to his physician with complaints of low back pain for the past 4 months. The pain is sharp and burning and radiates down the back of his left leg to the bottom of the foot. There is a tingling and occasional numbness on the sole of his foot. He has tried taking nonsteroidal anti-inflammatory agents (NSAIDs) with minimal benefit, and finally decided it was time to get the pain checked as golf season was around the corner, and he did not want it to impact his game. A magnetic resonance imaging (MRI) scan is performed and reveals a small central left paracentral disc herniation at L5-S1, which partially effaces the ventral thecal sac.

At this point, the physician recommends conservative management, including pharmacological treatment, along with physical therapy (PT) and exercises and instructs the patient to follow-up in 4–6 weeks.

However, the patient is not very happy with this news as he would like more rapid results in order to be able to compete in the inaugural golf outing. He mentions that his friend experienced similar pain symptoms, which dramatically improved after 2 epidural steroid injections (ESI). The patient insists to have an ESI performed.

The majority of patients who are seen in the primary care setting with low back pain and mild intermittent radicular symptoms generally exhibit rapid improvement over the course of the first month, with further gradual improvement for up to 3 months [1]. In those who have ongoing pain, such as the patient in question, a more in-depth history and physical examination are necessary, along with imaging tests, which may reveal different types of lumbar spine pathology, with disc herniation being frequently diagnosed.

The intervertebral disc sits between the vertebral bodies and is responsible for providing flexibility and acting as an absorber of spinal column loads. It is composed of 4 concentric layers, ranging from the nucleus pulposus in the center, to the outermost layer of the annulus fibrosus. In a healthy disc, the nucleus acts to distribute forces equally throughout the annulus. With normal ageing, the discs change volume, shape, and composition. Disc herniation is multifactorial, with degenerative and mechanical processes making up the majority of causes. Degeneration of the annulus is believed to be the most common inciting cause of lumbar disc herniation. However, mechanical events such as bending and stretching of the spine, as well as spinal rotation exercises or abrupt postural changes work synergistically with the degenerative changes [2]. The type of pain and associated symptoms depend largely on the site and degree of herniation, with the herniation occurring most frequently at L4-L5 and L5-S1 [3].

Both physical therapy and epidural steroid injections have been known to have an acceptable role in the management of low back pain with radicular symptoms.

Question

Epidural steroid injection or physical therapy for lumbosacral radiculopathy due to disc herniation?

PRO Physical Therapy: Multiple treatment options for subacute and chronic low back pain are available. They are typically divided into pharmacologic, noninterventional, nonsurgical interventional therapy, and surgery. For our patient with radicular pain, there is often no clear guideline as to when nonsurgical interventional therapy should be considered, but most physicians would agree that exhausting pharmacological and physical therapy modalities first would be a good approach.

R.T. Gualtier (✉)
Department of Anesthesiology, New York University Langone Medical Center, 550 First Avenue, New York, NY 10016, USA
e-mail: Ryan.gualtier@nyumc.org; Ryan.Gualtier@med.nyu.edu; rgualtie@gmail.com

C.S. Scher et al. (eds.), *You're Wrong, I'm Right*, DOI 10.1007/978-3-319-43169-7_100

An interesting observation from Cohen et al. is that more than 70 % of patients with radiculopathy will recover within 6 months, while a similar proportion will resorb their herniated discs within 1 year of presentation [4]. This may have important implications, as those who have received an ESI will be able to heal naturally while their acute discomfort is treated. Whether or not physical therapy plays a role in this process is debatable, but it sure cannot hurt.

A number of types of exercises are commonly utilized with chronic low back pain. The most common PT programs that are emphasized in literature include: core strengthening, flexion/extension movement, aerobic exercise, meditation, and functional restoration programs. In general, exercise therapy is safe, and patients should be advised to remain as active as possible.

PRO Epidural Steroid Injection: Yes, it "cannot hurt", but studies regarding physical therapy as a treatment for lumbosacral radicular pain commonly lack the structure and detail that is seen with interventional pain procedures and surgery. There also tends to be an inconsistent follow-through with PT regimens prescribed, and the patient education can widely vary depending on the patient's understanding. One of the major limitations of systemic reviews of exercise therapy is the inability to compare the innumerable types of activities that can be classified as exercise.

The PT is structured on multiple sessions and requires significant patient compliance and time. The results are not immediate and may even cause an initial worsening in pain.

The ESI requires fewer encounters, less time out of the patient's schedule, and results in a faster onset of symptom relief. These are endpoints that our patient is looking for and would benefit from in order to be ready for the golf season.

PRO Physical Therapy: Exercise has been shown to have some benefit in patients with subacute and chronic low back pain [5]. It improves short-term pain relief and function, with results that may last upwards of 1–3 years. The maximum benefit seems to be achieved when the exercise plan includes the following elements: individualized regimens, supervision, stretching, and strengthening.

With this in mind, there is a general consensus that PT is a relatively safe modality for the treatment of lumbosacral radicular pain and does have several advantages. Patient's that participate in PT are able to utilize less opioids, which are associated with their own set of negatives, including nausea, vomiting, respiratory depression, sedation, and constipation to name a few. In addition, PT allows patients to avoid invasive interventional pain procedures and surgery. Interventions generally require the patient to undergo diagnostic MRI, which can be very costly, in addition to exposure to fluoroscopic radiation. There is a risk for bleeding, infection, nerve damage, and possibility of making the pain worse. In addition, the US Food and Drug Administration (FDA) has brought attention to the rare but serious side effects associated with ESI (stroke, paralysis, death, etc.) [6]. When taking these side effects into account, PT is an excellent first choice in many patients as the benefits far outweigh the risks.

PRO Epidural Steroid Injection: As part of a comprehensive nonsurgical approach, epidural steroids should be considered in the management of back pain with radicular symptoms. ESI is among the most frequently performed procedures in pain clinics throughout the United States [7]. It is widely acknowledged to work best for radicular pain, although it has historically been used for all types of neuraxial pain. Manchikanti et al. [7] found high-quality evidence in a Cochrane review, demonstrating that epidural steroid injections have short-term benefits in terms of alleviating radicular pain and disability from disc herniation.

There have been few studies that compare ESI to other treatments, and only one in which blinded controls were used. In an underpowered 6-month study by Koc et al. [8], 29 patients were randomized to receive high-volume ESI or 2 weeks of physical therapy, and a control group was untreated. At follow-up, all of the groups improved in most measures, however, the only statistically significant differences in pain and function were noted at 2 weeks in which ESIs were superior to the non-injection groups [8]. Overall, the findings seem to be consistent with systemic reviews that found moderate evidence for short-term but inconsistent evidence for long-term benefit with ESI.

Regardless of the fact that there are few studies comparing ESI to other nonsurgical treatments, what we do know is that there have been more reviews and randomized controlled studies (greater than 45) that have evaluated epidural steroid injections for radicular pain than for any other treatment [4]. It seems to be a general consensus across all specialties that ESI provides at least short-term relief in properly selected patients. This short-term relief may be all that is necessary for some patients to get back on their feet and decrease the disability and health care costs associated with conservative treatment modalities.

Summary

The clinical course of low back pain with radicular symptoms is considered favorable for most patients. At this time, the indication for a specific treatment as a first-line therapy (physical therapy and/or epidural steroid injections) has only limited or inconclusive evidence, suggesting that more structured and specific studies are needed to effectively guide decision-making. Currently available conservative treatments such as PT may decrease pain without modifying the long-term clinical course of the disc herniation. On the other hand, numerous recent studies investigating the effects of epidural steroid injections for disc herniation suggest there are beneficial effects on pain and disability in the short term (3–6 weeks), but no long-term effect, including return to work and use of surgery [9]. Ultimately, it comes down to the patient and their doctor weighing the risks versus benefits of choosing one treatment plan over the other. As more standardized trials are performed, the hope is for both patients and physicians to be well informed about up to date evidence and expected outcomes in all the treatment options.

References

1. Chou R, Atlas S, Rosenquist E. Subacute and chronic low back pain: nonsurgical interventional treatment. UpToDate. 2015;1–10.
2. Choi J, Lee S, Hwangbo G. Influences of spinal decompression therapy and general traction therapy on the pain, disability, and straight leg of patients with intervertebral disc herniation. J Phys Ther Sci. 2015;27:481–3.
3. Hsu PS, Armon C, Levin K, Shefner JM, Dashe JF. Lumbosacral radiculopathy: pathophysiology, clinical features, and diagnosis. UpToDate. 2015;1–16.
4. Cohen SP, Bicket MC, Jamison D, Wilkinson I, Rathmell JP. Epidural steroids: a comprehensive, evidence-based review. Reg Anesth Pain Med. 2013;38(3):175–200.
5. Atlas S, Aronson M, Park L. Exercise-based therapy for low back pain. UpToDate. 2015;1–11.
6. Manchikanti L, Candido KD, Singh V, Gharibo CG, Boswell MV, Benyamin RM, et al. Epidural steroid warning controversy still dogging FDA. Pain Physician. 2014;17(4):E451–74.
7. Manchikanti L, Benyamin RM, Falco FJ, Kaye AD, Hirsch JA. Do epidural injections provide short- and long-term relief for lumbar disc herniation? A systemic review. Clin Orthop Relat Res. 2015;473(6):1940–56.
8. Koc Z, Ozcakir S, Sivrioglu K, Gurbet A, Kucukoglu S. Effectiveness of physical therapy and epidural steroid injections in lumbar spinal stenosis. Spine. 2009;34(10):985–9.
9. Valat JP, Giraudeau B, Rozenberg S, Goupille P, Bourgeois P, Micheau-Beaugendre V, et al. Epidural corticosteroid injections for sciatica: a randomized, double blind controlled clinical trial. Ann Rheum Dis. 2003;7:639–43.

Should a Trial of Epidural Steroid Injections Be Done Before Considering Spine Surgery? 101

Lori Russo

Case

Thanksgiving dinner each year consists of a house full of family members picking on cheese and crackers while anxiously awaiting the good news: The turkey is done cooking! Every year my Uncle Ricky would move briskly to his chair at the head of the dinner table and promptly reach for the serving fork to assure that he had first access to the best looking pieces of turkey. This year, however, was different. Uncle Ricky didn't get there first. I questioned him regarding his slow pace over to the feast.

He replied, "Oh you know, I'm getting old, everything hurts, mostly my back, and things just don't work the way they used to. I had an MRI done, which showed a bulging disc in my lumbar spine".

As a curious anesthesiologist, I then questioned him about his plans to rectify the situation. He informed me that his doctor had recommended a trial of epidural steroid injections (ESIs). Uncle Ricky had never been the type to speak much of his health conditions but he figured now that it was public information, he would go ahead and ask several questions. I stopped him from saying more as I recalled a discussion between 2 colleagues of mine: a pain management physician and a neurosurgeon. It seemed that the utility of epidural steroid injections has been a topic of hot debate. I asked my Uncle Ricky to write his questions down on a piece of paper and the next day I contacted my 2 colleagues. I requested that they review the literature on epidural steroid injections and to meet with me the following week to discuss my Uncle's questions.

Question #1 from Uncle Ricky

Is this a normal part of aging? Is it normal to feel like this?

L. Russo (✉)
Department of Anesthesiology, NYU Langone Medical Center, New York, NY 10016, USA
e-mail: Lori.Russo.Umdnj@gmail.com

Pain Management Physician: While chronic pain is typically not normal per se, unfortunately, it seems to be an epidemic. As per the Medical Expenditure Survey, approximately 100 million Americans are suffering from chronic pain. It is believed that the prevalence of chronic pain lies between 2 and 40 % and the median is 15 % [1].

Neurosurgeon: I agree that it's become an epidemic. However, let's not focus on just the prevalence but how it is affecting our country. This is a matter of lost quality of life, lost productivity from disability, and the effects that it has on health care dollars is monumental. As per Gaskin et al., productivity lost to chronic pain in 2010 was estimated to fall between 299 and 335 billion dollars, which is more than that of diabetes, cancer, or heart disease. The study also showed that the average health care expenditure of a patient without pain was $4475 while the expenditure for a patient with moderate pain was approximately $4500 higher. In the severe pain population, the expenditure was approximately $3200 higher than the moderate group [1].

Question #2 from Uncle Ricky

Are these epidural injections safe? What side effects and risk do they have?

Pain Management Physician: In a retrospective study by McGrath et al., 4265 injections from a 7-year period were assessed and of those there were zero "major" complications. Worsened pain, pain at the site of epidural injection, and numbness were the most frequent complications and, in my opinion, these are relatively minor issues and usually temporary. Epidural steroid injections are safe and I'm glad that your Uncle Ricky's physician recommended them! [2].

Neurosurgeon: ESIs are not entirely without risk. Both major and minor complications have been noted in the literature. For example, let's dig into the ASA Closed Claims

C.S. Scher et al. (eds.), *You're Wrong, I'm Right*, DOI 10.1007/978-3-319-43169-7_101

Project, which includes the review of cases from 1970 through 1999. Forty percent of claims related to management of chronic pain were related to ESIs. The most common complaints were related to injury to nerves, headache, and infection. There are 6 cases of paraplegia, 1 case of quadriplegia, 12 cases of meningitis, 7 cases of abscess in the epidural space, 3 cases of osteomyelitis, and 9 cases of death/brain damage all from epidural steroid injections. These are devastating complications and it's not correct to say that these are entirely safe procedures [3].

Question

At this point, I jumped in as I had a question of my own for my colleagues:

Nerve roots can become inflamed when injured disks or narrowing of foramen occur leading to radicular pain. For this reason, steroid injections near the site of inflammation have been helpful in controlling the inflammation. Historically, the popular belief has been superiority of TFESI (transforaminal epidural steroid injections) over ILESI (interlaminar epidural steroid injections) as the transforminal approach allows for more anterior spread of the injectate. In fact, because of this hypothesis, the Center for Medicare and Medicaid Services has reported an increase in TFESI by 20.4 % per year while only 2 % for ILESI [4]. What is your take on it?

Pain Management Physician: In 2006, Schaufele et al. published an analysis of patients receiving TFESI vs. ILESI and their pain control immediately after the injection and 2–3 weeks out (follow-up) by using the verbal numerical rating scale (VNRS) (0–10) pain scale [5]. Pre-injection pain scores were 5.9 for the TFESI group and 7.3 for the ILESI. For the TFESI group, immediately after injection pain reduced to 2.9 and at follow-up was at 3.2. For the ILESI group, immediately after injection pain was reduced to 3.1; however, at follow-up it was 5.9. Therefore, the mean change from pre-injection to follow-up was 2.7 for the TFESI while it was only 1.4 for the ILESI group. Only 10 % of the TFESI from this study went on to require surgery while 25 % went on to require it in the ILESI group [5]. The literature supports the long-standing hypothesis that the transforaminal approach is superior to the interlaminar approach.

Neurosurgeon: In a literature search by Chang-Chien, the primary outcome of relief of pain after TFESI vs. ILESI was studied as well as a secondary outcome of improvement of functional status [4]. Ultimately, they found that TFESI had improved control of pain at 2-week follow-up when compared to ILESI. However, they failed to show improvement at 1 or 6 months. The literature search showed that patients that had undergone ILESI had greater improvement in functionality than the TFESI. Additionally, Chang Chien feels that the risks associated with the transforaminal approach are considerably more devastating than the interlaminar approach. This includes intravascular injections, which can ultimately lead to paralysis from infarction of the spinal cord. Additionally, the transforminal approach does not decrease the likelihood of the known complications that can occur with ILESI including puncture dural/subdural puncture, cauda equina, or spinal cord hematoma. In my opinion, epidural steroid injections are a poor choice for chronic back pain management regardless of the approach! [4].

Question #3 from Uncle Ricky

These steroid injections should save me from having to have surgery?

Pain Management Physician: Yes! That's why we do them. Riew et al. performed the only prospective, randomized, controlled, double-blinded study that addresses whether ESI prevent progression to surgery. While surgery may be curative in some cases, it does carry risk of morbidity and mortality that I believe is higher than ESI. Additionally, it is costly and can likely be avoided by the less invasive ESI. Riew's study compares bupivacaine epidural injection versus bupivacaine with steroid injection. Of the patients that received only bupivacaine, approximately 67 % went on to require surgery, while of the patients who received the steroid in their epidural injection approximately 29 % went on to require surgery. I believe this literature proves that ESIs are the way to go! [6].

Neurosurgeon: I recall that study. They only had 55 patients. That's hardly enough to show significance! Bicket et al. put together a lovely, compact meta-analysis and systematic review of randomized controlled trials. The primary outcome was avoiding surgery. The literature here shows that there may be a slight decrease in need for surgery in the ESI population but only when considering the short term, which they have defined as less than 12 months. Long term, or greater than 12 months, however, there appears to be no significant difference between the rate of progression to surgery between the ESI and control groups. It sounds like your Uncle Ricky shouldn't wait around and hope that these silly injections work. He needs surgery and I know just the guy! [7].

Summary

After listening to the compelling arguments from both of my colleagues, I promptly head over to my Uncle Ricky's to discuss the meeting. He asks one final question, "What do you think I should do?"

Feeling as though this is the million dollar question, I responded to my uncle that while I am considerably more knowledgeable on the subject after the meeting, it remains controversial. It seems that ESI may be more cost-effective and less invasive than surgery. However, exposing a patient to these risks would be a tough decision as it is unclear if they prevent the need for more invasive measures such as surgery in the long run.

References

1. Gaskin DJ, Richard P. The economic costs of pain in the United States. J Pain. 2012;13(8):715–24.
2. McGrath JM, Schaefer MP, Malkamaki DM. Incidence and characteristics of complications from epidural steroid injections. Pain Med. 2011;12(5):726–31.
3. Fitzgibbon DR, Posner KL, Domino KB, Caplan RA, Lee LA, Cheney FW, American Society of Anesthesiologists. Chronic pain management American Society of Anesthesiologists Closed Claims Project. Anesthesiology 2004;100(1):98–105.
4. Chang-Chien GC, Knezevic NN, McCormick Z, Chu SK, Trescot AM, Candido KD. Transforaminal versus interlaminar approaches to epidural steroid injections: a systematic review of comparative studies for lumbosacral radicular pain. Pain Physician. 2014;17(4):E509–24.
5. Schaufele MK, Hatch L, Jones W. Interlaminar versus transforaminal epidural injections for the treatment of symptomatic lumbar intervertebral disc herniations. Pain Physician. 2006;9(4):361–6.
6. Riew KD, Yin Y, Gilula L, Bridwell KH, Lenke LG, Lauryssen C, Goette K. The effect of nerve-root injections on the need for operative treatment of lumbar radicular pain. A prospective, randomized, controlled, double-blind study. J Bone Joint Surg Am. 2000;82-A(11):1589–93.
7. Bicket MC, Horowitz JM, Benzon HT, Cohen SP. Epidural injections in prevention of surgery for spinal pain: systematic review and meta-analysis of randomized controlled trials. Spine J. 2015;15 (2):348–62.

Epidural Steroid Injection for Unilateral Radicular Pain: Is the Transforaminal Approach Superior to Interlaminar Injection?

102

Lucia Daiana Voiculescu, Tomas J. Kucera, and Angela Zangara

Case

A 35-year-old male patient with new onset left buttock pain radiating to the left lower extremity comes for evaluation and treatment. The pain started 4 weeks ago when the patient was walking his dog and slipped on ice. His pain was not severe at first; he was able to get up and walk home with only mild soreness in the left lower back. Over the next few days, however, the symptoms became increasingly severe, limiting his daily activities. The pain began radiating down the left lateral aspect of the leg to the top of the foot with associated burning and numbness. The patient presented to his local hospital emergency department and was given a prescription for ibuprofen, 600 mg every 6 h as needed, and cyclobenzaprine, 10 mg 3 times daily.

A lumbar magnetic resonance imaging (MRI) scan demonstrates the following: disc extrusion at the L4/L5 level in the left paracentral region, producing stenosis of the left lateral recess, impinging the downgoing left L5 nerve root. The disc material migrates inferiorly by about 3 mm. No evidence for neural foraminal narrowing was observed. Facet joints are preserved with no apparent arthropathy.

On physical examination, the patient is in significant discomfort, ambulating with difficulty, grimacing, and changing position frequently. A straight leg test is positive on the left side. There is no allodynia, and no sensory or motor deficit. Reflexes are normal.

L.D. Voiculescu (✉) · A. Zangara
Department of Anesthesiology, Perioperative Care and Pain Medicine, New York University School of Medicine, 550 First Avenue, New York, NY 10016, USA
e-mail: lucia.voiculescu@nyumc.org

A. Zangara
e-mail: angelamzangara@gmail.com

T.J. Kucera
Attending Physician, Advanced Pain Management, 4131 West Loomis Road #300 Greenfield, Madison, WI 53221, USA
e-mail: tomasjkucera@gmail.com

C.S. Scher et al. (eds.), *You're Wrong, I'm Right*, DOI 10.1007/978-3-319-43169-7_102

The patient states he is interested in epidural steroid injection (ESI) for pain management because a friend who fell skiing had one and it really helped his pain. The attending agrees that epidural steroid injection would be beneficial at this point and recommends a two-level transforaminal approach, left L4 and L5, as being more effective for the patient's unilateral radicular symptoms. The fellow, however, having recently attended a workshop where the efficacy and safety of the transforaminal approach was discussed, poses the following question:

Question

Epidural steroid injection for unilateral radicular pain: Is the transforaminal approach superior to interlaminar injection?

FELLOW: I am very concerned about the rare but devastating complications potentially associated with transforaminal steroid injection. The presence of the radicular artery in proximity to the nerve root in the neural foramen makes it vulnerable to unintentional needle penetration.

Events such as cord infarction followed by paralysis, permanent neurologic deficit, and even death can result from embolization of inadvertently injected steroid particles or from direct vascular injury, arterial spasm, or thrombosis [1, 2].

There are multiple case reports of transforaminal epidural steroid injections, mainly in the cervical region, that resulted in devastating neurologic complications including stroke, paralysis, and death. Cases have been reported in the lumbar region as well; however, at this level, they are very rare [2–7]. However, it is known that there is a high incidence of intravascular (arterial and venous) needle placement during lumbosacral transforaminal procedures [1, 8].

The transforaminal steroid injection is performed very close to the nerve root and the spinal segmental artery, increasing the risk for intra-arterial injection or needle-induced vascular or radicular injury. The artery of Adamkiewicz (arteria radicularis magna) originates at variable levels, in 85 % of the cases entering the spinal canal on the left side, between T9 and L2. An abnormally low-lying artery of Adamkiewicz (even as low as S1) has been documented, thus increasing the risk for associated complications at this level [4].

Avoiding proximity to these structures, the interlaminar approach reduces the risk of neurologic damage due to arterial injury or embolization and subsequent cord infarction.

ATTENDING: These are isolated, very rare events described only in case reports and reviews of malpractice claims [9]. The exact incidence is unknown. So far, only 16 thoracolumbar spinal cord infarctions have been reported following lumbosacral transforaminal epidural steroid injections [10]. Millions of epidural injections are performed annually. Between 2000 and 2011, the number of these increased 130 % in Medicare patients, with the highest increase (665 %) being recorded for lumbosacral transforaminal epidural injections [11, 12].

Transforaminal injections are safely performed under digital subtraction angiography (DSA) with contrast [6, 8]. A non-particulate steroid formula [9] and/or alternative approaches to the traditional technique for transforaminal injection [1] can be used to further decrease the risk of complications.

FELLOW: According to Chang-Chien et al. [13], who published a systemic review of studies comparing transforaminal to the interlaminar technique, there is no statistically significant difference in pain or functional improvement between the 2 approaches. While there are a few studies that report that the transforaminal approach may produce better results [14–16], no study has proven that the transforaminal is better than an interlaminar approach.

ATTENDING: Yes, this is true. Unfortunately, these studies suffer from a low number of subjects and low power. However, it is also worth noting that none of the recent studies show that transforaminal injections are less effective. Some studies have suggested the superiority of the transforaminal approach in reducing radicular pain over both short and long terms [14–16].

A prospective, randomized, blinded study by Gharibo et al., comparing the clinical effectiveness of interlaminar and transforaminal epidural steroid injection in subacute low back pain with radiculopathy, concluded that "patients may experience greater subjective relief, at least initially, from transforaminal epidural steroid injections over interlaminar" [15].

I believe that given the degree of acuity and intensity of his pain, this patient would benefit from a transforaminal injection targeting the specific level of pathology in the anterior epidural space and in close proximity to the dorsal root ganglion. While there is a paucity of data to support this, from clinical experience, I believe this is the best approach for him.

FELLOW: The interlaminar approach is typically faster and thus will expose you and the patient to less radiation. According to Manchikanti et al. [17], exposure to radiation is ~ 3 times as much with the transforaminal approach. A multitude of biological effects, both stochastic and deterministic, has been described as a result of radiation exposure. While the occasional exposure to low-dose medical radiation does not produce significant effects on patients, interventional pain physicians and operating room personnel are subject to its cumulative effects [18].

ATTENDING: Yes, this is true. But the overall exposure to radiation is minimal, less than that of an average two-view chest X-ray [17]. A skilled practitioner, abiding by safety radiation protocols, is able to perform a transforaminal epidural injection with minimal exposure, making it as safe as an interlaminar epidural [17, 18].

Summary

Despite a continuous and significant increase in the number of epidural steroid injections performed for radicular symptoms associated with disc pathology [11], there is no consensus regarding the compared efficacy and safety of the two most frequently used approaches. Interlaminar injections have the advantage of being fast, well tolerated, and associated with less potential for cord infarction. Transforaminal injections can be performed safely as well by experienced practitioners. There is no evidence that this approach is less effective than the interlaminar approach. The transforaminal approach targets the nerve root at the level and laterality of the pathology, which may contribute to better short-term analgesia, as demonstrated by multiple studies [15, 16]. As with many aspects of medicine, the final decision on treatment of a patient relies on a careful and complex evaluation that is unique to each patient's symptoms and pathology.

A practitioner's training, expertise, and knowledge of the risks and benefits associated with the two techniques should guide his or her decisions.

References

1. Atluri S, Glaser SE, Shah RV, Sudarshan G. Needle position analysis in cases of paralysis from transforaminal epidurals: consider alternative approaches to traditional technique. Pain Phys. 2013;16:321–34.
2. Lyders EM, Morris PP. A case of spinal cord infarction following lumbar transforaminal epidural steroid injection: MR imaging and angiographic findings. Am J Neuroradiol. 2009;30:1691–3.
3. Glaser SE, Falco F. Paraplegia following a thoracolumbar transforaminal epidural steroid injection. Pain Phys. 2005;8:309–14.
4. Houten JK, Errico TJ. Paraplegia after lumbosacral nerve root block: report of three cases. Spine J. 2002;2:70–5.
5. Kennedy DJ, Dreyfuss P, Aprill CN, Bogduk N. Paraplegia following image-guided transforaminal lumbar spine epidural steroid injection: two case reports. Pain Med. 2009;10:1389–94.
6. Patil M, Huntoon M. Interlaminar and transforaminal therapeutic epidural injections. In: Benzon H, Rathmell JP, Wu CL, Turk DC, Argoff CE, Hurley RW, editors. Practical management of pain. 5th ed. Philadelphia, PA: Elsevier Mosby; 2014. p. 805–15.
7. Somayaji HS, Saifuddin A, Casey AT, Briggs TW. Spinal cord infarction following therapeutic computed tomography-guided left L2 nerve root injection. Spine. 2005;30:E106–8.
8. Furman O'Brien EM, Zgleszewski TM. Incidence of intravascular penetration in transforaminal lumbosacral epidural steroid injections. Spine. 2000;25:2628–32.
9. Department of Health and Human Services: Centers for Medicare and Medicaid Services. https://www.cms.gov/Outreach-and-Education/Medicare-Learning-Network-MLN/MLNMattersArticles/downloads/SE1102.pdf. Accessed 6 April 2015.
10. Manchikanti L, Pampati V, Falco FJE, Hirsch JA. Assessment of the growth of epidural injections in the Medicare population from 2000 to 2011. Pain Phys. 2013;16:E349–64.
11. Dietrich T, Sutter R, Frolich J, Pfirrmann C. Particulate versus non-particulate steroids for lumbar transforaminal or interlaminar epidural steroid injections: an update. Skeletal Radiol. 2015;44:149–55.
12. Chang-Chien GC, Knezevic NN, McCormick Z, Chu SK, Trescot AM, Candido KD. Transforaminal versus interlaminar approaches to epidural steroid injections: a systematic review of comparative studies for lumbosacral radicular pain. Pain Phys. 2014;17:E509–24.
13. Rathmell JP, Benzon HT, Dreyfuss P, Huntoon M, Wallace M, Baker R, et al. Safeguards to prevent neurologic complications after epidural steroid injections. Consensus opinions from a multidisciplinary working group and national organizations. Anesthesiology. 2015;122:974–84.
14. Ackerman WE 3rd, Ahmad M. The efficacy of lumbar epidural steroid injections in patients with lumbar disc herniations. Anesth Analg. 2007;104:1217–22.
15. Gharibo CG, Varlotta GP, Rhame EE, Liu EC, Bendo JA, Perloff MD. Interlaminar versus transforaminal epidural steroids for the treatment of subacute lumbar radicular pain: a randomized, blinded, prospective outcome study. Pain Phys. 2011;14:499–511.
16. Schaufele MK, Hatch L, Jones W. Interlaminar versus transforaminal epidural injections for the treatment of symptomatic lumbar intervertebral disc herniations. Pain Phys. 2006;9:361–6.
17. Manchikanti L, Cash KA, Moss TL, Pampati V. Radiation exposure to the physician in interventional pain management. Pain Phys. 2002;4:385–93.
18. Zhou Y, Singh N, Abdi S, Wu J, Crawford J, Furgang FA. Fluoroscopy radiation safety for spine interventional pain procedures in university teaching hospitals. Pain Phys. 2005;8:49–53.

103 Is a Tricyclic Antidepressant the Best First-Line Agent in Treating Neuropathic Pain?

Dalia H. Elmofty

Case

A 72-year-old man with a 7-year history of type 2 diabetes presented with persistent burning pain in his lower and upper extremities that made daily activities challenging. He admitted that he had not felt as well as usual and that walking was becoming more difficult. His family also noted that he seemed to be stumbling more frequently. His primary care physician referred him to the pain clinic for treatment of diabetic peripheral neuropathy.

He is obese [body mass index (BMI) 33 kg/m^2] with a blood pressure of 138/85 mm Hg and a resting pulse of 80 beats/minute. An examination of the lower extremities shows normal skin pigmentation, hyperesthesia of the feet, easily palpable dorsalis pedis pulses, but decreased position sense and sensation to monofilament testing. He states that his glycemic control has never been optimal despite multiple insulin dose adjustments. Hemoglobin A_{1C} levels have typically been in the 8–9 % range for the past year. He takes gabapentin 100 mg three times daily, for neuropathic pain with minimal relief, and recently, his primary care physician added amitriptyline 50 mg to improve pain control. You recommend that the patient be sent for diabetes education and be given a diet and exercise program to help him lose weight and normalize his blood glucose levels. You also recommend discontinuing amitriptyline because of the adverse effects of tricyclic antidepressants (TCAs) in older patients. You suggest gradually increasing the dose of gabapentin and trying topical agents such as capsaicin cream or a lidocaine 5 % patch.

D.H. Elmofty (✉)
Department of Anesthesia and Critical Care, University of Chicago, 5841 S. Maryland Ave, Chicago, IL 60637, USA
e-mail: delmofty@dacc.uchicago.edu

Question

Should TCAs be administered for the management of neuropathic pain in older patients?

PRO: In the Western world, diabetes is the leading cause of peripheral neuropathy. Most of the diabetic population has some form of neuropathy, ranging from barely detectable to a severe, disabling, and painful disease, which can be distressing and difficult to treat. Neuropathic pain is defined by the International Association for the Study of Pain as pain "caused by a lesion of the somatosensory nervous system." Neuropathic pain has a negative impact on mental and physical health as well as the quality of life. I agree that we must take better measures to prevent neuropathic pain from developing. The Diabetes Control and Complication Trial and epidemiologic studies suggest that controlling blood sugar can prevent diabetic peripheral neuropathy. A diet and exercise program is a good idea to help the patient lose weight and improve glycemic control. But I disagree with discontinuing amitriptyline. TCAs were initially introduced in the 1950s as antipsychotics but have been found to be effective in numerous randomized, blinded, placebo-controlled trials for the treatment of neuropathic pain [1]. The exact mechanism of action of the analgesic effect is still unclear. TCAs inhibit reuptake of norepinephrine and serotonin and enhance descending antinociception in the central nervous system. They are also antagonistic at the N-methyl-D-aspartate receptor and may block sodium channels. These pharmacological properties make TCAs beneficial in the treatment of neuropathic pain.

CON: TCAs can help in treating neuropathic pain such as diabetic peripheral neuropathy in certain patient populations. Amitriptyline is a tertiary amine. These agents tend to cause considerable side effects in the elderly. The major effects are anticholinergic (altered mental status, dry mouth, and mydriasis); they also act on the central nervous system (myoclonus, syncope), heart (tachycardia, orthostatic hypotension), and gastrointestinal system (decreased bowel

C.S. Scher et al. (eds.), *You're Wrong, I'm Right*, DOI 10.1007/978-3-319-43169-7_103

motility). Caution is necessary when TCAs are prescribed for the elderly or patients with cardiovascular comorbidities. An electrocardiogram is recommended before initiating therapy for any patient older than 40 years. TCAs can be dangerous in older patients if they provoke or exacerbate cognitive impairment or disturb gait and increase the risk of falling. Maybe we can consider nortriptyline or desipramine, secondary amines that have less dangerous side effects. But keep in mind that the secondary amines can cause irritability and disturbed sleep.

PRO: Should we consider starting at a lower dose and gradually titrating upwards? I can schedule the patient for frequent follow-up visits to assess therapeutic effect and monitor for adverse reactions. TCAs have been recommended for the treatment of neuropathic pain. Several medical groups (the Neuropathic Pain Special Interest Group of the International Association for the Study of Pain, the Canadian Pain Society, and the European Federation of Neurological Societies) have published evidence-based clinical guidelines for the pharmacological treatment of neuropathic pain, which include TCAs as a first-line treatment option [2–4].

CON: Treatment of neuropathic pain in the elderly poses several challenges. Most of the current guidelines for the management of neuropathic pain were developed based on evidence generated from younger cohorts. The use of evidence-based medicine in combination with individualizing treatment options is recommended. "One size does not fit all" especially when it comes to TCAs and elderly patients. Aging is associated with a host of changes that affect drug metabolism, along with physiological alterations to the liver, kidneys, blood, and fat. Clinicians must be aware of potential drug–drug interactions and the central nervous system side effects associated with TCAs. Adverse drug reactions are a major public health problem in elderly patients, resulting in hospital admissions and additional health care costs.

The American Geriatric Society recommends against prescribing TCAs to patients older than 60 years because of the side effect burden. The pharmacological management of neuropathic pain in older patients has been described [5]. Gabapentinoids may be better suited to older patients because of fewer drug–drug interactions. Other agents such as capsaicin cream and lidocaine 5 % have minimal systemic side effects or drug–drug interactions and are a good option for elderly patients.

Summary

The management of neuropathic pain in the elderly is challenging for physicians because of the physiological changes and associated comorbidities in many patients. Understanding the pharmacology and patient-specific factors and monitoring for adverse effects can help to optimize outcomes. Age-targeted trials to develop clinical guidelines are needed to facilitate safe and effective pain control in this population.

References

1. Saarto T, Wiffen PJ. Antidepressants for neuropathic pain. Cochrane Database of Systematic Reviews 2007, Issue 4. Art. No.: CD005454. doi: 10.1002/14651858.CD005454.pub2.
2. Dworkin RH, O'Connor AB, Backonja M, Farrar JT, Finnerup NB, Jensen TS, et al. Pharmacologic management of neuropathic pain: evidence-based recommendations. Pain. 2007;132:237–51.
3. Moulin DE, Clark AJ, Gilron I, Ware MA, Watson CP, Sessle BJ, Canadian Pain Society, et al. Pharmacological management of chronic neuropathic pain—consensus statement and guidelines from the Canadian Pain Society. Pain Res Manag. 2007;12(1):13–21.
4. Attal N, Cruccu G, Baron R, Haanpää M, Hansson P, Jensen TS, European Federation of Neurological Societies, et al. EFNS guidelines on the pharmacological treatment of neuropathic pain: 2010 revision. Eur J Neurol. 2010;17(9):1113–23.
5. McGenney BE. Pharmacological management of neuropathic pain in older adults: an update on peripheral and central acting agents. J Pain Symptom Manag. 2009;38(2 Suppl):S15–27.

What are the Risks and Benefits of Spinal Cord Stimulators and Intrathecal Pumps? 104

Magdalena Anitescu and Nirali Shah-Doshi

Case

A 56-year-old male is evaluated during a scheduled follow-up appointment in the pain clinic for back and radicular pain that persists after an L3-5 laminectomy 2 years ago. His analgesic regimen is oxycodone controlled release, 60 mg BID (twice a day), with oxycodone immediate release, 15 mg TID (3 times a day), as needed, along with gabapentin, amitriptyline, and lidocaine patches. The patient is not satisfied with this regimen, because his pain prevents him from returning to work. He asks to have the dose of controlled release oxycodone increased because its efficacy has decreased over time. Lumbar epidural steroid injections and medial branch nerve blocks have not helped. Physical therapy offers only minimal pain relief. The patient consults with a psychiatrist for mild depression. After a recent consultation, he was offered a revision procedure by an orthopedic spine surgeon, but the patient is reluctant to accept, given the poor outcome from the first surgical intervention. The resident evaluating the patient is unsure of the next step: increase opioids? Repeat surgery? Other treatment options?

Question

Should this patient be considered for an implantable device?

PRO: Because other interventions have had limited results, an implantable device trial should be the next step. Increasing opioid dosage will not give him lasting pain relief but will increase side effects. Failed back surgery syndrome (FBSS) is the most common indication for either a spinal cord stimulator (SCS) or an intrathecal drug delivery system (IDDS). Because the success rate decreases with every subsequent back surgery, reoperation should be avoided. Conservative treatment with medication, physical therapy, and epidural steroid injections has failed, a clear indication that a trial with an implantable device, either SCS or intrathecal pump, is appropriate.

CON: I am not completely sold on the idea of implantable devices. Studies that compare patients with SCS to those who have had reoperation show that fewer narcotics are required for pain relief, but there is no change in functional status, work status, or activities of daily living.

PRO: Even if functional status is not affected, pain scores are significantly lower in patients with implantable devices for post-laminectomy syndromes. Outcomes were better with SCS placement than after reoperation in a small cohort of 50 patients followed up to 3 years after the intervention [1]. Of SCS patients, 9 of 19 compared to 3 out of 26 patients with reoperation had more than 50 % pain relief. There was less of a crossover rate to the other treatment from the SCS group compared to the reoperation group (5 of 24 vs. 14 of 26).

CON: In general, FBSS has been the main indication for placement of an SCS, but careful patient selection is the only measure that ensures success. SCS is more effective for radicular pain than musculoskeletal or discogenic back pain. This patient also shows signs of depression, and psychiatric disease decreases the efficacy of SCS. Patients with little relief from an SCS trial (less than 50 % pain reduction) have higher scores on the Minnesota Multiphasic Personality Inventory (MMPI) Depression and Mania subscales. Those with successful trials have better scores and higher energy levels.

PRO: The presence of back pain should not limit the use of implantable devices. Although SCS may be better to treat the

M. Anitescu (✉)
Department of Anesthesia and Critical Care, University of Chicago Medicine, 4851 S. Maryland Ave, MC 4028, Chicago, IL 60637, USA
e-mail: Manitescu@dacc.uchicago.edu

N. Shah-Doshi
Department of Anesthesia and Critical Care, The University of Chicago Medical Center, 5840 S. Maryland Ave, MC4028, Chicago, IL 60637, USA

C.S. Scher et al. (eds.), *You're Wrong, I'm Right*, DOI 10.1007/978-3-319-43169-7_104

neuropathic pain of radiculopathy, an intrathecal drug delivery system may be a good option for nociceptive back pain. Depression levels can improve remarkably with pain relief following SCS implantation. A thorough psychiatric evaluation is still indicated, but it should be considered as part of a comprehensive evaluation of a candidate for SCS implantation.

CON: I agree that a complete evaluation is needed before proceeding with a trial for either SCS or IDDS for non-cancer pain. However, there are risks with a device beyond conservative management or reoperation. A systemic review of SCS revealed an average overall adverse event rate of 36 % [2]. The most frequent complications were lead migration or breakage, comprising 22 % of complications. The infection rate was 3–4 %, unwanted stimulation was 2 %, and pain at the site was 8 %. There is also the potential for neurologic injury after implantation of leads in the epidural space [2].

Not only are there risks from the procedure and the device, but the patient also is signing on for future surgeries to replace batteries if the SCS fails or if a non-rechargeable internal pulse generator is chosen. The patient is excluded from evaluation with magnetic resonance imaging (MRI). Given these risks, I wonder if a surgical revision before an SCS trial may avoid some of the potential complications.

PRO: Many manufacturers have been working on equipment designs to reduce adverse events from implantable systems. New pliable leads decrease migration and limit breakage. With MRI safe technology at 1.5T, diagnostic images are possible with an implantable device in place. When infections occur, the system is removed and the infection is treated with antibiotics. Neurologic injuries associated with lead implantation are rare. They may be prevented with imaging studies to identify correctable spine pathology before lead placement. Patients also fare better if the SCS is implanted within 2 years of pain onset; the success rate in this group can be up to 85 % compared with only 9 % SCS effectiveness in pain reduction if the pain is long-standing (15 years or more) [3].

CON: We have not touched upon narcotic requirement. Given the patient's high doses and the combination of nociceptive and neuropathic pain, maybe we should discuss other management options. Larger doses of oxycodone have failed to provide adequate pain relief. Does this patient have side effects from narcotics? One option before implanting a device is opioid rotation or even an opioid holiday. This strategy may decrease his pain to a tolerable level, preventing the need for repeat surgery or device implantation.

PRO: The patient's opioid requirement is indeed concerning. However, an IDDS would likely solve the problem since it will minimize opioid side effects by acting on the primary site of analgesia, opioid receptors in the substantia gelatinosa.

An opioid holiday would also be of benefit in this case. Patients who were weaned off oral opioids weeks before intrathecal therapy experienced better results. Even weaning off half the opioids before intrathecal trial followed by complete discontinuation before a permanent implant has shown benefit.

CON: It is unclear whether discontinuing opioids and starting at a low intrathecal dose would have lasting benefits on the side effects. Patients with permanent IDDS also use oral opioids. At 6 months, compared to baseline, 65 % of the patients in one study had decreased or discontinued systemic opioids, but at 12 months, the percentage was only 43 %, meaning that almost half of the patients still took oral opioids despite the implantable device [4]. Most likely, if patients do not restart systemic opioids, they will need greater intrathecal doses. There is an average 2.6-fold to 7.4-fold increase from the initial dose at 24 months [4]. These data suggest that IDDSs decline in efficacy as time progresses. With SCS or IDDS, there is no significant increase in the number of patients returning to work.

Like SCS, implants can result in complications from the procedure and the device itself. Potential complications of an IDDS are urinary retention requiring catheterization, pain at the injection site, and postural (spinal) headache. With a permanent IDDS, complications include wound infection, meningitis, pump malposition, nausea/vomiting, urinary retention, and pruritus. There are also catheter-related complications, such as migration and granuloma formation. Battery revision is needed usually every 4–7 years. Several deaths have been reported from massive intrathecal morphine overdoses mistakenly injected into an access port connected directly to the cerebrospinal fluid. During frequent pump refills (every 2–3 months), subcutaneous morphine injection also is possible. The physiologic side effects of intrathecal opioids include hypogonadism, amenorrhea, decreased libido, and erectile dysfunction [5].

Summary

Implantable devices are useful therapeutic options for the right medical indication. Careful patient selection is essential in ensuring the success of these devices, whether SCS or IDDS such as pumps. SCS may be more effective in residual radicular neuropathic pain, and the IDDS, in nociceptive pain. Since these devices are considered "permanent," every patient considered for an implantable device should undergo a comprehensive evaluation: detailed medical history, physical examination, imaging studies, and psychiatric testing. Pain reduction of greater than 50 % is considered a successful trial for both devices. Implantation of either an SCS or IDDS carries risks of complications; therefore, patients should be well informed before making a commitment to the therapy.

References

1. North RB, Kumar K, Wallace MS, Henderson JM, Shipley J, Hernandez J, et al. Spinal cord stimulation versus re-operation in patients with failed back surgery syndrome: an international multicenter randomized controlled trial (EVIDENCE study). Neuromodulation. 2011;14(4):330–5 (discussion 335–6).
2. Veizi E, Hayek S. Interventional therapies for chronic low back pain. Neuromodulation. 2014;17:31–45.
3. Kumar K, Taylor RS, Jacques L, Eldabe S, Meglio M, Molet J, et al. Spinal cord stimulation versus conventional medical management for neuropathic pain: a multicentre randomised controlled trial in patients with failed back surgery syndrome. Pain. 2007;132(1–2):179–88.
4. Wilkes D. Programmable intrathecal pumps for the management of chronic pain: recommendations for improved efficiency. J Pain Res. 2014;7:571–7.
5. Turner J, Sears J, Loeser J. Programmable intrathecal opioid delivery systems for chronic noncancer pain: a systemic review of effectiveness and complications. Clin J Pain. 2007;23:180–95.

How Do You Determine If a Patient has Opioid-Induced Hyperalgesia?

105

Dalia H. Elmofty

Case

A 40-year-old Caucasian female with metastatic rectal cancer underwent an abdominoperineal resection with posterior vaginectomy and flap reconstruction. She had undergone several rounds of chemotherapy and radiation before the procedure. The patient complains of severe, constant, rectal pain, worse with bowel movements and sitting. She is taking morphine sulfate extended release 200 mg twice daily. Because of sudden, severe onset of pelvic pain and right foot drop, she has been hospitalized. Computed tomographic scan revealed extensive spread of cancer in the abdominal and pelvic cavity with tumor compressing the lumbosacral plexus. Surgery, chemotherapy, and radiation were no longer options. Efforts to control her pain with escalating doses of oral and intravenous opioids were unsuccessful. Because of this lack of efficacy, a decision was made to begin a trial of intrathecal infusion with morphine, which was titrated over several days without pain relief. Additional oral and intravenous hydromorphone was administered for breakthrough pain. Over the next 24 h, her pain continued to escalate. At this point, she was receiving 30 mg per day of intrathecal morphine. Her pain and suffering were extreme. She complained of whole body pain, accompanied by episodes of agitation and confusion. You suspect that the patient may be suffering from opioid-induced hyperalgesia. You recommend reducing the opioid dosage and starting a sub-anesthetic, low-dose ketamine infusion because, as an *N*-methyl-D-aspartate (NMDA) receptor antagonist, it may offset the hyperalgesia. Your hospice/palliative care colleague believes this is a case of opioid-induced tolerance and prefers to continue to escalate the dose of intrathecal morphine. He states that there is insufficient evidence to support the existence of opioid-induced hyperalgesia in humans.

D.H. Elmofty (✉)
Department of Anesthesia and Critical Care, University of Chicago, 5841 S. Maryland Ave, Chicago, IL 60637, USA
e-mail: delmofty@dacc.uchicago.edu

Question

Does opioid-induced hyperalgesia exist or is it a hypothetical phenomenon?

PRO: The history of medicine considers the existence of opioid-induced hyperalgesia. In the 1870s, Sir Thomas Clifford Allbutt, an English physician, questioned the benefits of intravenous morphine for pain control. He said, "Does morphia tend to encourage the very pain it pretends to relieve?" Opioid-induced hyperalgesia has become an area of interest, and more research is being conducted to understand the disorder. In this paradoxical phenomenon, the intensity of pain is increased rather than decreased in response to opioid administration. Hyperalgesia is defined by the International Association for the Study of Pain as increased pain from a normally painful stimulus. Allodynia is pain from a stimulus that does not normally provoke pain. Both hyperalgesia and allodynia indicate a hypersensitized state in patients with opioid-induced hyperalgesia. Studies have shown the existence of hyperalgesia in postoperative pain, cancer pain, chronic nonmalignant pain, and in experiments on healthy subjects [1].

CON: Evidence to support opioid-induced hyperalgesia in humans is insufficient. In the studies of postoperative pain and experiments in healthy subjects, a short-acting opioid was administered, and testing for opioid-induced hyperalgesia was conducted after the opioid was discontinued [1]. The increase in pain could have been from opioid withdrawal or even acute tolerance. There are multiple factors to explain why the patient is experiencing a deterioration in pain control even with escalation of her dose. In general, cancer patients suffer severe and intensifying pain from progression of the disease. Imaging has revealed extensive progression of the patient's cancer. She also has been taking long-acting opioids for several months. She could be developing tolerance and may require larger quantities of drug to achieve an acceptable level of analgesia. Opioid-induced tolerance is a physiological process in which a progressive lack of response to opioids requires an increase

C.S. Scher et al. (eds.), *You're Wrong, I'm Right*, DOI 10.1007/978-3-319-43169-7_105

in dose to produce the same effect. There is a shift to the right of the dose-response curve. During pharmacokinetic changes, up-regulation of the metabolic process is responsible for increased elimination of the drug. Pharmacodynamic changes result in down-regulation of the opioid receptor or desensitization. The opioid receptor is linked to a G-protein, which, when activated, produces a decrease in cyclic adenosine 3', 5'-monophosphate and inhibits Na^+ and Ca^{++} influx. Over time, changes in G-protein function can lead to desensitization and development of opioid tolerance. The increase in pain associated with opioid administration may therefore simply be attributed to reduced efficacy of the opioid because of pharmacological or even genetic effects. We should increase the dose or administer a different opioid.

PRO: Although chronic opioid exposure can lead to opioid-induced tolerance, it also can cause opioid-induced hyperalgesia. Clinical differentiation between them can be challenging. The patient continues to suffer exacerbation of pain, which has now become widespread, despite an increase in the dose of intrathecal morphine. If this were a case of opioid-induced tolerance, her pain should have improved in response to dose escalation and remained localized to its original site. With opioid-induced hyperalgesia, patients experience an increase of pain despite rapid opioid escalation. This paradoxical effect is a state of hypersensitivity that appears as hyperalgesia and allodynia—an abnormal sensation that is quantitatively different from normal pain sensation and differently localized from the site of the original complaint. She clearly has opioid-induced hyperalgesia because her pain is no longer located in the pelvic area, but rather is "whole body pain."

CON: I am not completely convinced. A structured evidence-based review showed that there is insufficient evidence to support the existence of opioid-induced hyperalgesia in humans [2]. The mechanism of opioid-induced hyperalgesia is not even fully understood. And if the mechanism is not fully understood, then how would you justify the treatment?

PRO: You are correct. The exact mechanism of opioid-induced hyperalgesia is unknown, just as are the mechanisms of many other painful disease states. But there is a growing body of evidence from basic science supporting the proposed pathophysiological mechanisms that contribute to opioid-induced hyperalgesia: involvement of the central glutaminergic system, spinal dynorphins, descending facilitation, genetic influence, and enhanced response to nociceptive neurotransmitters [3]. The central excitatory neurotransmitter glutamate activates the NMDA receptor. Prolonged exposure to morphine was shown to cause neurotoxicity by inducing NMDA receptor-mediated cell death in the dorsal horn. Prolonged exposure to μ(mu)-receptor agonists increased levels of spinal dynorphins, which increase the release of excitatory neuropeptides [3]. Activation of descending facilitation from the rostral ventromedial medulla can activate spinal nociceptive processing and increase excitatory neuropeptides [3]. The genetic variability of catechol-O-methyltransferase may also affect central pain processing [3]. Opioid-induced hyperalgesia and opioid tolerance are two distinct phenomena resulting in pain that is difficult to control. The initial response by most practitioners is to escalate the opioid dose. If no response is observed, opioid-induced hyperalgesia should be considered. Pain can be reduced by discontinuing or lowering opioid dosage. Opioid rotation also has been recommended; an agent such as methadone has unique properties that might mitigate opioid-induced hyperalgesia. NMDA receptor antagonists such as ketamine also have been suggested.

Summary

Opioid-induced hyperalgesia may be a cause of non-responsiveness to opioid dose escalation. Evidence to support this clinical phenomenon in humans is still lacking. The few studies that have been published could not be reproduced. This lack of reproducibility may be attributed to the absence of a clear set of clinical criteria for diagnosing opioid-induced hyperalgesia. Diagnostic criteria must thus be specified before clinical trials can be undertaken.

References

1. Eisenberg E, Suzan E, Pud D. Opioid-induced hyperalgesia (OIH): a real clinical problem or just an experimental phenomenon? J Pain Symptom Manag. 2014;49(3):632–5.
2. Fishbain DA, Cole B, Lewis JE, Gao J, Rosomoff RS. Do opioids induce hyperalgesia in humans? An evidence-based structured review. Pain Med. 2009;10(6):829–39.
3. Lee M, Silverman S, Hansen H, Patel V, Manchikanti L. A comprehensive review of opioid-induced hyperalgesia. Pain Physician. 2011;14:145–61.

Can Acute and Chronic Postsurgical Pain Be Decreased with Perioperative Neuropathic Agents?

106

Omar Rashid Qureshi and Sheetal Patil

Case

A 55-year-old nurse presents for a bilateral mastectomy with reconstruction for breast cancer. She failed treatment with chemoradiation and is now here for surgery. After developing chronic tenderness from her radiation therapy, she did some research on PubMed. In her hands is a printout of a recent article from the journal *Pain Medicine* stating that up to 60 % of women will develop chronic pain after a mastectomy [1].

Minimizing acute and chronic postsurgical pain is a challenging task that is the responsibility of both anesthesiologists and surgeons. Your (obviously well-informed) patient asks you, "Can my acute and chronic postsurgical pain be reduced with the perioperative administration of gabapentin?"

You aren't sure, so you approach 2 colleagues, Dr. Hypnos and Dr. Narkos, who are collegially arguing in the hall (a frequent occurrence), both experts in pain management, but whose views frequently differ.

Question

Does gabapentin reduce postoperative opioid consumption?

PRO: Dr. Hypnos jumps up to answer first, "Neural changes that are seen in both neuropathic and postsurgical pain may be prevented by gabapentin administration. Gabapentin binding to the α(alpha)-2 δ(delta) subunit of voltage-gated calcium channels decreases the release of nociceptive neurotransmitters such as glutamate, substance P, and norepinephrine. Anything that helps to cut down on the use of opioids is going to help your patient. As you know, opioids can lead to hypopnea, nausea, vomiting, and constipation, which limits their use. Additionally, opioid-induced hyperalgesia from chronic use has further deterred clinicians from relying too heavily on them. Clearly, opioids are a double-edged sword.

"A study in Istanbul analyzed 60 patients undergoing an abdominal hysterectomy, randomized into 3 groups: placebo, 1200 mg of gabapentin preoperatively, and ketamine intraoperatively as an infusion. The end point was patient-controlled analgesic (PCA) consumption of morphine. The patients who had received preoperative gabapentin used 42 % less morphine than the placebo group and also experienced fewer opioid-related adverse effects such as nausea, vomiting, pruritus, and constipation [2]."

CON: Dr. Narkos retorts, "That study only contained 60 patients [2]. You should not change your practice based on a study with such a small sample size. And those results were refuted when gabapentin was studied in patients undergoing total hip arthroplasty! Clarke et al., in Toronto, analyzed 126 patients randomized to 3 groups in a double-blind study: placebo only, gabapentin preoperatively, or gabapentin postoperatively. Everyone received acetaminophen, celecoxib, and dexamethasone. Patients were given a morphine PCA on the floor. Neither group that received 600 mg gabapentin had a decrease in the consumption of morphine or in pain scores [3].

"Paul et al. asked whether continuing gabapentin postoperatively would reduce opioid consumption. A group of 102 patients undergoing a total hip arthroplasty were randomized to receive a dose of gabapentin 600 mg preoperatively followed by 200 mg 3 times daily for 2 days or a placebo. They found no significant difference in the 72-h morphine consumption in both groups; in fact, they found a higher satisfaction rate in the placebo group [4]! Obviously,

O.R. Qureshi (✉)
Department of Anesthesia and Critical Care, University of Chicago Medical Center, 5841 S. Maryland Ave, MC 4028, Chicago, IL 60637, USA
e-mail: orqureshi@gmail.com

S. Patil
Department of Anesthesia and Pain Management, University of Chicago, 5841 S. Maryland Ave, MC 4028, Chicago, IL 60637, USA
e-mail: spatil@dacc.uchicago.edu

C.S. Scher et al. (eds.), *You're Wrong, I'm Right*, DOI 10.1007/978-3-319-43169-7_106

these are small sample sizes as well. The definitive large study has yet to be done!"

Question

You then ask, "Well, does gabapentin really reduce the incidence of chronic postsurgical pain (CPSP)?"

PRO: Dr Hypnos quickly responds, "Absolutely. When CPSP occurs, it can have a detrimental impact on a patient's entire quality of life. Thus, it is our job to make every effort to prevent CPSP. It is now thought that the same neural mechanisms implicated in neuropathic pain are responsible for the development of chronic postsurgical pain [5]. So gabapentin, which has been repeatedly shown to effectively treat neuropathic pain, has been used to prevent and treat CPSP as well.

"Even a single dose of gabapentin preoperatively can reduce its incidence, as shown in multiple studies! Sen et al., also published in *Pain Medicine*, analyzed the incidence of postsurgical pain at the 1-, 3-, and 6-month marks after an abdominal hysterectomy. They found that a 1200 mg dose of gabapentin prior to surgery led to a significant reduction in chronic postsurgical incision pain [2]. We see CPSP incisional pain patients in clinic all the time. So trust me, prevention is far easier than treating this condition after it occurs. Brogly et al. studied the incidence of CPSP in 50 patients undergoing a total thyroidectomy. Patients who received a single dose of gabapentin were significantly less likely to develop chronic pain issues at 6 months than patients in the placebo group (4 vs. 30 %) [6]!

"In fact, I even recall a study where gabapentin was effective for CPSP in breast surgery patients. Fassoulaki et al. demonstrated that patients who received 1200 mg of gabapentin for 8 days after breast cancer surgery were less likely to develop chronic pain 3 months after surgery (82 vs. 45 %) [7]."

CON: You see Dr. Narkos rolling his eyes. "I am not convinced," he firmly states. "While gabapentin is effective in treating neuropathic pain, its role in chronic postsurgical pain is not well established. Many of the studies validating its use in preventing CPSP are flawed because they combine gabapentin with other analgesic modalities such as nerve blocks or non-steroidal anti-inflammatory agents (NSAIDs). So you cannot just assume it is the gabapentin that helped. And again, that study by Sen et al. had 60 patients. These are hardly large randomized controlled trials we are looking at here! Ucak et al. analyzed the development of CPSP in patients undergoing coronary artery bypass graft surgery with median sternotomy and found no difference in the incidence of chronic pain at the 1- and 3-month marks in patients who received gabapentin [8]. I had a referral the other day for a patient that was on 3 times daily dosing of gabapentin before and after surgery and still developed severe post-sternotomy chronic pain. A similar result was found in another study that analyzed the effect of a single 1200 mg dose of gabapentin on the development of chronic pain in patients undergoing a total hip arthroplasty. The study found no difference in the incidence of chronic post-surgical pain or anxiety and depression scores after the administration of gabapentin [3]."

PRO: Dr. Hypnos responds, "Well I'm not throwing the baby out with the bathwater! Just because gabapentin didn't help for bone pain doesn't mean that it won't work for surgeries involving soft tissue. Although we don't have the science to prove this yet, perhaps slightly different receptors or pathways are involved in these two types of pain."

Question

Does gabapentin administration reduce the incidence of opioid-induced adverse effects after surgery?

PRO: Dr Hypnos quickly responds, "Well remember that the alternative would be using opioids to control her pain. In comparison, gabapentin has a more favorable, generally less dangerous side effect profile. A study analyzing the use of gabapentin for patients undergoing coronary artery bypass surgery found that gabapentin was very well-tolerated in the postoperative time period, with the most common complaint being mild nausea and vomiting that was easily treated [8]. Turan et al. found that a single dose of preoperative gabapentin actually reduced some of the side effects associated with morphine, such as urinary retention and vomiting [9]."

CON: Dr Narkos chimes in, "But you are failing to mention that gabapentin does have significant dose-limiting side effects, which often prevents the development of therapeutic levels. I see this in the pain clinic all the time. The most commonly reported adverse effects are somnolence and dizziness, which can not only impact quality of life but can also be particularly dangerous in elderly patients. This fear has discouraged many clinicians from using gabapentin in the perioperative time period [10].

"Let's look at a large meta-analysis, which, second to huge database studies, is the best form of evidence we have. Clivatti et al. looked at 26 randomized controlled trials and evaluated the effects of gabapentin in patients who received it preoperatively only versus both preoperatively and postoperatively. With only a preoperative dose, some studies demonstrated an increase in nausea, vomiting, and sedation. In patients receiving gabapentin both preoperatively and postoperatively, there were higher rates of sedation and dizziness [11]. Looking at gabapentin versus placebo, Compton et al. found that the incidence of nausea and dizziness was significantly higher in the gabapentin group [12].

"And don't forget the withdrawal syndrome that occurs after abrupt discontinuation [13]. The symptoms often mimic those seen with benzodiazepine and alcohol withdrawal: agitation, anxiety, and seizures [14]. Therefore, it is recommended to taper the dose in patients who receive long-term gabapentin [15]."

Summary

I ponder all this information as I wander back toward my patient. I know gabapentin has had a long-standing role in the treatment and prevention of neuropathic pain. It appears that it may also have a role in prevention of chronic postsurgical pain. While the exact mechanisms of how it reduces CPSP still remain unclear, numerous studies have validated its efficacy in reducing opioid consumption and opioid-related side effects, as well as reducing pain scores several months after the operation. Its use is limited by some noteworthy adverse effects, although many of these are well tolerated and I could inform my patient of these risks.

The data supporting gabapentin's use for both acute and chronic postsurgical pain are still in the early stages, and further research is warranted. It is important to keep in mind that many of these results will be potentially confounded by the use of additional analgesics in addition to gabapentin. Despite this, I believe perioperative administration of gabapentin may play an important role in reducing both acute and chronic postoperative pain and may be worth trialing for my patient today. I confidently approach her bedside, now equipped with more answers to her questions.

References

1. Fecho K, Miller NR, Merritt SA, Klauber-Demore N, Hultman CS, Blau WS. Acute and persistent postoperative pain after breast surgery. Pain Med. 2009;10(4):708–15.
2. Sen H, Sizlan A, Yanarates O, Emirkadi H, Ozkana S, Dagli G, et al. A comparison of gabapentin and ketamine in acute and chronic pain after hysterectomy. Pain Medicine. 2009;109(5):1645–50.
3. Clarke H, Pereira S, Kennedy D, Andrion J, Mitsakakis N, Gollish J, et al. Adding Gabapentin to a multimodal regimen does not reduce acute pain, opioid consumption or chronic pain after total hip arthroplasty. Acta Anaesthesiol Scand. 2009;53:1073–83.
4. Paul J, Nantha-Aree M, Buckley N, Shahzad U, Cheng J, Thabane L, et al. Randomized controlled trial of gabapentin as an adjunct to perioperative analgesia in total hip arthroplasty patients. Can J Anesth. 2015;62(5):476–84.
5. Melemeni A, Staikou C, Fassoulaki A. Gabapentin for acute and chronic post-surgical pain. Signa Vitae. 2007;2(1):42–51.
6. Brogly N, Wattier JM, Andrieu G, Peres D, Robin E, Kipnis E, et al. Gabapentin attenuates late but not early postoperative pain after thyroidectomy with superficial cervical plexus block. Anesth Analg. 2008;107:1720–5.
7. Fassoulaki A, Triga A, Melemeni A, Sarantopoulos C. Multimodal analgesia with gabapentin and local anesthetics prevents acute and chronic pain after breast surgery for cancer. Anesth Analg. 2005;101:1427–32.
8. Ucak A, Onan B, Sen H, Selcuk I, Turan A, Yilmaz A. The effects of gabapentin on acute and chronic postoperative pain after coronary artery bypass graft surgery. J Cardiothorac Vasc Anesth. 2011;25(5):824–9.
9. Turan A, Karamanlioğlu B, Memiş D, Hamamcioglu MK, Tükenmez B, Pamukçu Z, et al. Analgesic effects of gabapentin after spinal surgery. Anesthesiology. 2004;100(4):935–8.
10. Beal B, Moeller-Bertram T, Schilling JM, Wallace MS. Gabapentin for once-daily treatment of post-herpetic neuralgia: a review. Clin Interv Aging. 2012;7:249–55.
11. Clivatti J, Sakata RK, Issy AM. Review of the use of gabapentin in the control of postoperative pain. Rev Brasil Anestesiol. 2009;59 (1):87–98.
12. Compton P, Kehoe P, Sinha K, Torrington MA, Ling W. Gabapentin improves cold-pressor pain responses in methadone-maintained patients. Drug Alcohol Depend. 2010;109 (1–3):213–9.
13. Norton JW. Gabapentin withdrawal syndrome. Clin Neuropharmacol. 2001;24(4):245–6.
14. Barrueto F, Green M, Howland A, Hoffman RS, Nelson LS. Gabapentin withdrawal presenting as status epilepticus. J Toxicol. 2002;40(7):925–8.
15. Tran KT, Hranicky D, Lark T, Jacob NJ. Gabapentin withdrawal syndrome in the presence of a taper. Bipolar Disord. 2005;7 (3):302–4.

Is Urine Drug Testing a Good Idea for Patients on Chronic Opioid Therapy? 107

Chirag D. Shah, M. Fahad Khan, and David S. Cheng

Case

Mr. Anderson is a 46-year-old gentleman who presents to your pain clinic for an initial evaluation. He has had chronic low back pain for the past 10 years but is now complaining of new, electric, or "shooting pains" down his leg. He tells you that he underwent several epidural steroid injections years ago. They provided momentary relief initially, but now he is in constant discomfort. His primary care physician (PCP) has been providing him with Percocet (oxycodone and acetaminophen), which helps to abate these symptoms. He recently moved close to your hospital and is hoping to establish care with you instead.

You are a newly minted pain physician, first year out of fellowship, in a very busy practice. You learned that Mr. Anderson works for a high-end private equity firm and travels frequently. Both the stress of his job and the travel appear to exacerbate his symptoms. He is not particularly keen on seeing his current PCP given the long commute. He is also in the process of finding a new PCP, but asks that you prescribe his Percocet in the interim. While reviewing his intake sheet, you notice that he has tried many pain medications in the past such as ibuprofen, tramadol, and acetaminophen with codeine. He found these medications to be ineffective or intolerable. He insists that oxycodone/acetaminophen is the "only thing that works."

You decide to discuss your concerns with your colleague Dr. Brown, who also happens to be the managing partner. In particular, you ask about the logistics of obtaining a urine drug screen, knowing that this is not a standard practice within the group. Dr. Brown discourages you from ordering this test, stating that it is unnecessary. He reassures you that the office clientele is trustworthy and reliable. Moreover, ordering urine drug tests routinely would be too time-consuming. He contends that it would be bad for business as some patients may find this off-putting and potentially insulting.

Question

Should a urine drug screen be done prior to the prescribing of opioid medications for chronic pain patients?

PRO: Any time a new patient is seen to establish outpatient care for any specialty service, it is simply good practice to obtain as much information about the patient and his presenting condition. Sometimes, this can be as simple as talking to the patient and asking him about his symptoms or the reason he has been referred. Other times this fact-finding mission can involve reading through operative reports, reviewing radiographic tests, or interpreting complex electrodiagnostic studies. The reason for such thoroughness is to provide the best care possible.

Prescribing opioid medications to a patient should not be considered lightly. It should be done with thoughtful consideration and deliberation as these medications can be potentially harmful to the patient and others around him. Therefore, before prescribing this class of drug, I want to be as thorough as possible. Obtaining a urine drug screen would be an important tool for my practice.

CON: I do not disagree that urine drug screens can provide helpful information. However, stating that obtaining as much

C.D. Shah (✉)
Department of Physical Medicine and Rehabilitation, Rush University Medical Center, 1725 West Harrison Street, Suite 118, Chicago, IL 60612, USA
e-mail: Cdshah3@gmail.com

M. Fahad Khan
Department of Anesthesiology, Perioperative Care and Pain Medicine, New York University School of Medicine, 240 East 38th Street, 14th Floor, New York, NY 10016, USA
e-mail: fahad.khan@nyumc.org

D.S. Cheng
Department of Orthopedic Surgery/Physical Medicine and Rehabilitation, Rush University, 1611 West Harrison Street, Suite 300, Chicago, IL 60612, USA
e-mail: David.cheng@rushortho.com

C.S. Scher et al. (eds.), *You're Wrong, I'm Right*, DOI 10.1007/978-3-319-43169-7_107

information as possible is good practice may be reaching. Is a lumbar magnetic resonance imaging (MRI) scan ordered for every patient with uncomplicated low back pain? Are electrodiagnostic studies performed for everyone with leg numbness or tingling? No one will argue that these tests are valuable in the right setting; however, routine tests are excessive, time-consuming, and cost-prohibitive. With my patients, I would only order a test if it might change my medical management.

Logistical issues aside, urine drug test interpretation is not always straightforward. False-positive (and negative) findings are frequently seen. As such, changing management based on these findings is challenging. I have also found that it places a strain on the physician–patient relationship, which is especially critical in pain medicine.

Going back to Mr. Anderson, clearly there are many yellow flags in his case. A state-sponsored prescription monitoring program can be a useful resource to track his recent medications. If you feel uncomfortable with prescribing Percocet to him now, I don't think a "clean" urine drug screen would necessarily help you.

PRO: Among the guiding principles of prescribing opioid medications, are the "4 A's" of opioid prescribing. Specifically, this refers to: (1) analgesia, (2) adverse drug effects, (3) ability to perform activities of daily living (ADL), and (4) aberrant behavior.

While there are many tools to screen for aberrant behavior, urine drug screens are a relatively easy and objective measure. Alternatively, one can administer a patient-specific screening questionnaire, such as a Screener and Opioid Assessment for Patients with Pain (SOAPP) or an Opioid Risk Tool (ORT).

While obtaining a urine drug screen does indeed increase the overall cost of care, I think this needs to be balanced with protection for the patient and the prescriber. With law enforcement and other regulatory agencies pursuing prescribers as well as perpetrators in drug diversion, I think urine drug screens are a good way to avoid unnecessary risk.

CON: Those are all good and valid points. I know that times are different and there are probably new evidence and recommendations since I finished my fellowship. I know you are just trying to help. It's going to take a lot to convince our other partners to change their practice. Can you take some time to look at the current literature on this?

Follow-Up

After doing some reading at the medical library, you return the next day to share your findings.

PRO: I did some research last night and found that physicians often fall victim to what is known as the "truth bias." Physicians feel they have no reason not to believe their patients. This view has been scrutinized in numerous peer-reviewed studies. Interestingly, pain patient reports of illicit and non-prescribed controlled substances are often unreliable [1]. Taking patients at their word makes us liable. Clinicians instead are advised to use objective data in addition to subjective observations before initiating chronic opioid therapy (COT). These data include pill counting, prescription monitoring programs, watching for aberrant behavior (e.g., frequently losing medications), psychological evaluation, and baseline/random urine drug screens (UDS). A retrospective study was conducted to analyze the correlation of positive urine drug screens for illicit drugs or non-prescribed medications and behavioral red flags: 21 % of patients with no behavioral issues were found to have an inconsistent UDS. Conversely, of those with consistent UDS for medications prescribed, 14 % were found to have behavioral issues [2]. Thus, using all of these methods together provides the physician with the information to make the best clinical decisions [1].

CON: Thanks for looking this up. Hope it didn't take up your entire evening, but how much time can we spend on each patient? Shouldn't implementing some of these tests alone be enough to determine if a patient is going to abuse opioids?

PRO: There are lots of different psychological tests out there, but the best studied psychological test is the SOAP-R. This has been able to correctly identify 70–77 % of patients who would eventually be discharged. Unfortunately, it was unable to identify the other 23–30 % [1]. However, when used with UDS as well as other objective data, this percentage can be lowered. In this manner, UDS can help to narrow the gap on potential or eventual patient discharges from the practice.

CON: Is UDS implementation truly necessary for every patient? Is this cost-effective?

PRO: The cost of opioid abuse in the USA was recorded at $9.5 billion in 2005 [1]. After looking at different pain clinic models across the country, we can use the aforementioned tests to stratify patients into low-risk, moderate-risk, and high-risk groups. These groups can be assigned to varying frequencies of random UDS regimens. The high-risk patients would obviously be screened more frequently than the low-risk group. Based on these test results, patient groupings can be adjusted over time [3]. By stratifying patients, you are effectively spending healthcare costs specifically on patients who require closer supervision. Also, structured algorithms for chronic opioid therapy can help to identify abusers and decrease the complications of medications. This ultimately helps to decrease healthcare costs overall. Unfortunately, no data on cost-effectiveness are available.

CON: Another concern of mine is that abruptly adding UDS to our practice may jeopardize the patient–physician relationship and established trust. Wouldn't asking patients to take random UDS make them feel like drug addicts?

PRO: I agree that UDS can be off-putting, but if introduced in the appropriate fashion, this can be overcome. If we outline the rules of the practice early and clearly and explain that they are a part of our opioid agreement, then there should be no surprises [3]. This has been shown to reduce aggression, violence, and nightly calls. Once UDS was implemented, patient satisfaction also dramatically improved [4]. Additionally, patients may feel a stronger bond to their physicians if they perform well and stay true to the treatment plan. On the other hand, if the patient refuses to undergo a UDS, then this may constitute suspicious behavior [1].

CON: Can you tell me about the validity of UDS? What do we do about false positives?

PRO: There are several ways that we can try to avoid false positives. Prior to initiating a baseline UDS, we ask the patient which prescribed medications were taken last and what other medications were taken that week. If the UDS results are inconsistent, we can take steps to figure out why. It is important to be aware of the laboratory used for UDS as well as the type of test ordered. It is true that enzyme immunoassay (EIA), a commonly ordered UDS, is less accurate. However, EIA is cheap and fast. Its major limitation is that it cannot distinguish between drugs in the same class [1].

The gold standards for UDS are either gas chromatography/mass spectroscopy (GC/MS) or liquid chromatography (LC), which are generally reserved for confirmation [3]. In this model, we can order an EIA first then proceed to GC/MS only if necessary. That way, we are allocating expenses more efficiently. Physicians should develop a good understanding of metabolites and cutoff values, as well as creatinine concentration analysis [5]. This will prevent unnecessary testing. UDS can be expensive, ranging from $300 to $2,500 for an EIA test followed by confirmatory tests [6].

CON: Is gathering all of this information really necessary? I just don't see this changing my medical management all that much. What is the standard of care in our community? If we don't do this, is it a legal liability?

PRO: If we use UDS consistently and systematically, it can provide us with useful and accurate information that can potentially alter medical management. Additionally, if medications are prescribed to high-risk patients who are misusing them, then you may have to justify your medical management to the legal system. If clinicians are following a standardized approach that meets the community standard, this helps to mitigate legal scrutiny.

Summary

Medicolegal litigation in this area is still in the process of developing precedents. Physician negligence is often the crux of medical malpractice suits. In order to prove negligence, the prosecution needs to establish several elements. These include the existence of a duty between the physician and the patient, that the physician deviated from the standard of care owed the patient, that said deviation led to the patient's injury, and that there truly was an injury to the patient. Defenses to these claims and caveats to the burden of proof vary by state. In most cases, the legal system will not prosecute a physician who follows guidelines set out by the medical society or what is considered the standard of care. Although the number of studies and evidence supporting the use of UDS testing is scant, it is endorsed by pain and addiction experts, professional societies, and regulatory agencies as the standard of care for patients undergoing COT for greater than three months [7]. It may be argued that since there is little evidence to support these guidelines, they do not need to be followed. This will, however, be a difficult defense to stand on when it goes against the current "standard" of care. Moreover, there are still instances where physicians may be held liable when the benefit of a test outweighs the cost, regardless of the guidelines. For example, if a test is cheap and easy to do, like UDS, and can provide information to prevent abuse, medication complications, and overdose potentially leading to death, then a physician may still be held liable for not ordering the test. Thus, it appears that ordering UDS is a more legally sound medical decision as well. There only needs to be one bad outcome for a physician to lose his license and livelihood.

The question of obtaining a urine drug screen prior to prescribing opioid medications to a chronic pain patient can be a tricky one. It is not completely straightforward as there is a lack of consensus or practice mandate. When considering this screening test, physicians must seek to be thorough without being wasteful or indiscriminate.

Urine drug screening tests can be a useful tool to assess for some of the "4 A's" when prescribing opioid medications.

Furthermore, if these tests are presented to the patient in an appropriate, meaningful, and conscientious manner, they can actually serve to solidify rather than undermine the patient–physician relationship.

Finally, as long as the prescriber remains cognizant of the issues that may complicate the interpretation of urine drug screening tests (i.e., false positives and negatives), these tools will enhance the safety of opioid prescribing for the patient. They can also provide medicolegal protection for the prescriber.

References

1. Owen GT, Burton AW, Schade CM, Passik S. Urine drug testing: current recommendations and best practices. Pain Phys. 2012; 15(3 Suppl): ES119–33.
2. Katz NP, Sherburne S, Beach M, Rose RJ, Vielguth J, Bradley J, et al. Behavioral monitoring and urine toxicology testing in patients receiving long-term opioid therapy. Anesth Analg. 2003;97: 1097–102.
3. Peppin JF, Passik SD, Couto JE, Fine PG, Christo PJ, Argoff C, et al. Recommendations for urine drug monitoring as a component of opioid therapy in the treatment of chronic pain. Pain Med. 2012;13:886–96.
4. Sampson JM, Achololnu WW Jr. Reducing patient aggression and hostility in primary care with urine drug testing. South Med J. 2004;97:916–7.
5. Abadie J. How can the clinical picture guide appropriate laboratory drug testing in the treatment of pain clinic patients with opioid analgesics? Pain Med. 2012;13:857–9.
6. Schonwald G. What is the role of Urine Drug Testing (UDT) in the management of chronic non-cancer pain with opioids? Pain Med. 2012;13:853–6.
7. Starrels JL, Becker WC, Alford DP, Kapoor A, Williams AR, Turner BJ. Systematic review: treatment agreements and urine drug testing to reduce opioid misuse in patients with chronic pain. Ann Intern Med. 2010;152:712–20.

Dexamethasone: To Use or Not To Use—That is the Question

108

Lucia Daiana Voiculescu and Rahul Pathak

Case

Recently, during a busy office day, I received a phone call from Dr. P, one of my former colleagues who is now practicing pain management in Canada. Dr. P was concerned about his father-in-law, a 76-year-old successful lawyer in New York, who recently injured his back after playing 9 holes of "terrible golf". He has type 2 diabetes, borderline hypertension, and a remote history of L4–L5 disk disease that was treated 15 years ago with laminectomy and discectomy. He is very active and was symptom-free until the bad golf day. Now he experiences severe lumbosacral pain that radiates to the lateral aspect of his right leg. It is accompanied by electric shock sensations, tingling, and numbness of the dorsum of his foot. The lumbar magnetic resonance imaging (MRI) demonstrates L4–L5 grade 1 anterolisthesis with prior posterior decompression and a new free disk fragment extending inferiorly and compressing the right L5 nerve root.

He is very reluctant to consider another spine surgery. After discussing different therapeutic options, we decided to proceed with right L4 and L5 transforaminal epidural steroid injection (TFESI).

I called my colleague to let him know that the injection was planned for the same day.

Dr. P agreed and asked what steroid formula will be used. "Methylprednisolone acetate" I answered. As one of the 5 injectable corticosteroids (along with hydrocortisone, dexamethasone, betamethasone, and triamcinolone) methylprednisolone in particulate formula has been used extensively for decades in epidural injections. However, at the other end of the phone my colleague's voice did not sound happy. He suggested that the non-particulate dexamethasone is safer for transforaminal injections, and should replace the particulate steroids.

L.D. Voiculescu (✉) · R. Pathak
Department of Anesthesiology, Perioperative Care and Pain Medicine, New York University School of Medicine, 550 First Avenue, New York, NY 10016, USA
e-mail: lucia.voiculescu@nyumc.org

R. Pathak
e-mail: rahulpathakmd@gmail.com

Question

Dexamethasone: To use or not to use, that is the question.

PRO (Dr. P): As you know, there is increased concern about the use of particulate corticosteroids in the epidural space, especially with the transforaminal technique. Stroke, cord ischemia, quadriplegia, and other severe neurologic complications, including death, were reported subsequent to the epidural injection of steroids. Most of these catastrophic neurologic events followed the administration of different particulate corticosteroid formulas.

Particulate steroids are poorly soluble in water. If inadvertently injected into radicular or radiculomedullary arteries, the particles or aggregates have the potential to embolize and occlude small arterial and capillary vessels, resulting in cord ischemia. In a study on pigs, methylprednisolone acetate, a particulate steroid, injected into the vertebral artery produced irreversible neurologic injuries and death. The animals receiving a non-particulate formula (prednisolone sodium succinate or dexamethasone sodium phosphate) survived without sequelae [1]. The severity of some rare complications reported in humans after using suspension steroids for epidural injections prompted a recent consensus reaction from experts, who recommended the use of dexamethasone as a "first-line" agent for transforaminal injections at all lumbar levels [2].

CON (Dr. V): Indeed, these are devastating but also very uncommon events. Since 2002, only 16 cases of lumbosacral TFESIs complicated with cord ischemia have been described [3]. These reports should be analyzed in the context of millions of epidural steroid injections performed every year.

C.S. Scher et al. (eds.), *You're Wrong, I'm Right*, DOI 10.1007/978-3-319-43169-7_108

It is very important to remember that direct causality between the use of particulate steroids and cord infarction has not been categorically demonstrated. Embolic ischemia is only one of the suggested mechanisms. Arterial spasm, thrombosis, or dissection by direct needle injury, neurotoxicity, or vasospasm due to chemical irritation and prolonged vascular compression by the injected volume are other possible mechanisms, unrelated to the steroid particles and their size, and inferred by the variable timeline of complication onset.

Dexamethasone may be safer if injected intra-arterially. However, there is an increasing body of data regarding dexamethasone's neurotoxicity and possibly limited clinical efficacy [4–7].

Dr. Williams' research demonstrated a time- and concentration-dependent neurotoxicity when ropivacaine was combined with dexamethasone [4]. Applied perineurally, dexamethasone alone was shown to reduce the blood flow in normal nerves and in normal dorsal root ganglia at the threshold for ischemic changes [7]. This vasoconstrictive effect may become important in certain clinical circumstances, patients with diabetes (such as your father-in-law) representing one susceptible category. Experts agree that the lowest dose of dexamethasone should be used in order to avoid neurotoxicity. Further studies need to be done to define epidural dexamethasone's therapeutic and safety profile.

PRO (Dr. P): It is true that dexamethasone's efficacy has not been shown to be superior to other steroids. However, a non-inferiority profile has been outlined by multiple studies. A recent double-blind randomized controlled trial (RCT) compared outcomes (pain, function, and complications) after transforaminal injections with dexamethasone and betamethasone. It demonstrated similar pain relief and functional improvement after both particulate and non-particulate injections [3]. Although this study was underpowered, its conclusions parallel the results obtained earlier by other authors. In 2013, a retrospective observational study on a cohort of 2634 patients by El-Yahchouchi et al. concluded that there is "no evidence that dexamethasone is less effective than particulate steroids in lumbar TFESIs performed for radicular pain with or without radiculopathy" [8].

CON (Dr. V): As you know, methodological inconsistencies have raised questions regarding some of these "non-inferiority" studies [9]. It is really important for your father-in-law, as for most patients with his condition, to minimize the number of injections and avoid surgery. Spine surgery in general and failed back surgery in particular can be associated with a multitude of complications [10, 11]. Post-surgical complication rates vary greatly, for some types of spine surgery ranging from 10 % to more than 80 % [11]. Each subsequent reoperation for failed back syndrome has a lower probability of success. I totally understand your father-in-law's desire to avoid further interventions and maximize nonoperative alternatives.

In small studies, particulate steroids have been shown to be more effective than dexamethasone for lumbar radiculopathy [12], producing longer-term pain relief with fewer injections and referrals for surgery [13, 14]. These clinical results may be explained by the differences in the corticosteroids' pharmacokinetics. Being poorly soluble in water, suspension steroids are released slowly in the surrounding tissues. The ester must be hydrolyzed to the active form by an endogenous esterase, thus increasing their presence in the epidural space, and perhaps prolonging their effects. Methylprednisolone acetate is a depot suspension, with extended release and prolonged action. Therefore, Dr. P, is not the slightly higher risk of complications from a single TFESI with particulate steroid outweighed by the larger risk of an operation or repeated injections with non-particulate steroid?

Concession from PRO In the end, we all agreed that methylprednisolone may be a better choice for Dr. P's father-in-law. The decision was based on the lack of solid evidence in favor of dexamethasone's therapeutic and safety superiority, and the patient's desire to maximize nonsurgical, non-opioid options. The procedure was performed in the radiology suite, using real-time fluoroscopy and contrast for injectate localization.

Summary

Devastating cord infarction is still a rare risk associated in most cases with the transforaminal injection of steroids. Particulate steroids have been used in all of the reported cases, but no absolute causality has been established so far. Although the routine use of non-particulate formulations for TFESIs has been suggested [15], the evidence that dexamethasone has a superior safety and therapeutic profile is yet to be presented.

In 2014, the US Food and Drug Administration (FDA) warned that "the safety and effectiveness of epidural administration of corticosteroids have not been established, and corticosteroids are not approved for this use" [16]. The advisory applies to all injectable steroids, dexamethasone included.

The practitioner's experience, use of contrast under real-time fluoroscopy, and the particularities of each case should be decisive in selecting a specific corticosteroid.

References

1. Okubadejo GO, Talcott MR, Schmidt RE, Sharma A, Patel AA, Mackey RB, et al. Perils of intravascular methylprednisolone injection into the vertebral artery. J Bone Joint Surg Am. 2008;90:1932–8.
2. Rathmell J, Benzon HT, Dreyfuss P, Huntoon M, Wallace M, Baker R, et al. Safeguards to prevent neurologic complications after epidural steroid injections. Anesthesiology. 2015;5:974–84.
3. Denis I, Claveau G, Filiatrault M, Fugère F, Fortin L. Randomized double-blind controlled trial comparing the effectiveness of lumbar transforaminal epidural injections of particulate and nonparticulate corticosteroids for lumbosacral radicular pain. Pain Med. 2015;16:1697–708.
4. Williams BA, Hough KA, Tsui BY, Ibinson JW, Gold MS, Gebhart GF. Neurotoxicity of adjuvants used in perineural anesthesia and analgesia in comparison with ropivacaine. Reg Anesth Pain Med. 2011;36:225–30.
5. Williams BA, Schott NJ, Mangione MP, Ibinson JW. Perineural dexamethasone and multimodal perineural analgesia: how much is too much? Anesth Analg. 2014;118:912–4.
6. Rahangdale R, Kendall MC, McCarthy RJ, Tureanu L, Doty R Jr, Weingart A, et al. The effects of perineural versus intravenous dexamethasone on sciatic nerve blockade outcomes: a randomized, double-blind, placebo-controlled study. Anesth Analg. 2014;118:1113–9.
7. Shishido H, Kikuchi S, Heckman H, Myers RR. Dexamethasone decreases blood flow in normal nerves and dorsal root ganglia. Spine. 2002;27:581–6.
8. El-Yahchouchi C, Geske JR, Carter RE, Diehn FE, Wald JT, Murthy NS, et al. The noninferiority of the nonparticulate steroid dexamethasone vs the particulate steroids betamethasone and triamcinolone in lumbar transforaminal epidural steroid injections. Pain Med. 2013;14:1650–7.
9. Rajan R, Shatia A. Particulate and non-particulate steroids in lumbar transforaminal epidural injections. Pain Med. 2014;15:877–8.
10. Kim SS, Michelsen CB. Revision surgery for failed back surgery syndrome. Spine (Phila Pa 1976). 1992;17:957–60.
11. Smith JS, Shaffrey CI, Lafage V, Schwab F, Scheer JK, Protopsaltis T, et al. International Spine Study Group comparison of best versus worst clinical outcomes for adult spinal deformity surgery: a retrospective review of a prospectively collected, multicenter database with 2-year follow-up. J Neurosurg Spine. 2015;5:1–11.
12. Park CH, Lee SH, Kim BI. Comparison of the effectiveness of lumbar transforaminal epidural injection with particulate and nonparticulate corticosteroids in lumbar radiating pain. Pain Med. 2010;11:1654–8.
13. Kennedy DJ, Plastaras C, Casey E, Visco CJ, Rittenberg JD, Conrad B, et al. Comparative effectiveness of lumbar transforaminal epidural steroid injections with particulate versus nonparticulate corticosteroids for lumbar radicular pain due to intervertebral disc herniation: a prospective, randomized, double-blind trial. Pain Med. 2014;15:548–55.
14. Kim D, Brown J. Efficacy and safety of lumbar epidural dexamethasone versus methylprednisolone in the treatment of lumbar radiculopathy: a comparison of soluble versus particulate steroids. Clin J Pain. 2011;27:518–20.
15. Rathmell JP. Toward improving the safety of transforaminal injection. Anesth Analg. 2009;109:8–10.
16. FDA Briefing Document. Anesthetic and Analgesic Drug Products Advisory Committee Meeting. November 24–25, 2014. Epidural steroid injection (ESI) and the risk of serious neurologic adverse reactions. http://www.fda.gov/downloads/AdvisoryCommittees/CommitteesMeetingMaterials/Drugs/AnestheticAndAnalgesicDrugProductsAdvisoryCommittee/UCM422692.pdf. Accessed 2 Aug 2015.

Should Opioid Analgesics Be Used for Managing Pain in a Patient with a Drug Addiction?

109

Tiffany Sou

Case

A 45-year-old man presents for his initial appointment to your pain clinic with chronic hip pain. The pain started after a total hip arthroplasty about 2 years ago for a right femoral neck fracture. Oxycodone for pain was prescribed by his orthopedic surgeon. All subsequent evaluations have been negative.

A couple of months ago, his surgeon abruptly stopped prescribing oxycodone and switched him to non-steroidal anti-inflammatories (NSAIDs). When he told his surgeon that they were not helping and asked for something stronger, he was told that an opioid prescription could only come from a pain specialist.

The patient is visibly in distress. He states he has been to many doctors and no one believes he is in pain. As you conduct the initial interview, you ask him about his history of substance abuse. He hesitates but admits that he has a remote history of intravenous drug abuse; however, he has been clean for the last 10 years. When you finish the interview, you tell the patient that you generally do not prescribe narcotics on the first visit as you need more information first. You ask him to have his orthopedist fax any and all workup to your office and to schedule a follow-up appointment after this is done.

After the patient leaves, you are typing up the visit note when your colleague peeks his head into your office and says, "Wow, with his history of drug abuse, he sounds like a drug seeker to me!"

Questions

Do patients with a history of substance abuse have an increased risk of opioid misuse? Do the benefits of effective pain management outweigh the morbidity and mortality risk if the patient were to take more than prescribed? How can adequate pain relief be provided to the patient while minimizing risk of drug abuse?

CON Your colleague continues on to say, "I really don't think this patient should be prescribed opioids. Two recent reviews of the literature supports the conclusion that people with preexisting substance use disorders and/or substance-related legal problems may be at higher risk for opioid misuse" [1, 2].

PRO "Both of these reviews admit that the evidence is limited and more research is needed. Oftentimes it's hard to say whether the patient's substance abuse disorder developed as a result of undertreated pain or whether his substance abuse preceded his chronic pain and increased his risk of opioid abuse. Also, just because someone has a positive risk factor doesn't mean he will definitely misuse the prescription."

CON "I think the potential for harm is significant in these patients. Consequences of opioid abuse could be devastating, including overdose and death. Didn't we take an oath as physicians to do no harm?"

PRO "Yes and I agree that we must deliver care in the patient's best interest. On that same note I think that every patient has a right to effective treatment of pain and people with a history of substance abuse should not be treated any differently. Morasco et al. found that 'chronic non-cancer pain patients with history of substance use disorder report poorer pain-related functioning and are less likely to experience clinically significant improvements from usual pain treatment' [3]. It seems that these patients need more intensive treatment for their pain and yet they rarely receive it. Pain is debilitating and destructive and opioids are very effective for relief of pain and suffering. It would be unethical to withhold adequate treatment for any patient

T. Sou (✉)
Department of Anesthesiology, New York University Langone Medical Center, 550 First Avenue, New York, NY 10016, USA
e-mail: Tiffany.Sou@nyumc.org; tsou333@gmail.com

C.S. Scher et al. (eds.), *You're Wrong, I'm Right*, DOI 10.1007/978-3-319-43169-7_109

complaining of severe pain and if this means incorporating opioids into the treatment plan for this patient, then so be it!"

CON "What you are saying is to apply the beneficence principle. Based on this principle you would have to prescribe opioids in a safe way to minimize abuse. I recently read a systematic review by Starrels et al. who found 'relatively weak evidence supporting the effectiveness of opioid treatment agreements and urine drug testing in reducing opioid misuse by patients with chronic pain' [4]"

PRO "Actually, small studies showed that interventions such as structured checklists, motivational interviewing and randomized drug tests can reduce aberrancy in high-risk pain patients [5]. For the patient with a substance use disorder, on top of the precautions you mentioned, I would also adopt an interdisciplinary approach to his care, which reduces misuse of opioids in many patients over time [6]. Goulay et al. affirmed that 'if an addictive disorder dominates, aggressive treatment of an underlying pain problem will likely fail if not coordinated with treatment for the concurrent addictive disorder' [7]".

Summary

There are limited data on the risk of abuse of medically prescribed opioids in the substance abuse patient. More research is needed, which will ideally support the development of better guidelines for opioid prescribers.

References

1. Turk D, Swanson K, Gatchel R. Predicting opioid misuse by chronic pain patients: a systematic review and literature synthesis. Clin J Pain. 2008;24:497–508.
2. Chou R, Fanciullo GJ, Fine PG, Miaskowski C, Passik SD, Portenoy RK. Opioids for chronic noncancer pain: prediction and identification of aberrant drug-related behaviors: a review of the evidence for an American Pain Society and American Academy of Pain Medicine clinical practice guideline. J Pain. 2009;10(2):131–46.
3. Morasco BJ, Corson K, Turk DC, Dobscha SK. Association between substance use disorder status and pain-related function following 12 months of treatment in primary care patients with musculoskeletal pain. J Pain. 2011;12:352–9.
4. Starrels JL, Becker WC, Alford DP, Kapoor A, Williams AR, Turner BJ. Systematic review: treatment agreements and urine drug testing to reduce opioid misuse in patients with chronic pain. Ann Intern Med. 2010;152(11):712–20.
5. Jamison RN, Ross EL, Michna E, Chen LQ, Holcomb C, Wasan AD. Substance misuse treatment for high-risk chronic pain patients on opioid therapy: a randomized trial. Pain. 2010;150:390–400.
6. Holmes CP, Gatchel RJ, Adams LL, Stowell AW, Hatten A, Noe C, et al. An opioid screening instrument: long-term evaluation of the utility of the pain medication questionnaire. Pain Pract. 2006;6:74–88.
7. Gourlay DL, Heit HA, Almahrezi A. Universal precautions in pain medicine: a rational approach to the treatment of chronic pain. Pain Med. 2005;6:107–12.

Is Sympathetic Blockade Useful in Complex Regional Pain Syndrome (CRPS)? 110

Tomas Kucera and Floria Chae

Case

A 22-year-old soccer player presents to the pain clinic with right ankle pain. He was kicked in the right ankle during a soccer match 6 weeks prior. Since the injury, he has had increasing pain, swelling, abnormal perspiration, color changes and has been unable to bear weight due to pain. He went to see an orthopedic sports medicine physician for evaluation. Magnetic resonance imaging (MRI) and X-ray of the foot were negative for fracture or any other soft tissue injury. Infection was ruled out, and no surgical intervention was indicated. He tried physical therapy but was unable to tolerate it due to pain. Gabapentin and nortriptyline only provided minimal improvement. The sports medicine physician diagnosed him with complex regional pain syndrome (CRPS) Type I and referred him to the pain clinic for consideration of lumbar sympathetic nerve block. Today's pain is 8/10 in the right ankle. He describes the pain as burning, sharp, and gnawing. Aggravating factors include movement, socks. Relieving factors include gabapentin.

On examination, there is edema, hyperalgesia, and allodynia of the right ankle. Compared to the left ankle, the skin on the right ankle appears to be mottled and clammy. There is decreased range of motion of right plantar and dorsiflexion due to pain. Strength is otherwise 5/5 in all other extremities.

Question

Is sympathetic blockade useful in complex regional pain syndrome (CRPS)?

T. Kucera (✉)
Advanced Pain Management, 4131 West Loomis Road #300, Greenfield, Wisconsin 53221, USA
e-mail: tomasjkucera@gmail.com

F. Chae
Department of Anesthesiology, Perioperative Care and Pain Medicine, New York University Langone Medical Center, 550 First Avenue, New York, NY 10016, USA
e-mail: floriachaemd@gmail.com

PRO CRPS is a chronic disorder characterized by debilitating pain, vasomotor, sudomotor, and motor disturbances. The pathophysiology of CRPS is multifactorial. The mechanism can vary from patient to patient and can even change in the same patient over time [1]. Accepted mechanisms include autonomic nervous system dysfunction, neurogenic inflammation, central sensitization, glial activation, and alterations in the somatosensory cortex [2]. Local anesthetic sympathetic blockade has been traditionally recognized as an important procedure that has both diagnostic and therapeutic utility. It allows the diagnosis of sympathetically mediated pain as there is increasing evidence to the importance of the sympathetic nervous system in CRPS [3].

CON That being said, you don't need to perform a sympathetic block to diagnosis CRPS. According to the revised Budapest criteria, which have been accepted by the International Association for the Study of Pain, there is no diagnostic laboratory test for CRPS. Instead, it is based on history, symptoms, physical examination, and the exclusion of other causes [4]. Furthermore, CRPS can be sympathetically independent pain or sympathetically mediated pain. The evidence and latest Cochrane review by Stanton in 2013 states that "from the existing evidence, it is not possible to draw firm conclusions regarding the efficacy or safety of this intervention but the limited data available does not suggest that local anesthetic sympathetic block is effective for reducing pain in CRPS." [5].

PRO Yes, this is true. However, it is important to note that the Cochrane review included 12 studies (combined $n = 386$). Only 2 trials ($n = 23$) compared placebo to sympathetic nerve block [5]. That is severely underpowered, and there is not enough evidence to definitively say it does not work. This patient has tried and failed multiple modalities. It's worth a try.

C.S. Scher et al. (eds.), *You're Wrong, I'm Right*, DOI 10.1007/978-3-319-43169-7_110

CON Why would you expose this patient to these risks if there is no evidence of benefit? Sympathetic nerve blocks carry risk of arterial injection, organ injury, bleeding, infection, hypotension, and local anesthetic toxicity to name a few.

PRO A skilled physician using ultrasound or fluoroscopic guidance can minimize the likelihood of adverse effects. According to the Cochrane review, only five studies reported minor adverse effects and there was no permanent injury [5]. Again, this patient has tried and failed multiple modalities. This could possibly benefit the patient, aid in diagnosis of sympathetically mediated pain, and enable him to participate in physical therapy.

CON OK, fine. Let's say you do the sympathetic nerve block with bupivacaine. How do you know if the block is successful? There are no guidelines or definition of a successful block. Schurmann et al. demonstrated the clinical difficulty in the correlation of temperature elevation, Horner's syndrome, and complete sympathetic block [6]. Malmqvist et al. defined success as 4 out the 5 following criteria: Horner's syndrome increased skin temp, increased skin blood flow, and abolished response to ulnar and radial; only 15 out of 54 blocks successfully met his criteria, which indicates the relatively high rate of partial or incomplete block [7].

PRO True, there is no agreement on what is determined as a clinically successful block. This makes studies and the lack of evidence difficult to interpret as the block being efficacious or not. However, that being said, do you need a complete sympathetic block for it to work? Can a partial block be efficacious? Price et al. demonstrated that lidocaine/bupivacaine sympathetic blockade had a mean of 3 days 18 h of analgesia versus 19 h in saline (placebo) group [8]. Price monitored for signs of autonomic block, which were variable.

CON The sympatholysis will be short lived and temporary. How does this help the patient and what will you do next?

PRO Yes, it is short lived. However, if the block provides good analgesia, then repeat blocks in conjunction with physiotherapy have been advocated by consensus expert recommendations to be beneficial [9].

CON Well it seems to me that the evidence is scare. With new modalities such as neuromodulation and spinal cord stimulation (SCS), why perform a sympathetic nerve block at all?

PRO Yes, the patient should have a multimodal approach, but interventions such as SCS have risks as well. The current guidelines advocate for a comprehensive and individualized plan for each patient. Sympathetic nerve block still remains a part of the multimodal approach for the difficult treatment of CRPS.

Summary

While there is very limited high-quality evidence, lack of standardization of what constitutes a successful block, and lack of good studies comparing to placebo, a local anesthetic sympathetic block remains clinically important as it can facilitate pain relief, improve function, and allow the patient to better tolerate rehabilitation techniques. Therefore, local anesthetic sympathetic blockade remains in most CRPS treatment algorithms in order to differentiate between sympathetically mediated pain and sympathetically independent pain [5]. A promising trial compared bupivacaine plus botulinum toxin versus bupivacaine alone in nine patients undergoing lumbar sympathetic block for CRPS. The trial found that botulinum toxin prolonged the duration of analgesia from a mean of 10–71 days. [10].

References

1. Shah A, Kirchner JS. Complex regional pain syndrome. Foot Ankle Clin N Am. 2011;16:351–66.
2. Bussa M, Guttilla D, Lucia M, Mascaro A, Rinaldi S. Complex regional pain syndrome type I: a comprehensive review. Acta Anaesthesiol Scand. 2015;59(6):685–97.
3. Harden RN, Oaklander AL, Burton AW, Perez RS, Richardson K, Swan M, et al. Complex regional pain syndrome: practical diagnostic and treatment guidelines, 4th edition. Pain Med. 2013;14(2):180–229.
4. Harden RN, Bruehl S, Stanton-Hicks M, Wilson PR. Proposed new diagnostic criteria for complex regional pain syndrome. Pain Med. 2007;8:326–31.
5. Stanton TR, Wand BM, Carr DB, Birklein F, Wasner GL, O'Connell NE. Local anaesthetic sympathetic blockade for complex regional pain syndrome. Cochrane Database Syst Rev. 2013;8: CD004598.
6. Schürmann M, Gradl G, Wizgal I, Tutic M, Moser C, Azad S, Beyer A. Clinical and physiologic evaluation of stellate ganglion blockade CRPS Diagnostic and Treatment Guidelines for complex regional pain syndrome type I. Clin J Pain. 2001;17:94–100.
7. Malmqvist EL, Bengtsson M, Sorensen J. Efficacy of stellate ganglion block: a clinical study with bupivacaine. Reg Anesth. 1992;17:340–7.

8. Price D, Long S, Wilsey B, Rafii A. Analysis of peak magnitude and duration of analgesia produced by local anesthetics injected into sympathetic ganglia of complex regional pain syndrome patients. Clin J Pain. 1998;14:216–26.
9. Stanton-Hicks MD, Burton AW, Bruehl SP, Carr DB, Harden RN, Hassenbusch SJ, et al. An updated interdisciplinary clinical pathway for CRPS: report of an expert panel. Pain Pract. 2002;2:1–16.
10. Carroll I, Clark JD, Mackey S. Sympathetic block with botulinum toxin to treat complex regional pain syndrome. Ann Neurol. 2009;65:348–51.

Part XIII
Trauma

Is Pulse Pressure Variation More Accurate Than Central Venous Pressure (CVP) or Pulmonary Artery Pressure (PAP) for Volume Resuscitation?

111

Corey S. Scher

Case

A 48-year-old man on postoperative day 2 is recovering in the surgical intensive care unit (SICU) from an extensive retroperitoneal sarcoma resection. The case was complicated by transfusion of 12 U of packed red blood cells (PRBCs), 6 U of fresh frozen plasma (FFP), and two packs of platelets. Due to the nature of his operation and the likely stormy postoperative course, it is decided to keep the patient sedated, intubated, and mechanically ventilated.

From the beginning of his stay in the SICU, the retroperitoneal drain puts out an abundance of serosanguinous fluid. The surgeon orders equivolemic replacement with intravenous Normosol-R. The output on the day of surgery is 1500 mL. Postoperative day 1 output is 1200 mL. Toward evening, the patient becomes unstable with a blood pressure of 70/40, a pulse of 120, and a distended abdomen. Likely, more fluid is trapped inside the retroperitoneal cavity. The critical care team is clearly behind on fluid resuscitation.

Question

Is pulse pressure variation more accurate than central venous pressure (CVP) or pulmonary artery pressure (PAP) for volume resuscitation?

CON: The mL for mL replacement is ridiculous. The actual fluid loss can be much higher, as the raw surgical surface from the resection is generating retroperitoneal fluid that simply may not be near the drain. I would start out by giving a liter of a balanced salt solution and replacing the Foley catheter that was removed yesterday. I would also get blood drawn for electrolytes. Assuming that the labs were OK, I would hang a second liter of a balanced salt solution. While I was administering these fluids, I would support the circulation with phenylephrine to keep the pressure up until the intravascular space was filled—as evidenced by a stable blood pressure.

PRO: I would prefer to place an arterial line to guide resuscitation.

CON: What for? We do this kind of resuscitation all the time without an arterial line. We give some "neo" (phenylephrine) and just fill the patient up with intravenous fluids.

PRO: The ultimate goal of fluid resuscitation is to restore a normal stroke volume. Since he is intubated, we could put in a trans-esophageal echocardiogram (TEE) probe to measure stroke volume and titrate fluid administration to optimal cardiac hemodynamics. However, no hospital has the resources to have a TEE in every operating room (OR). Pulse pressure variation is a decent surrogate for stroke volume [1]. Pulse pressure is the difference between the systolic and diastolic pressures. The pulse pressure is considered to be "low" or "narrow" when it is <25 % of the systolic pressure. The most common cause of a narrow pulse pressure is a decrease in stroke volume.

CON: I cannot imagine where you are going with this. At the end of the day, is your management any different than mine?

PRO: My style cannot differ more. When you look at the arterial trace, you will notice that the peak of the systolic wave will vary with the ventilation cycle. When a positive pressure breath is given, the entire arterial line tracing will move up. This is even more visible if you change the sweep speed on your monitor to the lowest level possible (from 25 to 6.5 mm/s). This will make the respiratory variation of the arterial line more obvious. On many monitors, there is a button that says "activate the cursor." With this cursor,

C.S. Scher (✉)
Department of Anesthesiology, Perioperative Care and Pain Medicine, New York University School of Medicine, New York, NY 10016, USA
e-mail: coreyscher@gmail.com

C.S. Scher et al. (eds.), *You're Wrong, I'm Right*, DOI 10.1007/978-3-319-43169-7_111

measure from the height of the highest arterial line trace during a breath to the lowest height at end-expiration. Calculate the percentage difference between the two. If the difference is >13 %, you are on the steep portion of the Starling curve and therefore very amenable to hydration or, better stated, your stroke volume is down. Give intravenous fluids until this number reaches 13 %, and at that point, you are close to a normal stroke volume. This technique, looking at pulse pressure variation, correlates well with direct stroke volume measurements utilizing a TEE. If you give too much intravenous fluid, and the pulse pressure variation sinks below 13 %, there is a risk of pulmonary edema and congestive heart failure [2].

CON: I think the CVP is much more useful for volume assessment. A CVP of 2 tells me to give fluid while a CVP of 12 means the patient is well hydrated.

PRO: CVP is deceptive because it depends on vein distensibility. If a vein is very distensible, with a lot of elastin in the walls, hydration will distend the vein but not necessarily increase the CVP. If a vein is not distensible, even small and inadequate volumes of fluid will increase the pressure in the vein and the CVP will still not reflect volume status. And how do you interpret a number that is in-between, such as a CVP of 6? The days of CVP have already passed. There are many clinicians who like to use it for trending. I think that is ridiculous. Pulse pressure variation is better because it does not rely on a trend. Pulse pressure variation tells you when to give fluid and when to stop.

CON: The pulmonary artery (PA) catheter is my go-to when I need an assessment of volume status. I can get a cardiac output, systemic vascular resistance, pulmonary vascular resistance, and above all, pulmonary capillary wedge pressure, which reflects pressure in the left heart. You may have heard that left heart pressure is what most of the world calls volume status.

PRO: The pulmonary artery catheter only measures the pressure in the pulmonary artery; the wedge pressure is subject to the same controversies as the CVP [3].

CON: The big issue I have with pulse pressure variation is that you need to be (1) intubated and (2) you must have an arterial line.

PRO: Pulse oximetry tracings also can be used to measure pulse pressure variation, although more research needs to be done. Besides, the way I look at it, if fluid therapy is clearly needed, as it is in blunt trauma, organ transplantation, cardiac surgery, major vascular surgery or any case where hemorrhage is expected, you will have an arterial line and an intubated patient anyway.

CON: Why don't you just follow the 4–2–1 formula that we all memorize on the first day of residency?

PRO: The true origin of fluid replacement goes back to the 1800s. Shires, through his laboratory, perpetuated the concept that hydration should include the intravascular space, the extravascular space, and the "third space" [4]. There is not a soul on the planet who knows where the third space is, but the myth has been somehow passed down from generation to generation. The 4–2–1 guidelines have no relevance to the modern day practice of anesthesia; the studies supposedly validating this guideline had a very small number of patients [5]. For some reason, the 4–2–1 rule went viral and became the basis of anesthesia practice.

CON: In practice, we end up giving fluid based on the heart rate and blood pressure for patients with significant blood loss. In non-blood loss surgery, we just toss in a liter or 2.

PRO: I would agree. Your comment is essentially what we do when pulse pressure variation cannot be used.

CON: I still hear from very experienced clinicians that they would use some colloid in order to expand the intravascular space without making the patient completely edematous. Do you do that? [6].

PRO: In multiple trials compared in the Cochrane Database [6], there is no evidence in severely ill patients that colloids are better than crystalloids, and the recommendations indicate that because crystalloids are cheaper they should be the go-to fluid. Despite the overwhelming evidence of parity between the two, I do ignore these findings and use colloid, because I still find in my own practice that this leads to less fluid given and less edema. I clearly do not follow every study or guideline.

Summary

In hyperacute cases, fluid resuscitation should be guided by TEE findings or pulse pressure variation. If the case is not acute, I would give fluids based on clinical judgment. In a case with no excitement, such as a sleeve gastrectomy or a hip fracture, it does make sense to replace fluids from fasting and insensible losses by giving a liter or 2. For blunt trauma, use the arterial line tracing to measure pulse pressure variation and guide fluid administration, with or without TEE backup.

References

1. Auler JO Jr, Galas FR, Sundin MR, Hajjar LA. Arterial pulse pressure variation predicting fluid responsiveness in critically ill patients. Shock. 2008;30(Suppl 1):18–22.
2. Auler JO Jr, Galas F, Hajjar L, Santos L, Carvalho T, Michard F. Online monitoring of pulse pressure variation to guide fluid therapy after cardiac surgery. Anesth Analg. 2008;106(4): 1201–6.
3. Schwann NM, Hillel Z, Hoeft A, Barash P, Möhnle P, Miao Y, et al. Lack of effectiveness of the pulmonary artery catheter in cardiac surgery. Anesth Analg. 2011;113(5):994–1002.
4. Shires T, Williams J, Brown F. Acute changes in extracellular fluids associated with major surgical procedures. Ann Surg. 1961;154:803–10.
5. Moore FD, Shires T. Moderation. Ann Surg. 1967;166:300–1.
6. Perel P, Roberts I, Ker K. Colloids versus crystalloids for fluid resuscitation in critically ill patients. Cochrane Database Syst Rev. 2013;28(2):000567.

What Is the Best Management Strategy for Venous Air Embolism?

112

Amit Prabhakar and James Riopelle

Case

A tall, slender 24-year-old male sustained a single gunshot wound to the upper abdomen while attempting to wrestle his bicycle from a thief. On arrival to the emergency department, he was pale, unconscious, and flaccid with a heart rate on telemetry of 160 beats per minute and barely palpable carotid pulses. He was rushed to the operating room, moved to the operating table in a supine position, ventilated with 100 % oxygen, and tracheally intubated. Breath sounds were equal and clear. The patient was placed on volume-control mechanical ventilation with 600 ml tidal volumes and peak inspiratory pressures of 23 mm Hg. Scopolamine 0.6 mg and pancuronium 8 mg were the only drugs administered.

Despite the presence of a scaphoid abdomen, intraperitoneal and retroperitoneal bleeding was quickly ruled out during an emergency exploratory laparotomy. A left thoracotomy revealed tense pericardial tamponade. The pericardium was incised, and the pumping hole in the anteroinferior right ventricle was closed with a purse string suture. Circulatory function immediately returned permitting administration of normal doses of intravenous and inhalational anesthetic agents (fentanyl, isoflurane). An arterial line was inserted with the first blood gas showing normal oxygenation and a 12 mEq base deficit. The latter was treated with 200 mEq sodium bicarbonate.

The head surgeon breathed a sigh of relief and quickly moved on to the surgical exploration for bleeding vessels prior to chest closure. Less than 10 min later, the normal-appearing, vigorously contracting heart suddenly began to dilate and lose all efficacy at pumping blood. End-tidal carbon dioxide ($CO2$) dropped precipitously from 36 to 5 mm Hg. Inhalation anesthesia was discontinued. Equal bilateral breath sounds were auscultation, and normal inspiratory pressures were confirmed. No new surgical bleeding was identified.

Although the telemetry monitor showed normal sinus rhythm, the arterial pressure waveform was flat at 25 mm Hg and no carotid pulses could be palpated. Open chest cardiac massage was begun and epinephrine 1 mg administered intravenously. Despite vigorous manual squeezing of the heart, arterial systolic pressure remained below 40 mm Hg. Additional doses of epinephrine were not effective in elevating the arterial pressure, and carotid pulsations remained absent.

The anesthesiology resident said. "Let's use the Advanced Cardiovascular Life Support (ACLS) algorithm for causes of cardiac arrest, the '5 Hs and 4 Ts': Hypoxia, Hyperkalemia, Hypothermia, Hypoglycemia, H+ (acidosis), Trauma, Tension pneumothorax, and Thrombus (cardiac or air)' [1]. We haven't yet addressed the possibility of air embolism."

Saying "It's worth a try," the surgeon picked up a sterile 30-ml syringe with an 18-gauge needle attached. The needle was inserted into the right ventricle with subsequent evacuation of 60 cc of air, followed by aspiration of blood. The arterial pressure waveform immediately returned to normal. No source for air entrainment was identified.

Chest closure, chest tube placement, and patient transfer to the intensive care unit (ICU) were uneventful. The patient was stable overnight. The patient was later transferred to a neighboring private facility for continued rehabilitation and was thought to be lost to follow-up. However, 6 months later, he walked into the ICU to thank all those who had cared for him. He apologized for not coming sooner, his excuse being that he needed to first successfully pass all his examinations for engineering graduate school.

A. Prabhakar (✉)
Department of Anesthesiology, Louisiana State University Health Sciences Center, 1542 Tulane Ave., Suite 653, New Orleans, LA 70112, USA
e-mail: Amitprabhakar7@gmail.com; aprab1@lsuhsc.edu

J. Riopelle
Department of Clinical Anesthesiology, Louisiana State University Health Sciences Center, 1542 Tulane Avenue, 6th Floor, New Orleans, LA 70112, USA
e-mail: jriope@lsuhsc.edu

C.S. Scher et al. (eds.), *You're Wrong, I'm Right*, DOI 10.1007/978-3-319-43169-7_112

Question

What is the best management strategy for venous air embolism?

PRO If you want to know the best management strategy for venous air embolism, it is imperative to first know what situations you can expect to see it in. VAE is classically associated with neurosurgical procedures performed in the sitting position, and occurs secondary to a gravitational gradient in 76 % [2].

CON That's great but just like anything in medicine, it is not always so cut and dry. Venous air embolism is not always associated with these common high-risk surgeries. Laparoscopic and minimally invasive procedures use gas for insufflation and exposure of the surgical field, leading to a risk for injection or entrainment of this gas into the venous system [1]. As an anesthesiologist, you have to be prepared for uncommon occurrences in common situations. This case is a prime example of that. Here, there was no clear source for introduction of air into the venous system. But, as is common in trauma cases such as this one, you may not have the time to fully identify the extent of the patient's injuries prior to the operating room. Especially in life-threatening hemorrhagic trauma, every second matters.

PRO One good thing about VAE is that it seldom results in clinically significant hemodynamic compromise; however, it naturally follows that many episodes occur without clinician awareness. While the majority of research has been done using animal models, the consensus is that clinically significant VAE in humans occurs between 3–5 ml/kg and 200–300 ml of air [2]. The rate of air accumulation is a key determinant in clinical significance [2]. Prompt identification of VAE is key. Currently, transesophageal echocardiography is the most sensitive monitoring device available with the ability to detect as little as 0.02 ml/kg of air [3]. Precordial Doppler has been shown to be the most sensitive noninvasive monitor for VAE detection [4].

CON The odds of you actually having the time or accessibility to use those methods in a situation in which venous air embolism is not suspected are slim to none. You can't lean on technologies that will waste time and delay proper treatment. The importance of the time from the onset of hemodynamic compromise to treatment can't be overstated. In this situation, the clinician successfully used clinical signs such as a drop in $ETCO_2$ and loss of arterial waveform to successfully identify the problem. A drop of 2 mmHg of $ETCO_2$ can signify VAE [2].

PRO Treatment of VAE is best accomplished by lowering the operative site below the level of the heart, flooding the operative field to prevent further air entry, and positioning the patient left side down and in Trendelenburg [5]. This helps to prevent further air entrainment into the venous system. The patient should also be placed on 100 % oxygen. Other rescue maneuvers include the initiation of cardiopulmonary resuscitation and chest compressions.

CON Actually, recent studies have refuted this conventional method of thinking [6]. Animal studies failed to show that repositioning to the left lateral position improved hemodynamic performance [6]. Keeping the patient in the supine position may actually be better for the patient because it allows for better access to perform chest compressions and other rescue maneuvers [6]. This case shows that the life-saving treatment is not always the one that is written about or studied the most in textbooks and papers. The quick actions of the anesthesiologist and surgeon allowed for rapid evacuation of the air embolus from the right ventricle and saved the young man's life.

Summary

Venous air embolism is an under-recognized and often insignificant event. However, when VAE leads to hemodynamic compromise, the clinician often only has seconds to identify the source (Table 112.1) and formulate a plan for treatment. More research needs to be done in order to

Table 112.1 Gremlids: anesthetic catastrophes, often assumed to be simple accidents, are actually the work of gremlids (anesthesia goblins)

Gremlids
Oxygen insufficiency (hypoxic mixture of inhaled gases)
Absolute versus relative to an individual patient's needs
Obstruction of the breathing system or the patient's airway
Anesthesia machine or circuit (peep valve, soda lime, HME, exhaust tubing, draeger muffler)
Upper airway (teeth, tongue, nasal turbinates, redundant pharyngeal tissue)
Larynx: epiglottis pushed down by oral airway or LMA tip; laryngospasm
Tracheal tube or LMA (mucus, blood, clot)
Trachea or major bronchus (mucus, blood, clot, tumor of airway or anterior mediastinum)
Distal airways: bronchospasm, air trapping
Overdosage or other drug administration error
Wrong inhalational or intravenous agent; exaggerated drug reaction; more concentrated drug (ketamine, lidocaine); look-alike drug
Intolerance (including allergic reaction) to drugs given by anesthesia, surgeon, perfusionist (including irrigation, methyl methacrylate, etc.)
Hypoventilation
Ventilator turned off
Major disconnection or breathing circuit leak
Tracheal extubation
Disconnection or major leak at corrugated circuit connection to machine or tracheal tube
Pop-off (APL) valve wide open during mechanical ventilation (older machines)
Soda lime canister seals not correctly mated
Gastric tube (Salem sump) in trachea, especially if connected to suction
Shock
Hypovolemic
Dehydration
Hemorrhage (especially concealed hemorrhage)
Cardiogenic
Myocardial infarction
Cardiac tamponade
Pharmacologic/toxicologic (local or general anesthetic overdose, beta blocker, methyl methacrylate, acidosis)
Arrhythmia (V-Tach—sux, ischemia, ↕K^+, SVT or rapid atrial fib, bradycardia, heart block)
Obstructive (physical obstruction to circulation)
Cardiac tamponade (blood, effusion, air; e.g., from jet ventilation in presence of upper airway closure)
Inferior vena cava compression (pregnant uterus) or portal compression (surgeon)
Tension pneumothorax or air trapping from inadequate exhalation time
Embolism [air/other gas, (venous) thromboembolism]
Distributive/cytotoxic
Septic
Anaphylactic (drugs, blood product, latex)
Neurogenic (high spinal/epidural anesthesia, spinal cord injury, brainstem herniation)
Endocrine/metabolic (Addisonian crisis, thyroid storm, hypothyroidism/myxedema, carcinoid), ↓ ionized [Ca ++]—e.g., due to blood product administration, especially in patients with liver hypofunction: cirrhosis/thoracic aortic crossclamp)
Amniotic fluid embolism
Pharmacologic/toxicologic (IV or inhaled anesthetic agent, vasodilator, methyl methacrylate, acidosis)
Hyperthermia/hypothermia
Malignant hyperthermia

(continued)

Table 112.1 (continued)

Passive hyperthermia/hypothermia (e.g., massive transfusion with cold blood, especially with blood warmer off)
Hyperthyroid/hypothyroid
Intubation catastrophe
Esophageal intubation
Submucosal placement of nasal tube
Mediastinal intubation via perforation of pyriform sinus or airway tumor
Pre-tracheal misplacement of tracheostomy tube
Tension pneumothorax or other pulmonary catastrophe
Pneumothorax from disease, surgery, airway instrumentation, ventilator barotrauma/jet ventilation, subclavian puncture
Atelectasis (secretions, bronchial intubation, microatelectasis)
Aspiration (e.g., of gastric contents)
Asthma/bronchospasm/air trapping
Pulmonary edema (fluid overload, cardiogenic, non-cardiogenic; e.g., negative pressure)

The presence of a gremlid in the operating room can be deduced when, during the administration of a general anesthetic, the patient suddenly and unexpectedly becomes cyanotic, hypotensive, or difficult to ventilate
HME heat and moisture exchanger, *LMA* laryngeal mask airway, *APL* adjustable pressure limiting, *V-Tach* ventricular tachycardia, *K* potassium, *SVT* supraventricular tachycardia, *Ca* calcium, *IV* intravenous

validate a definitive treatment for clinically significant venous air embolism.

References

1. Neumar RW, Otto CW, Link MS, Kronick SL, Shuster M, Callaway CW, et al. Part 8: adult advanced cardiovascular life support: 2010 American Heart Association guidelines for cardiopulmonary resuscitation and emergency cardiovascular care. Circulation. 2010;122(18 Suppl 3):S729–67.
2. Mirski MA, Lele AV, Fitzsimmons L, Toung TJK. Diagnosis and treatment of venous air embolism. Anesthesiology. 2007;106:164–77.
3. Furuya H, Suzuki T, Okumura F, Kishi Y, Uefuji T. Detection of air embolism by transesophageal echocardiography. Anesthesiology. 1983;58:124–9.
4. Chang JL, Albin MS, Bunegin L, Hung TK. Analysis and comparison of venous air embolism detection methods. Neurosurgery. 1980;7:135–41.
5. Durant TM, Long J, Oppenheimer MJ. Pulmonary (venous) air embolism. Am Heart J. 1947;33:269–81.
6. Simon G. Management of venous air embolism. Letter to editor. Anesth Analg. 2014;119(1):215–6.

Does Cerebral Oximetry Have an Important Role in Trauma?

113

Corey S. Scher

Case

A 29-year-old man decided to slide down the newly placed bannister in Grand Central Station. During his ride down, he lost his balance and fell. Observing commuters commented to emergency medical services (EMS) that he landed on his head. He was unconscious, and his Glasgow coma score was 5–6. There were no obvious fractures, and his abdomen was soft to palpation. Cardiopulmonary auscultation at the train station was normal. He appeared to only have a closed head injury or traumatic brain injury (TBI). He was transported to the nearest hospital, and his low Glasgow coma score led to an endotracheal intubation without incident.

An immediate computed tomography (CT) scan was done and demonstrated diffuse axonal injury (DAI). The criteria for DAI include CT findings of the following: (1) single or multiple small intraparenchymal hemorrhages in the cerebral hemispheres (<2 cm in diameter); (2) intraventricular hemorrhage; (3) hemorrhage in the corpus callosum; (4) small focal areas of hemorrhage adjacent to the third ventricle (<2 cm in diameter); and (5) brain stem hemorrhage.

When he arrives at your hospital, one of the medical students asks you, "I've seen cerebral oximetry used intraoperatively in patients at risk for stroke, could it be useful here as well?"

Question

Does cerebral oximetry have an important role in trauma?

PRO This diagnosis carries a high mortality, and every monitor and treatment available should be used.

CON Cerebral oximetry won't help you in a patient with diffuse axonal injury. There are three stages of axonal degeneration, all of which are determined microscopically. Stage 1 is defined as the "occurrence of diffuse damage to axons in the cerebral hemispheres, the corpus callosum, the brain stem and sometimes the cerebellum resulting from head injury" [1]. Stage 2 requires corpus callosum damage, and Stage 3 includes all of the above plus brain stem injury. Other than serial scanning or magnetic resonance imaging (MRI) studies, there are no monitors for this dreaded diagnosis. Essentially, it is a deceleration injury where the white matter is sheared off the gray matter. There is no use for any treatment other than time.

PRO I do agree that in the case presented, cerebral oximetry gives very little information as blood flow disturbance is spotty and the oximeter cannot measure oxygenation in deeper brain structures. I agree that this monitor is more useful in detecting perioperative neurologic injury, which may be related to an imbalance in regional to cerebral microcirculation, which can be monitored by the cerebral oximeter [2].

CON I am very familiar with the oximeter. It is very different from pulse oximetry. The leads or stickers are placed symmetrically on the frontal lobe. The frontal lobe cortex is quite vulnerable to changes in oxygen supply and demand. Cerebral oximetry differs from the pulse oximeter by using two photodetectors allowing sampling at a specified depth. Near-field (scalp and skull) is subtracted from far-field (scalp, skull, and brain) reading to provide a measurement of brain oxygenation beyond a predefined depth [2]. It is essential to know that the blood monitored is 75 % venous and 25 % arterial. Therefore, the normal cerebral oximeter saturation is around 70 %. When the readings from one side of the frontal lobe are different from the other side, there is almost nothing that an anesthesiologist can do to get the lower reading back to normal [2].

C.S. Scher (✉)
Department of Anesthesiology, Perioperative Care and Pain Medicine, New York University School of Medicine, New York, NY 10016, USA
e-mail: coreyscher@gmail.co

C.S. Scher et al. (eds.), *You're Wrong, I'm Right*, DOI 10.1007/978-3-319-43169-7_113

PRO A cerebral oxygen saturation below 50 % is a call for clinical action by increasing cerebral circulation with appropriate vasopressors or increasing oxygen-carrying capacity with a blood transfusion.

CON Let's say the cerebral oxygen saturation is 70 % on one side of the frontal lobe and 60 % on the other side. Do I ignore that? There are very few guidelines or clinical algorithms that describe when to intervene or if the interventions that you describe have any value. The surgeons want the mean arterial pressure (MAP) low to decrease blood loss, especially in situations in which the patient may be coagulopathic. You want the MAP high to improve any difference in the venous saturation. An argument will break out. In a severe blunt trauma with a head injury and a hemorrhaging patient, it is difficult problem. If we did not put on the cerebral oximetry stickers, we would not know the difference. I think dealing with the massively bleeding patient takes priority.

PRO There are some very distinct clinical settings where the oximeter is helpful. For years, in the cardiac anesthesia world, the oximeter has detected patients suffering from an intraoperative stroke. In carotid endarterectomy procedures, if the cerebral oxygen saturation decreases while the carotid is clamped, the team can take steps such as raising the blood pressure or limiting clamp time in order to decrease the possibility of a stroke. The cerebral oximeter can also be useful in cases that require unusual positioning that leads to the possibility of altered cerebral perfusion, such as the beach chair for posterior fossa tumors or deep reverse Trendelenburg for laproscopic bariatric cases.

CON Really: Do you use the cerebral oximeter in laparoscopic bariatric cases where the operating room table is placed in severe reverse Trendelenburg? There are subsets of patients undergoing this procedure who have decreased venous return with resultant intracranial hypoperfusion. If you believe in the cerebral oximeter, why don't you use it in these cases? Do these patients have any neurocognitive loss?

PRO I have never used the oximeter in the bariatric arena and am unaware of neurocognitive changes when I see these patients on postoperative day 1.

CON How could you possibly know if these patients have neurocognitive changes, as most patients on post-op day 1 on narcotics develop a low-grade systemic inflammatory response or simply are exhausted from the whole event of surgery? Neurocognitive changes are diagnosed with complex examinations that are validated and reliable.

PRO I think that during a cardiac arrest, if you apply cerebral oximetry and are able to maintain oxygen saturation around 50 %, this may predict return of spontaneous circulation and better neurologic outcomes.

CON What you think is not true as this has been looked at in several studies. Adequate cerebral saturations during a cardiac arrest do not predict return of circulation or better neurologic outcomes. This was studied prospectively in Japan only a year ago [3]. The oximeter is not helpful for advanced cardiac life support (ACLS).

PRO While I know that you think that is a monitor looking for a place, I can think of one clinical scenario where it is essential. We have a large bariatric service as Medicaid now reimburses well for these cases. The patient population presenting for these cases differs widely with respect to geography. Patients in states such as Mississippi and Louisiana are significantly larger than those in New York. At our public hospital, women weigh around 220 lb, but from my experience in the Deep South, 400 and 500 lb patients were not unusual. In all laparoscopic gastric sleeve and gastric bypass cases, the operating room bed is put in the deepest reverse Trendlenburg possible. In very obese patients, blood pools in their lower extremities and systemic blood pressure drops precipitously. I have done a small pilot study that is now turning into a real institutional review board (IRB) investigation where cerebral oximetry measures venous saturations supine and then in steep reverse Trendlenburg. Seven of the 10 patients who became hypotensive had cerebral oximetry changes from a baseline of 70 % to around 50 %. This is an incredible finding. I wonder if there are any cognitive changes with prolonged venous saturations at 50 % or below.

CON While I believe the venous saturations you are describing are real, finding cognitive changes with all of the variables that affect a patient in the perioperative period will be almost impossible.

PRO The "Beach Chair Study" was reported in *Anesthesia and Analgesia* in January of 2015 by Laflam et al. Patients in this position for surgery had an impairment in autoregulation of the brain without changes in cognition or biomarkers of brain injury [4]. Low blood pressure did occur in the beach chair position, which was treated with vasopressors, which restored the cerebral oxygen saturation to its original values [4]. What I take away from these studies is that if you do not specifically measure cerebral oximetry but you do treat the hypotension, the venous saturation is restored. The bottom line is that at least according to this study, the beach chair position did not really have an impact on patient care. The bariatric patient is entirely different, and I do expect a clinically significant desaturation rate.

Summary

Other than the obvious use for the cerebral oximeter in carotid endarterectomies, there is very little evidence that the cerebral oximeter improves outcomes. Yet, I believe that it is a monitor that is slowly increasing in utility to make our patients safe. There is so much room for further clinical investigation to determine when the cerebral oximeter improves patient safety and well-being.

References

1. de Lanerolle NC, Kim JH, Bandak FA. Neuropathology of traumatic brain injury: comparison of penetrating, nonpenetrating direct impact and explosive blast etiologies. Semin Neurol. 2015;35(1):12–9.
2. Scher C. Chapter 5: general principles of intraoperative management of the severe blunt or polytrauma patient: the resuscitative phase. In: Scher C, editor. Anesthesia for Trauma. New York: Springer; 2014. p. 95–6.
3. Fukuda T, Ohashi N, Nishida M, Gunshin M, Doi K, Matsubara T, et al. Application of cerebral oxygen saturation to prediction of the futility of resuscitation for out-of-hospital cardiopulmonary arrest patients: a single-center, prospective, observational study: can cerebral regional oxygen saturation predict the futility of CPR? Am J Emerg Med. 2014;32(7):747–51.
4. Laflam A, Joshi B, Brady K, Yenokyan G, Brown C, Everett A, et al. Shoulder surgery in the beach chair position is associated with diminished cerebral autoregulation but no differences in postoperative cognition or brain injury biomarker levels compared with supine positioning: the anesthesia patient safety foundation beach chair study. Anesth Analg. 2015;120(1):176–85.

Should New Trauma Paradigms Be Used in the Care of the Severe Trauma Patient?

114

Corey S. Scher

Case

A 32-year-old male who works for the United Parcel Service is leaving a building in Manhattan after dropping off a package. A few steps past the revolving door, a car, clearly out of control, pins the UPS worker against the outside wall of the building. He is now bleeding from an open pelvic fracture, and there is no evidence of head injury.

Someone calls 911 and within moments 2 fire trucks arrive. One team of paramedics is designated to take care of the driver and the other to care for the UPS delivery man. The driver appears on initial examination to be uninjured. The smell of alcohol on his breath is more than noticeable. Within 3 min, the car is pulled off the delivery man by the firefighters. A cervical collar is placed on both the driver and the victim.

A team of paramedics places the UPS worker on a spine board, inserts an IV, places a non-rebreathing oxygen mask, and calls the nearest Level I trauma center to report. Initial vital signs are a blood pressure (BP) of 75/40, pulse at 120 beats per minute (bpm), and temperature of 34.9 °C. Oxygen saturation is 88 %.

In the emergency room (ER), the trauma team does a complete initial assessment of the UPS delivery man. The FAST (Focused Assessment with Sonography in Trauma) examination is positive for blood in the abdomen. Due to his hemodynamic instability and likely full stomach, a rapid sequence induction with etomidate and succinylcholine, and intubation with manual in-line stabilization, is performed before transport to the operating room (OR). The cervical collar is re-applied. Vital signs are now BP 60/40 with a pulse of 140 bpm. An initial arterial blood gas (ABG) sample reveals combined metabolic and respiratory acidosis. The lactate is 8.

The trauma anesthesia team consists of 4 residents and 2 attendings.

Questions

Should new trauma paradigms be used in the care of the severe trauma patient? Are blood products and hypertonic saline better than vasopressors for treating hypotension in trauma patients?

CON: The first attending says, "Give me a syringe of phenylephrine stat!"

PRO: The second attending shouts back, "No! The pressure is not only fine but that is what we want. Just give him blood if you have it or 5 % saline if you don't. Activate the massive transfusion protocol!"

CON: "I have been involved with trauma care for 30 years and this is ridiculous. I am giving 200 micrograms of phenylephrine. He is, until proven otherwise, a closed head injury and hypotension could result in a poor neurological outcome!"

PRO: "You must be kidding me. Phenylephrine is a terrible vasopressor for critically ill patients. Sure, in most cases there is not a big difference among pressors, but here it matters! If you have to use a pressor, choose vasopressin. There are no vasopressin receptors in the lung so the necessary low pulmonary vascular resistance is maintained while the systemic pressure goes up. I have never seen a patient in a surgical intensive care unit (SICU) on a phenylephrine infusion. Never! Even better would be to allow for deliberate hypotension until the blood products or 5 % saline arrives. The average age of a trauma patient is 29 and he fits right into the evidence that deliberate hypotension

C.S. Scher (✉)
Department of Anesthesiology, Perioperative Care and Pain Medicine, New York University School of Medicine, New York, NY 10016, USA
e-mail: coreyscher@gmail.com

C.S. Scher et al. (eds.), *You're Wrong, I'm Right*, DOI 10.1007/978-3-319-43169-7_114

corrects coagulopathy, acidosis, and hemorrhage [1]. Let the pressure be corrected with the appropriate blood products. His cerebral oximeter reading is 70 on both sides of the brain."

CON: "What? Since when did you become a threat to the patient? When did the cerebral oximeter become the gold standard for the entire brain?"

PRO: "I guess you are right about the oximeter. Let's look at overall outcomes, though. Research shows that permissive hypotension during initial resuscitation may improve trauma outcomes [1]. I believe that future studies will show that permissive hypotension may save lives."

CON: "What does the word 'may' mean? How is it that I have never heard of this? I will read the paper critically. What other center does this?"

PRO: "In the sentinel Morrison paper [1], utilizing deliberate hypotension works, particularly in our patient population, which is usually young and healthy. Patients undergoing laparotomy or thoracotomy for trauma that was either blunt or penetrating were enrolled if they had 1 or more episodes of low blood pressure (SBP < 90 mm Hg). The two groups were a goal mean arterial pressure (MAP) of 50 mm Hg (study group) versus a MAP of 65 mm Hg (control group). This project took place at Ben Taub, Baylor's trauma hospital. Ninety patients were enrolled. The data on transfusion requirements, correction of coagulopathy, and survival are impressive [1]."

CON: "Do you believe everything in a citable journal? Without reading the paper, the sample size is ridiculously low at 90. The institutional review board (IRB) must have been drunk to approve this study. You cannot compare any single trauma to any other trauma and therefore how are the cohorts made? How do you define blood loss in cases where our booties squish and squash when we walk in the room? A multivariate analysis to control all the variables in this study, while well done, may simply not be enough to convince the clinician. It is a very interesting idea but I am not changing my practice until I read the paper for myself."

PRO: "Even things that are far out have been proposed. In a planned project at the University of Pittsburgh, surgeons will drain a severe trauma patient's blood and replace it with freezing saltwater. With deep hypothermic circulatory arrest, the heart and brain will be put in suspended animation—the patients will be clinically dead. Then they will fix whatever they can. They have based this technique on animal models where there was no neurocognitive change. However, scientists have never tried anything like this in humans, and unconscious patients will not be able to consent to the procedure. Therefore, free bracelets are being given to any Pittsburgh citizens who do not want to be included in the study if they are in a trauma. The Department of Defense is providing the funding. The study will involve 20 subjects with 'catastrophic penetrating trauma' and cardiac arrest secondary to hemorrhage. There are no data yet, but something has to be done, as the prognosis in severe blunt trauma is not good."

> "Only 1 in 10 survives with your approach to these patients. I think the permissive hypotension study [1] is an attempt to quickly turn things around, and has more of a chance of changing practice than the Frankenstein attempt at Pittsburgh. Permissive hypotension didn't get a fair trial."

CON: "There is no way in just 20 patients this Pittsburgh study can account for the variables, and this study will take so long that other approaches may prevail."

PRO: "I read with great anticipation about a new initiative that should improve the 1 in 10 survival rate for severe trauma. The military has a project called the Prehosptial Air Medical Plasma (PAMPer) trial [2]. Severe hemorrhage and coagulopathy are the main players in early preventable death in both military and civilian trauma. Trauma centers advocate early plasma transfusion as it has consistently been shown to improve outcomes. Having plasma in the field shortly after the time of injury has demonstrated both feasibility and improved short-term outcomes. The PAMPer trial will look at both coagulation and immunological response to early plasma as well as 30-day mortality. The trial is ongoing and the original paper claims a very positive outcome in all areas being examined while at the same time referring to flaws in the trial's design, which are not very different from the usual trauma trials (Cannot be double-blind, examiner bias, etc.). Because universal donor plasma is blood type AB, the benefits of transfusion in the field outweighs the costs."

CON: "Great idea, but it seems way too complicated for the civilian population. Are first responders going to have thawed fresh frozen plasma (FFP) on their emergency vehicles and if they do, how long can each unit survive at room temperature? There could be a few vehicles specifically designed to go to every trauma with the exclusive goal of preparation and transfusion of FFP and any other procoagulants. Simply stated, I just do not see in happening and adopted so readily."

PRO: "Another very practical concept is having interventional radiology (IR) next to the trauma OR or, better, to have the radiology suite as part of the trauma operating room. Ideally, the computed tomography (CT) scan would be close by as well. Clinical logistics often influence care, and these arrangements would remove the difficulties of patient transport and lead clinicians down the best pathway: either damage control surgery with the risks of coagulopathy, acidosis, hypothermia and possible bleeding; or simple embolization of non-essential vessels that are responsible for hemorrhage [3]. Including whole body CT (WBCT) in the initial work-up of trauma patients leads to a higher radiation dose, during a shorter scan, as well as fewer add-on CT scans. WBCT takes 12 min, which might be too long if the aforementioned arrangement is not assembled. Traveling from CT to IR to OR could be more than the 'Golden Hour' would allow."

Summary

All of the new trauma approaches are actually used today. They may or may not work in the culture of the level 1 trauma center. Use of low blood pressure to minimize coagulopathy and to control bleeding has been adopted by many well-known centers. The administration of FFP in the field is a great idea if the logistics and investigations pan out. Having the OR, IR, and CT scan in the same suite is a fantastic idea, but is used only in newer or planned hospitals. A universal algorithm for choosing IR over surgery or surgery over IR needs further investigation. The pro-con discussion here brings out the fact that an ongoing diversity of practice is not going to change significantly in the near future.

References

1. Morrison CA, Carrick MM, Norman MA, Scott BG, Welsh FJ, Tsai P, et al. Hypotensive resuscitation strategy reduces transfusion requirements and severe postoperative coagulopathy in trauma patients with hemorrhagic shock: preliminary results of a randomized controlled trial. J Trauma. 2011;70(3):62–3.
2. Brown JB, Guyette FX, Neal MD, Claridge JA, Daley BJ, Harbrecht BG, et al. Taking the blood bank to the field: the design and rationale of the prehospital air medical plasma (PAMPer) trial. Prehosp Emerg Care. 2015;19(3):343–50.
3. Gordic S, Alkadhi H, Hodel S, Simmen HP, Brueesch M, Frauenfelder T, et al. Whole-body CT-based imaging algorithm for multiple trauma patients: radiation dose and time to diagnosis. Br J Radiol. 2015;88(1047):20140616.

Part XIV
Perioperative

Do Herbal Supplements Create Unnecessary Risk for Patients?

115

Mark R. Jones, Francisco Calixto, and Alan David Kaye

Case

As the resident anesthesiologist preparing for a scheduled total thyroidectomy on a Friday morning, I hurried into the preoperative ward to assess my patient. We were already behind on the day, and a palpable angst hung thick in the operating room (OR) as we headed into a holiday weekend. I ran through the patient's medications with her at the bedside. Her past medical history included coronary artery disease with a bare metal stent (BMS) placed a little over a year ago. She assured me that, as instructed, she hadn't taken her aspirin or clopidogrel for 7 days. When she reached into her purse for the slip of paper with her medication timetable, I noticed a green prescription bottle with what appeared to be tables of indications, adverse reactions and the like listed upon it.

"What's in that bottle?" I asked her.

"Oh, that's garlic," she replied. "My sister said it's good for your heart."

Concerned, I dug for some more information. I learned that she had been taking 1000 mg of powdered garlic capsules daily for the past 2½ weeks, with her last dose just this morning. The patient's preoperative assessment form, completed 3 weeks ago in the preoperative clinic, did not indicate any supplement use. I asked why she had failed to mention her usage of herbal supplements, to which she simply stated, "No one had ever asked me about it. It's not a drug. It's natural."

M.R. Jones
Department of Surgery, Harvard Medical School, Brigham and Women's Hospital, Boston, MA 02115, USA

F. Calixto
Department of Anesthesiology, Tulane Medical Center, 1415 Tulane Ave, New Orleans, LA 70112, USA
e-mail: fcalixto@tulane.edu

A.D. Kaye (✉)
Department of Anesthesiology, Louisiana State University Health Sciences Center, Room 656, 1542 Tulane Ave, New Orleans, LA 70112, USA
e-mail: alankaye44@hotmail.com

I knew that garlic can act synergistically with other medications such as warfarin, heparin, and aspirin to increase bleeding time, but I wasn't sure how much of a risk it posed for this potentially bloody procedure [1]. To confuse matters further, she admitted to taking 600 mg of ginseng a day as well to increase her physical stamina. I recalled that ginseng has antiplatelet properties as well [2]. Once more, she nonchalantly brushed off the gap in her medication record, repeating that the supplements are "natural and harmless." I hurried off to find the staff anesthesiologist who planned on starting the case with me.

We nearly collided as he careened around the corner. He was running 2 rooms that day—1 with a critically ill patient undergoing a coronary artery bypass graft. He cut me off midway through my question.

No. It's fine. Garlic and ginseng are perfectly fine. Go ahead with the case.

Question

I remained concerned. Did these herbal supplements create unnecessary risk for the patient?

After the staff gave me the OK, I finished prepping the room for the case. My phone rang shortly after; my attending informed me he was caught up in the heart case and had paged one of his colleagues to come start the thyroidectomy with me.

The new staff anesthesiologist met us as we were rolling the patient back. I greeted her and handed over the preoperative evaluation.

"Everything looks good," she remarked. "Anything else I need to know?"

CON: I told her about the herbal medications, and that the original anesthesiologist scheduled for the case had said not to worry about it. In his experience, garlic and ginseng did not present an issue. The antiplatelet effects of both herbs are modest at most [3].

C.S. Scher et al. (eds.), *You're Wrong, I'm Right*, DOI 10.1007/978-3-319-43169-7_115

"Yes, that's true. They can increase bleeding. But, judging by her normal coagulation panel, there's no cause for concern about overt bleeding," said the new staff anesthesiologist.

"Those coags were run 3 weeks ago," I said.

At this point we had reached the room. The nurses, scrub tech, and surgery resident were finishing up their preparations. The staff anesthesiologist had a nervous look about her, and asked me to go through the patient's history with her once more. I told her that the patient had a bare metal stent placed roughly a year ago, hence the clopidogrel and aspirin. While she had stopped those 7 days prior to surgery, we now had new information: the herbal medications that she had begun after her preop labs were run.

PRO: "This is inappropriate," my staff exclaimed. "We have a non-emergent surgery without an accurate assessment of this patient's bleeding risk. This new information renders the coags we have on her irrelevant. We haven't properly measured her platelet function as it stands right now."

She explained that, while not common, she had seen thyroidectomies bleed extensively. She went on, "Garlic leads to antiplatelet activity via inhibition of thromboxane synthesis by direct non-competitive inhibition with the COX enzyme [4]. In 1 study, after 26 weeks of consuming a clove of fresh garlic a day, thromboxane A2 levels went down by 80 % [4]."

This was no trivial matter, and we needed to postpone the case.

While she ran off to find the surgeon and deliver the news, I decided to look up the American Society of Anesthesiologists (ASA) guidelines on herbal medications [5]. Sure enough, the ASA recommends that all herbal medications be discontinued at least 2 weeks before an elective procedure. I also took a look at the literature, and found recent information on a second mechanism leading to bleeding: Garlic leads to a decrease in the number of functional GPIIb/IIIa receptors on platelets, decreasing the binding of fibrinogen and vWF, and inhibiting platelet aggregation [1].

I could hear the case being discussed outside the room.

CON: Naturally, the surgeon was upset. "I've performed hundreds of these cases, and you know what? Sometimes the patient is taking an herbal supplement. There's never going to be a perfect scenario, and there will always be risk involved in surgery." He motioned to the operating room, all ready to go. "You want to waste all this time and money? That's a big expense to write off, don't you think?"

PRO: "The bottom line," the staff anesthesiologist explained, "is that we had no way of immediately assessing this patient's risk. Compounding the risk was the fact that this patient has also been taking ginger, which exhibits significant antiplatelet action via inhibition of the arachidonic acid pathway and by decreasing thromboxane synthetase, thereby prolonging bleeding time [6, 7]."

With this procedure we had to consider not only the intraoperative bleeding involved, but also the increased risk of airway collapse with postoperative hematoma formation. On top of it all, this elderly patient had multiple risk factors and comorbidities, which further increased her risk status [8, 9]. I gave her the ASA guidelines on my phone, which supported what I told her. She showed these recommendations to the surgeon and referenced the literature that enforced the risk of increased bleeding time associated with these supplements [1–4, 6–8, 10, 11].

While we were all disappointed to cancel the case, we could not allow our eagerness to overwhelm what was the correct course of action. In all likelihood, we would have been able to perform this case and get away with it. But shooting from the hip in the face of the unknown is not proper medicine, and we knew that. The surgeon begrudgingly accepted, and agreed to postpone the case for a later date.

Summary

The dietary supplement industry has seen a vast proliferation in recent years, propelled largely by unsubstantiated promises of health benefits and "natural" cures for many ubiquitous medical conditions. Whether they be herbals, vitamins, minerals, amino acids, or enzymes, these seemingly benign supplements do, in fact, have important pharmacokinetic and pharmacodynamic implications. Given the right setting, they can easily and ultimately provoke serious perioperative complications. To further exacerbate the situation, while it is estimated that more than 55 million US adults report using supplements in their lifetime, as many as 70 % of these patients do not disclose their use of these supplements if they are not specifically asked [9, 12]. Thus, it is imperative for the anesthesiologist to be thorough during the preoperative evaluation, and to explicitly inquire about all potential dietary supplements consumed by the patient. This will help to eliminate the confusion often encountered by patients who misconstrue what is necessary to disclose medication-wise. Likewise, it is essential for the practitioner to understand the multifaceted implications of each supplement listed, particularly the potential effect on the patient's perioperative hemodynamics, coagulation status, central nervous system function and endocrine system. The American Society of Anesthesiologists currently recommends that all dietary supplements be discontinued 2 weeks prior to an elective surgical procedure.

The anesthesiologist must be vigilant regarding some of the more common supplements that may affect blood loss, such as: bilberry, bromelain, dong quoi, feverfew, fish oil, flax seed oil, garlic, ginger, gingko biloba, grade seed extract, saw palmetto, chamomile, dandelion root, horse chestnut, vitamin K, and vitamin E [5].

References

1. Bordia A. Effect of garlic on human platelet aggregation in vitro. Atherosclerosis. 1978;30:355–60.
2. Kuo SC, Teng CM, Lee JC, Ko FN, Chen SC, Wu TS. Antiplatelet components in Panax ginseng. Planta Med. 1990;56(2):164–7.
3. Amico AP, Terlizzi A, Damiani S, Ranieri M, Megna M, Fiore P. Immunopharmacology of the main herbal supplements: a review. Endocr Metab Immune Disord Drug Targets. 2013;13(4):283–8.
4. Ali M, Thomson M, Afzal M. Garlic and onions: their effect on eicosanoid metabolism and its clinical relevance. Prostaglandins Leukot Essent Fatty Acids. 2000;62(2):55–73.
5. Apfelbaum JL, et al. American Society of Anesthesiologists. Practice guidelines for perioperative blood management. An updated report by the American Society of Anesthesiologists Task Force on Perioperative Blood Management. Anesthesiology. 2015;122(2):241–75.
6. Backon J. Ginger: inhibition of thromboxane synthetase and stimulation of prostacyclin: relevance for medicine and psychiatry. Med Hypotheses. 1986;20:271–8.
7. Nurtjahja-Tjendraputra E, Ammit AJ, Roufogalis BD, Tran VH, Duke CC. Effective anti-platelet and COX-1 enzyme inhibitors from pungent constituents of ginger. Thromb Res. 2003;111(4–5):259–65.
8. Tachjian A, Maria V, Jahangir A. Use of herbal products and potential interactions in patients with cardiovascular diseases. J Am Coll Cardiol. 2010;55(6):515–25.
9. de Souza Silva JE, Santos Souza CA, da Silva TB, Gomes IA, Brito Gde C, de Souza Araújo AA, et al. Use of herbal medicines by elderly patients: a systematic review. Arch Gerontol Geriatr. 2014;59(2):227–33.
10. Apitz-Castro R, Badimon JJ, Badimon L. Effect of ajoene, the major antiplatelet compound from garlic, on platelet thrombus formation. Thromb Res. 1992;68(2):145–55.
11. Kaye AD, Sabar R, Vig S, Ricaldi C, Kaye AM, Hofbauer R, Heavner JE. Nutraceuticals—current concepts and the role of the anesthesiologist. Part 2. Panax ginseng, kava kava, feverfew and ma huang. Am J Anesthesiol. 2000;27(8):467–71.
12. Kaye AD, Clarke RC, Sabar R, Vig S, Dhawan KP, Hofbauer R, Kaye AM. Herbal medicines: current trends in anesthesiology practice—a hospital survey. J Clin Anesth. 2000;12(6):468–71.

How Much Evaluation of the Airway Is Essential Prior to Anesthesia?

116

Levon M. Capan, Sanford M. Miller, and Corey S. Scher

Case

A 60-year-old man, 165 cm tall and weighing 90 kg, is scheduled for sigmoid colectomy. He has no history of cardiac, respiratory, or other vital organ disease, allergies, or licit or illicit drug use. He complains of pain in his joints. Four years ago he underwent an inguinal herniorrhaphy with general anesthesia, apparently, as he states, without any anesthetic problem.

The preoperative anesthetic evaluation is performed by the CA1 anesthesia resident scheduled to administer the anesthetic under the supervision of an anesthesiologist the next day. His airway evaluation consists of the patient's Mallampati score, which reveals a visible uvula, and measuring a thyromental distance, which is 4 cm. Upon the resident's presentation of the case, his supervising attending asks for additional airway evaluation findings.

Question

Should your airway evaluation be limited to the Mallampati score and the thyromental distance?

PRO: Yes. I do not think we need any further airway evaluation with our current airway algorithms and technologies. In the past 30 years, we have seen the widespread use of intubating supraglottic airways (SGAs), such as the laryngeal mask airway (LMA), flexible fiber-optic bronchoscopes, videolaryngoscopes, bougies, and sophisticated stylets. Obviously, it is important to look at and examine the patient, but I am not totally convinced that extensive evaluation beyond the Mallampati score and thyromental distance measurement, and even those two tests, specifically provide us with clinically useful information.

CON: I disagree and will try to explain the reason for my disagreement, but can you first tell me about the evidence behind your statements?

PRO: Numerous existing studies show that the tests designed to predict difficult intubation may predict easy intubation (specificity) better than difficult intubation (sensitivity), but they are not 100 % sensitive or specific. The reason was succinctly explained by Yentis [1] in a 2002 editorial: Because of the overlap in features between the easy and difficult intubation populations, there is no existing test capable of separating these patients with absolute accuracy. The best these tests can do is to separate them into discrete groups, but there is enough overlap to result in a much less than absolute sensitivity, specificity, and positive and negative predictive values for the difficulty of intubation. Then, the clinician has 2 choices: either to consider subjecting some of the predicted but not actually difficult patients to special airway management maneuvers, or to do the opposite by applying conventional management techniques to some of the predicted easy but actually difficult patients, which may result in disastrous complications.

When airway management techniques were limited to Macintosh or Miller blades and flexible fiber-optic bronchoscopes, airway evaluation was very important. Failing to secure the airway with conventional blades meant that your only other options were fiber-optic bronchoscopic guidance

L.M. Capan (✉) · C.S. Scher
Department of Anesthesiology, Perioperative Care and Pain Medicine, New York University School of Medicine, 560 First Avenue, New York, NY 10016, USA
e-mail: Levon.Capan@nyumc.org

C.S. Scher
e-mail: coreyscher@gmail.com

S.M. Miller
New York University School of Medicine, New York, NY, USA
e-mail: sanfordmmiller@gmail.com

S.M. Miller
Department of Anesthesiology, Bellevue Hospital Center, 27th Street and First Avenue, New York, NY 10016, USA

C.S. Scher et al. (eds.), *You're Wrong, I'm Right*, DOI 10.1007/978-3-319-43169-7_116

either asleep or awake, or a surgical airway. Converting to an awake fiber-optic intubation, however, involves significant additional preparation, time loss, and risk in the presence of edematous airway structures after multiple laryngoscopy attempts. Now, failed intubation with conventional direct laryngoscopy can in some cases be rescued without a long preparation—with a videolaryngoscope or a supraglottic airway with the endotracheal tube then successfully directed under direct vision with the videolaryngoscope or blindly through the supraglottic airway. So I believe that a detailed airway evaluation in a patient with normal-looking facial anatomy, and without a history of disease that would contribute to difficult intubation, will not necessarily improve outcomes, given the current advances in airway management.

CON: I believe this matter is not that simple. Obtaining an adequate airway history and examination is essential. For example, aspiration, obstructive sleep apnea (OSA), and morbid obesity are 3 common causes of morbidity and mortality irrespective of the technique used. Regurgitation or vomiting resulting in aspiration of gastric contents, and the potential for aspiration pneumonitis, is more likely in patients with a history of gastroesophageal reflux disease (GERD) and factors that delay gastric emptying such as opioid use, pregnancy, or diabetes. Obviously, recent food intake increases the likelihood of aspiration as well. Ultrasonographic evaluation of gastric contents by examining the diameter of the gastric antrum may be able to determine the presence of a full stomach [2]; however, further studies are needed to establish diagnostic reliability. Patients with obstructive sleep apnea (OSA) will likely have symptoms of frequent awakening and gasping for air during sleep or snoring loud enough to be heard through a door. Also, a short questionnaire, the STOP-Bang algorithm can be used [3]. Although some patients with OSA are not obese, those with obesity may be more likely to be difficult to ventilate by mask or supraglottic airway (SGA), or to be difficult to intubate by conventional laryngoscopy. A history of easy airway management during a previous surgery does not necessarily eliminate the possibility of a difficult intubation. A patient may have gained weight, or underlying disease such as jaw arthritis or a tumor impinging on the airway may have worsened, or head and neck radiation may have distorted the airway anatomy.

Determining the inter-incisor gap provides definitive information, if it is less than 2 cm, it will be impossible to introduce either a conventional or a videolaryngoscope, and an awake fiber-optic intubation will be required. I agree that the conventional airway evaluation measures such as thyromental distance, Mallampati score, chin protrusion, compliance of mandibular space, length and thickness of the neck, and neck range of movement are less useful in providing information about the ease or difficulty of intubation with videolaryngoscopy [4]. Nevertheless, a thorough airway examination should be performed in case conventional laryngoscopy will be used. It should be added that even in patients with a normal airway examination and unremarkable history, laryngoscopy may be impossible. This is often due to the presence of lingual tonsillar hypertrophy blocking the glottis opening, which cannot typically be determined on history or physical.

PRO: As you mentioned, with the exception of mouth opening, the rest of the airway examination does not apply to videolaryngoscopy. Also, airway evaluation measures for laryngoscopy with conventional blades are not highly predictive. Why not use a videolaryngoscope routinely then to improve the success rate and also to eliminate the need for a pre-intubation examination?

CON: Although the available evidence suggests that intubation with a videolaryngoscope results in greater success than with conventional blades, the videolaryngoscope is by no means an absolute guarantee of successful intubation [5]. In fact, there are instances when intubation fails with videolaryngoscopy but is successful using conventional blades [6, 7]. Similarly, a supraglottic airway is an outstanding rescue device, and can often be used as a guide to facilitate fiber-optic intubation, but also will fail in some cases. If there is any question that a case could become a "can't intubate, can't ventilate" situation, an awake intubation, or non-general anesthetic technique when possible (regional or local anesthesia) should be used.

True, the sensitivities and specificities of individual airway assessment tests may be low, but their usefulness increases when they are combined. For example, multifactorial risk assessment for difficult intubation using conventional airway evaluation tests have sensitivities of 60–95 % and specificities of 65–92 %, which, given a 2–3 % difficult intubation rate, results in a low positive predictive value (18 %) but a high negative predictive value (99 %) [8]. Thus, by performing a thorough evaluation we can improve our prediction of easy intubation with conventional laryngoscopy. Preoperative airway evaluation is performed to plan for airway management. The preoperative evaluation not only is used to guide our evaluation of intubation difficulty, but also to determine whether mask ventilation will be feasible, and if a supraglottic airway is appropriate. Risks increase in patients with a full stomach or in circumstances when the head of the patient will be away from the anesthesiologist. Additionally, in patients with a potential difficult airway, it may be appropriate to have an additional fully trained anesthesiologist in the room for induction and extubation. In the Fourth National Audit Project of the United Kingdom (NAP4) performed by the Royal College of Anaesthetists, one of the causes of undesirable airway outcomes in critical care and emergency department units (although not in elective operating room patients) was inadequate airway evaluation and planning [9]. Thus I believe proper airway evaluation is essential prior to attempting any airway management.

PRO: I am still somewhat surprised that videolaryngoscopy is not considered a default intubation technique in most institutions. Most of the currently available videolaryngoscopes have a lens or video chip attached to the distal end of the blade and are capable of transmitting the magnified images to a display screen. Thus, they permit a direct view of the glottic opening by the operator and also by others in the room. They are easy to use in the operating room and also in remote locations, including the prehospital setting, and require minimal setup time. Appropriately sized videolaryngoscopes can rescue failed direct laryngoscopy in both adults and children, they can be used in sedated awake patients when the airway is anesthetized with topical anesthetics, they provide a better view with less vertebral movement in immobilized patients with cervical spine disease, and they allow more successful intubation by individuals less trained in airway management [10]. Unlike conventional laryngoscopy, which requires establishment of a straight line between the operator's eye and the glottis, videolaryngoscopes, can look "around the corner," and do not require force on the soft tissues or unusual head and neck positioning. Thus, trauma to the supraglottic structures is probably less likely and less severe [10].

CON: Most of the advantages you mentioned for videolaryngoscopy are true. Indeed, the success rate of intubation is close to 100 % (98 %) and the rescue rate by these scopes after failed direct laryngoscopy is about 94 % [5]. However, directing the endotracheal tube into the larynx may be difficult for several reasons. The path of the tube requires a much sharper curve than the conventional "hockey stick" tip deflection. Thus, unless a stylet with almost the same curve as the videolaryngoscope blade is used, directing the tube to the larynx may become difficult. Also, the bulk of the videolaryngoscope blade leaves little room to manipulate the tube toward the larynx, especially if there is a space-occupying lesion, such as a malignancy, extensive infection, or fixation of the oropharyngeal soft tissue as occurs in patients with prior radiotherapy to the head and neck [5]. Additionally, blood or secretions in the oropharynx, even in small quantities, may obstruct the view by smudging the lens of the videolaryngoscope. It is not possible to remove such secretions with a flexible suction catheter as the catheter often does not follow the curve of the blade and thus cannot be directed accurately [10]. Intraoral blood and secretions do not cause obstruction of the view as easily during conventional laryngoscopy, and due to the direct line between the anesthesiologist's eye and the vocal cords, can often be suctioned out with a standard suction catheter.

Summary

Traditional airway assessment performed for conventional laryngoscopy, and intubation is the standard of care and must be performed routinely irrespective of the type of airway management device or technique used. Although airway assessment methods used for conventional laryngoscopy are little help for videolaryngoscopic or supraglottic airway facilitated intubation, they should be performed routinely; in case, there is a need to rescue a failed videolaryngoscopic intubation with conventional laryngoscopy. If ventilation or intubation may be impossible, an alternate anesthetic technique (local or regional) should be used when possible. If general anesthesia is needed, an awake intubation should be performed. Routine use of the videolaryngoscope for airway management is a controversial issue, and there is a need for further scientifically rigorous study results to embark on such decisions.

References

1. Yentis SM. Predicting difficult intubation—worthwhile exercise or pointless ritual. Anaesthesia. 2002;57:105–9.
2. Perlas A, Chan VWS, Lupu CM, Mitsakakis N, Hanbidge A. Ultrasound assessment of gastric content and volume. Anesthesiology. 2009;111:82–9.
3. Chung F, Subramanyam R, Liao P, Sasaki E, Shapiro C, Sun Y. High STOP Bang score indicates a high probability of obstructive sleep apnoea. Br J Anaesth. 2012;108:768–75.
4. Saleem MM, Ahmed-Nusrath A. Should videolaryngoscopes be used in difficult airways? Br J Hosp Med. 2012;73:478.
5. Aziz MF, Healy D, Kheterpal S, Fu RF, Dillman D, Bambrink AM. Routine clinical practice effectiveness of the Glidescope in difficult airway management: an analysis of 2004 GlideScope intubations, complications, and failures from two institutions. Anesthesiology. 2011;114:34–41.
6. Cavus E, Callies A, Doerges V, Heller G, Merz S, Rösch P, et al. The C-MAC videolaryngoscope for prehospital emergency intubation: a prospective multicenter, observational study. Emerg Med J. 2011;28:650–3.
7. Brown CA, Bair AE, Pallin DJ, Laurin EG, Walls RM, National Emergency Airway registry (NEAR) investigators. Improved glottis exposure with the video macintosh laryngoscope in adult emergency department tracheal intubations. Ann Emerg Med. 2010;56:83–8.

8. Anderson J, Klock PA. Airway management. Anesthesiol Clin. 2014;32:445–61.
9. Cook TM, Woodall N, Harper J, Benger J. Fourth national audit project; Major complications of airway management in the UK: results of the Fourth National Audit Project of the Royal College of Anaesthetists and Difficult Airway Society. Part 2: intensive care and emergency departments. Br J Anaesth. 2011;106:632–42.
10. Rothfield KP, Russo SG. Videolaryngoscopy: should it replace direct laryngoscopy? A pro-con debate. J Clin Anesth. 2012;24:593–7.

Are There Concerns with Using Droperidol for Sedation for an Awake Fiberoptic Intubation?

117

Corey S. Scher

Case

A 60-year-old patient with a history of squamous cell carcinoma on the floor of his mouth presents for esophageal dilation, which is needed after his radiation, chemotherapy, and surgery. The tumor was completely resected and he has a flap to his face and neck to cover an extensive wound. Of late, he has had a problem eating solid food as a result of a narrowed esophageal lumen. It is hoped that the dilation will allow him to eat and maintain his current weight. From the airway examination and history, it is obvious that an awake fiberoptic intubation is the safest course of action. Due to what appears to be a treacherous airway, a second attending anesthesiologist is asked to join the resident and assigned anesthesiologist.

Attending 1 explains, "There are 3 components to the awake fiberoptic intubation that are essential for success: excellent nerve blockade, outstanding sedation that does not compromise respiration, and a detailed preprocedure discussion that makes each step crystal clear so the patient never panics."

"So, what is your sedation plan?" the resident asks.

"I start with 10–15 mg of droperidol, an infusion of 0.7 mcg/kg/h of dexmedetomidine with a small dose of ketamine (10–20 mg). With dexmedetomidine alone, patients arouse very easily. I do not give fentanyl ever or any other drug that is a respiratory depressant as once he becomes apncic wc could casily lose the airway."

C.S. Scher (✉)
Department of Anesthesiology, Perioperative Care and Pain Medicine, New York University School of Medicine, New York, NY 10016, USA
e-mail: coreyscher@gmail.com

Question

Is droperidol a good choice for sedation during an awake fiberoptic intubation?

CON (Attending 2): Ten to 15 mg of droperidol! You must be crazy. He will sleep forever. Also, the drug has a black box warning, because it could prolong the Q–T interval and make the patient at risk for torsades de pointes. Should you not get an electrocardiogram (EKG), to obtain a baseline Q–T interval before giving a drug that could increase the QT interval further?

PRO: If I said haldol and not droperidol, would that make a difference? We give haldol to disruptive patients in similar doses and keep going until the patient is calm. We do not seem to care, yet it does not impact the Q–T interval any differently than droperidol. Psychiatrists prescribe both atypical and classic antipsychotics all the time without an EKG or concern for the Q–T interval. I am not sure that this is even an issue. In a study by Calver et al. [1], more than 1000 patients in the emergency room were given high-dose droperidol for sedation. Many of these patients were taking medications known to increase the Q–T interval, yet none experienced torsades. That study was published in 2015.

CON: The black box warning did not come from outer space, and despite your claim or personal feelings, droperidol is still on the list. There is no indication that it is going to be taken off. I have been successful with midazolam and fentanyl and have never had a patient go apneic. I also use the spray-as-you-go technique as I move down the airway with a syringe of 2 % lidocaine attached to the port on the fiberoptic scope.

PRO: Several recent studies from the past 3 years strongly declare that what I do with droperidol is safe in regard to the Q–T interval and avoiding torsades [2–4]. Macht et al. [2]

C.S. Scher et al. (eds.), *You're Wrong, I'm Right*, DOI 10.1007/978-3-319-43169-7_117

found that in 532 agitated patients given haloperidol or droperidol outside of the hospital, no significant difference existed in QTc prolongation, adverse events, or need for repeat sedation between the groups who were given haloperidol and those administered droperidol. The mean droperidol dose in this study was 7.9 mg [2]. Nuttall et al. [3] found that low-dose droperidol does not increase the incidence of polymorphic VT or death when used in a dose of 0.625 mg to treat postoperative nausea and vomiting in the surgical population, in a large population study of 20,122 patients who received 35,000 doses of droperidol.

Torsades is triggered by a prolongation of cardiac repolarization [4]. The contribution of many anesthetic drugs to "torsadogenicity" has been studied and detailed in a review article by Staikou et al. (Table 117.1) [4].

As you can see, most of what we use each day might induce torsades. Droperidol is just one of many drugs on the list. We don't worry about torsades every time we turn on the desflurane.

CON: Why would you use 10–15 mg though?! The patient will sleep forever.

PRO: Full effect could take 30 min with a lower dose. Anesthesiologists do not like to wait. When the full effect is achieved, the patient becomes "chemically handcuffed" and will do whatever is asked of him or her. This translates into opening his mouth and taking a deep breath, which results in open vocal cords. The patient will hold his breath for long enough that you can do the fiberoptic intubation. The only downside is that maximum sedation may occur after a short case is over.

CON: I get great sedation with my technique. I can reverse the fentanyl and the midazolam. You cannot reverse the droperidol if the case is short and you may wait over an hour for the patient to wake up. I am not changing my technique; or better stated, I am not making any changes when I teach a student fiberoptic intubation.

Table 117.1 Anesthetic drugs and electrocardiogram (ECG) signs of torsadogenicity

Drug	QT interval	QT corrected for HR (Qtc)	Transmural dispersion of repolarization
Isoflurane		++	
Desflurane		++	
Sevoflurane		+	∅
Propofol		Min or −	Min
Fentanyl		∅	
Alfentanil		∅	
Remifentanil		∅	
Sufentanil	+ at high doses		
Succinylcholine		+, lessened by opioids, β(beta)-blockers	
Non-depolarizing neuromuscular blockers		∅	
Anticholinesterase–anticholinergic agents together (neuromuscular blockade reversal)		++	
Sugammadex		∅ in low or high doses	
Local anesthetics		∅	
Subarachnoid sympathetic block		+ if extensive	
Thoracic epidural anesthesia		−	−
Midazolam		∅	∅
Droperidol, domperidone, 5-HT3 antagonists		++	

Based on information from [4]
+ = prolongs that interval
++ = "significantly" prolongs that interval
∅ = No effect
Min = minimal effect
− = decreases that interval

PRO: The next time I do a fiberoptic intubation, I will grab you to show you how smooth the procedure is with droperidol.

CON: I still maintain it is a muddled topic. I do agree that anti-emetic doses of droperidol are safe, but I am not convinced that a larger dose is OK.

PRO: The paper where droperidol was given in a mean dose of 8 mg in the emergency room says it all [2]. Any sensible literature on the topic will look at QT corrected for heart rate (QTc). Obviously, the QT interval increases when the heart rate slows, making any study that looks only at the QT interval worthless.

CON: If I was taking the oral boards, I would never bring up the topic of droperidol at the doses you suggest. Perhaps high doses are safe, but since I have been fortunate to use my midazolam/fentanyl combination with great success, I have no reason to get into this muddled zone. I have looked at PubMed, and I see that you are citing only the prodroperidol paper and ignoring the countless papers that conclude there remains a significant danger with those drugs that increase the QT interval.

PRO: Once you turn on your inhaled anesthetics and give ondansetron, you are back in the muddled zone. Why are you OK with sevoflurane and ondansetron when the QT prolongation is more than significant? When have you seen or heard of a psych patient given haldol go into torsades? It is ridiculous.

CON: Again, you may be right but I have no place in my practice for large doses of droperidol.

Summary

With the current ongoing drug shortages, many hospitals no longer have first-line drugs for fiberoptic intubation such as dexmedetomidine and ketamine, and clinicians have become experts with other drugs that do not depress ventilation such as droperidol. While I am certain that high-dose droperidol is safe, as demonstrated in the old days with the use of Innovar (combination of droperidol and fentanyl), I no longer use it. It is not available in our practice and may never be back in our anesthesia carts. I have moved on for practical reasons to other medications for sedation for the awake fiberoptic. I am no longer in mourning for droperidol.

References

1. Calver L, Page CB, Downes MA, Chan B, Kinnear F, Wheatley L, et al. The safety and effectiveness of droperidol for sedation of acute behavioral disturbance in the emergency department. Ann Emerg Med. 2015;66(3):230.e1–238.e1.
2. Macht M, Mull AC, McVaney KE, Caruso EH, Johnston JB, Gaither JB, et al. Comparison of droperidol and haloperidol for use by paramedics: assessment of safety and effectiveness. Prehosp Emerg Care. 2014;18(3):375–8.
3. Nuttall GA, Malone AM, Michels CA, Trudell LC, Renk TD, Marienau ME, et al. Does low-dose droperidol increase the risk of polymorphic ventricular tachycardia or death in the surgical patient? Anesthesiology. 2013;118(2):382–6.
4. Staikou C, Stamelos M, Stavroulakis E. Impact of anesthetic drugs and adjuvants on ECG markers of torsadogenicity. Br J Anaesth. 2014;112(2):217–30.

Do Special Measures—Such as Postoperative CPAP, a Prolonged PACU Stay, and PACU EtCO2 Monitoring—Improve the Outcome in a Patient with Obstructive Sleep Apnea?

118

Brent J. Luria

Case

As the anesthesiologist in charge, I was kept informed of all complications in the post-anesthesia care unit (PACU). Most, when investigated, were isolated incidents and not systemic PACU deficiencies. However, over a few weeks last January, a man was found with an oxygen saturation of 89 % requiring opioid reversal, and then a woman had a full respiratory arrest resulting in reintubation. Three similar cases in February set all of us on edge. With some detective work and analysis, one commonality was discovered: All carried a preoperative diagnosis of obstructive sleep apnea (OSA). Was this coincidence or connection? The department chairman wisely asked me to look into the issue and to suggest solutions. My mission was to decide whether patients with OSA should be treated differently in the PACU and to implement new policies to improve patient safety (and not unduly utilize resources).

As a faculty member at a teaching hospital, I, of course, turned this into a teaching opportunity. I found two eager residents, each to investigate and debate one side of the topic. A few days later, we sat down together:

Question

Do special measures such as postoperative continuous positive airway pressure (CPAP), a prolonged PACU stay, and PACU end-tidal carbon dioxide (EtCO2) monitoring improve outcomes in patients with OSA?

B.J. Luria (✉)
Department of Anesthesiology, Perioperative Care and Pain Medicine, New York University Langone Medical Center, 550 First Avenue, New York, NY 10016, USA
e-mail: Brent.luria@nyumc.org

PRO: Dr. Luria, I reviewed the literature and considered this topic and one thing is abundantly clear to me: The only safe option to minimize respiratory complications is to implement new measures for all patients with OSA in the PACU. Specifically, continuous positive airway pressure (CPAP), end-tidal carbon dioxide (EtCO2) monitoring, and a prolonged stay in the PACU or other fully monitored setting. Every patient who walks in the door should be screened for sleep apnea, and a positive result should trigger these measures even if they haven't received a formal diagnosis.

CON: I too have reviewed the literature, and I believe that my fellow resident goes too far. Sure, these precautions are reasonable in patients with known severe sleep apnea. But it is drastic and a misallocation of hospital resources to take these measures on ALL patients with known or suspected sleep apnea without taking into account that the patient could have only a minor degree of OSA, and the procedure could be just a nevus excision with local and a squirt of midazolam. Clinical judgment is required, not another imposed policy.

PRO: I understand that you are more concerned with saving the hospital money than with providing the safest care for our patients, but let me explain where I'm coming from.

First, we can relatively easily identify patients that are at risk of sleep apnea in the preoperative setting with the STOP-Bang survey, which takes 30 s for eight questions (Table 118.1) [1]. Answering yes to three or more questions means likely OSA, and yes to 6 is suspicious for severe OSA [1].

Second, postoperative respiratory complications and likely associated cardiac complications are more common in OSA patients [2].

Third, not only is the percentage of the population with documented OSA rising, but there is a higher prevalence of OSA among patients presenting for surgery than in the general population [2].

C.S. Scher et al. (eds.), *You're Wrong, I'm Right*, DOI 10.1007/978-3-319-43169-7_118

Table 118.1 STOP-Bang questionnaire [1, 7]

1. Snoring Do you snore loudly (louder than talking or loud enough to be heard through closed doors)?
2. Tired Do you often feel tired, fatigued, or sleepy during daytime?
3. Observed Has anyone observed you stop breathing during your sleep?
4. Blood Pressure Do you have or are you being treated for high blood pressure?
5. Body mass index: more than 35 kg/m^2
6. Age over 50 years old?
7. Neck circumference greater than 40 cm? (measured by staff)
8. Gender male?

High risk of OSA answering yes to 3 or more items
Low risk of OSA answering yes to fewer than 3 items

Increasing patient safety regarding OSA is achievable! We can take various preemptive measures with these patients and significantly cut down on the number of postoperative complications.

CON: It's not clear that OSA patients have a much higher risk of respiratory complications in the postoperative period. Most of the studies showing increased risk were small, single-institution, retrospective studies [2]. A meta-analysis used to create the Society for Ambulatory Anesthesia's consensus statement on OSA patients in outpatient settings found absolutely no increased risk of ventilatory assistance, reintubation, or death in patients with OSA [3].

PRO: Perhaps you have fallen behind in your reading. A newer large meta-analysis published in 2014 extracted data from more than 530,000 patients undergoing total hip or total knee arthroplasty at 400 institutions [3]. After controlling for confounding factors, the authors concluded that patients with documented sleep apnea had a higher risk of respiratory complications and a much higher risk of emergent reintubation in the immediate postoperative period.

CON: OK, I will concede that patients with significant, documented obstructive sleep apnea are at an increased risk of a small number of postoperative complications for these two specific surgical procedures. I would like to see studies like this expanded to other surgical procedures before we decide to generalize the findings to all the surgical services. And where's the proof that implementing these extreme new measures in the PACU will decrease complications? Are there any prospective, randomized controlled trials showing that CPAP, EtCO2 monitoring, and prolonged recovery room admissions will cut down on these complications? Just because we have identified a problem does not mean that the measures being proposed here are the perfect or even the best solution.

PRO: Well, you make a valid point. I admit that the data are limited right now. However, given the problems we are having at this institution and the data that are out there, I think that it is a reasonable step to institute these measures. So far we have been pretty lucky. While there have been a few small complications, we have not seen death or permanent disability. But do we really want to wait until something terrible happens before we take preventative measures?

CON: Of course I don't want to see anyone suffer terrible complications as a result of their OSA. But medicine is all about evaluating the risks and benefits of a given test or intervention. In this case, I agree that the interventions you proposed are fairly low risk. But you cannot necessarily predict the poor outcomes that would result from unnecessary utilization of these limited resources. Furthermore, CPAP is not well tolerated by many patients. In fact, it is probably one of the least adhered-to therapies in all of medicine! [4] I can envision patients who are already discombobulated from their surgical procedure, and anesthetic becoming quite agitated if they are forced to wear a CPAP mask while still recovering from anesthesia in the postoperative setting.

PRO: That doesn't mean we shouldn't still try it. Some patients would be willing to endure short-term discomfort for their long-term health. Certainly, I think most patients would prefer wearing a CPAP mask for a few hours to being reintubated in the PACU! Also important to consider is that sleep apnea is underdiagnosed. So many patients in the "no OSA" group in these studies actually do have some symptoms of OSA, are at an increased risk of postoperative complications, and therefore bias the data. If you put the patients with diagnosed and undiagnosed OSA into one group, and those patients exhibiting none of the symptoms of OSA into the other group, I believe that you would see an even bigger difference in the postoperative complication rate.

CON: Given the expense and lack of evidence, let's start with less extreme measures. For example, the Society for Ambulatory Anesthesia consensus statement advises limiting the patients, procedures, and anesthetic techniques in ambulatory settings. Specifically, they advise avoidance of very painful procedures (necessitating a heavy opioid-based anesthetic) or airway procedures on OSA patients as outpatients. Also, patients with OSA whose medical comorbidities are not well-managed are not optimal candidates for ambulatory centers [5]. Instituting these measures at our ambulatory facilities would allow us to meet the standards set by our national organizations without imposing excessive and unnecessary restraints on our patients and overworking our PACU staff.

PRO: I agree that those would be prudent, easily implemented measures. Encouraging opioid-sparing anesthetic techniques is beneficial in both the ambulatory and non-ambulatory settings. However, I don't think that this is sufficient. Is there a set of interventions that would protect our OSA patients from avoidable perioperative complications yet not deplete our resources for little or no benefit?

CON: There are definitely some less labor-intensive interventions we could employ. Let's ask patients who use CPAP at home to bring their equipment or mask for PACU use if they show signs of respiratory insufficiency. Not all OSA patients will need this, but isn't CPAP preferable to reintubation? [6]. I also think that it would be reasonable to institute EtCO2 monitoring in patients requiring oxygen via nasal cannula or face mask in the recovery room. As you know, many of our patients, even those with OSA, are able to maintain their arterial hemoglobin saturation at or near 100 % without supplemental oxygen. I really don't think it is necessary to monitor EtCO2 if the patient is not requiring additional opioid doses and has maintained a high arterial oxygen saturation (SaO2) for >30 min. However, in OSA patients requiring supplemental oxygen in the PACU, monitoring EtCO2 as a method to identify airway obstruction seems to be a simple measure to implement. Obviously, we still need more evidence that these interventions will actually decrease our complication rate, but cost is low and potential is high to improve outcomes without unduly burdening the PACU staff.

PRO: Well, I'm glad that we have been able to reach a compromise on these issues. I would like to do a better job of identifying patients with undiagnosed OSA and apply some of these changes in those patients as well, but I understand that the literature does not yet support this broad of a policy change. What do you think of extending the mandatory PACU length of stay for patients with OSA?

CON: I disagree with writing a policy mandating a longer PACU stay for patients with OSA. We know that some OSA patients are going to recover from anesthesia just as quickly as patients without OSA. What I propose is to do a better job of educating our perioperative staff about OSA. Specifically, I would like to organize a lecture about perioperative management of patients with OSA for our anesthesiologists, the NPs staffing the recovery room, and the PACU nurses. Once we know what signs and symptoms to look for in patients with OSA in the PACU, we can avoid utilizing a "one-size-fits-all" approach.

PRO: I definitely agree. Let's take the next step in research as well.

Summary

Recent literature suggests that obstructive sleep apnea puts patients at an increased risk of postoperative problems, especially respiratory. There are now well-validated tools to identify patients at risk of sleep apnea who have not yet received a formal diagnosis. These tools should be utilized in the preoperative period so that anesthesiologists can use the information to help guide intraoperative and postoperative management. Ensuring that patients with suspected or confirmed OSA are anesthetized in a non-ambulatory setting and utilizing opioid-sparing anesthetic techniques are both low-cost interventions that could be implemented quickly. More resource intensive are the use of postoperative CPAP, EtCO2, and prolonged PACU stays, but these options should at least be available, and consideration should be given to utilizing these for every OSA patient. Further research is needed to determine how to maximize safety while not unnecessarily increasing costs. As an anesthesiologist, volunteering your time to teach educational sessions for all clinicians caring for OSA patients perioperatively should be a priority.

References

1. Chung F, Yang Y, Liao P. Predictive performance of the STOP-Bang score for identifying obstructive sleep apnea in obese patients. Obes Surg. 2013;23(12):2050–7.
2. Memtsoudis S, Liu SS, Ma Y, Chiu YL, Walz JM, Gaber-Baylis LK, Mazumdar M. Perioperative pulmonary outcomes in patients with

sleep apnea after noncardiac surgery. Anesth Analg. 2011;112: 113–21.
3. Memtsoudis SG, Studner O, Rasul R, Chiu YL, Sun X, Ramachandran SK, et al. The impact of sleep apnea on postoperative utilization of resources and adverse outcomes. Anesth Analg. 2014;118:407–14.
4. Weaver TE, Grunstein RR. Adherence to continuous positive airway pressure therapy: the challenge to effective treatment. Proc Am Thorac Soc. 2008;5(2):173–8.
5. Joshi GP, Ankichetty SP, Gan TJ, Chung F. Society for Ambulatory Anesthesia Consensus Statement on preoperative selection of adult patients with obstructive sleep apnea scheduled for ambulatory surgery. Anesth Analg. 2012;115:1060–8.
6. Mutter TC, Chateau D, Moffatt M, Ramsey C, Roos LL, Kryger M. A matched cohort study of postoperative outcomes in obstructive sleep apnea. Anesthesiology. 2014;121:707–18.
7. The American Sleep Apnea Association (US). STOP-Bang Questionnaire. http://www.sleepapnea.org/assets/files/pdf/STOPBANG%20Questionnaire.pdf. Accessed 25 Apr 2015.

Part XV
Professionalism

Do not Resuscitate: What Does that Mean Perioperatively?

119

Elizabeth A.M. Frost

Case

You are running a little late this morning. That could be a problem as today's surgeon is not known for his patience. Glancing at the schedule you see it is a "redo" heart. You meet your patient in the holding area and review his chart, and the preanesthetic assessment completed by a colleague a few days ago. He is a 69-year-old man who has undergone several stent placements over the past 5 years, an aortic valve replacement 3 years ago, and a coronary artery bypass 2 years ago. He still has severe angina and is very limited in his daily activities. He has several comorbidities including diabetes, retinopathy, and end-stage renal disease, requiring dialysis.

As you are explaining your anesthetic plan to the patient, he hands you a completed advance directive and says he wants it followed.

You approach the surgeon and telling him that this document must be reviewed. He replies, "You may not realize it but it is already 7:30 and I have 2 more cases to do today, so let's just forget about it and get on with things."

Question

Do the consequences of anesthesia and surgery allow automatic suspension of do not resuscitate (DNR) orders perioperatively?

PRO: Look, I am a surgeon. When I was training we had none of this nonsense. DNR stuff was simply suspended when the patient signed consent, which means that he has agreed to surgery and all that goes with it. Sure there is a risk. There is a risk in every minute that you breathe. The only hope this guy has is if I can improve the blood flow to his myocardium. Then, his angina will go away and he will be fine.

CON: True, back in the 1990s we did suspend orders. For witnessed intraoperative arrests, closed chest massage was applied to any patient in cardiopulmonary arrest. In fact, dying in the hospital meant cardiopulmonary resuscitation (CPR) for everyone, no matter their wishes. But, you know, as long ago as the mid-1970s decisions not to resuscitate were formalized by the American Heart Association (AHA) [1]. Some 20 years later, it was more officially recognized that patients' autonomy and self-determination were compromised in order to qualify for surgery. The American Society of Anesthesiologists (ASA) drew up a policy of "required reconsideration" that has been updated several times [2]. And what's more, even with your brilliant surgery, he still has lots of other comorbidities that will not improve.

PRO: You don't know when this thing was written, if it has been updated, and what his condition was at that point. With whom did he discuss it? Who wrote it? Was he given accurate prognostic information? He never discussed any of this with me so I don't think he knows what he is talking about.

CON: It is dated as of last week. I guess he talked to his primary care physician and cardiologist. There are lots of notes about his condition in the chart from those two. They note he is "optimized" but even at that he is pretty sick. But, given this "clearance" I imagine his doctors expect him to survive. I would make him an ASA 4. I do think we must talk to him together to find out exactly what he wants.

PRO: Yes, well you better. After all you are the one who is going to take him to the brink of death, paralyze him, breathe for him, probably drop his blood pressure to almost nothing, or make it so high that he bleeds, leave him in severe pain

E.A.M. Frost
Icahn Medical Center at Mount Sinai, 1 Gustav L Levy Place, New York, NY 10029, USA

E.A.M. Frost (✉)
2 Pondview West, Purchase, NY 10577, USA
e-mail: elzfrost@aol.com; elizabeth.frost@mountsinai.org

C.S. Scher et al. (eds.), *You're Wrong, I'm Right*, DOI 10.1007/978-3-319-43169-7_119

afterward and vomiting his head off…unless you overdose him and he stays on a ventilator forever and gets pneumonia. Or maybe you are scared and don't give him enough anesthesia so he remembers everything. Any way around, you are the one he should be most scared of.

CON: Anesthesia is a controlled state of unconsciousness. With all the monitors I intend to use, I can ensure that he will be adequately and appropriately anesthetized. But what if his disease is such that you cannot get him off bypass and his myocardial function is insufficient for spontaneous return? You must explain the risks and see what he understands and how much resuscitation beyond the routine reversal of drug action, mine and yours, he wants, including a period of vasopressor infusions.

PRO: As you just outlined, operating room (OR) management is very different from ward care. We have all the drugs and means and training to keep the patient alive, or at least his heart going. Have you even considered what it is like to have a death in the OR? As Ewanchuk and Brindley pointed out, death in the OR means huge time delays, long debriefing of the staff, no time for the relatives to see the patient to say good-bye, no religious rights can be observed [1]. It is absolutely clear… just keep him going no matter what and take him to the intensive care unit (ICU) where they can take him off life support in a controlled manner. That way, he died because the drugs didn't work anymore. It was not a surgical death. Anyway, you don't know that he won't miraculously wake up and do fine.

CON: The ICU staff doesn't appreciate having a patient who is dying or brain dead dumped on them. It is even more traumatic for them as they feel they are being used. We must talk to the patient's relatives after we find out what he wants and make sure they are also on the same page and understand and are prepared for what might happen. He can see a religious leader in the holding area if he wishes…they are all on call and available.

PRO: I don't believe that this hospital has a policy for allowing DNR orders to stay in place… I know that the other place where I work never gives me a hard time like this.

CON: This hospital does have a policy, drawn up by the ethics committee, which has representation from the departments of anesthesia and surgery and was approved several years ago by the hospital board. But I know what you are saying. Sadly, Hardin and Yusufaly did a study and found that 68 % of physicians made decisions inconsistent with advanced directives [3]. And these findings were confirmed more recently by Byrne and others when they recognized that many health care providers do not recognize the complexity and significance of the DNR order [4]. Moreover, Maxwell and others showed that DNR status is associated with worse outcomes in just the type of surgery you are planning today [5].

PRO: But all orders are not the same are they? Can we still ignore this one?

CON: True and not true. An advance directive is written or verbal instructions from the patient before his illness or surgery. It may include a health care proxy, DNR order, and a living will, and it must be followed intraoperatively. As long as the patient is conscious, the decision rests with him. A DNR order instructs the medical staff not to try to revive a patient in cardiopulmonary arrest. It may be requested by all adults if 2 witnesses are present and may be applicable to minors in some cases. It may also be ordered by a health care proxy who has been appointed as a health care agent and gives him or her signatory rights. The health care proxy must be identified by signature on the applicable form. A written will specifies instructions about medical care and is evidence of the patient's wishes if he is too ill to communicate. It does not require a health care proxy but must be adhered to perioperatively.

Concession from PRO: Communication with the patient and his family followed. The patient was well aware of the effects of anesthesia and the necessary steps it entailed. He told the surgeon that if he could not be removed successfully from bypass after 3 attempts, nothing further should be done. Regarding anesthesia and continued intubation, he reiterated that if he required assisted ventilation after 36 h, the endotracheal tube was to be removed. It could be replaced only once for a further 36 h and then he was to be extubated. These instructions were spelled out in the advanced directive. The patient did not want any part of the document to be rescinded. The family was in agreement. Complete documentation was made in the chart and signed by the surgeon, anesthesiologist, and the nurse witness.

Summary

Although guidelines have been presented, policies implemented, and laws passed acknowledging the rights of patients to decision making and autonomy, physicians still have difficulty adhering to them and essentially "doing nothing." While the surgical team may agree in principle to withholding treatment, putting theory into practice is difficult. For the anesthesiologist, it is especially hard to define where anesthesia ends and resuscitation begins. But only the patient alone can gauge his quality of life and what is sustainable for him.

References

1. Ewanchuk M, Brindley PG. Ethics review: Perioperative do-not-resuscitate orders–doing "nothing" when "something" can be done. Crit Care. 2006;10(4):219–23.
2. American Society of Anesthesiologists. Ethical guidelines for the anesthesia care of patients with do-not- resuscitate orders or other directives that limit treatment. Approved by the ASA House of Delegates on October 17 2001 and last amended on October 16, 2013. http://www.asahq.org/~/media/Sites/ASAHQ/Files/Public/Resources/standards-guidelines/ethical-guidelines-for-the-anesthesia-care-of-patients.pdf. Accessed 26 Mar 2015.
3. Hardin SB, Yusufely YA. Difficult end-of-life decisions; do other factors trump advance directives? Arch Intern Med. 2004;164(14):1531–3.
4. Byrne SM, Mulcahy S, Torres M, Catlin A. Reconsidering do-not-resuscitate orders in the perioperative setting. J Perianesth Nurs. 2014;29(5):354–60.
5. Maxwell BG, Lobato RL, Cason MB, Wong JK. Perioperative morbidity and mortality of cardiothoracic surgery in patients with a do-not-resuscitate order. Peer J. 2014;22(2):e245.

Should a Trainee Be Allowed to Return to Anesthesiology After Narcotic Diversion and Presumed Addiction?

120

Corey S. Scher

Case

Strong rumors quickly solidified when a resident who was suspected of diverting narcotics was caught in the men's locker room by his co-residents, injecting a drug in a "hep lock" intravenous line that was placed in his left saphenous vein. The resident confessed that he was injecting fentanyl and begged the residents not to "rat him out." Although the residents agreed to his face, 2 went to the Chair's office to report this issue immediately. The Chair grabbed a senior attending to serve as a witness in confronting the resident. Apparently, the Chair had experience with this ongoing issue. I was also asked to witness the event. Although I had been a program director for many years in the Deep South, this issue had never come up before in my career.

When we all arrived in the locker room, the resident in question was making an attempt to plea with his classmates to not disclose what he had done. He had tears in his eyes and was quietly sobbing with each sentence. The Chair arrived and simply stated, "You have a choice. You can go straight to Rehab or go to the police station to confess these activities as a felon."

Hospital security was called in case the present atmosphere degenerated.

There was an open drug rehabilitation bed in Pennsylvania, and the resident went straight from the Chair's office to wait for the hospital vehicle for the 2-h drive. The other senior attending asked what the long-term plan was for the resident. The Chair said he would be inpatient for a year and then be transitioned to outpatient treatment, before being slowly reintroduced into the residency program. Was the Chair's plan the right thing to do?

C.S. Scher (✉)
Department of Anesthesiology, Perioperative Care and Pain Medicine, New York University School of Medicine, New York, NY 10016, USA
e-mail: coreyscher@gmail.com

Question

Should a trainee be allowed to return to anesthesiology after narcotic diversion and presumed addiction?

PRO: The Chair pointed out that it was possible for a resident to return to anesthesiology consistent with the school of medicine bylaws and the rules of the Accreditation Council for Graduate Medical Education (ACGME) with American Board of Anesthesiologist's guidance.

CON: I tried not to show the incredible disbelief that the plan included a return to anesthesia.

I spoke out, "This seems parallel to placing an alcoholic in a bar."

There are several unique features to anesthesiology that made me lash out at this plan. "No other specialty has easier access to needles and syringes than anesthesiologists. No other specialty has the highest grade of proficiency at putting in an intravenous line. No other specialty has access to potent opioids and other controlled substances related to severe addiction. This sounds like a disaster in the making. If your kid were an anesthesia resident, would you want him to return from rehab when this often results in a return to drug use and death? Small doses of opioid lead to large doses and finally to an overdose. Addiction is a chronic disease, with multiple relapses. It is rarely cured, and requires a lifetime of treatment."

This plan made no sense. "There must be data on this issue and we should examine it before a professional life plan is offered to the resident."

PRO: The Chair spoke out, "Each drug abuser is treated on a case-by-case basis instead of having a global policy for all."

C.S. Scher et al. (eds.), *You're Wrong, I'm Right*, DOI 10.1007/978-3-319-43169-7_120

CON: I could not restrain myself. "Why don't we offer him a spot in another field that has a much lower rate of substance abuse, like pediatrics, or a medicine subspecialty like neurology? He will have dignity and a meaningful professional life with less temptation to return to drug use."

I made my way over to my office and signed into PubMed. According to Collins et al. [1], relapse is common with a rate of 46 % upon reentry into an anesthesia training program. Death from overdose is not uncommonly the first sign of diversion [1]. This dismal outcome reinforced my logic on this sensitive issue. My search in the literature, however, was frustrating as it addressed mostly residents, and was contradictory and inconclusive. Even the classic notion that "white male anesthesia residents" are the number one offenders was disputed.

Regrettably, attendings that abuse anesthetic drugs can easily return to the operating room with few consequences. After a period of rehab, an attending physician could potentially move elsewhere in the country without a new employer having knowledge of previous substance abuse. The field of anesthesia itself could be a factor in making susceptible individuals into drug addicts. Research into this area is difficult, especially for attendings that choose rehab, because there is no way to track the long-term outcomes of these individuals. The bottom line is that we do not know what happens to what I would say is the majority of anesthesiologists in training or after training after they have succumbed to addiction. I had a colleague in our department years ago who was addicted to meperidine. He was found in the locker room with a needle in his arm. With stimulation, he woke up and ran to the parking lot. Five years passed until he was found practicing in the state of Washington. We have no idea whether he went to rehab or whether he ran into legal problems. Simply stated, he vanished in a way that I do not think is that uncommon.

While the Chair felt that reentry into anesthesiology must be viewed as a case-by-case basis, why bother? If relapse is common, why increase the odds of trouble by allowing these individuals to return? The temptation must be brutal.

PRO: The Chair stepped into my office. He conceded that half of the risk of addiction is not modifiable because it is due to genetics [2] and that the literature on actual outcomes is, as I thought, weak. He said that his approach, however, was based on the evidence that the other half of the risk of addiction was due to causes that could be treated, such as depression, anxiety, and poor coping skills [2]. He went through the list of names, over the last 10 years of residents and attendings who were addicted to fentanyl. All 10 of the people he named were back in the department and were successful in their anesthesia careers. Since relapse commonly occurs in the first year after intensive recovery, he assimilates residents into the anesthesia training program by having them work in the hospital (teaching through simulation, giving lectures) for a year before immersion back into anesthesia. Every day since their "crash" is a day further away from relapse.

CON: While this is a great outcome, it is a small sample. If the next 2 addicts relapse, there will be a 1/6 failure rate, which would be awful.

Concession from CON: Although anecdotal, the Chair's comments reflect a unique and admirable approach.

Summary

Although this remains a heated topic that has an enormous impact on our field, guidance by data may not be possible. As the specialty of anesthesia changes, there will be a continued evolution in the ways in which the stress from our profession impacts the individual who is genetically susceptible to a chronic disease-like addiction.

Although there have been significant improvements in the utilization of surveys in medical research, there remain numerous obstacles to obtaining significant data from addicts who are thought to represent some of the most unreliable patients in medicine. My Chair did not agree at all with my bias and chose to treat every addict on a case-by-case basis. We will rarely agree on this issue. Providers who are addicts and have "recovered" are at an increased risk for return to drug use if they return to specialties where access is easy. We can only hope that a valid and reliable means to collect a robust number of cases is developed to give a true answer to what appears to be an unanswerable question.

References

1. Collins GB, McAllister MS, Jensen M, Gooden TA. Chemical dependency treatment outcomes of residents in anesthesiology: results of a survey. Anesth Analg. 2005;101(5):1457–62.
2. Schonwald G, Skipper GE, Smith DE, Earley PH. Anesthesiologists and substance use disorders. Anesth Analg. 2014;119(5):1007–10.

Should Anesthesia Personnel Be Subject to Mandatory Drug Testing?

121

Thor Lidasan and Judy Chang

Case

Dr. A, a CA-2 resident, was considered outstanding. He belonged to the top echelon of his medical school class, passed his examinations with high scores, and worked well with his co-residents and attendings. He was concerned about his patients and vigilantly watched over them while they were in his care. He was known as a very meticulous and hardworking resident. However, he also lived a double life. He was an addict.

His fascination with drugs started when he was a college student. Ritalin and coffee kept him awake for those long nights preparing for his examinations. After the examinations, prescription Ambien helped him to recover from the effects of stimulants and rested his weary mind and body. In medical school, he honed his understanding of the pharmacology of stimulants and benzodiazepines. Anatomy, physiology, and pharmacology were his favorite courses as a medical student. He decided that anesthesiology was the career he wanted to pursue, thinking it was a natural progression of his interests.

As an anesthesiology resident, he felt he was in the most demanding but rewarding stage of his life. The hours were long but he loved what he was doing. However, the stress of learning new things, taking care of patients, and working every day under the direct supervision of his attendings slowly took its toll on his psyche. At first, alcohol helped him during the weekends and Ambien to recover from the long calls of his resident life. But he could only take so much alcohol. In fact, he never liked being drunk. What he wanted was being able to go to sleep and wake up as if nothing had happened.

Every time he saw his patients drift off to sleep during induction, it reminded him of how benzodiazepines also helped him in the past. The benzodiazepine recall kept coming back. He kept brushing off those thoughts and coped with his resident life the best he could.

One day, as he was emptying the pockets of his scrubs, he found a vial of fentanyl. Next thing he knew, he was euphoric. He discovered how powerful opiates are, much more powerful than what he dabbled in before. That night began his descent into the world of addiction. Six months later, he was found dead in the on-call room of his hospital with a syringe and an empty vial of sufentanil at his bedside. His colleagues were shocked when they heard the news. They never suspected that Dr. A was using opiates. They had worked with him every day and never saw any signs that he might be using.

Questions

How prevalent is drug use among anesthesia residents? When does the highest risk of drug-related death occur among anesthesia providers? How effective are the current measures to detect and prevent drug use among anesthesia providers in training? Should anesthesia personnel be subject to mandatory drug testing?

PRO: A survey of 111 anesthesia programs revealed that 80 % of programs have had anesthesia residents abusing opioids [1]. Nineteen percent of those programs reported at least 1 death from drug overdose or suicide [1]. It is estimated that the incidence of substance use is 1.6 % among anesthesia residents [2]. That is a concerning statistic. Imagine airline pilot schools reporting that 80 % of their programs have pilot trainees using drugs while learning to fly and that 1.6 % of their trainees who later become pilots abuse drugs. How would you react? Pilots, military

T. Lidasan (✉)
Department of Anesthesiology, Perioperative Care and Pain Medicine, Bellevue Hospital Center, 462 First Avenue, Suite 11N34, New York, NY 10016, USA
e-mail: Thor.lidasan@nyumc.org

J. Chang
Department of Anesthesiology, Perioperative Care and Pain Medicine, New York University Langone Medical Center, 560 First Avenue, New York, NY 10016, USA

C.S. Scher et al. (eds.), *You're Wrong, I'm Right*, DOI 10.1007/978-3-319-43169-7_121

personnel, and postal workers are randomly tested for drug abuse, shouldn't anesthesia providers in training be tested too?

CON: I agree that compared to residency programs in other specialties, anesthesiology residents are overrepresented in rehabilitation programs by a factor of 7; in fact, 35 % of impaired residents in one state that monitored physicians are anesthesia residents [3]. However, some programs have strong substance abuse prevention protocols in place to detect and identify trainees who might be diverting drugs. For example, there are automated drug dispensing systems currently available that are able to analyze atypically high usage of drugs dispensed to specific providers, raising the suspicion of diversion. No research has shown that random, suspicion-less drug testing prevents drug use. Drug testing "for cause" is relevant and more effective. Are you advocating drug testing as a deterrent or as a solution in preventing drug use? Why residents only? Why not randomly drug test all anesthesia providers and all medical providers?

PRO: Why specifically anesthesia trainees? Let's look at the studies. The types of drugs that are typically abused are potent agents. Fentanyl and sufentanil have short half-lives and produce earlier functional deterioration in the disease process of addiction. There is also a study showing that the highest cause-specific risk for drug-related death of an anesthesia resident occurs in the first 5 years after graduation from medical school [4]. What I propose is adding random drug screening to the current strict medication controls and analysis of administration of controlled agents. The precautions currently in place are not enough. An impaired anesthesia provider can go through months of diversion before any discrepancy is noticed. It has been shown repeatedly that anesthesia providers are uncovered at the downward spiral of their impairment and that they have been diverting for weeks or months before discovery. Random drug screening should be part of an active approach to detect diversion at the stage of the highest risk for drug use among residents, along with the current protocols. It is a shift from "for cause" drug testing that is currently done in the majority of academic institutions. In addition, a survey among anesthesia department chairmen showed that 61 % favor random drug screens for their trainees [5].

CON: I do agree that strong measures have to be in place to detect diversion and impairment. However, you also have to protect the privacy, dignity, and work ethic of the 99 % of the residents who are unlikely to divert and abuse substances. Drug screens are for that 1 % of the resident population who are at a higher risk for substance use and impairment [6]. Random drug screens work when used in a setting where 100 % of the population tested are known substance abusers, like a treatment monitoring program. However, in a population where 99 % are unlikely to be substance abusers, it would be difficult to implement such a protocol [6]. There are also issues we have to deal with that are specific to the clinical environment of anesthesiologists. For example, we cannot just pull out an anesthesia provider in a middle of a case to provide a sample. How much time does the resident have to give a sample when notified to do so? An immediate response will create logistical problems in implementation. Meanwhile, if you extend the window for submitting the sample to 24–36 h, this would allow enough time for someone who wants to invalidate the test to do so. An individual can acquire a sample from someone else, an adulterant can be added, or even just diluting the urine can invalidate a test [6]. A successful drug testing program depends on compliance of the tested population and the integrity of the drug testing methodology.

PRO: Programs that have initiated random drug screening as part of their substance abuse prevention protocol have dealt specifically with those issues and managed to implement random drug testing in their institutions [7]. Random testing is not utilized simply to identify positive drug screens. It is more valuable as a tool to increase resident and patient safety. Earlier detection of anesthesia providers who might be using and abusing drugs increases both patient and resident safety. Drug treatment will also be instituted earlier for the impaired provider. Approximately 20 % of individuals with known drug dependence escape discovery if using behavioral detection alone [6]. With random drug screens, individuals who do not exhibit behavioral signs of drug dependence may be identified much earlier.

CON: There are already systems in place that allow early detection of drug diversion and use. Computerized records are readily available and can provide real-time evidence of high wastage, high use, and transactions recorded on canceled cases. A responsive anesthesia information management system can be configured to analyze patterns of drug diversion and providers who exhibit suspicious record keeping can be easily identified and asked to explain their documentation. A monthly report of their transactions can also be generated and examined for drug diversion. "For cause" drug testing can then be done if their records cannot be explained adequately. This is the opposite of random drug testing where individuals are pulled out of operating rooms to submit urine samples. The approach should be a calibrated response to an event or a series of events, not randomly selecting providers for drug screening just because their number is up. We also have to take into account the possibility of a false-positive test on an innocent provider [8]. The effect of a false positive on an individual is devastating. There is a potential loss of employment, loss of licensure, and public humiliation.

PRO: It is impossible to eliminate human and technical errors in mandatory random drug testing. A program that includes random drug testing as part of its drug use prevention protocol should have in place support systems for the possibilities of false-positive and false-negative results. Collection and testing of specimens should follow the strictest standards. The result of the drug test must also stand the scrutiny of a court challenge, since it can be used as evidence in case a provider challenges a positive result. The program should provide safeguards for the participating providers against loss of employment, loss of licensure, and assurances that their privacy is protected while an initial positive screen is undergoing validation.

CON: The practice of anesthesiology is unique among all medical specialties in the sense that we deal with potent, highly addictive, readily available lethal agents. A momentary lapse of judgment in the form of self-medication can have profound and devastating results. Hence, anesthesiologists, regardless of whether in training or after residency, should always maintain a high level of awareness regarding addiction issues. This level of awareness should be instituted at the earliest stage of the anesthesiologist's career in the form of teaching during residency, stringent record keeping, monitoring of usage/wastage of drugs, and constant reinforcement of the inherent danger of drug use in our specialty.

Summary

Substance abuse is more frequent among anesthesia providers than those in other specialties, as shown by data from rehabilitation centers and various state physician health committees. Addiction as a disease may be devastating not only to the afflicted physicians but also to the unsuspecting patients that impaired physicians take care of. It is still a major issue in the anesthesia workplace, and despite advances in pharmacy information systems and strict monitoring of controlled substances, there are still physicians who die from drug abuse [4]. This is not surprising. Anesthesiologists have access to highly addictive drugs. An impaired physician can easily divert small quantities of controlled drugs for personal use. The high-stress environment in which anesthesiologists work predisposes individuals with underlying comorbidities and poor personal stress management mechanisms to start medicating themselves with substances that are easily available to them. Recent clinical investigations also posited that exposure in the workplace sensitizes the reward pathways in the brain and thus promotes substance abuse [3].

Substance abuse is the most serious occupational safety issue in the field of anesthesiology. The effectiveness of random drug screening as part of an active strategy to prevent the problem still remains to be proven. However, what is more important is that a program to prevent and detect substance abuse should always be a priority for any anesthesia department in caring for the safety of its own providers and in ensuring the safety and best possible care of its patients.

References

1. Collins GB, McAllister MS, Jensen M, Gooden TA. Chemical dependency treatment outcomes of residents in anesthesiology: results of a survey. Anesth Analg. 2005;101:1457–62.
2. Booth JV, Grossman D, Moore J, Lineberger C, Reynolds JD, Reves JG, Sheffield D. Substance abuse among physicians: a survey of academic anesthesiology programs. Anesth Analg. 2002;95:1024–30.
3. Bryson EO, Silverstein JH. Addiction and substance abuse in anesthesiology. Anesthesiology. 2008;109:905–17.
4. Alexander BH, Checkoway H, Nagahama SI, Domino KB. Cause-specific mortality risks of anesthesiologists. Anesthesiology. 2000;93:922–30.
5. Bryson EO. Should anesthesia residents with a history of substance abuse be allowed to continue training in clinical anesthesia? The results of a survey of anesthesia residency program directors. J Clin Anesth. 2009;21(7):508–13.
6. Brock MF, Roy CR. Random urine drug testing. Anesth Analg. 2009;108(2):676–7.
7. Fitzsimons MG, Baker KH, Lowenstein E, Zapol WM. Random drug testing to reduce the incidence of addiction in anesthesia residents: preliminary results from one program. Anesth Analg. 2008;107(2):630–5.
8. Fitzsimons MG, Ishizawa Y, Baker KH. Drug testing physicians for substances of abuse: case report of a false-positive result. J Clin Anesth. 2013;25:669–71.

Does Returning a Recovered Addicted Physician to Active Anesthesiology Practice Do More Harm Than Good?

122

Judy Chang and Thor Lidasan

Case

Dr. Edwards was a gifted anesthesiologist. He graduated top of his medical school, and after completing his residency at a major academic center, he stayed on in the department as a junior attending. He was well liked at work; often taking on extra-shifts and offering to give breaks. However, unbeknownst to others, he had become addicted to fentanyl. He started to have mood swings and explosive episodes of anger. Over time, Dr. Edwards would go to increasingly incredulous lengths to obtain his drug of choice. Occasionally, a colleague might become suspicious after Dr. Edward's patient reported a large amount of pain in the recovery room despite liberal narcotic use documented on the patient's chart. Finally, during one shift, Dr. Edwards was discovered rummaging through a sharps container for unused narcotic. He admitted to other troubling behaviors such as replacing narcotics intended for patients with saline or esmolol and to using up to 1000 μg of fentanyl in a single injection to relieve his withdrawal symptoms.

The young physician appeared relieved to have been discovered and voluntarily agreed to immediately enter a drug treatment facility. After he completed the 8-week program where he was "cooperative and compliant," a long-term extended care program was instituted, which involved group therapy sessions and urine monitoring.

After a year, Dr. Edwards approached his former chairman about returning to clinical anesthesia practice. Although the state allows physicians to return to work after inpatient treatment, his chairman and several other colleagues in the department expressed conflicted opinions.

J. Chang
Department of Anesthesiology, Perioperative Care and Pain Medicine, New York University Langone Medical Center, 560 First Avenue, New York, NY 10016, USA

T. Lidasan (✉)
Department of Anesthesiology, Perioperative Care and Pain Medicine, Bellevue Hospital Center, 462 First Avenue, Suite 11N34, New York, NY 10016, USA
e-mail: Thor.Lidasan@nyumc.org

Question

Does returning a recovered addicted physician to active anesthesiology practice do more harm than good?

PRO: Reentry of highly motivated individuals can be effective. During my time as chairman over the past 10 years, I have seen multiple residents and attendings that were addicted to narcotics, underwent rehabilitation, and went on to be successful in their anesthesia careers. In fact, the possibility of a resident returning to anesthesiology is consistent with our school of medicine bylaws and the rules of the Accreditation Council for Graduate Medical Education (ACGME) with American Board of Anesthesiologist's guidance. Nonetheless, the decision to allow reentry to clinical anesthesia practice remains a controversial topic. A 2007 survey of program directors of ACGME accredited residencies showed that 43 % believed that residents in recovery should be allowed to return and 30 % disagreed [1]. Program directors who had a history of successful rehabilitation of residents were more likely to answer positively, whereas the opposite was true for the latter.

Despite the debate, very few studies out there examine the prognosis for a recovering drug-addicted anesthesiologist [2, 3]. Historically, the consensus was that most anesthesiologists who completed therapy were allowed to return to work. This is also frequently the recommendation of addiction medicine and psychiatry.

CON: The reentry of a former addict into anesthesia practice has an unacceptably high risk of relapse and death. Anesthesiologists make up 5 % of the total number of physicians, but disproportionately make up 13–15 % of persons receiving management and monitoring for drug addiction [4]. Also, anesthesiologists are more likely to use major opioids (fentanyl, sufentanil, morphine, and other injectable narcotics) whereas other physicians had an inclination for alcohol abuse [4]. There are several factors proposed to

C.S. Scher et al. (eds.), *You're Wrong, I'm Right*, DOI 10.1007/978-3-319-43169-7_122

explain the high incidence of drug abuse in anesthesiologists: proximity to large quantities of addictive drugs, relative ease of diverting, high-stress work environment, and a chronic low level exposure in the workplace that sensitizes reward pathways in the brain [5].

While it is true that it has not been shown that anesthesia providers who return to clinical practice after successful treatment are at greater risk for relapse than the general population, it is very alarming that they are at increased risk of death in the event of relapse [6, 7]. Due to these high stakes, Berge et al. argue that the "one strike, you're out" approach should be implemented throughout our specialty [8].

PRO: Has it actually been proven that there is increase in risk of death?

CON: A widely quoted report from 2009 by Menk et al. followed anesthesia residents who abused opioids [7]. The study showed a high rate of relapse (66 %) and 16 % mortality in the subgroup that was allowed to reenter residency. Unfortunately, death was the first sign of relapse in that subgroup. Again, very similar results were seen in a 2005 report by Collins et al. that showed 46 % successful residency completion among reentry, but a 9 % mortality rate [6]. If your kid were an anesthesia resident, would you want him to return to such a work environment when this often results in a return to drug use and death?

PRO: That is a good point, but not all rehabilitated physicians will relapse. In your hypothetical scenario, my kid could be one of the successful ones.

CON: There is some belief that physicians who fall victim to drug abuse have a genetic or biochemical predisposition to addiction. There has been considerable amount of research done in mice that suggests a genetic basis for addiction. Many genes have been postulated to have a role, but only a few have their mechanisms identified.

PRO: No, addiction cannot be blamed entirely on genetics, you have to also take into account other environmental factors as well. Several coexisting factors have been noted by the Washington Physicians Health Program (PHP) when they reviewed their data from working with physicians over a 10-year period [9]. Rate of relapse is significantly increased in the setting of major opioid use, a family history of substance abuse, or a coexisting psychiatric disorder. A patient with all 3 risk factors was found to have a 13.25-fold increase in relapse risk [9]. Perhaps each individual should be evaluated on a case-by-case basis instead of having a global policy for all. If an individual has other risk factors making them at higher likelihood of relapse, we can be more hesitant about the possibility of reentry into anesthesia practice.

CON: What kind of treatments are out there? Are some more effective than others?

PRO: Treatment for the drug-addicted physician involves admission to an inpatient facility specializing in treatment of physicians, followed by long-term abstinence monitoring, receptor antagonists, self-help groups, professional behavioral observation, and individual and group psychotherapy. The physician is regularly tested by a variety of methods including urine analysis, hair analysis, and naltrexone testing (to verify compliance with receptor antagonist treatment).

A subset of Physicians Health Programs (PHP) that incorporate aggressive monitoring have significantly decreased relapse rates. Remarkably, these results describe similar outcomes for anesthesiologist and other types of physicians [10].

CON: But despite the various treatments available, the assessment of their long-term effectiveness is very difficult because these physicians are often lost to follow-up. An attending physician could potentially move elsewhere in the country without a new employer having knowledge of previous substance abuse. We could offer Dr. Edwards a spot in another field that has a much lower risk of substance abuse, for example, pediatrics or internal medicine. He could still maintain dignity and a meaningful professional life with less temptation to return to drug use. And yet, one finds the same issue of a lack of data. No one knows whether anesthesia providers who go on to other specialties are less likely to relapse since they are almost always lost to follow-up.

PRO: Well that is true, but also keep in mind that there are federal laws (such as the Americans with Disabilities Act) and state civil right laws that offer protection to physicians who are actively involved in chemical dependency treatment programs as well as recovering addicts. These laws require "reasonable accommodation" be made for the physician and job protection during a medical leave for addiction treatment. If an addiction psychiatrist recommends reentry into anesthesia, the Americans with Disabilities Act places the burden of responsibility on the employer to prove the patient is unable to perform responsibilities. Generally, employers can impose restrictions on employment in a work reentry contract.

CON: I see all the points that you are making, but I think that ultimately there is the legal and ethical issue of allowing a potentially disabled physician to have responsibility over patient care. Dire consequences can occur with any lapse of judgment. There is also the issue of informed consent. Certainly, all of us would want to know whether our anesthesia provider had a history of drug addiction.

Summary

Although this remains a heated topic that has an enormous impact on our field, guidance by data may not be possible. There have been significant improvements in the utilization of surveys in medical research; however, there remain numerous obstacles to obtaining significant data from addicts who are thought to represent some of the most unreliable patients in medicine.

Additionally, as the specialty of anesthesia changes, there will be a continued evolution in the ways in which the stress from our profession impact the individual who is genetically susceptible to a chronic disease like addiction.

This anesthesia department will have to decide if they will go with the "case-by-case basis" approach or the "one strike, you're out" approach. We will rarely come to a consensus on this highly emotional issue. Providers who are addicts and have "recovered" may be at increased risk for relapse to drug use and death if they return to specialties where access is easy. We can only hope that a valid and reliable means to collect a robust number of cases is developed to guide us to an answer to what appears to be an unanswerable question.

References

1. Bryson EO. Should anesthesia residents with a history of substance abuse be allowed to continue training in clinical anesthesia? The results of a survey of anesthesia residency program directors. J Clin Anesth. 2009;21:508–13.
2. Oreskovich MR, Caldeiro RM. Anesthesiologists recovering from chemical dependency: can they safely return to the operating room? Mayo Clin Proc. 2009;84(7):576–80.
3. Schonwald G, Skipper GE, Smith DE, Earley PH. Anesthesiologists and substance use disorders. Anesth Analg. 2014;119 (5):1007–10.
4. Berge KH, Seppala MD, Schipper AM. Chemical dependency and the physician. Mayo Clin Proc. 2009;84(7):625–31.
5. Bryson EO, Silverstein JH. Addiction and substance abuse in anesthesiology. Anesthesiology. 2008;109:905–17.
6. Collins GB, McAllister MS, Jensen M, Gooden TA. Chemical dependency treatment outcomes of residents in anesthesiology: results of a survey. Anesth Analg. 2005;101(5):1457–62.
7. Menk EJ, Baumgarten RK, Kinsley CP, Culling RD, Middaugh R. Success of reentry into anesthesiology training programs by residents with a history of substance abuse. J Am Med Assoc. 1990;263(22):3060–2.
8. Berge KH, Seppala MD, Lanier WL. The anesthesiology community's approach to opioid- and anesthetic-abusing personnel. Anesthesiology. 2008;109:762–4.
9. Domino KB, Hornbein TF, Polissar NL, et al. Risk factors for relapse in health care professionals with substance use disorders. J Am Med Assoc. 2005;293(12):1453–60.
10. McLellan AT, Skipper GS, Campbell M, DuPont RL. Five year outcomes in a cohort study of physicians treated for substance use disorders in the United States. Br Med J. 2008;4(337):a2038.

Does Disruptive Behavior Among Anesthesia Care Providers Decrease Patient Safety? 123

Sergey Pisklakov

Case

Over the last few years, Andrew, an anesthesiology faculty member, has been doing primarily high-profile case assignments and taking a significant amount of overnight call. He has been extremely helpful and attentive to his colleagues, patients, needs of the department, and requests of the surgeons. Andrew's demeanor is jovial and friendly with members of the department and operating room (OR) staff. Over the last 2 months, however, he has called out sick several times and he has stopped teaching residents. As a director of the OR, you learn that one of your fellow anesthesiologists, Nicholas, often makes derogative and humiliating comments to Andrew in regard to his clinical abilities and rapport with surgeons. The situation has been made worse as others appear entertained by Andrew's ordeal.

Question

What is happening to Andrew? Why does he look depressed? Do you see symptoms of burnout or substance abuse, depression, or personality disorder? Is he simply reacting to the hostile disruptive environment at his workplace?

PRO: Stress, family issues, separation from a significant other, and lack of a supportive community can lead to depersonalization, exhaustion, inefficacy, and poor clinical and academic performance [1, 2]. The American Psychological Association defines disruptive behavior as an aggressive demeanor intended to cause distress. There is a disparity of power or strength between the aggressor and the victim. The individual at the receiving end has difficulty in defending himself or herself against these actions [3].

S. Pisklakov (✉)
Department of Anesthesiology, Montefiore Medical Center, Albert Einstein College of Medicine, 111 East 210th Street, Bronx, NY 10467, USA
e-mail: SPISKLAK@montefiore.org; spisklakov@hotmail.com

CON: Burnout can be easily mistaken for substance abuse, depression, or personality disorder. Key features of depression and substance abuse can include persistent sadness, anxious mood, hopelessness, quietness, aloofness, restless irritability, feelings of guilt and worthlessness, disinterest in work-related activities, sleep problems, and medical errors. However, in the case of burnout the symptoms are job-site related and more about dissatisfaction, rather than hopelessness and withdrawal, as is in cases of substance abuse and/or depression.

Question

Is there a reliable and professional way to approach a bullying problem among adults, especially physicians?

PRO: Aggressive and disruptive behavior in the workplace is fueling a nationwide legislative effort to draft and enforce policies aimed at stopping it [4]. Disruptive behavior is blamed for creating high cost, turnover, insurance claim, and thwarting productivity [5]. It is a patient safety issue. Preventive methods include providing educational materials and communication skills training for residents, staff, and educators [6]. These initiatives should promote inclusive language and a culture of collegiality and respect for all faculty, staff, and trainees [7]. Other preventive measures should rely in part on clear reporting mechanisms, so that any occasion of abusive or discriminatory language or behavior can be addressed as soon as it arises. Disruptive behavior needs both decisive intervention and help [8]. Approaches should be educational and organizational. Psychotherapy may be indicated for the perpetrator, to help them realize their internal motives and causes behind their antagonistic actions and inappropriate bullying. This therapy should also comprise work on self-awareness and interpersonal skills so that the perpetrator can explore and adopt alternative ways of behaving [9].

C.S. Scher et al. (eds.), *You're Wrong, I'm Right*, DOI 10.1007/978-3-319-43169-7_123

CON: In the meantime, and until further data confirm or deny the concerns identified here, we should be duly vigilant. The recent and universal focus on professionalism in medical education and professional behavior of physicians in practice will also help us to eradicate this unacceptable behavior [5].

Question

Should the department intervene? What is the role of the department, chief, or colleagues?

PRO: Aggression underlies disruptive behavior. Children show this with physical violence. Adults are more practiced, and their bullying is often not obvious to a supervisor, due to their often indirect and sophisticated methods. Violations are unchecked and bad behavior occurs at the expense of others [9, 10]. Disruptive behavior during training is also a part of the experience of many early career doctors, medical students, and residents [11].

Approaches should be both educational and organizational. Work with the individual accused may include psychotherapy to explore the reasons for bullying or aggressive behavior. Work on interpersonal and self-awareness skills also needs to be done so that the bully can explore and adopt alternative ways of behaving [9]. The organizational culture needs to change as well. Many commercial companies have put in place clearly defined written policies to prevent bullying and harassment at work [10], and these policies should be given a higher profile. Continuous vigilance is needed, however, to make sure that these policies are not underhandedly used to perpetuate more bullying [12]. For example, "incident reports," intended to improve quality by letting leadership know about problems, at some hospitals are used as weapons against other personnel. Strong leadership, with good judgment when these policies are implemented, is necessary to truly prevent bullying. A combination of good policies and outstanding implementation by strong leaders should encourage victims to come forward so that individual bullies can be identified [13].

CON: Disruptive behavior needs both decisive intervention and help [8, 14]. Often victims do not report these events because they do not recognize that how they are being treated is disruptive behavior. Poor self-esteem can result in a person accepting bullying treatment as normal, although the person may still suffer the negative consequences such as depression and worsened work performance [13, 15, 16]. Hospitals, departments, and individual personnel need to develop a higher level of awareness. Victims should approach their line manager or the human resources department. They could also approach their professional association for advice and support [9].

We know little about how disruptive behavior and bullying is triggered and how it might be prevented [17]. In the meantime, and until further data confirm or deny the concerns identified here, we should be duly vigilant. The recent and universal focus on professionalism in medical education and professional behavior of physicians in practice will also help us to eradicate this unacceptable behavior.

Summary

Physicians experiencing disruptive behavior often do not see any hope of positive change in their situations. A new standard from The Joint Commission [formerly the Joint Commission on Accreditation of Healthcare Organizations (JCAHO)] was implemented in January 2009. Mandatory for hospitals is "a code of conduct that defines acceptable, disruptive, and inappropriate staff behaviors" and for "leaders [to] create and implement a process for managing disruptive and inappropriate staff behaviors. Leaders must address disruptive behavior of individuals working at all levels of the [organization], including management, clinical and administrative staff, licensed independent practitioners, and governing body members." Included as problematic are "uncooperative attitudes" and "condescending language or voice intonation and impatience with questions."

A solution may be a better detection system, more responsiveness to patient complaints, or more training for employees on how to respond professionally yet compassionately to difficult patient or staff situations [18, 19]. The lack of action against disruptive and aggressive behavior can lead to serious liabilities since these incidents usually constitute not only bullying, but also sometime sexual harassment and discrimination [20]. Intimidating, condescending, off-putting, or discouraging behavior by the physician inhibits positive teamwork. Disruptive behavior by any member of the team, including the physician, nurse, or supervisor, will impair the quality of care, endangering patient safety. Hospitals need to create a workplace conduct policy forbidding disruptive and aggressive behavior, bullying or harassment. In addition to comprehensive training courses for all physicians [21], smart and strong leaders must exist, who will evaluate each issue individually, and make decisions based on the overall picture of what is best for the patients and employees.

Disruptive behavior occurs across many types of providers. Physician behavior, however, may have the greatest impact because of the position of authority that doctors hold as members of the healthcare team [11, 20]. A team member may, from fear of intimidation, hesitate to speak up when they see a potentially dangerous situation [5].

References

1. Campbell D, Sonnad S, Eckhauser F, Campbell K, Greenfield LJ. Burnout among American surgeons. Surgery. 2001;130:696–702 (discussion 702–5).
2. Ramirez A, Graham J, Richards M, Cull A, Gregory W. Mental health of hospital consultants: the effects of stress and satisfaction at work. Lancet. 1996;347:724–8.
3. Einharsen S, Raknes BI, Mathiesen SB. Bullying and harassment at work and their relationships to work environment quality: an exploratory study. Eur Work Organ Psychol. 1994;4(4):381–404.
4. Yamada DC. Workplace bullying and American employment law: a ten-year progress report and assessment. Comp Labor Law J. 2010;32(1): SSRN. http://ssrn.com/abstract=1908465.
5. Rosenstein A, O'Daniel M. Disruptive behavior and clinical outcomes: Perceptions of nurses and physicians. Am J Nurs. 2005;105:54–64.
6. Baldwin D, Daugherty S, Eckenfels E. Student perceptions of mistreatment and harassment during medical school: a survey of ten U.S. schools. West J Med. 1991;155:140–5.
7. Quine L. Workplace bullying in NHS community trust: staff questionnaire survey. Br Med J. 1999;318:228–32.
8. Cohen J, Leung Y, Fahey M. The happy docs study: a Canadian Association of Interns and Residents well-being survey examining resident physician health and satisfaction within and outside of residency training in Canada. BMC Res Notes. 2008;1:105.
9. Houghton A. Tips on dealing with bullies. Br Med J Career Focus. 2005;330:201–2.
10. Paice E, Aitken E, Houghton A, Firth-Cozens J. Bullying among doctors in training: cross sectional questionnaire survey. Br Med J. 2004;329:658–9.
11. Quine L. Workplace bullying in junior doctors: questionnaire survey. Br Med J. 2002;324:878–9.
12. Duffy M. Preventing workplace mobbing and bullying with effective organizational consultation, policies, and legislation. Consult Psychol J Pract Res. 2009;61(3):242–62.
13. Bosk C. Forgive and remember: managing medical failure. Chicago: University of Chicago Press;1979.
14. Stratton T, McLaughlin M, Witte F. Does students' exposure to gender discrimination and sexual harassment in medical school affect specialty choice and residency program selection? Acad Med. 2005;80:400–8.
15. Kozlowska K, Nunn K. Adverse experiences in psychiatric training. Aust N Z J Psychiatry 1997;31:641–52.
16. Firth Cozens J. Depression in doctors. In: Katona C, Robertson MM, editors. Depression and physical illness. Chichester: Wiley;1997. p. 95–111.
17. Farrell G. Aggression in clinical settings: nurses' views: a follow-up study. J Adv Nurs. 1999;29:532–41.
18. The Joint Commission. Accreditation requirements. 2009. http://www.jointcommission.org/NR/rdonlyres. Accessed 9 Jan 2009.
19. Joint Commission. Sentinel Event Alert—behaviors that undermine a culture of safety. Issue 40, 9 July 2008.
20. Porto G, Lauve R. Disruptive clinician behavior: a persistent threat to patient safety. http://www.psqh.com/julaug06/disruptive.html. Accessed 8 Feb 2009.
21. Institute for Safe Medication Practices (ISMP): Survey on workplace intimidation. 2003. http://ismp.org/Survey/surveyresults/Survey0311.asp. Accessed 5 Feb 2009.

Is Burnout Among Anesthesiologists a Humbug or a Real Entity?

124

Sergey Pisklakov

Case

Nicholas is a member of your anesthesiology faculty. Over the last 2 months, he called out sick a few times. His passion for mountain skiing and spending time outdoors is well known to the department, but he has almost stopped talking about these activities over the past 6 months. He has stopped teaching residents, and there has been no further development with his research project. It was noted by several members of the operating room (OR) team that Nicholas has become overly argumentative with surgeons and nurses. He even expressed that he is dissatisfied with his career choice and that he is "considering quitting this once and for all and looking for a place in healthcare administration," complaining that sometimes he feels that his patients treat him like an impersonal object and only remember their surgeons.

The chairman, Dr. D, asks you to look into Nicholas' problem. You find that Nicholas' narcotic record keeping is excellent with patient narcotic usage not out of the ordinary. You meet with Nicholas to ask him about his problems and offer your help. Nicholas tells you that he has no specific stressors in his life. Mountain skiing had become boring for him over the last couple of years so he lost interest. He says he is extremely tired, and despite his insistence that he still has a passion for anesthesiology and critical care, he complains that work has become a routine and he is "desperate for a change."

Question

What happened to Nicholas? What went wrong with his professional practice? Is he simply tired and burned out? Or are his problems due to substance abuse, depression, or even a psychiatric issue?

PRO: Burnout occurs when one feels overwhelmed and unable to meet constant demands. As the stress continues, you begin to lose interest or motivation [1]. Burnout is a known concern for many large companies and corporations, leading to staff rotation and decreased retention. The epidemic of burnout has spread and has not left health care untouched—especially critical care specialties. Significant burnout rates have been found among emergency medicine physicians, anesthesiologists, and obstetricians. A high incidence of burnout was recently reported among anesthesiology residents and academic chairpersons [2–6]. Individual factors, stress, family issues, separation from a significant other, and lack of supportive community are all reported, which can lead to depersonalization, exhaustion, and finally to inefficacy and poor clinical and academic performance [4, 6].

CON: Burnout can be mistaken for substance abuse, depression, or a personality disorder. Key features of depression and substance abuse can include persistent sadness, anxious mood, hopelessness, quietness, aloofness, restless irritability, feelings of guilt and worthlessness, disinterest in work-related activities, sleep problems, and medical errors. The same signs and symptoms may be present in cases of burnout [7]. However, in burnout, the symptoms are job-site related and more about dissatisfaction, rather than the hopelessness and withdrawal that occur in substance abuse and/or depression. Being burned out means feeling empty and devoid of motivation, and beyond caring. Physicians experiencing burnout often do not see any hope of positive change in their situations. If excessive stress is like drowning in responsibilities, burnout is like being all dried up. There is one other difference between stress and burnout: While you are usually aware of being under a lot of stress, you do not always notice burnout when it happens [8, 9].

S. Pisklakov (✉)
Department of Anesthesiology, Montefiore Medical Center, Albert Einstein College of Medicine, 111 East 210th Street, Bronx, NY 10467, USA
e-mail: SPISKLAK@montefiore.org; spisklakov@hotmail.com

C.S. Scher et al. (eds.), *You're Wrong, I'm Right*, DOI 10.1007/978-3-319-43169-7_124

Question

Can we help him? What is the role of the department, either the chief, colleagues, or both?

PRO: A meeting with a burned out colleague can begin with an informal one-on-one assessment of his/her needs, while also taking the needs of the department into account. The individual's goals can be achieved through a carefully formulated series of questions to fully understand any issues that he or she is experiencing. Only then can an initial assessment be made as to what form the stress management help will take. Burned out physicians can be taught the essentials of stress management, such as getting social support, developing positive self-talk, and demanding less perfection for yourself, as well as be shown techniques that will enable them to deal with stress, making it manageable and thereby increasing performance and value to the department [10].

CON: Prevention of emotional exhaustion is probably the best way to prevent burnout. Utilizing recommendations initially developed for commercial pilots and flight attendants [1] and modified for emergency room physicians, we can make recommendations for Nicholas. Simple things such as exercise, a hobby, and availability of significant others would be the best advisable preventers of burnout [11]. The department's role is to enforce a respectful, safe, and fair environment at the work place and to shield members of the department from those who are unfair and abusive. Every time there is a destructive force interfering with job performance, satisfaction, and personal safety, it is in the department's best interest and responsibility to intervene and protect its members.

Question

Can we do anything to prevent burnout?

PRO: To alleviate and to prevent further burnout we can advise Nicholas to:

1. Balance stress and recovery to achieve best performance: When feeling emotionally exhausted, push yourself beyond your usual maximums and then allow yourself adequate means to recover. In this way, your limits will expand. Just like physical exercise, if you push a bit more each time, your capacity will grow [11].
2. Create a ritual of disconnecting: Technologies such as smart phones and social networking sites make it easy for us to never truly disconnect. It is not unusual for many people to bring work phones and laptops on vacation and check e-mails and take phone calls the entire time. This is socially sanctioned, but the logic of "living life as a long distance runner" is faulty [11].
3. Create healthy breathing, eating, sleeping, and exercising habits.

Breathing is an easy way to relax and prevent burnout throughout the day. Make a habit of inhaling to a count of 3 and exhaling to a count of 6 for several minutes.

Eat small meals at regular intervals (5–6 times a day), in amounts that are satisfying but not overfilling or under-filling [11].

Sleep for at least 7–8 h per night (some individuals may need more sleep).

Exercise regularly and add or keep some form of sports or training in your routine.

"Simple things such as exercise, a hobby, and availability of significant others are the best advisable preventers of burnout" [11].

CON: Many large corporations have established special programs to prevent burnout and to provide help to those who have fallen victim to it. This approach seems to be missing in the field of anesthesiology. In some departments, a Clinical Practice Committee takes the lead.

The importance of bullying and abuse as contributors to burnout cannot be understated. Abuse is characterized by lack of respect for coworkers. It is sometimes obvious, but can be disguised. Subtle forms of bullying often cause the most damage and can be responsible for increased absenteeism, more individuals who quit, unsatisfied workers, unmotivated employees, no trust, and no teamwork. It is the department's duty to listen, to interfere, and to be proactive in such cases [12].

The most obvious tangible benefit of the department's, chairperson's, and/or colleague's interference is an enhancement of the anesthesiologist's personal productivity, since he can then focus his attention on patient care.

Summary

Too much stress over a long period of time leads to burnout, which is defined as exhaustion—mentally, emotionally, and physically. For many years, employers and entrepreneurs have realized that on-the-job factors significantly affect workers' ability to perform their duties appropriately and to be productive and successful. Prevention is the best way to prevent burnout. The department needs to assume a certain responsibility for its members and can help by establishing a fair system for case assignments, on-call schedules, and vacation distribution and by enforcing mutual respect and a collegial environment.

References

1. Freudenberger H. The staff burn-out syndrome in alternative institutions. Psychother Theory Res Pract. 1975;12(1):73–82.
2. Hall K, Wakeman M, Levy R, Khoury J. Factors associated with career longevity in residency-trained emergency physicians. Ann Emergy Med. 1992;21:291–7.
3. Fields A, Cuerdon T, Brasseux C, Getson P, Thompson A, Orlowski J, Youngner S. Physician burnout in pediatric critical care medicine. Crit Care Med. 1995;23:1425–9.
4. Hyman S, Michaels D, James M, Schildcrout J, Mercaldo N, Weinger M. Risk of burnout in perioperative clinicians: a survey study and literature review. Anesthesiology. 2011;114:194–204.
5. De Oliveira G, Ahmad S, Stock M, Harter R, Almeida M, Fitzgerald P, McCarthy R. High incidence of burnout in academic chairpersons of anesthesiology: should we be taking better care of our leaders? Anesthesiology. 2011;114(1):181–93.
6. Campbell D, Sonnad S, Eckhauser F, Campbell K, Greenfield L. Burnout among American surgeons. Surgery. 2001;130:696–702 (discussion 702–5).
7. Ramirez A, Graham J, Richards M, Cull A, Gregory W. Mental health of hospital consultants: the effects of stress and satisfaction at work. Lancet. 1996;347:724–8.
8. Spickard A, Gabbe S, Christensen J. Mid-career burnout in generalist and specialist physicians. JAMA. 2002;288:1447–50.
9. Brooke D, Edwards G, Taylor C. Addiction as an occupational hazard: 144 doctors with drug and alcohol problems. Br J Addict. 1991;86:1011–6.
10. McCray L, Cronholm P, Bogner H, Gallo J, Neill R. Resident physician burnout: is there hope? Fam Med. 2008;40:626–32.
11. Nyssen A, Hansez I. Stress and burnout in anaesthesia. Curr Opin Anaesthesiol. 2008;21:406–11.
12. Kivimaki M, Elovainio M, Vahtera J, Ferrie J. Organizational justice and health of employees: prospective cohort study. Occup Environ Med. 2003;60:27–33.

The Tumor Is Inoperable: Tell the Patient or Punt to the Surgeon?

125

Elizabeth A.M. Frost

Case

You were somewhat acquainted with the lady. After all you had met her several times at the nail salon. She was probably in her early 40s and she had children about the same age as yours. You talked about them. They were only a couple of grades apart in the same school. In fact, after you told her you were an anesthesiologist and sometimes your cases ran late, she offered to pick up your children and bring them to her house until you got home. So perhaps it was not surprising that she asked you about the indigestion she was getting, and the bloating feelings, and the vague pains. You suggested that she should try some antacids and some nonsteroidal anti-inflammatories. When that did not work, you gave her the name of a gastroenterologist friend of yours.

You met her again some 3 weeks later and she said that the doctor did not find anything but thought she should see a general surgeon and perhaps have a laparoscopic procedure just to look around and check things out. She really trusted you and wanted to come to your hospital where you could take care of her. Again, you gave her the name of a general surgeon that you liked. He saw her, agreed that laparoscopy was reasonable, and told her it should be an ambulatory case.

The following week you met her in the holding area. She was nervous but felt reassured because you were there. After an uneventful induction, the surgeon remarked that he suspected a tumor of some sort. Because he really had no idea what was wrong he had opted to be very positive as she was so young. So he had reassured her she would probably go home that evening. You continued the case with sevoflurane and remifentanil.

As soon as the surgeon inserted the ports, it became clear that there was a major disease. To get a better understanding of the problem, the case was converted to an open procedure. Considerable ascites was encountered. The diagnosis appeared to be ovarian carcinoma with lesions throughout the peritoneal cavity and in the liver. The surgeon tried to page a gynecologist without success. Given the extent of the pathology, he decided to take several biopsies and close the abdomen.

Your patient awoke quickly and was transferred to the postoperative care unit (PACU). The surgeon still had a long list of cases to complete at another hospital. He had written his postoperative orders, reassured her that she was stable, and left. The patient was happy to see that you were still with her and asked immediately, "So, what did they find?"

The nurse was still with you and she quickly said to the patient, "Take it easy, you are just waking up… your surgeon will be right in to talk to you."

The patient turned to you, "My tummy hurts… what did they do? I can see the clock… I was asleep for more than 3 h —that is too long for just a little look."

Again the nurse told her that the case was not nearly that long; she was just sleeping and as soon as she was fully awake, the surgeon would be in to see her.

You excused yourself and went off to order some morphine and patient-controlled analgesia (a PCA) for her. You attempted to call the surgeon but he was already scrubbed in at another hospital some distance away. Through the circulating nurse, he advised you to be vague and that he would work it out later that evening. You asked if he had arranged for a bed for her. He admitted that that item had escaped his memory and asked you to call admitting for him and tell the patient she would be staying overnight. You suggested that was a task for his physician assistant but that person had gone home with a bad cold.

You returned to the patient's bedside. The nurse had left and the PACU nurse told you that the patient was really asking for a diagnosis. "You can't tell her, of course," she

E.A.M. Frost
Icahn Medical Center at Mount Sinai, 1 Gustav L Levy Place, New York, NY 10029, USA

E.A.M. Frost (✉)
2 Pondview West, Purchase, NY 10577, USA
e-mail: elzfrost@aol.com; elizabeth.frost@mountsinai.org

C.S. Scher et al. (eds.), *You're Wrong, I'm Right*, DOI 10.1007/978-3-319-43169-7_125

said, "that is not your job. It is for the surgeon to say what the problem is!"

Again the patient reached for your hand. "Tell me what is going on. Don't you know? Were you not in the operating room as you promised? And when can I go home?"

As a medical student, and long before that, you had learned that honesty was the best policy. You had also been taught to "first do no harm." Would you harm your patient/friend if you told her the truth [1]? What if you were wrong and it was not inoperable cancer? But you had seen the operative field; you had heard the surgeon's expressions of despair and his attempts to get a more qualified surgeon. You had read his operative note, describing a surgically hopeless situation, amenable to nothing more than tissue biopsies.

And she is your friend and she trusted you. Have you somehow let her down because you cannot help her now? Or can you? Is it guilt? Sadness? Her 3 young girls: one in middle school and two just started high school?

But do you really know what she wants to hear? Is she still under the effects of anesthesia although you did not give her any benzodiazepines? Should you speak to her family first or ask them to join you? But would that infringe on patient confidentiality? Does she want her family there at this time? What would you want to hear under the circumstances?

Would it be an alternative to sit with your friend, hold her hand, and say, "We found that surgery is not the answer for you right now. The surgeon took several specimens and sent them to other specialists so we can work out what is the best treatment for you…and there are several options. We think it is best that you stay in the hospital tonight because we hope to have more information for you tomorrow. Would you like me to get your family?"

Question

What do you say?

PRO: Telling the truth and honesty should be a hallmark of the doctor/patient relationship. That the patient is a friend further demands a degree of trust. Promises were made. The team is well aware of the diagnosis and the procedures that were done. The operative report is in the chart and the patient has a right to see it.

CON: It is easier to make the relaying of unpleasant information someone else's responsibility. Traditionally, surgeons have been the ones to convey findings after surgery. Often they are not in the postoperative care unit. The patient may still be under the effects of anesthesia and will not understand or misunderstand what is said. Histology may prove the suspected diagnosis wrong. Patients' understanding and reaction to unwanted news are unpredictable.

Searching for a solution is difficult.

Reference

1. Drane JF, Reich GH. Honesty in medicine: should doctors tell the truth? Am J Bioeth. 2002;2:14–7.

What Is the Role of Pain Physicians in the Opioid Epidemic?

126

Nicholas J. Bremer

Case

A 35-year-old male construction worker presents to his family physician a week after "tweaking" his back while on the job. He has some lumbar back pain bilaterally, but what really concerns him is the pain that goes down his right thigh, crosses his knee, and goes down to his toes. He denies any bowel or bladder dysfunction, saddle anesthesia, or new focal neurologic deficits.

On the right, he has a positive straight leg raise sign, but normal lower extremity reflexes and motor strength. A lumbar magnetic resonance imaging (MRI) is ordered, and after checking the state's opioid prescription monitoring Web site, the patient is placed on ibuprofen and combined oxycodone/acetaminophen pills.

Follow-up on the MRI reveals a right-sided L4-5 nucleus pulposus herniation. The family physician tells the patient that the pain will likely resolve on its own within a few months, and his medication regimen is changed to long-acting oxycodone 10 mg twice daily for basal dosing, with short-acting oxycodone 5 mg every 4 h for breakthrough pain, in addition to a referral to physical therapy. At the 2-week follow-up appointment, the patient states that the "only thing that helps the pain is the oxycodone" and requests dose escalation, which the family physician views as reasonable and prescribes. After all, the patient is motivated to get well, attending every physical therapy appointment and focusing on an expeditious return to work to support his family.

A similar conversation occurs at every 2-week visit for the next 2 months until the patient is on long-acting oxycodone 40 mg twice daily and short-acting oxycodone 20 mg every 4 h. The family physician does not access the state's opioid prescription monitoring Web site every visit, since he now knows the patient well.

A week later, the family physician receives a call from an emergency department (ED) because his patient presented with respiratory depression and was admitted for management of an opioid overdose. He quickly checks the state's opioid monitoring program Web site and sees that his trusted patient was obtaining opioids from 2 other physicians in the state. He calls the newly opened interventional pain group in town to establish a relationship and to ask for guidance on how to manage this situation and for guidance on appropriate opioid prescribing.

Question

Where is the role of pain physicians in the opioid epidemic?

PRO: In discussing the case, the family physician points out that the patient had "real" pain, likely from a structural defect caused by an injury at work, and that opioids were appropriate in his view. He states that he trusted the patient and did not feel compelled to check at every visit. He states that there is an "unlimited opioid ceiling" and dose escalation is appropriate until pain is controlled. He states that pain is the "fifth vital sign" and he can be sued for not addressing pain as such.

CON (Pain Specialist): I am happy that the family physician reached out to me, but I realize I have my work cut out for me. I took this opportunity to briefly educate the family physician on the current state of affairs in pain medicine. I agree that this patient's pain would have probably ameliorated with a tincture of time and physical therapy. Even massive disk herniations can be treated conservatively, with the expectation of complete and sustained recovery in upward of 87 % of patients at 2 years [1].

N.J. Bremer
Division of Pain Medicine, Department of Anesthesiology, Columbia University Medical Center, 622 West 168th Street (PH 5-Stem), New York, NY 10032, USA

N.J. Bremer (✉)
600 West 169th St, Apt. 1, New York, NY 10032, USA
e-mail: Nicholas.Bremer.MD@gmail.com; njbremer@gmail.com

C.S. Scher et al. (eds.), *You're Wrong, I'm Right*, DOI 10.1007/978-3-319-43169-7_126

"Avoiding opioids altogether in this case is possible and desirable," I tell the family physician. "I would have managed this patient by performing epidural steroid injections (ESIs), which can decrease pain to the extent that the patient can participate meaningfully in physical therapy. A major trial even showed that ESIs reduce the need for spine surgery [2]. Sometimes this type of pain completely resolves with a single or several injections, especially in a young, healthy, motivated patient. In my practice, I rarely prescribe opioids for any reason."

PRO: The family physician says, "What type of PAIN doctor doesn't prescribe opioids!? I was hoping you were going to take over all the patients I started and have maintained on opioids!"

CON: I realize I have a long way to go with this particular physician. I respectfully articulate that family physicians are the single largest source of all opioid prescriptions and furthermore are associated with the greatest incidence of fatalities due to overdose [3]. I explain how the field of pain medicine evolved away from the "unlimited opioid ceiling" model, as dangers became clear over time.

"From 1999 to 2007, the prime years that model was touted, death rates from legitimate opioid prescriptions rose 127 % [4]," I tell the family physician. "Recent data also suggest that many of these deaths are dose-dependent and occur secondary to prescriptions given legitimately to patients with chronic pain [5]. At the current time, standard practice is to limit outpatient opioids to 100 mg of morphine (or equivalent) daily. Modern pain medicine focuses more on functional status than the numerical pain rating scale ('pain score') as a 'fifth vital sign.' The American Pain Society (1996) [6] and the Joint Commission (2000) [7] sought to achieve better inpatient pain control and advocated the 'fifth vital sign' in the inpatient setting; this inadvertently led to unintended increased opioid use in outpatient settings. Also important to note is that the numerical 'pain score' was never validated for chronic pain."

PRO: He says, "What about the risks of ESIs? Infection and nerve damage? Do they even work?"

CON: "While all pain medicine interventions certainly carry risks, they are small. With ESI, I quote patients that they have a 1/100 risk of headache—due to post-dural puncture (which I can typically relieve with an epidural blood patch, although after at least 24 h), and a greater than 1/100,000 of bleeding, infection, or nerve damage [8].

"In 2011, the Centers for Disease Control (CDC) cited 16,917 deaths from opioids [9]. In comparison, deaths from all interventional pain techniques over 20 years were 131 patients (excluding the multistate fungal outbreak). The multistate fungal meningitis outbreak that led to more than 130 deaths was the result of the negligence of a single pharmaceutical compounding company. ESI is endorsed by the North American Spine Society [10]. Cervical/thoracic/lumbar interlaminar ESIs are low risk and effective; lumbar transforaminal ESI is moderate risk and effective, and cervical transforaminal ESI is high risk and not effective [11]."

PRO: "While all this is interesting, what about my patients whose pain does not get better? Like the patients I have on standing opioids for 10 years? Most of the patients I send to the spine surgeon end up with open diskectomies and multilevel fusions. They have long recovery times, and in the end return the same or worse than before, with the spine surgeons offering more surgery to provide additional relief. I started referring to a different spine surgeon who often says he cannot offer any surgical remedy. I am out of options and frustrated by the lack of options for my patients. What can you offer them?"

CON: "One well-established therapy is spinal cord neurostimulation, which, according to the neurosurgery literature in multiple high-quality trials, achieves much better results than a second surgery, thereby obviating the need for more and more surgery [12–14]. In fact, when the odds of a successful surgical outcome are uncertain (at an overall cost of $89,000), spinal cord neurostimulation could even be considered as a primary treatment option [15]. Our percutaneous leads can be inserted and implanted in an outpatient setting, with no hospital stay, and are removable if the patient does not achieve the desired result. This procedure may make sense to some patients who want to avoid an operation that carries significant surgical and anesthetic risk, with an associated inpatient hospital stay, pain, and an extended outpatient recovery period. Research in pain management is ongoing."

Summary

A multidisciplinary approach using multimodal and multimechanistic methods and techniques can achieve the end result of pain relief. Pain physicians often reduce or eliminate opioids prescribed by other physicians. While pain physicians are certainly knowledgeable—arguably the most knowledgeable physicians on the topic of opioids—pain physicians use opioids discretely, judiciously, and appropriately. Thus, it is clear that pain physicians are part of the solution to the opioid epidemic problem.

References

1. Benson RT, Tavares SP, Robertson SC, Sharp R, Marshall RW. Conservatively treated massive prolapsed discs: a 7-year follow-up. Ann R Coll Surg Engl. 2010;92(2):147–53.
2. Radcliff K, Hilibrand A, Lurie JD, Tosteson TD, Delasotta L, Rihn J. The impact of epidural steroid injections on the outcomes of patients treated for lumbar disc herniation: a subgroup analysis of the SPORT trial. J Bone Joint Surg Am. 2012;94(15):1353–8.
3. Porucznik CA, Johnson EM, Rolfs RT, Sauer BC. Specialty of prescribers associated with prescription opioid fatalities in Utah, 2002–2010. Pain Med. 2014;15(1):73–8.
4. Dunn KM, Saunders KW, Rutter CM, Banta-Green CJ, Merrill JO, Sullivan MD, et al. Opioid prescriptions for chronic pain and overdose: a cohort study. Ann Intern Med. 2010;152(2):85–92.
5. Bohnert ASB, Valenstein M, Bair MJ, Ganoczy D, McCarthy JF, Ilgen MA, et al. Association between opioid prescribing patterns and opioid overdose-related deaths. JAMA. 2011;305(13):1315–21.
6. The American Pain Society and the National Pharmaceutical Council. Section II: assessment of pain. http://americanpainsociety.org/uploads/education/section_2.pdf. Accessed 14 March 2016.
7. The Joint Commission on Accreditation of Healthcare Organizations (JCAHO) and the National Pharmaceutical Council. Improving the quality of pain management through measurement and action. March 2003. http://www.npcnow.org/system/files/research/download/Improving-the-Quality-of-Pain-Management-Through-Measurement-and-Action.pdf. Accessed 14 March 2016.
8. Turnbull DK, Shephard DB. Post-dural puncture headache: pathogenesis, prevention and treatment. Br J Anaesth. 2003;91:718–29.
9. Chen LH, Hedegaard H, Warner M. Drug-poisoning deaths involving opioid analgesics: United States, 1999–2011. NCHS Data Brief, vol 166. September 2014. http://www.cdc.gov/nchs/data/databriefs/db166.pdf. Accessed 14 March 2016.
10. Cervical epidural steroid injections. Review and recommendation statement. North American Spine Society. March 2011. https://www.spine.org/Documents/ResearchClinicalCare/CESIReviewRecStatement.pdf. Accessed 14 March 2016.
11. Cohen SP, Bicket MC, Jamison D, Wilkinson I, Rathmell JP. Epidural steroids. A comprehensive, evidence-based review. Reg Anesth Pain Med. 2013;38(3):175–200.
12. North RB, Ewend MG, Lawton MT, Kidd DH, Piantadosi S. Failed back surgery syndrome: 5-year follow-up after spinal cord stimulator implantation. Neurosurgery. 1991;28(5):692–9.
13. North RB, Campbell JN, James CS, Conover-Walker MK, Wang H, Piantadosi S, et al. Failed back surgery syndrome: 5-year follow-up in 102 patients undergoing repeated operation. Neurosurgery. 1991;28(5):685–90 (discussion 690–1).
14. North RB, Kidd DH, Farrokhi F, Piantadosi SA. Spinal cord stimulation versus repeated lumbosacral spine surgery for chronic pain: a randomized, controlled trial. Neurosurgery. 2005;56(1):98–106.
15. North RB, Kidd D, Shipley J, Taylor RS. Spinal cord stimulation versus reoperation for failed back surgery syndrome: a cost effectiveness and cost utility analysis based on a randomized, controlled trial. Neurosurgery. 2007;61(2):361–8.

Index

C.S. Scher et al. (eds.), *You're Wrong, I'm Right*, DOI: 10.1007/978-3-319-43169-7

D

E

F